Y0-BZG-186

Series Editors:
Steven F. Warren, Ph.D.
Joe Reichle, Ph.D.

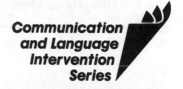

**Communication
and Language
Intervention
Series**

Volume 7

Transitions in
Prelinguistic Communication

Also in the Communication
and Language Intervention Series:

**Communication
and Language
Intervention
Series**

Volume 7
Transitions in
Prelinguistic Communication

Edited by

Amy M. Wetherby, Ph.D.
Professor
Department of Communication Disorders
Regional Rehabilitation Center
Florida State University
Tallahassee

Steven F. Warren, Ph.D.
Professor
Department of Special Education
Department of Psychology and Human Development
George Peabody College
Vanderbilt University
Nashville, Tennessee

and

Joe Reichle, Ph.D.
Professor of Communication Disorders
and Special Education
Department of Communication Disorders
University of Minnesota
Minneapolis

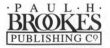

·P A U L·H·
BROOKES
PUBLISHING Co

Baltimore • London • Toronto • Sydney

Paul H. Brookes Publishing Co.
Post Office Box 10624
Baltimore, Maryland 21285-0624

Typeset by Signature Typesetting & Design, Baltimore, Maryland.
Manufactured in the United States of America by
Thomson-Shore, Inc., Dexter, Michigan.

Library of Congress Cataloging-in-Publication Data

Transitions in prelinguistic communication / edited by Amy M. Wetherby, Steven F.
  Warren, Joe Reichle.
     p.   cm. — (Communication and language intervention series ; 7)
  Includes bibliographical references (p.   ) and index.
  ISBN 1-55766-262-2
  1. Language acquisition.   2. Language disorders in children.   I. Wetherby,
Amy M.   II. Warren, Steven F.   III. Reichle, Joe, 1951–   .   IV. Series.
P118.T72   1998
401'.93—dc21   97-23955
                                                                   CIP

British Library Cataloguing in Publication data are available from the British Library.

Contents

Series Preface

THE PURPOSE OF THE *Communication and Language Intervention Series* is to provide meaningful foundations for the application of sound intervention designs to enhance the development of communication skills across the life span. We are endeavoring to achieve this purpose by providing readers with presentations of state-of-the-art theory, research, and practice.

In selecting topics, editors, and authors, we are not attempting to limit the contents of this series to those viewpoints with which we agree or that we find most promising. We are assisted in our efforts to develop the series by an editorial advisory board consisting of prominent scholars representative of the range of issues and perspectives to be incorporated in the series.

We trust that the careful reader will find much that is provocative and controversial in this and other volumes. This will be necessarily so to the extent that the work reported is truly on the so-called cutting edge, a mythical place where no sacred cows exist. This point is demonstrated time and again throughout this volume as the conventional wisdom is challenged (and occasionally confirmed) by various authors.

Readers of this and other volumes are encouraged to proceed with healthy skepticism. In order to achieve our purpose, we take on some difficult and controversial issues. Errors and misinterpretations inevitably are made. This is normal in the development of any field and should be welcomed as evidence that the field is moving forward and tackling difficult and weighty issues.

Well-conceived theory and research on development of both children with and children without disabilities are vitally important for researchers, educators, and clinicians committed to the development of optimal approaches to communication and language intervention. For this reason, each volume in this series includes chapters pertaining to both development and intervention.

The content of each volume reflects our view of the symbiotic relationship between intervention and research: Demonstrations of what may work in intervention should lead to analyses of promising discoveries and insights from developmental work that may in turn fuel further refinement by intervention researchers.

An inherent goal of this series is to enhance the long-term development of the field by systematically furthering the dissemination of theoretically and empirically based scholarship and research. We promise the reader an opportunity to participate in the development of this field through the debates and discussions that occur throughout the pages of the *Communication and Language Intervention Series.*

Editorial Advisory Board

Contributors

The Editors

Amy M. Wetherby, Ph.D., Professor, Department of Communication Disorders, 107 Regional Rehabilitation Center, Florida State University, Tallahassee, FL 32306-1200. Dr. Wetherby also serves as the executive director of the Florida State University Center for Autism and Related Disabilities. Her research has focused on communicative and cognitive-social aspects of language problems in young children, and more recently, on the early identification of children with communicative impairments. She has published extensively on these topics and presents regularly at national conventions, and she is a co-author of the *Communication and Symbolic Behavior Scales* (with Barry M. Prizant [Applied Symbolix, 1993]).

Steven F. Warren, Ph.D., Professor, Department of Special Education and Department of Psychology and Human Development, Box 328, George Peabody College, Vanderbilt University, Nashville, TN 37203. Dr. Warren also is the deputy director of the John F. Kennedy Center for Research on Human Development at Vanderbilt University and the co-director of the center's Mental Retardation Research Training Program. He has conducted extensive research on communication and language intervention approaches.

Joe Reichle, Ph.D., Professor of Communication Disorders and Special Education, University of Minnesota, Minneapolis, MN 55495. Dr. Reichle has published extensively in the areas of communication intervention and augmentative communication system applications for people with moderate and severe disabilities. He is actively involved in preservice and in-service training of speech-language pathologists and special educators, and he serves as a reviewer for a number of scholarly journals.

The Chapter Authors

Lauren B. Adamson, Ph.D., Professor, Department of Psychology, and Associate Dean, College of Arts and Sciences, Georgia State University, Atlanta, GA 30303. Dr. Adamson's research interests include the development of shared attention during the first 3 years of life and patterns of atypical communication development.

Dianne G. Alexander, Ph.D., Clinical Director, Center for Autism and Related Disabilities, 107 Regional Rehabilitation Center, Florida State University, Tallahassee, FL 32306-1200. Dr. Alexander received her Ph.D. in Communication Disorders from Florida State University. Her clinical experience has been primarily with individuals with severe communication disorders. As the program director of the Center for Autism and Related Disabilities, she works with individuals with pervasive developmental disorders.

Lois Bloom, Ph.D., Edward Lee Thorndike Professor of Psychology and Education, Teachers College, Columbia University, 525 120th Street, Box 5, New York, NY 10027. Dr. Bloom is the Edward Lee Thorndike Professor of Psychology at Teacher's College, Columbia University. She received the American Speech-Language-Hearing Association Honors in 1992 and the G. Stanley Hall Award from Division 7, Developmental Psychology, of the American Psychological Association in 1997. She has written several books, and her most recent book, *The Transition from Infancy to Language: Acquiring the Power of Expression* (Cambridge University Press, 1993), was awarded the Eleanor Maccoby Book Award from the Developmental Psychology Division of the American Psychological Association in 1996.

Stephen N. Calculator, Ph.D., Professor and Chair, Department of Communication Disorders, University of New Hampshire, Durham, NH 03824-3563. Dr. Calculator is a professor and chair of the Department of Communication Disorders at the University of New Hampshire and an adjunct professor of Pediatrics at Dartmouth Medical School, Hanover, New Hampshire. His principal research and clinical activities have been related to the role of augmentative communication and assistive technology in fostering the inclusion of individuals with severe disabilities in their home communities.

Susan Ellis Chance, M.A., Doctoral Student, Department of Psychology, Georgia State University, Atlanta, GA 30303. Ms. Chance's interests include developmental psychopathology and applied clinical research.

Truman E. Coggins, Ph.D., Associate Professor, Speech and Hearing Sciences, Box 357920, Seattle, WA 98195. Dr. Coggins is an associate professor in the Department of Speech and Hearing Sciences at the University of Washington. He is also the head of speech-language pathology at the Center on Human Development and Disability. His research interests focus on assessing the social-communicative abilities of children and adolescents who are difficult to test.

Elizabeth R. Crais, Ph.D., Associate Professor, University of North Carolina, Campus Box 7170, Chapel Hill, NC 27599-7170. Dr. Crais is an associate professor in the Division of Speech and Hearing Sciences of the Medical School of the University of North Carolina at Chapel Hill. Her research and clinical interests have included examining the adequacy of personnel preparation of professionals for working with young children with special needs and their families and a focus on the role of families in child assessment. She is also investigating the emergence of gestures and words in infants and toddlers.

Mary M. Donegan, Ph.D., Assistant Professor, University of Michigan–Dearborn, 4901 Evergreen, Dearborn, MI 48128. Dr. Donegan is an assistant professor in early childhood education at the University of Michigan–Dearborn. Her professional interests include teaching and research in preparing early childhood teachers to work in inclusive settings. Prior to completing her doctorate in early childhood special education at the University of Illinois at Urbana-Champaign, she was an education coordinator and teacher of preschool children with speech and language disorders at North Shore University Hospital Preschool Development Program, Long Island, New York.

Erik Drasgow, Ph.D., Assistant Professor, University of South Carolina, 236-I Wardlaw, Columbia, SC 29208. Dr. Drasgow received his Ph.D. in Applied Behavior Analysis/Moderate and Severe Disabilities from the University of Illinois in 1996. He is the coordinator of the Severe Disabilities Program at the University of South Carolina, and he teaches courses in functional curriculum, direct instruction, and functional communication training for individuals with severe disabilities. His research has focused on generalization and language intervention with individuals with severe disabilities.

Glen Dunlap, Ph.D., Professor, Florida Mental Health Institute, University of South Florida, 13301 Bruce B. Downs Boulevard, Tampa, FL 33612. Dr. Dunlap is a professor in the Department of Child and Family Studies at the University of South Florida, where he serves as the director of the Division of Applied Research and Educational Support. Dr. Dunlap's principal activities and interests have been in the areas of autism and related disabilities, assessment and intervention for significant behavioral problems, early childhood development and intervention, and family perspectives and family supports.

Susan A. Fowler, Ph.D., Associate Dean and Professor, University of Illinois at Urbana-Champaign, 38 Education Building, 1310 South Sixth Street, Champaign, IL 61820. Dr. Fowler is a professor of special education and the associate dean for academic affairs in the College of Education at the University of Illinois at Urbana-Champaign. Her areas of research focus on service transitions for young children and their families, interagency coordination, and children's social development.

James W. Halle, Ph.D., Professor, Department of Special Education, University of Illinois at Urbana-Champaign, 1310 South Sixth Street, Champaign, IL 61820. Dr. Halle's research program focuses on communication and language learners with significant disabilities. The analysis of variables that comprise the social context of language and that mediate generalized use of language are central to his research focus. His research includes the assessment and intervention of communication form, function, and context of learners who communicate without language. He has published more than 50 articles and chapters and has completed a 3-year tenure as the editor of the *Journal of The Association for Persons with Severe Handicaps.* He serves as an associate editor for the *Journal of Applied Behavior Analysis.*

Jana M. Iverson, Ph.D., Postdoctoral Fellow, Department of Psychology, Indiana University, Tenth and Walnut Grove, Bloomington, IN 47405. Dr. Iverson works primarily in the area of cognition and cognitive development, with a particular focus on representational and perceptual-motor aspects of communicative processes in children and adults. Her work has focused on the nature, function, and development of gesture and its relationship to speech.

Kary S. Kublin, M.S., Doctoral Candidate, 107 Regional Rehabilitation Center, Florida State University, Tallahassee, FL 32306-1200. Ms. Kublin is a doctoral candidate in Communication Disorders at Florida State University. She has been involved with several research and clinically based early intervention efforts in Tallahassee, Toronto, and North Carolina, including the standardization of the *Communication and Symbolic Behavior Scales* (Wetherby & Prizant, Applied Symbolix, 1993). In 1995, she traveled to New Zealand on a Fulbright Grant to study the language and emergent literacy abilities of 4- and 5-year-old children.

Shirley V. Leew, M.A., Speech-Language Pathologist, Vanderbilt University, 311 Village at Vanderbilt, Nashville, TN 37212. Ms. Leew is a speech-language pathologist of 18 years who is working on a Ph.D. at Vanderbilt University. Her interests include early communication development in the context of responsive environments.

Karin Lifter, Ph.D., Associate Professor, Department of Counseling Psychology, Rehabilitation, and Special Education, Northeastern University, Boston, MA 02115. Dr. Lifter directs personnel preparation programs in early intervention and special education at Northeastern University. Her research interests center on descriptive studies of children's play and language and on intervention studies in which play activities—identified through an analysis of what children know—are taught to preschoolers with developmental disabilities to facilitate developments in cognition, language, and social competence.

Rebecca McCathren, Ph.D., Assistant Professor, University of Missouri, 813 Fairfax Drive, Columbia, MO 65201. Dr. McCathren's research interests are in the areas of early communication and language development and assessment.

Peter Mundy, Ph.D., Professor of Psychology, University of Miami, 5665 Ponce de Leon Boulevard, Coral Gables, FL 33146. Dr. Mundy is a professor of psychology, the director of the Center for Psychological Services, as well as the director of the Center for Autism and Related Disabilities at the University of Miami. His research focuses on the development of social, cognitive, and communication skills in the preschool period.

Robert O'Neill, Ph.D., Associate Professor, University of Utah, 221 Milton Bennion Hall, Salt Lake City, UT 84112. Dr. O'Neill is an associate professor of special education at the University of Utah. His primary research and teaching interests include functional assessment, teaching communication skills as alternatives to problem behaviors, community-based support strategies for children and adults who exhibit problem behaviors, and strategies for supporting teachers and caregivers working with such individuals.

Michaelene M. Ostrosky, Ph.D., Associate Professor, University of Illinois at Urbana-Champaign, 288 Education, 1310 South Sixth Street, Champaign, IL 61820. Dr. Ostrosky received her doctorate in education and human development with an emphasis on early childhood special education from Vanderbilt University. Her research has focused on the transitions of young children between multiple programs in which they are enrolled, the social and communicative interactions between children with and without disabilities, and parent-implemented language interventions.

Patsy L. Pierce, Ph.D. Director of Professional Services, North Carolina Infant-Toddler Program, 325 North Salisbury Street, Raleigh, NC 27603. Dr. Pierce directs North Carolina's Comprehensive System of Personnel Development. Prior to this position, she conducted research at the Center for Literacy and Disability Studies, formerly located at the University of North Carolina at Chapel Hill. She continues to promote developmentally appropriate practices that enhance literacy development in all young children.

Barry M. Prizant, Ph.D., CCC-SLP, Professor, Division of Communication Disorders, Emerson College, 168 Beacon Street, Boston, MA 02116. Dr. Prizant, a Fellow of the American Speech-Language-Hearing Association, developed and co-directs a family-centered program for newly diagnosed toddlers with autism/pervasive developmental disorders and their families. He has published extensively in the areas of communication and language development, and autism and other social-communicative disorders in young children and is an editorial consultant for six professional journals. His research and clinical interests include relationships between communication and social and emotional development, and identification and treatment of infants, toddlers, and preschool children at risk for social-communicative difficulties. He is co-author of the *Communication and Symbolic Behavior Scales* (with Amy M. Wetherby [Applied Symbolix, 1993]) and contributed to the *Handbook of Autism and Pervasive Developmental Disorders.*

Michelle S. Shannon, B.S.E., M.A., Research Associate, Arizona State University, Tempe, AZ 85287-1908. Ms. Shannon is a faculty research associate at Arizona State University. She has more than 10 years of experience in providing services to young children with communication disorders and their families.

Carol Stoel-Gammon, Ph.D., Professor of Speech and Hearing Sciences, University of Washington, 1417 NE 42nd Street, Seattle, WA 98105-6246. Dr. Stoel-Gammon's research is in the area of normal and phonological development in children. She is particularly interested in the relationship between babble and speech and also in early identification of toddlers with speech and language disorders.

Donna J. Thal, Ph.D., Professor, Department of Communication Disorders, and Director, Developmental Psycholinguistics Laboratory, San Diego State University, San Diego, CA 92182. Dr. Thal's research has focused on early prediction of language impairment, relationships between language and nonlinguistic cognition, and cross-population studies of brain–behavior relationships in at-risk infants and toddlers.

Bobbie J. Vaughn, Ph.D., Assistant Professor, Department of Child and Family Studies, DARES (Division of Applied Research and Educational Support), 13301 Bruce B. Downs Boulevard, MHC1-250A, Tampa, FL 33612-3899. Dr. Vaughn is Director of the Family Network Project, a 3-year, federally funded research project that provides positive behavioral supports to families of children with developmental disabilities. She has provided training and technical assistance to schools, families, and residential agencies and has conducted in-home consultation with individual families.

M. Jeanne Wilcox, Ph.D., Professor, Department of Speech and Hearing Sciences, Arizona State University, Post Office Box 871908, Tempe, AZ 85287-1908. Dr. Wilcox has established and directs the Infant Child Communication Research Programs at Arizona State University, a facility that provides early intervention services to families and their infants and young children and that also functions as a training site for graduate students in speech-language pathology. Dr. Wilcox is recognized for her expertise and scholarly activity in communication and language assessment and intervention for infants and young children with disabilities; she has published extensively, including articles, chapters, books, and treatment protocols and manuals; and she has been an invited speaker at numerous meetings and conferences. Her research program focuses on developing and determining the most effective methods for facilitating the acquisition of communication and language skills in infants and young children with disabilities.

Jennifer Willoughby, M.S., Graduate Student, Department of Psychology, Psychology Annex, University of Miami, Post Office Box 249229, Coral Gables, FL 33124-0721. Ms. Willoughby is a graduate student in child clinical/pediatric psychology at the University of Miami. Her research interests include early communication and social development in infants and toddlers who are at high risk.

Paul J. Yoder, Ph.D., Associate Professor, George Peabody College, Vanderbilt University, 21st Avenue, Nashville, TN 37203. Dr. Yoder has spent 14 years studying parent–child interaction as it relates to prelinguistic and linguistic communication development in children with and without disabilities. He has contributed to both the methodological and the substantive literature in this and related areas. His background is in special education, communication disorders, and developmental psychology.

Acknowledgments

Most of what I know about prelinguistic development I learned from Carol Prutting while I was a doctoral student. It was the end of a decade during which pragmatics was introduced to our field and prelinguistic communication was wholeheartedly recognized as making a significant contribution to language acquisition. Carol was much more than a mentor on language development. Her unexpected death in 1989 at the age of 48 is still an immense loss, and I continue to feel much gratitude that I had the opportunity to study with her. I also want to express gratitude to my daughter Rebecca, who was born while I was finishing my dissertation. She provided me with personal opportunities not only to observe the precise orchestration of events that unfold during early development but also to participate in the process as a caregiver and communicative partner. Finally, I want to express special recognition to Barry M. Prizant for his professional collaboration, personal support, and friendship, which spans over 2 decades. The foundational framework for this volume is rooted in the model that Barry and I have developed for the *Communication and Symbolic Behavior Scales* (Applied Symbolix, 1993), which is an assessment tool and framework for understanding and enhancing early communicative, social-affective, and symbolic development.

Amy M. Wetherby

I wish to acknowledge my ongoing debt to three people: to my first mentor, Don Baer, for his instruction in the art and science of critical thinking; to my incomparable colleague, Paul J. Yoder, the finest critical thinker I know; and to my own first language teacher, Ruth Warren.

Steven F. Warren

I wish to acknowledge Tom Longhurst, David E. Yoder, Jon Miller, and Robin Chapman. Each of these individuals significantly influenced my professional growth. Also, I wish to acknowledge my two co-editors for the insights that I have gained from our association.

Joe Reichle

1

Introduction to Transitions in Prelinguistic Communication

Amy M. Wetherby,
Steven F. Warren, and Joe Reichle

P RELINGUISTIC COMMUNICATION HAS RECEIVED INCREASING attention since the mid-1970s when Elizabeth Bates (1976) introduced the construct of pragmatics to the child language literature and delineated two major transitional points in the emergence of language: 1) movement from preintentional to intentional communication and 2) movement from presymbolic to symbolic communication. This volume addresses these two pivotal transitions in communication development for infants and toddlers who may be typically developing or at risk for communication delays as well as for older prelinguistic individuals who have moderate to severe disabilities. This volume critically examines theories on the emergence of intentional communication and symbolic communication, presents research findings on assessment and intervention approaches to move children toward intentional and/or symbolic communication and discusses the clinical and educational implications of these findings, and compares and contrasts findings on children who are chronologically between birth and 2 years of age and those who are developmentally functioning at prelinguistic levels.

Throughout this volume the term *children,* or learners, is used to refer to individuals who are chronologically or developmentally in the prelinguistic stage of language development. The literature has underscored the importance of clinical and educational practices that are developmentally and chronologically appropriate for both populations of prelinguistic individuals. The ramifications of using developmentally and chronologically appropriate practices for young children are quite different from those for older learners. The use of the term *nonlinguistic* as opposed to *prelinguistic* may be more accurate in reference to older learners with severe disabilities. However, both populations are included in one volume on prelinguistic communication because it is assumed that the underlying process of moving toward intentional and symbolic communication is similar, although the rate and potential for acquisition will differ. Many of the intervention principles, goals, and procedures for the transition toward inten-

1

tional and symbolic communication are similar, although the contexts in which they will be implemented are different. The chapters in Part I focus primarily on younger children to build a foundational framework. Part II addresses principles and practices for both populations. Chronologically older learners receive substantial attention in Part II, particularly in Chapters 11, 13, 14, 17, and 18, which cover special issues with older learners. This volume's contributors are brought together to bridge the literature on these two populations.

The theoretical framework underlying this volume is the transactional model of communication development. That is, communication development is viewed as a transactional process that involves a developmental interaction vis-à-vis the child and communicative partners. This perspective emphasizes the reciprocal, bidirectional influence of the communication environment, the responsiveness of communicative partners, and the child's own developing communicative competence. For example, this model assumes that the increasing readability or clarity of the child's communicative behavior may influence the parent's style and frequency of contingent responsiveness in ways that will further scaffold the child's developing competence during the transition to linguistic communication. The provision by the adult of linguistic mapping (i.e., naming things the child refers to) in response to clear communication acts is but one example of this process. The transactional model is described in much greater detail in Chapters 9, 12, and 15.

The child's transitions to intentional and symbolic communication were first delineated in the 1970s. Bates and associates (Bates, 1976; Bates, Camaioni, & Volterra, 1975) provided an instrumental developmental pragmatics framework to describe the emergence of communication and language, which has been embraced by researchers and clinicians. Pragmatics has its roots in speech-act theory, which describes the basic unit of communication as the *speech act*. A speech act consists of three components: the intention (illocution), the function (perlocution), and the proposition (locution) (Austin, 1962). Borrowing terminology from the speech-act theory of Austin, Bates and associates identified three stages in the development of communication. From birth, the infant begins in the perlocutionary stage. The infant's behavior systematically affects the caregiver, thus serving a communicative function, although the infant is not yet deliberately producing signals with the intention of accomplishing specific goals. Communicative interactions are rooted in early social and affective development in infants. Eye gaze, facial expression, body movement, and orientation are signals that inform the caregiver of a child's physiological and emotional state and thus guide the caregiver's responses to the infant to regulate social interactions. Early social interactions involving shared emotional experiences lead to the infant's awareness of the effect that his or her behavior can have on others (Bruner, 1981; Dore, 1986). The caregiver's interpretation of and contingent responsiveness to the infant's preintentional communicative signals play an important role in the development of intentional communication (Dore, 1986; Dunst, Lowe, & Bartholomew, 1990).

At about 9 months of age the typical child makes the transition to the illocutionary stage and begins to use preverbal gestures and sounds to communicate intentionally. The transition to intentional communication occurs when the child begins to deliberately use particular signals to communicate to others. Young children learn to communicate to accomplish a variety of intentions and functions before they begin to talk. Bruner (1981) suggested that there are three innate communicative intentions: 1) behavior regulation, to regulate another's behavior to request or protest an object or action; 2) social interaction, to draw another's attention to oneself for affiliative purposes; and 3) joint attention, to reference another's attention to comment on objects and events. Children are able to communicate for these purposes with preverbal gestures and sounds by the end of their first year of life (Wetherby, Cain, Yonclas, & Walker, 1988).

A distinction can be made between the terms *communicative intention* and *communicative function*. Communicative intention refers to the goal of the speaker, and communicative function refers to the effect on the listener (Wetherby & Prizant, 1989). Because communication involves a cooperative interaction between a speaker and a listener, the success of a communicative act depends on whether the speaker's intentions are interpreted appropriately by the listener. Effective communication is when the communicative intention of the speaker is the same as the communicative function interpreted by the listener. Numerous taxonomies exist to describe communicative intentions and functions. This volume uses the broad categories identified by Bruner (1981), that is, behavior regulation, social interaction, and joint attention, as well as more specific categories that fit into one of the broad categories. For example, proto-imperatives or requests are specific examples of behavior regulation, and proto-declaratives or comments are specific examples of joint attention. The same categories can be used to describe both communicative intentions and functions. The difference is in whether the decision is based on the inferred intention of the speaker and/or the interpretation of the listener.

At about 13 months of age the typically developing child begins to make the transition to the locutionary stage with the construction of propositions, that is, by communicating intentionally with referential words. Two major developmental principles are evident as children begin to encode meaning with words. First, communication development involves continuity from preverbal communication to the intentional use of language to communicate (Bates, 1979; Harding & Golinkoff, 1979). Words are mapped onto preverbal intentions, and the transition to using words referentially is a gradual one. Second, the capacity to symbolize or make one thing stand for and represent something else involves a complex interplay of emerging abilities in social-affective, communicative, cognitive, and language domains (Bates, 1979).

Thus, communication and language development can be conceptualized as a continuous three-stage ontogenetic process involving a transition from perlocutionary or preintentional communication to illocutionary or intentional preverbal communication and a transition to locutionary or symbolic communication used intentionally to communicate. In this volume, the term *prelinguistic communication* refers to that period of development before a child has a linguistic system for acquiring language. *Linguistic communication* begins with the emergence of a semantic-based system of learning word meanings and use. This volume focuses on children who are prelinguistic communicators expressively. Typically developing children are likely to reach a linguistic level of comprehension in advance of production. Learners with developmental disabilities who are at a prelinguistic stage of language production show a wide range of comprehension abilities. Some may have receptive abilities that are also at a prelinguistic level, whereas others may have the capacity for linguistic comprehension despite limited expressive abilities. Much of the focus in this volume is on production, although parallel developments in comprehension are addressed in Chapters 4 and 9.

OVERVIEW OF THIS VOLUME

Part I provides a description and discussion of the foundations of intentional, interpersonally directed behavior. Adamson and Chance (Chapter 2) offer evidence that shared attention changes qualitatively during the period of prelinguistic communication development. As infants learn to express object-focused intentions, they begin to coordinate their attention between other people and events of mutual attention. As toddlers, they increase their focus to include representations of past events. Spanning this period, the increasing sophistication of coordinated attention represents a dyadic achievement that provides a base for researchers to study in greater depth advances in joint attention that might correspond to milestones of first word acquisition and the child's initial vocabulary spurt. Additional areas highlighted in this chapter include the relationship among joint attention, emerging object exploration, and affect development.

Yoder, Warren, McCathren, and Leew (Chapter 3) review a body of growing research on the effects of responsiveness on communication and language development. They conclude that the effects of adult responsivity to children's communicative acts, although important, may have limitations. They discuss available data suggesting that responsiveness plays an important role in acquiring early vocabulary and moving from single- to multiple-word utterances. In addition, they discuss the indirect influence that responsivity may have on joint attentional focus and exploration, and the possible limitations of intervention strategies based solely on enhancing responsivity.

Iverson and Thal (Chapter 4) examine the modes used in receiving and expressing elements of an emerging communicative repertoire. They present a detailed review of the emergence of the production and comprehension of gestures and describe general patterns in the coordination of initial gestural and vocal repertoires. They also suggest that early gestural production appears to provide the child with means of producing progressively more complex communicative forms while reducing demands on developing speech production and cognitive skills.

Stoel-Gammon (Chapter 5) focuses on the link between prespeech and early speech development in typically developing children. She describes relationships among the onset of canonical babbling, consonant babble, and the onset of speech and the rate of subsequent lexical development and queries possible influences that partner responsivity may have on early vocal and verbal production. Furthermore, she reports that in some populations (e.g., those with Down syndrome), these events may be of less predictive value. Results of her review lead to a call for more research addressing the relationship between babbling and speech with those who have conditions such as autism, cerebral palsy, and otitis media. Together, Chapters 4 and 5 provide a depth of perspective into the development of early means of communicative expression.

Mundy and Willoughby (Chapter 6) echo the sentiments of Iverson and Thal (Chapter 4), who call for the careful study of nonverbal communicative development as a window to communication development. Mundy and Willoughby discuss possible relationships between social-cognitive and social-emotional aspects of development. Emphasizing achievements during the second year of life, they conclude that research supports a theoretical point of view that nonverbal communication development may reflect processes critical to maladaptive social-cognitive and social-emotional development among preschoolers. In developing a social-motivational model of joint attention, the authors propose that joint attention and attachment measures may be complementary but independent predictors of development.

Wetherby, Alexander, and Prizant (Chapter 7) focus on communication skills that enhance the negotiation of meaning once a miscommunication has occurred. These authors conclude that the ability to repair communicative breakdowns is a significant part of the ability to communicate intentionally. Their discussion provides an extension of Iverson and Thal's (Chapter 4) discussion of the interplay of gestural and vocal communicative modes. The gestural mode initially plays a critical role in repair attempts with a dramatically increasing role for vocal and verbal behavior. These authors conclude that the available data suggest that preverbal repairs have important implications for early identification and represent critical early intervention targets.

Lifter and Bloom (Chapter 8) explore the role that play serves in the development of an initial communicative repertoire. They offer a fresh perspective on social and representational aspects of play. The role that selecting and teaching play activities may have on enhancing the child's focus of attention and providing activities that children can talk about is discussed. These authors suggest that play creates a critical context for learning to produce and comprehend language.

Contrary to some conversational approaches, these authors build a case for using play as the focus for intervention. They describe play as a medium for self-expression and interpretation. Play results in revision and change in experiences that inform developments in cognition. This observation provides the rationale for the view that interventions designed to facilitate play can be implemented successfully. The authors also frame important areas to consider in examining the influence that culture has on the emergence of play.

Wetherby, Reichle, and Pierce (Chapter 9) summarize the transition to symbolic communication from a constructivist perspective in which children "construct" or build knowledge and shared meanings based on interactions with people and experiences in their environment. The authors consider vocal, gestural, and graphic mode development as they examine the emergence of expressive lexicon and parallel developments in the comprehension of meaning. In addition, current theories addressing the emergence of a communicative repertoire are discussed. The authors conclude that the provision of early intervention to increasingly younger children has created an impetus to view communication as a multimodal process. The authors emphasize the need for dynamic assessment strategies that carefully address vocal, graphic, and gestural modes. Correspondingly, the authors emphasize that intervention strategies must maximize children's opportunities to utilize the most efficient communicative means in the context of a wide range of environments. This, in turn, requires interventionists to consider a multimodal approach that coordinates gestural, graphic, and vocal modes.

The chapters in Part I collectively offer a rich picture of the knowledge regarding the emergence of early communicative behavior. Part II addresses the incorporation of this knowledge into assessment and intervention strategies that are theoretically sound and that can be empirically validated.

Coggins (Chapter 10) discusses how professionals gather evidence to reach informed decisions. This chapter emphasizes that assessment is a continuous process that begins with screening and continues through intervention planning and program evaluation. In discussing the types of assessment available, the author emphasizes the degree to which assessment conditions reflect those in which children are likely to operate. In selecting what to assess, Coggins addresses what is known about the stability of performance emitted by infants and toddlers and the predictive validity that certain classes of behavior may have on future communicative acquisitions. His discussion of an interactive and dynamic model of assessment serves as a springboard for amplification in Chapters 12 and 13. The case for assessment tasks that are flexible enough to fit contextually into the range of perspectives represented in a transdisciplinary team is the focus of elaboration in Chapters 13 and 17.

Crais and Calculator (Chapter 11) describe the importance of collaborative planning during the assessment and intervention process. Building consensus among the major stakeholders in the educative process yields a more cohesive, organized, and practical outcome. The authors conclude that a particularly critical aspect of collaborative planning is the involvement of family members. In addition to building consensus, family involvement is likely to enhance the social validity of assessment outcomes.

Careful attention to collaboration is the initial step in developing a dynamic assessment process delineated by Kublin, Wetherby, Crais, and Prizant (Chapter 12). These authors suggest that the use of dynamic assessment can be broadened to include not only the forms of behavior being assessed but also the number of communicative contexts, individualized repertoires of help and support, and shared decision making with families as to the purpose and content of assessment activities. The authors provide a substantial review of empirical support for the notion that a family-centered dynamic assessment process can help family members feel successful as caregivers and as advocates because their preferences for assessment activities, intervention procedures, and support services are supported. They hypothesize that, in the future, identifying children who are communicatively "at risk" may not be limited to linguistic factors that have only been examined in limited contexts. Instead, assessment may involve considering the role that a variety of contextual features have on a child's communicative abilities.

Perhaps one of the clearest examples of the value of a dynamic assessment approach is found in the efforts to determine the communicative intent of socially unacceptable behavior among children with very limited conventional communicative repertoires. O'Neill, Dunlap, and Vaughn (Chapter 13) offer an assessment logic that assumes that most challenging behavior is motivated to gain more desirable contexts or to escape or avoid less desirable contexts. These authors outline a process of functional assessment. The goal of functional assessment is to obtain information that will enable the collaborative development and implementation of effective support plans that can alter antecedents or consequences associated with problem behavior and/or establish functionally equivalent, socially acceptable communicative alternatives to achieve the social outcomes that result from challenging behavior. Although O'Neill and his colleagues come from a more behaviorally grounded theoretical base, and the authors of Chapter 12 are more developmentally grounded in their approach, the two chapters coordinate as a demonstration of the importance of considering performance in a variety of contexts and from a variety of perspectives. These authors emphasize the importance in designing a plan of coordinated assessment and intervention that represents a good contextual fit for all interested in improving the learner's quality of life.

Dunlap, Vaughn, and O'Neill (Chapter 14) provide a cohesive follow-up to O'Neill et al. (Chapter 13). This chapter takes the results of a functional assessment and describes viable proactive intervention strategies that lead to a plan of comprehensive behavioral support that can minimize the need for an individual to produce socially motivated challenging behavior. This chapter includes rich examples of the multicomponent elements of an overall intervention plan. The authors provide examples of the importance of collaborative planning and dynamic assessment in building a plan that requires the careful coordination of all assessment and intervention activities.

From the outset of the assessment process, consideration is being given to the communicative forms and functions that may be likely candidates for intervention. Warren and Yoder (Chapter 15) examine the importance of children's transition from preintentional to intentional communication. They make the case that this transition is pivotal in triggering transactional processes that ultimately lead to symbolic behavior. Consequently, they take the perspective that any substantial delay in this transition may cause other delays that may have devastating repercussions. These authors suggest that for children who are at risk for delayed communicative development, intervention should be intensive and focus on establishing frequent, clear prelinguistic communication as early in development as possible. They then describe the theoretical and empirical basis for and application of prelinguistic milieu teaching, an intervention approach they developed and have been investigating.

Wilcox and Shannon (Chapter 16) describe mechanisms for facilitating the transition from presymbolic to symbolic communication. These authors take the perspective that children's individual capabilities represent a critical component to a successful transition to linguistic communication. One important area of discussion focuses on behavioral and biological indicators that may identify critical points in development during which a child is most likely to benefit from language intervention. This chapter also addresses the efficacy of initial linguistic interventions in multicultural environments with a discussion of the role of contextual fit between intervention strategies and the supporting environment. Scrutinizing intervention efficacy involves evaluating intervention in a context larger than simple dependent measures of child performance in a single context.

Reichle, Halle, and Drasgow (Chapter 17) discuss issues involved in implementing graphic and gestural mode communication to supplement vocal mode communicative production. This chapter discusses traditional approaches to communication intervention that move an individual from perlocutionary communication to the beginning of locutionary communication. These authors summarize and discuss criteria often used in defining intentional communicative acts with individuals who have significant developmental disabilities. In teaching a beginning communicative repertoire, it is likely that individuals with severe disabilities will have a more extensive repertoire of idiosyncratic (and perhaps challenging) behavior that is used communicatively. Complementing the approach described by Warren and Yoder (Chapter 15), the authors propose that early intervention takes the form of adult responsiveness to a learner's communicative overtures. In selecting and implementing intervention objectives, the authors offer a discussion of response efficiency and its role in replacing idiosyncratic signals and symbols with more conventional alternatives.

Ostrosky, Donegan, and Fowler (Chapter 18) provide a cogent description of the challenges that dynamic assessment and program planning encounter when serving individuals across a range of environments. The numerous transitions that occur in the course of a daily routine require planning not only within one setting but often across three or more settings. This challenge to planning can involve interagency coordination at the systems level in addition to collaborative participants at the level of direct service delivery. Although preliminary evidence is extremely supportive of joint planning efforts, few systematic evaluations of multicomponent recommended practice strategies exist.

SOME CONCLUDING THOUGHTS

This volume provides a snapshot of the rich and rapidly expanding knowledge base on prelinguistic communication development and intervention. A comparison of this snapshot with one taken in the 1980s would surely reveal how much more focused and clear the picture of prelinguistic communication development has become. The drive to link levels of analysis (i.e., gene, cell, neuron, behavior, context) and domains of behavior (i.e., linguistic, social, cognitive, emotional) should further sharpen the developmental picture and lead to increasingly effective assessment and intervention options.

There are still many questions in need of investigation. The reader will encounter examples of these throughout the volume; a section toward the end of each chapter is devoted to identifying future research directions. The extent to which these questions are inherently embedded within other issues often will not be clear upon initial consideration. But these broad, extraordinarily important questions are never far in the background. How and to what extent is communication and language development a continuous or discontinuous process? How is socioemotional development related to the development of social interaction? How do the inevitable cultural biases cloud and distort professionals' understanding of prelinguistic development or impede the effectiveness of intervention efforts? Conversely, what are prelinguistic universals? Can they be significantly affected by intervention? And so on, and so on.

Communication development and cultural differences are inextricably linked in a multitude of ways. Gaining a solid understanding of these linkages and learning how to reliably separate the biases of the observer from enduring and important universal differences is of vital importance. Yet few challenges appear more daunting in the midst of a world in which formerly distinct cultures are colliding, merging, even collapsing at a dizzying rate—a world in which pure ethnic groups are dwindling, in which the Golden Arches are a worldwide symbol, and in which increasing socioeconomic variance ensures that the differences from top to bottom within cultures are often greater than the differences between cultures. Despite these challenges, in most chapters readers will find thoughtful discussions of relevant cultural issues, sometimes presented as a separate and distinct section of the chapter, sometimes in the form of an ongoing dialogue throughout the chapter. The complexity of cultural issues and their direct relevance to communication and language required an approach that embedded this dialogue throughout the volume, as opposed to isolating it to a single chapter on cultural issues, as is so often the case. However, in our effort to address multicultural issues, we were distressed over the lack of empirical research on most aspects of prelinguistic development with cultures other than mainstream Caucasian, middle-class American. This highlights a critical need that should be addressed in future research.

From our perspective, the ultimate value of theory and research on typical and atypical communication and language development can be defined by its relevance to the prevention and remediation of communication and language delays and disorders. In keeping with this perspective, most chapters include a discussion of the clinical and educational implications of the work being discussed. In some chapters in Part II, these implications are embedded throughout the discussion; in other chapters, a separate section is devoted to their consideration.

With 18 chapters, we believe this volume offers much to the reader in the way of both developmental theory and research and practical state-of-the-art applications to assessment and intervention. Yet there is much that is not covered here as is the inevitable weakness of any volume, edited or otherwise. Our intent is not to create a comprehensive volume but instead a thematically oriented, representative "work in progress" that will stimulate further theory development and research as well as more effective clinical and educational practice to the benefit of children and families.

REFERENCES

Austin, J. (1962). *How to do things with words.* Cambridge, MA: Harvard University Press.

Bates, E. (1976). *Language and context: The acquisition of pragmatics.* New York: Academic Press.

Bates, E. (1979). *The emergence of symbols: Cognition and communication in infancy.* New York: Academic Press.

Bates, E., Camaioni, L., & Volterra, V. (1975). The acquisition of performatives prior to speech. *Merrill-Palmer Quarterly, 21,* 205–226.

Bruner, J. (1981). The social context of language acquisition. *Language and Communication, 1,* 155–178.

Dore, J. (1986). The development of conversation competence. In R. Scheifelbusch (Ed.), *Language competence: Assessment and intervention* (pp. 3–60). San Diego, CA: College-Hill Press.

Dunst, C.J., Lowe, L.W., & Bartholomew, P.C. (1990). Contingent social responsiveness, family ecology, and infant communicative competence. *National Student Speech-Language-Hearing Association Journal, 17,* 39–49.

Harding, C., & Golinkoff, R. (1979). The origins of intentional vocalizations in prelinguistic infants. *Child Development, 50,* 33–40.

Wetherby, A., Cain, D., Yonclas, D., & Walker, V. (1988). Analysis of intentional communication of normal children from the prelinguistic to the multi-word stage. *Journal of Speech and Hearing Research, 31,* 240–252.

Wetherby, A., & Prizant, B. (1989). The expression of communicative intent: Assessment guidelines. *Seminars in Speech and Language, 10,* 77–91.

PART I

Emergence of
Intentional and
Symbolic Communication

2

Coordinating Attention to People, Objects, and Language

Lauren B. Adamson and Susan Ellis Chance

For talking to us she [Shinn's 11-month-old niece] used a wonderfully vivid and delicate language of grunts, and cries, and movements. She would point to her father's hat, and beg till it was given her; then creep to him and offer the hat, looking up urgently into her face, or perhaps would get to her feet at his side and try to put it on his head; when he put it on, up would go her little arms with pleading cries till he took her, and then she would point to the door and coax to be carried outdoors. (Shinn, 1900, p. 237)

As HUMAN INFANTS NEAR 1 year of age, they begin to communicate with their caregivers about objects and events in their immediate surroundings. The most notable parts of this nascent referential communication system are expressive behaviors such as Shinn's niece's "grunts, and cries, and movements." But there is also another crucial aspect of the system: the infant's attentional stream. Every cry and coax, and each point and offer, is deeply contextualized in a flow of attention toward the animate, the inanimate, and the symbolic realms.

Baby biographers from Darwin (1877) to Shatz (1994) have captured the attentional qualities of alertness, involvement, engagement, fascination, and even mindfulness that characterize early referential communication. However, attention itself has rarely been a focal topic, and behavioral scientists have often resisted the concept of attention. For example, James, who in 1890 defined attention as "the taking possession by the mind, in clear and vivid form, of one out of what seems several simultaneously possible objects or trains of thought" (p. 404), began his cogent chapter on attention with a plea to psychologists that they acknowledge that attention is central to experience despite its studied neglect by British empiricists. In 1979, Gibson and Rader urged their colleagues to overcome their aversion to a phenomenon that carries "an enormous burden of concealed assumptions" (p. 20) to renew efforts to understand attention and hence how "a motivated organism living and adapting to an environment ... searches for information that is necessary for performance" (pp. 6–7).

This chapter was supported by funding from a grant from the Chancellor's Initiative Fund of Georgia State University.

Since the 1980s, many researchers concerned with preverbal communication have tried to bring attention into the foreground. Their interest has been spurred by a renewed appreciation of traditional developmental perspectives such as Vygotsky's (1978) sociohistorical theory and Werner and Kaplan's (1963) organismic view, both of which place interactional processes at the cutting edge of cognitive development. From these perspectives, early communication development is best understood not only as a series of developmental milestones, such as smiles, points, and words, but also in terms of the construction of dialogues of actions and words between children and caregivers (Dore, 1985). Central to several studies of these dialogues has been the description of the flow of attention throughout a web of sites, including partners, shared objects and events, and language. By documenting attention during social interactions, investigators hope to address basic issues related to the development of behavioral and emotional regulation, the emergence of communicative intentions, and the acquisition of culturally specific forms of communication (Adamson & Bakeman, 1991).

This chapter surveys the research literature on the early development of attention during communication. One central developmental strand is singled out for consideration: the emergence and consolidation of an attentional structure called *coordinated attention*. During episodes of coordinated attention, a child's attention flows between different foci, such as people, objects, and symbols, within a communicative exchange. There are two particularly noteworthy aspects to the process of coordinating attention. First, such coordination may result in episodes of *joint attention*, that is, an attentional state during which the child and partner share a site of interest, such as an object or an event, in their immediate surroundings. This juxtaposition allows caregivers and infants to engage in referential communication during which the adult interprets and informs the child's experience with the environment (Adamson & McArthur, 1995). As Bruner maintained, "Joint attention is not just joint attention, but joint participation in a common culture" (1995, p. 11). Second, this coordination reflects the child's ability to share experiences of events with other people, a process often called *secondary intersubjectivity* (Trevarthen & Hubley, 1978). It is possible for a caregiver to support his or her infant's exploration of objects without the infant actively acknowledging the caregiver, thus achieving joint attention without coordinated attention on the part of the infant (Bakeman & Adamson, 1984). By the beginning of their second year, however, infants are often clearly active participants in episodes of joint attention as they alternate their gaze between their partner and their shared objects, a state of attention that Bakeman and Adamson (1984) labeled *coordinated joint engagement*.

This chapter's review of the literature related to coordinated attention is organized into three sections. First, we consider the developmental pattern of coordinated attention's emergence and chart its roots in earlier episodes of interpersonal attention and its fruits in the just-verbal child's first conversations. Second, we discuss the process of coordinating attention during the transitions to intentional communication and to symbolic communication. For each of these transitions, we cull the literature to locate normative events and informative variations in the way toddlers and their social partners modulate shared attention as new communicative abilities develop. Third, we discuss the implications of the research on coordinated attention for clinical intervention and for future study of communication development.

COORDINATING ATTENTION:
A DEVELOPMENTAL PERSPECTIVE

An infant's attention during social interactions is as varied as a newborn's wide-eyed stare, a 3-month-old's prolonged gaze at her partner's face, a 1-year-old's glances between parent and perplexing toy, and a 2-year-old's mention of a favorite object that is out of sight but not out of mind. From a developmental perspective, each of these manifestations appears as a milestone along a path comprising ways of selectively attending during a communicative episode. This section sketches this path to locate the emergence of coordinated joint attention and to discuss the significance of this placement.

Developmental Path of Shared Attention

During a child's first 2 years, the way he or she attends during social interactions undergoes fundamental changes. One way to summarize the developmental pattern of these changes is to note where infants of different ages typically focus when they communicate. Using such a frame, infancy can be divided into three periods (Adamson, 1996; Adamson & Bakeman, 1991): 1) an initial period when the infant develops patterns of attending to social partners; 2) a period from about 6–18 months during which an infant comes to maintain a shared attentional focus to objects and events with a variety of social partners; and 3) a transitional period out of infancy when a child begins to appreciate that symbols, including those contained in language, may bring represented as well as present objects and events into social interactions.

This division of infancy into three periods is a fairly standard practice (Adamson & Bakeman, 1991; also see Wellman's 1993 discussion of the developmental phases in the emergence of theory of mind). For our purposes, it is a useful exercise because it highlights an important developmental point: Coordinated attention to people and objects occupies a pivotal point during early communication development. It begins to emerge only after infants have devoted many weeks to a "fundamental education" (Spitz, 1972) during which they master the rudiments of sharing attention with a social partner. It is consolidated only many months later, at a time when children typically begin to make the transition from presymbolic to symbolic communication.

A Precursor to Coordinated Joint Attention: Attention to Social Partners
The first period of the development of shared attention is characterized by an

intense and predominant interest in the interpersonal realm. From birth on, typically developing newborns sustain episodes of shared attentiveness that occur when the infant maintains a state of quiet alertness within a social context. Although the baby does not yet fill shared moments with specific communicative acts, he or she is receptive to social contact and—as revealed in a fascinating experimental literature—social content (e.g., DeCasper & Fifer, 1980; for a review, see Adamson, 1996). By the end of the second month, infants' interests clarify as they begin to modulate their visual attention toward and away from interesting sights while producing interpretable emotional expressions. The preferred target of this selective attention is often another person who is acting in ways that draw and hold interest. Of particular note is the split-second timing with which a young infant can pace his or her expressive activities with those of a social partner (Brazelton, Koslowski, & Main, 1974; Stern, 1974; Tronick, Als, & Adamson, 1979).

The Emergence and Consolidation of Coordinated Joint Attention The second period in the development of shared attention is characterized by the mutual attention of social partners to objects and events in the immediate surrounding. This period begins at about 5–6 months of age when the infant enters "the era of handling things" (Shinn, 1900), which is also known to developmentalists as the stage of "secondary circular reactions" (Piaget, 1963). Between their fifth and sixth months, infants' prolonged focus on their social partner wanes as they turn single-mindedly to objects and events near at hand (Kaye & Fogel, 1980). The infant who just displayed finely tuned skills for modulating attention toward and away from another person suddenly appears unwilling or unable to shift attention away from an engaging object. Yet a partner may still influence periods of object focus. For example, a solicitous caregiver may join the infant's object engagement even if she is not explicitly invited to do so, as when a mother animates a doll her son is holding without her son shifting his gaze toward her and away from the interesting object. During such episodes, which Adamson and Bakeman (1991) labeled *supported joint engagement,* an infant's partner carries much of the burden of ensuring that a shared focus is maintained. These episodes fulfill one of the primary requirements of coordinated joint attention, that there be shared focus on an aspect of the object world, without fulfilling a second requirement, that the infant actively relate as well to his or her social partner.

For the purposes of this chapter, a central developmental shift occurs when an infant begins to actively integrate attention to people into some of his or her object-focused activities. Such coordinated attention to people and objects may take many forms. The infant may briefly glance at a partner to check if she is looking at the point of a pointing gesture (Butterworth & Grover, 1990; Leung & Rheingold, 1981); to seek information about an event or object that stirs uncertainty, a process called *social referencing* (Klinnert, Campos, Sorce, Emde, & Svejda, 1983); or to request help obtaining a desired object (Bruner, Roy, & Ratner, 1982). The coordination also may be sustained for minutes during the execution of a standardized format such as give-and-take or picture book reading (Bruner, 1982). Once an infant and partner consolidate a format, some of the format's subroutines (e.g., look at a picture then glance toward mother, glance at father and then release the ball) routinely pattern the flow of attention between objects and people.

The consolidation of coordinated joint attention spans several months. Its first manifestations occur at around 6 months of age when a baby switches his or her gaze between a caregiver and an object that lie in the same visual field (Newson & Newson, 1975). However, it is not until about 13 months of age that most infants maintain periods of sustained attention to both a caregiver and objects, and it may be several months more before they do so with less cooperative partners, such as peers (Bakeman & Adamson, 1984). By the middle of the second year, the coordination of attention to people and objects in the immediate surroundings is usually skillfully executed.

Changes in Coordinated Attention During the Transition to Language Although there is little research that focuses primarily on the coordination of attention after infancy, there are many hints that a major shift occurs as a child begins to penetrate the symbolic realm. To chart movement into this new domain, we have designated a third period, symbol-infused coordinated attention, along the developmental path of shared attention. The boundary with the second period is difficult to draw, in part because people often surround infants with language and act as if the infants understand their utterances (see, e.g., Rheingold & Adams, 1980) and in part because most children introduce speech only gradually into their social interactions (Bakeman & Adamson, 1986). Nevertheless, by the last half of the second year, symbols are clearly woven into the fabric of shared attention. For example, a child may confirm his or her partner's verbal command by acting in ways that specifically conform (or do not conform) to what the partner says, with or without glancing toward the partner. A child and his or her partner may also focus together on represented events, thus infinitely expanding the topics of their interactions to include shared memories, individual minds, and imaginary entities. Furthermore, they may concentrate concurrently on the symbolic code itself, as when one partner provides a name for an object or demonstrates a symbolic gesture.

Summary Throughout infancy, children clarify, add, and integrate different foci of attention. A newborn only rarely fixates his or her gaze, conveying the impression of just becoming oriented. The 18-month-old successively concentrates on an object and a person, shifting his or her attention smoothly between them. By skillfully drawing together the social and object realms, the infant constructs a psychological space for the meeting of intimate personal relationships and engaging environmental events. Once this construction is consolidated, the infant then begins to move his or her attention to represented as well as to present sites, preparing for the integration of symbols, including language, into ongoing social interactions.

**Developmental Placement of
Coordinated Attention to Partners and Objects**

From a developmental perspective, locating coordinated joint attention amid the path of shared attention entails more than merely placing it on a list of milestones; it also situates it within an intellectual tradition that predisposes researchers to entertain certain hypotheses about the relation between milestones and to adopt particular approaches to the description of early social interactions. Following Werner (1957), developmental researchers typically pose heuristic hypotheses that posit an ontogenetic relation between milestones such that later ones (e.g., coordinated joint attention) are viewed as more differentiated and hierarchically integrated versions of earlier-developing phenomena (e.g., engagement with people and supported joint exploration of objects). Furthermore, they consider how earlier milestones might serve as a springboard for the emergence of later milestones (e.g., symbol-infused coordinated attention) and how the proposed developmental path leads toward major accomplishments (e.g., the acquisition of language and of a theory of mind).

The developmental tradition also has influenced how researchers study coordinated attention by drawing their attention to the details of how adults and infants act during relatively brief episodes of object-focused interaction. This penchant for microanalysis was inspired by studies of attention modulation during the face-to-face social interactions of early infancy. It was in these studies (e.g., Brazelton et al., 1974; Kaye & Fogel, 1980) that investigators first gathered convincing evidence of the dynamic flow of attention during preverbal communication. This microanalytic approach to coordinated attention has several strengths. It acknowledges infants' sensitivity to the split-second timing of social interactions (Stern, Beebe, Jaffe, & Bennett, 1977; Watson, 1985), and it is readily amenable to the application of sequential analyses (Bakeman & Gottman, 1986) that can be used to abstract interactional patterns from behavioral particulars. Furthermore, it has helped researchers think about the development of shared attention within the broader perspectives of systems theory (Fogel & Thelen, 1987; Sander, 1977) and to articulate questions about how shared attention between infants and caregivers may frame communicative acts such as affective expressions and words (Adamson & Bakeman, 1985; Tomasello & Farrar, 1986).

However, it is also important to note a potential danger of microanalysis. A close focus on temporal textures may produce details taken out of a broader context, especially when pragmatic constraints demand that investigators narrow their focus to videotaped observations that last only minutes. To counteract this tendency, developmental psychologists have revived Vygotsky's (1978) concept of the zone of proximal development in the hope of guiding observations toward periods of shared attention that may play a particularly important role in early communication development. Within a zone, the developmental unit is the child in interaction with a developmentally more advanced partner. Both contribute to the structuring of interpersonal attention by engaging in complementary activities: the child as an active, organized seeker of information and the partner as a teacher who supports good learning that fosters developmental movement (see also Chapter 12).

There are two particularly noteworthy aspects to a Vygotskian approach to social interactions. First, it is fundamentally cultural. Caregivers are agents of culture (Trevarthen, 1988) who set an infant's nascent actions within an intimate setting that is deeply informed by the caregiver's cultural knowledge. Caregivers cannot help but view infants' expressions as meaningful within the human sphere of their own culture. Infants, in complement, are quintessential cultural apprentices who seek the guided participation of their elders (Rogoff, 1990).

Second, the notion of a zone of proximal development reveals a pattern of developmental change in which a phase of adult support precedes a phase of independent infant accomplishment. Each cycle begins with a newly displayed behavior, such as a smile, a visually directed reach, or a babble. The adult's reactions and interpretations transform the infant's emerging behavior into a social act. In essence, the child induces the adult to recruit the act for communication (Bakeman, Adamson, Konner, & Barr, in press). After many experiences of supported expression, the child gradually masters an action that is qualified with cultural meaning. The act has passed through the zone of proximal development during which the adult has educated the child in its use. This shift from supported emergence to active consolidation can be abstracted during each of the periods in the development of shared attention during infancy. In each, the emergence of a new form of shared attention (i.e., to people, objects, and symbols, respectively) involves a transactional pattern in which the caregiver initially provides and then gradually withdraws interpersonal support for an emerging pattern of the infant's interest in a particular aspect of his or her world.

In summary, from a developmental perspective, the emergence of coordinated joint attention appears as an integration of earlier emerging interests in people and in objects. The drawing together of people and objects into a single attentional field allows the infant to be educated by caregivers who may support and enculturate an infant's first forays into the inanimate world. Moreover, as infants consolidate the skill of attending simultaneously to people and to shared objects, a foundation is being laid for a developmental movement into the realm of symbols.

COORDINATING ATTENTION AND
THE EMERGENCE OF COMMUNICATIVE INTENTIONS

We now focus more specifically on attentional processes during two crucial points of change in early communication development, the transition to communicative intentions and the transition to symbolic modes. During early development, shared attention and communicative intention are inextricably intertwined.

(esp. language development)

Bruner (1983), drawing inspiration from Jakobson (1960), argued persuasively that certain structures of attention to people and objects are crucial for the communication of object-focused messages. As he noted, "The problems of how reference develops can be restated as the problem of how people manage and direct each others' attention" (Bruner, 1983, p. 68).

During the last months of their first year, most infants make major strides in coordinating different behaviors and, hence, acting intentionally. As Piaget (1963) argued, when an infant can sequence acts so that one serves as a means to the performance of another, it is reasonable to contend that the child is behaving intentionally. Although Piaget did not highlight the implications for communication development of the capacity to coordinate acts, he reported observations (e.g., Obs. 127 and 128, pp. 223–224) in which his child directs an action toward him (e.g., gently moving Piaget's hand) to produce a coveted result (e.g., having Piaget tap his cheek and drum on his eyeglasses).

Several other theorists (e.g., Bates, Camaioni, & Volterra, 1975) have extended Piaget's theory to the development of communicative intentions. They have retained his emphasis on the importance of the infant's emerging understanding of intentionality, "an awareness of the effect that a message will have on the addressee" (Bretherton, 1992, p. 60; for a contrasting view, see Moore & Corkum, 1994). Moreover, they find evidence for this budding awareness in the way infants pattern their actions toward people and with objects, rather than in the emergence of new behavioral forms per se. For example, already developed forms, such as the extension of an index finger, are often performed in new ways to serve emerging communicative intentions (Fogel & Thelen, 1987; Werner & Kaplan, 1963).

Preverbal object-focused communicative intentions can be divided into two basic categories: requesting (or imperatives) and commenting (or declaratives) (see Chapter 6). These have most often been discussed in terms of their behavioral forms (see, e.g., Bates, 1976), but it is also possible to abstract their attentional structure. Both entail a triadic arrangement between the infant, the partner, and an object, although what aspects are marked most predominantly vary as a function of communicative intent (Adamson, 1992). Requests typically focus foremost on the partner as the communicator tries to tell him or her what to do with an object. Comments, in turn, highlight a specific event that becomes a topic for shared contemplation.

It is difficult to date exactly when a child begins to pattern his or her attention in ways that support certain communicative messages. First, not all communicative intentions are mastered at the same time. Although requests often are noted by 9–10 months of age, comments are first observed at about 12 months (Bakeman & Adamson, 1986; Bates et al., 1975; for studies revealing a similar pattern of onset for the comprehension of commenting acts, see Butterworth & Grover, 1990). The relatively late emergence of commenting acts, such as pointing, may reflect in part the difficulty of displacing attention away from a partner and toward an object. Despite these logistical differences, both requesting and commenting are fundamentally dependent on an active attentional linking of the child, the partner, and the object. Second, the coordination of attention to people and objects is not a solitary accomplishment. It is a shared act, one that is fundamentally dependent on the mutual regulation of the partners' actions.

Zone of Proximal Development for Coordinated Joint Attention

A precise blending of partners' attention is needed for object-related communicative messages to flow within their social interaction, but both partners need not be equally responsible for the management of this attention. Throughout the last year of infancy, the balance shifts markedly as the infant passes through a zone of proximal development. When the infant is 6 months old, the adult appears to take all responsibility for ensuring that a triadic arrangement of self, infant, and object endures. By the age of 1½ years, infants and adults share management, albeit with different acts and aims.

Observational studies of attention management document how well adults can meet their infants within a zone of proximal development to bridge the gap between the emergence of infants' fascination with objects and their ability to coordinate attention to people and objects. There is little doubt that adults can support a joint attentional focus and that this support may be sensitively tuned to the ever-changing capacities of their infant partners. The research literature contains detailed accounts of maternal scaffolds, including narrative reports (e.g., Bruner, 1983; Trevarthen & Hubley, 1978) and systematic microanalytic studies (e.g., Adamson & Bakeman, 1984; Hodapp, Goldfield, & Boyatzis, 1984).

It is far more difficult to discern the infant's contributions. This point is well illustrated by an experiment conducted by Ross and Lollis (1987), who observed mothers and infants playing turn-taking games with objects. When the game was proceeding without a hitch, the mothers appeared to carry the joint attention management burden. The infants often appeared to be almost completely absorbed by the object of the shared game, such as the toppling of blocks or the beating of a drum, and to ignore their obliging partners. But when mothers, by experimental design, failed to take a turn, infants often showed that they were aware both of the adult and of the game's turn-taking structure: Nine-month-olds filled the unexpected pause with vocalizations and other communicative signals; whereas fifteen-month-olds actively prompted the adult to continue the game. Thus, infants rose to the occasion by taking a more active role in managing joint attention than they might usually take (see Chapter 7 for a discussion of preverbal repairs).

To view infants' developing capacities to negotiate attentional foci with their caregivers, it is helpful to look beyond the brief periods of object-focused play that are the typical fare of systematic studies of coordinated attention. One particularly revealing situation in middle-class Western culture involves the ubiquitous high chair, which elevates and confines the infant within the adult's visual field. In this position, infants typically display persistence and flexibility as they try to attract a caregiver's attention to themselves and to a specific referent, often in service of a communicative intention such as requesting an object. For example, when Golinkoff (1986) observed 1-year-old infants in their high chairs at lunchtime (a context she noted is "a naturally occurring infant-constructed 'test' of communicative capability," p. 472), she found that mothers did not understand the infants' goals in half of the infant-initiated episodes. However, infants stayed focused on conveying their goals, often through several cycles of negotiation during which they increasingly exaggerated and, by the middle of their second year, increasingly varied their communicative acts. Rogoff, Mistry, Radziszewska, and Germond (1992) observed even younger infants in the captive context of a high chair and also noted intentional requests for adult help with objects by the end of the first year. Rogoff and colleagues located the elements of object requests, such as attempts to establish eye contact, well before observers reliably coded intentional communication. Some observers found these early elements convincing, whereas others were less liberal interpreters. This suggests that there was ample time and substance for adults to help construct a zone of proximal development before infants had fully mastered ways to communicate intentionally.

One important cue for communicative intent may be the coordination of attention toward the partner and the desired objects. Although adults are often unaware of why they act as they do when interacting with infants (see, e.g., Papoušek & Papoušek, 1987, on intuitive parenting), it is possible to probe their reasons for ascribing intentionality by using nonverbal methods (Adamson, Bakeman, Smith, & Walters, 1987). For example, Yoder and Munson (1995) asked mothers to review videotapes of just-completed play sessions with their 10-month-old infants and to indicate by pushing a button each time they believed that the infant had communicated intentionally. The researchers found that there was a positive correlation between how often mothers attributed intentionality and how often their infants displayed coordinated attention. Yoder and Munson (1995) also documented temporal overlap: Mothers were most likely to ascribe communicative intent to acts that occurred when infants were coordinating their attention to people and objects.

Variations in Coordinating Attention to People and Objects

The strong central theme that emerges from consideration of the normative development of coordinated attention is one of directed movement through a zone of proximal development. However, it is important to consider variations in this theme to get a fuller sense of its boundaries and direction. Particularly revealing are descriptions of situations that differ qualitatively from the narrow range of parent–infant interactions that researchers usually examine. The study of non-Western cultures may provide some challenging observations. Child-rearing contexts that contrast with those prevalent in the United States can provide a new perspective on how adults and infants may contribute to the orchestration of coordinated attention. One important dimension of variation is the value placed on object possession and manipulation. In middle-class Western society, adults often encourage infants to explore objects in culturally designated ways; that is, they invite the infant into a zone of proximal development in which objects have a central place. Thus, researchers need to investigate if and when infants develop joint attention skills in cultures in which nurturing caregivers are relatively indifferent to objects and in which object-focused formats are relatively rare.

However, there are few studies. Those that are available support the claim that the timetable for the emergence of coordinated attention may be a developmental universal. For example, Bakeman, Adamson, Konner, and Barr (1990) systematically studied the emergence of object involvement by infants of the !Kung San in Botswana. Ethnographic reports indicate that the !Kung place relatively little emphasis on the object world, except during ritualized object exchange (Lee, 1979), and that !Kung San adults reportedly neither restrain nor encourage object manipulation (Konner, 1972). The !Kung San was a feasible group to study. During the 1970s, Konner created a large data archive of observations of !Kung San infants during everyday events using ~~ethological~~ methods. By *ethological* doing new analyses of this data set, Bakeman and colleagues revealed a pattern of shared attention development that is consistent with the picture of the development of coordinated joint attention drawn for Western infants. Thus, !Kung infants displayed sustained interest in other people during their first months; at about 4 months of age, they started to attend to objects; and, at about 8 months of age, they began to offer objects to others, a form of coordinated joint attention. Furthermore, Bakeman et al. (1990) found that although !Kung caregivers are often very attentive (see, e.g., Barr, Konner, Bakeman, & Adamson, 1991), they usually ignored infants when the infants played with objects with one exception: Caregivers were readily responsive whenever infants initiated an object offer. Thus, by the end of their first year, !Kung infants, like their American (as well as their Scottish and Yoruba [see Trevarthen, 1988]) counterparts, had begun to coordinate their attention to people and to objects of shared interest.

From observations such as these, it is reasonable to conclude that infants can achieve coordinated joint attention even without the extensive scaffolds erected by the caregivers whom researchers are most apt to study. The basic developmental trajectory is set by the infant. However, given the inherent intertwining of acts of coordinated attention and expressions of communicative intention, it would be misleading to assign primary responsibility only to the child. Even if adults do not actively attempt to share objects with infants, infants may act in ways to induce such sharing. Adults, in turn, may respond in ways that provide a culturally refined reading of the infant's universal display of interest in object sharing.

A second way to gain a broader view of the development of coordinated attention is to observe infants with developmental disabilities that affect their attention deployment. In rare cases, an infant may display so little interest in objects that establishing a joint attentional focus may be essentially precluded (e.g., Yoder & Farran, 1986). More common is the development of the basic attentional elements for coordinated engagement, but at an older age and with less frequency than typical. Such a delay has been documented in studies of infants with Down syndrome (for a review, see Berger, 1990) and of high-risk, prematurely born infants (Landry, 1995). Analyses of how coordinated joint attention develops when the developmental path is prolonged may reveal stumbling blocks that can hinder the development of object-focused communicative intentions. Several possible points of difficulty have been located along the normative path. For example, Legerstee and Bowman (1989) suggested that earlier attentional problems experienced by infants with Down syndrome during the period of interpersonal engagement might hamper movement to object engagement. Hyche, Bakeman, and Adamson (1992) speculated that the relative mutedness of these infants' earliest manifestation of object interest might make it more difficult for even experienced caregivers to read these actions and recruit them for communicative exchanges. A possible imbalance of people-focused and object-focused interests also has been considered. Infants with Down syndrome often display relatively strong interpersonal skills such as turn-taking and a concomitant deficit in object-requesting skills (Mundy, Sigman, Kasari, & Yirmiya, 1988), a pattern that some researchers (e.g., Krakow & Kopp, 1983) think might reflect problems meeting the cognitive demands of shifting attention from a partner to an object.

In some instances, the balance between interest in people and interest in objects is so askew that distortions in the basic structure of coordinated joint attention may persist. For example, a study of how one young child with Williams syndrome, a rare genetic disorder usually diagnosed well after infancy (Bellugi, Bihrle, Neville, & Doherty, 1992), deployed her attention during social interaction (Bertrand, Mervis, Rice, & Adamson, 1993) suggested that a persistent engagement with a partner's face may compete with the coordination of attention to people and objects. The child's attention during social interactions was first observed at 18 months of age; during this session, the proportion of time she devoted to coordinated joint engagement was comparable to that noted for typically developing toddlers (Bakeman & Adamson, 1984). However, there were two intriguing differences in how she modulated her attention during the observations made during the next year. First, she persistently focused on faces (be it on a person or an inanimate toy, especially if it was novel), gazing intently at them without producing communicative acts. Second, she sometimes simultaneously manipulated an object and stared intently at her partner, without actively combining these two foci. For example, at 22 months of age, she "flew" a toy airplane while looking expressionlessly toward her mother. Thus, the child's coordinated attention sometimes appeared qualitatively different from that observed in typical infants: The elements for coordination were displayed, but they were not always integrated into a single attentional structure.

Young children with autism display another form of imbalance between attention to people and to objects. An impairment in joint attention skills is one of autism's core symptoms (Loveland & Landry, 1986; Sigman & Kasari, 1995; Wetherby & Prutting, 1984) that appears early in its developmental course (Osterling & Dawson, 1994). This impairment is particularly pronounced when communication involves shared contemplation of objects. Children with autism rarely bring toys to their parents to see, look at their parents for approval, or perform social reference for the purpose of acquiring information (Sigman & Kasari, 1995). They may, however, seek help obtaining an object. Furthermore, they may never produce a point to share interest in or attention to an object (i.e., a "proto-declarative" point), but they may point to obtain an object (i.e., a "proto-imperative" point) or to identify one item as distinct from another (i.e., a "referential" point [Baron-Cohen, 1989; Goodhart & Baron-Cohen, 1993]).

Various explanations center the problem with shared reference in children with autism in different arenas. Some emphasize underlying neurological impairments in a module that specifically controls shared attention (e.g., Baron-Cohen, 1989) or in brain regions that serve attention shifting (e.g., Courchesne et al., 1994). Others stress arousal regulation difficulties that may result in problems with sustaining attention to unpredictable stimuli (e.g., Dawson & Lewy, 1989) or with integrating attention and cognition with affect (Mundy & Sigman, 1989). The difficulty a child with autism has in sustaining a joint attentional focus may profoundly affect early communication development and may limit reception of partners' immediate messages about objects. Moreover, it may also narrow the zone of proximal development so that the child misses out on many of the interactions that help a typical child consolidate the structure of coordinated attention. Thus, the young child with autism may have less access to cultural symbols, including language, that caregivers typically carry with them as they share objects with preverbal children (McArthur & Adamson, 1996). The recognition of the central importance of shared attention for subsequent development has opened avenues for early identification and intervention.

COORDINATING ATTENTION AND THE TRANSITION TO LANGUAGE

At about 18 months of age, infants readily reveal their ability to coordinate attention by gazing successively toward a partner and visible events and by producing communicative acts, such as points, to mark their interests. During the next several months, however, the flow of their attention becomes increasingly difficult to track as they begin to pay attention to distant and imaginary events as well as to what transpires in the here and now. Not only do toddlers coordinate their attention to people and objects on the overt plane of the present, they also focus attention on what transpires on the covert plane of symbols. As they explore this plane, they attend to aspects of communication, such as language, that afford infinite depth and scope to human communication. Toddlers also begin to act as if they have a rudimentary understanding (or theory) of their communicative partners' knowledge and intentions (Tomasello, 1995). For example, they are able to take into account their partner's intentions and attention when assigning novel words to referents, thus avoiding mapping errors that might result if they were simply to rely on the co-occurrence of words and objects (Baldwin, 1995).

By the middle of the second year, there are several indications that children are forming symbols (Piaget, 1962; Werner & Kaplan, 1963). This new cognitive capacity transforms attention deployment during communicative exchanges. For example, children now begin to follow an adult's gazes and points when they are directed toward sites that are not within their current environment (e.g., the area behind one's back) (Butterworth & Grover, 1990). Furthermore, they begin to rapidly acquire words that they can comprehend and produce in new communicative contexts (Reznick & Goldfield, 1992).

There has been little systematic research that specifically examines how coordinated attention is transformed as language is acquired. In part, this may be due to the difficulty of applying systematic observational methods to a process in which key elements are hidden from view. However, one aspect of this transformation—the infusion of language into periods of coordinated attention—has begun to stir interest. Although language is only part of the developmental story, it is the most complex and important chapter. It has been written about from many perspectives, including some that seek to view its acquisition as a social-pragmatic achievement (Bruner, 1983). From this vantage point, the influence of language on the flow of attention to current events can be examined, for example, to demonstrate that adults' talk about an object prolongs an infant's attention to it (Baldwin, 1995). How language provides a new way of framing attention so that it gains narrative continuity (Bruner, 1995) and how episodes of mutual attention are managed to support the infusion of language, particularly the learning of new words (Tomasello, 1995), also could be explored.

Joint Attention and Early Word Learning

There are several indications that joint attention and early word learning are related. Toddlers are most likely to produce their first words while they are attending to both their caregiver and objects (Bakeman & Adamson, 1986). Moreover, the more often they experience joint attention during a play session with their caregiver, the larger the toddler's early vocabularies are likely to be (e.g., Dunham & Dunham, 1992; Smith, Adamson, & Bakeman, 1988).

These general relations suggest that periods of object sharing may, at least for some caregivers and toddlers, become occasions for metalinguistic lessons. Observational studies indicate that adults and toddlers from middle-class Western culture often spontaneously engage in word-learning routines when they share an activity. Caregivers use a range of instructional strategies that guide the child's attention to the link between a word and a referent (Deffebach & Adamson, 1994). For example, they may call attention to the name of an object by pointing to the referent while providing its label ("That's a *bear*") or by prompting the child to provide a conventional label ("What is *this* [object shown] called?"). In addition, they may focus on the child by speaking for the child (*"Thank you, Mommy"*) or by cueing the child to speak ("Now what do you say?") to demonstrate how to use social-regulative words. Caregivers and children may even package these strategies into routines such as book reading that provide culturally standard ways of modulating attention to foster vocabulary acquisition (Bruner, 1982; Ninio, 1983).

Microanalyses of the flow of attention during metalingual lessons suggest that adults may most successfully teach nouns when they map their own attention onto their child's current focus. For example, Tomasello and Farrar (1986; see also Dunham, Dunham, & Curwin, 1993) demonstrated experimentally that a toddler is more likely to learn a new noun if an adult introduces it when the toddler is already focused on the referent (i.e., an attention-following strategy) than if the adult seeks to shift the toddler's attention to a new object and then provides a label (i.e., an attention-shifting strategy). Adults, however, may need to use a different strategy to optimize the teaching of verbs. Tomasello and Kruger (1992), for example, found that adults were most effective when they provided a new verb just before, rather than during, the occurrence of a to-be-labeled action (e.g., "Now I'm going to roll it" versus "Look, the ball is rolling").

Despite the clarity of these demonstrations that well-managed coordinated attention may facilitate word learning, two important issues remain unresolved. First, it is not clear what children must understand about the link between joint attention and words for language learning to occur. Baldwin (1995) stated the theoretical stakes involved by arguing that toddlers who are learning language not only engage in joint attention, they also display a newly emerging level of intersubjectivity that includes an awareness of their partner's focus and referential intent. Second, it remains unclear whether joint attention is necessary for the transition to language. Tomasello (1995) highlighted this issue by championing the bold hypothesis that "to acquire a new word—to learn to comprehend and produce it in conventionally appropriate contexts—the child must enter into a state of joint attentional focus with an adult" (p. 117).

Variations in Coordinating Attention to People, Objects, and Language

To probe outstanding issues about the relation between joint attention and language development, it is helpful to examine variations in the way language infuses social interactions. Enough different cultural arrangements for language teaching have been documented to rule out any singular notion of specific relation among people, objects, and words a toddler must experience to learn language (Schieffelin & Ochs, 1986). Furthermore, the study of children with disabilities that affect the infusion of language is raising important qualifiers to our understanding of what aspects of language are nurtured during episodes of joint attention. Research about communication development of children with autism provides a good case. If and when a child with autism acquires complex language, the impact of earlier-developing difficulties with joint attention may be confined to how language is used, not to its form. For example, Tager-Flusberg (1994) found that six verbal boys with autism spoke grammatically but had difficulty using language to serve the same communicative functions of declaring and sharing information that are also problematic during the development of coordinated attention.

However, these observations of language-learning children with autism do not preclude the possibility that a timely transition to language depends on the placement of language within periods of joint engagement. Approximately half of all children with autism do not speak, and their joint attention skills predict subsequent word learning (Mundy, Sigman, & Kasari, 1990). Moreover, although young deaf children do not seem to have undue difficulty mastering coordinated attention (Spencer & Kelly, 1993), they may have difficulty "uptaking" language unless their partners adjust their actions to suit the children's visual attention. Spencer and Lederberg (1997) report that deaf mothers often use strategies that introduce deaf infants to language (e.g., signing on or near the object the infant was looking at, waiting for the infant to look at her before signing) that hearing mothers of deaf infants, even when they try to sign, are less likely to display. They also found that for both hearing infants with hearing mothers and deaf infants with deaf mothers, but not for deaf children with hearing mothers, time spent in periods of coordinated joint engagement was significantly related to early word learning. Thus, whether coordinated attention provides a frame for language learning may depend on whether the adult and child can draw usable language into their shared activity.

EDUCATIONAL AND CLINICAL IMPLICATIONS

Our basic claim in this chapter is that attentional processes that draw together people, objects, and language are crucial for early communication development. We support this claim with observational and experimental literature. From this research, we abstract three phases in the development of shared attention during infancy. In narrowing our focus to joint attentional processes during the transitions to intentional communication and symbolic communication, we find both a wealth of rich descriptions and several open issues. This section briefly evaluates our understanding of the development of coordinated attention to people, objects, and language.

The study of shared attentional processes during infancy underscores that communication development involves more than the mastery of specific actions. Infants also must master ways of interrelating their own interests with those of their social partners, of forming and conveying intentions, and of learning cultural conventions. There are several implications of this complex view of communication development for the early identification of communication problems and for the design and assessment of intervention programs.

Several efforts are already well under way to incorporate research related to coordinated attention into diagnostic tools for early assessment. For example, Wetherby and Prizant (1992) considered the normative development of joint attention in their construction of the Communication and Symbolic Behavior Scales (Wetherby & Prizant, 1993), an instrument that provides a profile of a child's mastery of communicative skills that typically emerge between 8 and 24 months of age. Several parameters of attention deployment are measured, including the production of communicative acts that establish joint attentional focus and the presence of gaze shifts back and forth between people and objects. Baron-Cohen, Allen, and Gillberg (1992) also devised a screening instrument, the Checklist for Autism in Toddlers, that includes questions related to joint attention and proto-declarative pointing and appears to have good predictive validity.

In concert with early identification, early intervention programs are being designed to foster joint attention skills in young children (see Chapters 15 and 16). Of particular note are intensive programs that specifically target children with autism and other pervasive developmental disorders in hopes of igniting the children's interest in people and structuring shared attention to objects (see, e.g., Greenspan, 1992; Klinger & Dawson, 1992). There are also less extensive ways that consideration of attentional processes might inform intervention efforts. For example, the initial vocabulary for an augmentative device to be used by a nonspeaking child might be broadly selected so that the child is provided both labels for marking objects and social-regulative terms (e.g., "I want") to highlight the alignment of partners' interests (Adamson, Romski, Deffebach, & Sevcik, 1992).

DIRECTIONS FOR FUTURE RESEARCH

The study of attentional processes during early development is now at an exciting juncture. A basic developmental path has been laid out, and several issues have been articulated about the relation between shared attention and the transitions to intentional and symbolic communication. Researchers are well positioned to focus their studies on specific sites along this path, such as the milestones of the first word and of the vocabulary spurt (e.g., Bloom, 1993). Furthermore, they are beginning to probe more deeply into a child's emerging appreciation of how his or her partner's attentional patterns may convey messages about intentions (e.g., Baldwin, 1995; Tomasello, 1995).

Further research is also needed to explore the boundaries of the well-charted developmental path. Systematic observations of the development of coordinated attention by infants in different cultural contexts and in different contexts within one culture would both enrich the appreciation of the diversity of infants' experiences and inform ongoing discussions of mechanisms of development. The longitudinal studies can provide an important test of claims that certain attainments in attention management, such as the consolidation of coordinated joint attention, are crucial to later-developing achievements, including language and new levels of intersubjectivity such as a "theory" of other people's minds. There is also much work to be done to articulate how the development of coordinated attention to objects, people, and language is related to other developmental streams, including attention deployment during solitary object exploration (see, e.g., Ruff, 1986) and the expression of affect (see Chapter 6).

CONCLUSION

Shared attention changes qualitatively during major transitions in prelinguistic communication. As infants begin to express object-focused intentions, they also begin to coordinate attention to people and events of mutual interest. As toddlers begin to form symbols, they also start to focus with partners on the representation of past events, on entities with no more immediate substance than the contents of a partner's mind or an imaginary object, and on the system of language itself. The orchestration of these new patterns of shared attention is a dyadic accomplishment. As infants display new interests and new integrative capacities, caregivers provide culturally informed support that helps to structure and guide the infants' attention.

REFERENCES

Adamson, L.B. (1992). Variations in the early use of language. In L.T. Winegar & J. Valsiner (Eds.), *Children's development within social context: Vol. 1. Metatheory and theory* (pp. 123–141). Hillsdale, NJ: Lawrence Erlbaum Associates.

Adamson, L.B. (1996). *Communication development during infancy.* Boulder, CO: Westview.

Adamson, L.B., & Bakeman, R. (1984). Mothers' communicative acts: Changes during infancy. *Infant Behavior and Development, 7,* 467–478.

Adamson, L.B., & Bakeman, R. (1985). Affect and attention: Infants observed with mothers and peers. *Child Development, 56,* 582–593.

Adamson, L.B., & Bakeman, R. (1991). The development of shared attention during infancy. In R. Vasta (Ed.), *Annals of child development* (Vol. 8, pp. 1–41). London: Jessica Kingsley Publishers, Ltd.

Adamson, L.B., Bakeman, R., Smith, C.B., & Walters, A.S. (1987). Adults' interpretation of infants' acts. *Developmental Psychology, 23,* 383–387.

Adamson, L.B., & McArthur, D. (1995). Joint attention, affect, and culture. In C. Moore & P.J. Dunham (Eds.), *Joint attention: Its origin and role in development* (pp. 205–221). Hillsdale, NJ: Lawrence Erlbaum Associates.

Adamson, L.B., Romski, M.A., Deffebach, K., & Sevcik, R.A. (1992). Symbol vocabulary and the focus of conversations: Augmenting language development for youth with mental retardation. *Journal of Speech and Hearing Research, 35,* 1333–1343.

Bakeman, R., & Adamson, L.B. (1984). Coordinating attention to people and objects in mother–infant and peer–infant interaction. *Child Development, 55,* 1278–1289.

Bakeman, R., & Adamson, L.B. (1986). Infants' conventionalized acts: Gestures and words with mothers and peers. *Infant Behavior and Development, 9,* 215–230.

Bakeman, R., Adamson, L.B., Konner, M., & Barr, R.G. (1990). !Kung infancy: The social context of object exploration. *Child Development, 61,* 794–809.

Bakeman, R., Adamson, L.B., Konner, M., & Barr, R.G. (in press). Sequential analyses of !Kung infant communication: Inducing and recruiting. In E. Amsel & A. Renninger (Eds.), *Change and development.* Hillsdale, NJ: Lawrence Erlbaum Associates.

Bakeman, R., & Gottman, J.M. (1986). *Observing interaction: An introduction to sequential analysis.* New York: Cambridge University Press.

Baldwin, D.A. (1995). Understanding the link between joint attention and language. In C. Moore & P.J. Dunham (Eds.), *Joint attention: Its origin and role in development* (pp. 131–158). Hillsdale, NJ: Lawrence Erlbaum Associates.

Baron-Cohen, S. (1989). Joint-attention deficits in autism: Towards a cognitive analysis. *Development and Psychopathology, 1,* 185–189.

Baron-Cohen, S., Allen, J., & Gillberg, C. (1992). Can autism be detected at 18 months? The needle, the haystack, and the CHAT. *British Journal of Psychiatry, 161,* 839–843.

Barr, R.G., Konner, M., Bakeman, R., & Adamson, L.B. (1991). Crying in !Kung San infants: A test of the cultural specificity hypothesis. *Developmental Medicine and Child Neurology, 33,* 601–611.

Bates, E. (1976). *Language and context: The acquisition of pragmatics.* New York: Academic Press.

Bates, E., Camaioni, L., & Volterra, V. (1975). The acquisition of performatives prior to speech. *Merrill-Palmer Quarterly, 21,* 205–226.

Bellugi, U., Bihrle, A., Neville, H., & Doherty, S. (1992). Language, cognition, and brain organization in a neurodevelopmental disorder. In M. Gunnar & C. Nelson (Eds.), *Developmental behavioral neuroscience: The Minnesota symposium* (pp. 201–232). Hillsdale, NJ: Lawrence Erlbaum Associates.

Berger, J. (1990). Interactions between parents and their infants with Down syndrome. In D. Cicchetti & M. Beeghly (Eds.), *Children with Down syndrome: A developmental perspective* (pp. 101–146). Cambridge, England: Cambridge University Press.

Bertrand, J., Mervis, C., Rice, C.E., & Adamson, L.B. (1993, March). *Development of joint attention by a toddler with Williams syndrome.* Paper presented at the Gatlinburg Conference, Gatlinburg, TN.

Bloom, L. (1993). *The transition from infancy to language.* Cambridge, England: Cambridge University Press.

Brazelton, T.B., Koslowski, B., & Main, M. (1974). The origins of reciprocity: The early mother–infant interaction. In M. Lewis & L.A. Rosenblum (Eds.), *The effect of the infant on its caregiver* (pp. 49–76). New York: John Wiley & Sons.

Bretherton, I. (1992). Social referencing, intentional communication, and the interfacing of minds in infancy. In S. Feinman (Ed.), *Social referencing and the social construction of reality in infancy* (pp. 57–77). New York: Plenum.

Bruner, J. (1982). The formats of language acquisition. *American Journal of Semiotics, 1,* 1–16.

Bruner, J. (1983). *Child's talk: Learning to use language.* New York: Norton.

Bruner, J. (1995). From joint attention to the meeting of minds: An introduction. In C. Moore & P.J. Dunham (Eds.), *Joint attention: Its origins and role in development* (pp. 1–14). Hillsdale, NJ: Lawrence Erlbaum Associates.

Bruner, J., Roy, C., & Ratner, N. (1982). The beginnings of request. In K.E. Nelson (Ed.), *Children's language* (Vol. 3, pp. 91–138). Hillsdale, NJ: Lawrence Erlbaum Associates.

Butterworth, G., & Grover, L. (1990). Joint visual attention, manual pointing, and pre-verbal communication in human infancy. In M. Jeannerod (Ed.), *Attention and performance XIII* (pp. 605–624). Hillsdale, NJ: Lawrence Erlbaum Associates.

Courchesne, E., Townsend, J.P., Akshoomoff, N.A., Yeung-Courchesne, R., Press, G.A., Marakami, J.W., Lincoln, A.J., James, H.E., Saitoh, O., Egaas, B., Haas, R.H., & Schreibman, L. (1994). A new finding: Impairment in shifting attention in autistic and cerebellar patients. In S.H. Broman & J. Grafman (Eds.), *Atypical cognitive deficits in developmental disorders: Implications for brain function* (pp. 101–137). Hillsdale, NJ: Lawrence Erlbaum Associates.

Darwin, C. (1877). A biographical sketch of an infant. *Mind, 2,* 285–294.

Dawson, G., & Lewy, A. (1989). Arousal, attention, and the socio-emotional impairments of individuals with autism. In G. Dawson (Ed.), *Autism: Perspectives on nature, diagnosis, and treatment.* New York: Guilford Press.

DeCasper, A.J., & Fifer, W.P. (1980). Of human bonding: Newborns prefer their mothers' voices. *Science, 208,* 1174–1176.

Deffebach, K., & Adamson, L.B. (1994). Teaching referential and social-regulative words to toddlers: Mothers' use of metalingual language. *First Language, 14,* 249–261.

Dore, J. (1985). Holophrases revisited: Their "logical" development from dialog. In M. Barrett (Ed.), *Children's single-word speech* (pp. 23–58). New York: John Wiley & Sons.

Dunham, P.J., & Dunham, F. (1992). Lexical development during middle infancy: A mutually driven infant–caregiver process. *Developmental Psychology, 28,* 414–420.

Dunham, P.J., Dunham, F., & Curwin, A. (1993). Joint-attentional states and lexical acquisition at 18 months. *Developmental Psychology, 29,* 827–831.

Fogel, A., & Thelen, E. (1987). Development of early expressive and communicative action: Reinterpreting the evidence from a dynamic systems perspective. *Developmental Psychology, 23,* 747–761.

Gibson, E., & Rader, N. (1979). Attention: The perceiver as performer. In G.A. Hale & M. Lewis (Eds.), *Attention and cognitive development* (pp. 1–21). New York: Plenum.

Golinkoff, R.M. (1986). "I beg your pardon?": The preverbal negotiation of failed messages. *Journal of Child Language, 13,* 455–476.

Goodhart, F., & Baron-Cohen, S. (1993). How many ways can the point be made? Evidence from children with and without autism. *First Language, 13,* 225–233.

Greenspan, S.I. (1992). *Infancy and early childhood: The practice of clinical assessment and intervention with emotional and developmental challenges.* Madison, CT: International Universities Press.

Hodapp, R.M., Goldfield, E.C., & Boyatzis, C.J. (1984). The use and effectiveness of maternal scaffolding in mother–infant games. *Child Development, 55,* 772–781.

Hyche, J.K., Bakeman, R., & Adamson, L.B. (1992). Understanding communicative cues of infants with Down syndrome: Effects of mothers' experience and infants' age. *Journal of Applied Developmental Psychology, 13,* 1–16.

Jakobson, R. (1960). Linguistics and poetics. In T.A. Sebeok (Ed.), *Style in language* (pp. 350–377). New York: John Wiley & Sons.

James, W. (1890). *The principles of psychology* (Vol. 1). New York: Holt.

Kaye, K., & Fogel, A. (1980). The temporal structure of face-to-face communication between mothers and infants. *Developmental Psychology, 16,* 454–464.

Klinger, L.G., & Dawson, G. (1992). Facilitating early social and communicative development in children with autism. In S.F. Warren & J. Reichle (Eds.), *Communication and language intervention series: Vol. 1. Causes and effects in communication and language intervention* (pp. 157–186). Baltimore: Paul H. Brookes Publishing Co.

Klinnert, M.D., Campos, J.J., Sorce, J.F., Emde, R.N., & Svejda, M. (1983). Emotions as behavior regulators: Social referencing in infancy. In R. Plutchik & H. Kellerman (Eds.), *Emotion: Theory, research and experience* (Vol. 2, pp. 57–86). New York: Academic Press.

Konner, M. (1972). Aspects of the developmental ethology of a foraging people. In N. Blurton Jones (Ed.), *Ethological studies of child behavior* (pp. 285–304). Cambridge, England: Cambridge University Press.

Krakow, J.B., & Kopp, C.B. (1983). The effects of developmental delay on sustained attention in young children. *Child Development, 54,* 1143–1155.

Landry, S.H. (1995). The development of joint attention in premature low birth weight infants. In C. Moore & P.J. Dunham (Eds.), *Joint attention: Its origin and role in development* (pp. 223–250). Hillsdale, NJ: Lawrence Erlbaum Associates.

Lee, R.B. (1979). *The !Kung San: Men, women, and work in a foraging society.* Cambridge, England: Cambridge University Press.

Legerstee, M., & Bowman, T.G. (1989). The development of responses to people and a toy in infants with Down syndrome. *Infant Behavior and Development, 12,* 465–477.

Leung, E.H.L., & Rheingold, H.L. (1981). Development of pointing as a social gesture. *Developmental Psychology, 17,* 215–220.

Loveland, K.A., & Landry, S.H. (1986). Joint attention and language in autism and developmental language delay. *Journal of Autism and Developmental Disorders, 16,* 335–349.

McArthur, D., & Adamson, L.B. (1996). Joint attention in pre-verbal children: Autism and developmental language disorder. *Journal of Autism and Developmental Disorders, 26,* 481–496.

Moore, C., & Corkum, V.L. (1994). Social understanding at the end of the first year of life. *Developmental Review, 14,* 349–372.

Mundy, P., & Sigman, M. (1989). The theoretical implications of joint-attention deficits in autism. *Development and Psychopathology, 1,* 173–183.

Mundy, P., Sigman, M., & Kasari, C. (1990). A longitudinal study of joint attention and language development in autistic children. *Journal of Autism and Developmental Disorders, 20,* 115–128.

Mundy, P., Sigman, M., Kasari, C., & Yirmiya, N. (1988). Nonverbal communication skills in Down syndrome children. *Child Development, 59,* 235–249.

Newson, J., & Newson, E. (1975). Intersubjectivity and the transmission of culture. *Bulletin of the British Psychological Society, 28,* 437–446.

Ninio, A. (1983). Joint book reading as a multiple vocabulary acquisition device. *Developmental Psychology, 19,* 445–451.

Osterling, J., & Dawson, G. (1994). Early recognition of children with autism: A study of first birthday home videotapes. *Journal of Autism and Developmental Disorders, 24,* 247–257.

Papoušek, H., & Papoušek, M. (1987). Intuitive parenting: A dialectic counterpart of the infant's integrative competence. In J.D. Osofsky (Ed.), *Handbook of infant development* (2nd ed., pp. 669–720). New York: John Wiley & Sons.

Piaget, J. (1962). *Play, dreams, and imitation in childhood.* New York: Norton. (Originally published in 1945 as *La formation de symbole.*)

Piaget, J. (1963). *The origins of intelligence in children.* New York: Norton. (Originally published in 1936.)

Reznick, J.S., & Goldfield, B.A. (1992). Rapid change in lexical development in comprehension and production. *Developmental Psychology, 28,* 406–413.

Rheingold, H.L., & Adams, J.L. (1980). The significance of speech to newborns. *Developmental Psychology, 16,* 397–403.

Rogoff, B. (1990). *Apprenticeship in thinking: Cognitive development in social context.* New York: Oxford University Press.

Rogoff, B., Mistry, J., Radziszewska, B., & Germond, J. (1992). Infants' instrumental social interaction with adults. In S. Feinman (Ed.), *Social referencing and the social construction of reality in infancy* (pp. 323–348). New York: Plenum.

Ross, H.S., & Lollis, S.P. (1987). Communication within infant social games. *Developmental Psychology, 23,* 241–248.

Ruff, H.A. (1986). Components of attention during infants' manipulative exploration. *Child Development, 57,* 105–114.

Sander, L.W. (1977). The regulation of exchange in the infant–caretaker system and some aspects of the context–content relationship. In M. Lewis & L.A. Rosenblum (Eds.), *Interaction, conversation, and the development of language* (pp. 133–156). New York: John Wiley & Sons.

Schieffelin, B.B., & Ochs, E. (Eds.). (1986). *Language socialization across cultures.* Cambridge, England: Cambridge University Press.

Shatz, M. (1994). *A toddler's life: Becoming a person.* New York: Oxford University Press.

Shinn, M.W. (1900). *The biography of a baby.* Boston: Houghton Mifflin.

Sigman, M., & Kasari, C. (1995). Joint attention across contexts in normal and autistic children. In C. Moore & P.J. Dunham (Eds.), *Joint attention: Its origin and role in development* (pp. 189–203). Hillsdale, NJ: Lawrence Erlbaum Associates.

Smith, C.B., Adamson, L.B., & Bakeman, R. (1988). Interactional predictors of early language. *First Language, 8,* 143–156.

Spencer, P.E., & Kelly, A.B. (1993, March). *Deaf infants' coordination of attention to persons and objects.* Paper presented at the Society for Research in Child Development, New Orleans.

Spencer, P.E., & Lederberg, A.R. (1997). Different modes, different models: Communication and language of young deaf children and their mothers. In L.B. Adamson & M.A. Romski (Eds.), *Communication and language acquisition: Discoveries from atypical development* (pp. 203–230). Baltimore: Paul H. Brookes Publishing Co.

Spitz, R. (1972). Fundamental education: The coherent object as a developmental model. In M. Piers (Ed.), *Play and development* (pp. 43–63). New York: Norton.

Stern, D.N. (1974). Mother and infant at play: The dyadic interaction involving facial, vocal and gaze behaviors. In M. Lewis & L.A. Rosenblum (Eds.), *The effect of the infant on its caregiver* (pp. 187–213). New York: John Wiley & Sons.

Stern, D.N., Beebe, B., Jaffe, J., & Bennett, S.L. (1977). The infant's stimulus world during social interaction: A study of caregiver behaviors with particular reference to repetition and timing. In H.R. Schaffer (Ed.), *Studies in mother–infant interaction* (pp. 177–202). New York: Academic Press.

Tager-Flusberg, H. (1994). Dissociation in form and function in the acquisition of language by autistic children. In H. Tager-Flusberg (Ed.), *Constraints on language acquisition: Studies of atypical children* (pp. 175–194). Hillsdale, NJ: Lawrence Erlbaum Associates.

Tomasello, M. (1995). Joint attention as social cognition. In C. Moore & P.J. Dunham (Eds.), *Joint attention: Its origins and role in development* (pp. 103–130). Hillsdale, NJ: Lawrence Erlbaum Associates.

Tomasello, M., & Farrar, M.J. (1986). Joint attention and early language. *Child Development, 57,* 1454–1463.

Tomasello, M., & Kruger, A.C. (1992). Joint attention on actions: Acquiring verbs in ostensive and non-ostensive context. *Journal of Child Language, 19,* 311–333.

Trevarthen, C. (1988). Universal co-operative motives: How infants begin to know the language and culture of their parents. In G. Jahoda & I.M. Lewis (Eds.), *Acquiring culture: Cross cultural studies in child development* (pp. 37–90). London: Croom Helm.

Trevarthen, C., & Hubley, P. (1978). Secondary intersubjectivity: Confidence, confiding and acts of meaning in the first year. In A. Lock (Ed.), *Action, gestures and symbol* (pp. 183–229). London: Academic Press.

Tronick, E., Als, H., & Adamson, L.B. (1979). The communicative structure of early face to face interaction. In M. Bullowa (Ed.), *Before speech: The beginnings of interpersonal communication* (pp. 349–372). Cambridge, England: Cambridge University Press.

Vygotsky, L.S. (1978). *Mind in society: The development of higher psychological processes.* Cambridge, MA: Harvard University Press.

Watson, J.S. (1985). Contingency perception in early social development. In T.M. Field & N.A. Fox (Eds.), *Social perception in infants* (pp. 157–176). Norwood, NJ: Ablex.

Wellman, H.M. (1993). Early understanding of mind: The normal case. In S. Baron-Cohen, H. Tager-Flusberg, & D.J. Cohen (Eds.), *Understanding other minds: Perspectives from autism* (pp. 10–39). New York: Oxford University Press.

Werner, H. (1957). The concept of development from a comparative and organismic point of view. In D. Harris (Ed.), *The concept of development* (pp. 125–148). Minneapolis: University of Minnesota Press.

Werner, H., & Kaplan, B. (1963). *Symbol formation.* New York: John Wiley & Sons.

Wetherby, A.M., & Prizant, B.M. (1992). Profiling young children's communicative competence. In S.F. Warren & J. Reichle (Eds.), *Communication and language intervention series: Vol. 1. Causes and effects in communication and language intervention* (pp. 217–251). Baltimore: Paul H. Brookes Publishing Co.

Wetherby, A.M., & Prizant, B.M. (1993). *Communication and Symbolic Behavior Scales (CSBS): Normed ed.* Chicago: Applied Symbolix.

Wetherby, A., & Prutting, C. (1984). Profiles of communicative and cognitive-social abilities in autistic children. *Journal of Speech and Hearing Research, 27,* 364–377.

Yoder, P.J., & Farran, D.C. (1986). Mother–infant engagements in dyads with handicapped and nonhandicapped infants: A pilot study. *Applied Research in Mental Retardation, 7,* 51–58.

Yoder, P.J., & Munson, L.J. (1995). The social correlates of coordinated attention to adult and objects in mother–infant interaction. *First Language, 15,* 219–230.

3

Does Adult Responsivity to Child Behavior Facilitate Communication Development?

Paul J. Yoder, Steven F. Warren,
Rebecca McCathren, and Shirley V. Leew

Many early intervention models assume that social responsiveness to young children's behavior and communicative acts facilitates their communication and language development. What is meant by "responsiveness," however, is often vague or narrowly defined (Martin, 1989). Some scholars suggest that the actual effects of social responsiveness on language development are quite limited (e.g., Pinker, 1994; Rosenburg & Abbeduto, 1993). Others have shown that there even may be periods during child development when too much of a particular type of responsivity may have a negative effect on particular aspects of development and adaptation (Belsky, Rovine, & Taylor, 1984; Harding, 1983; Hubbard & van Ijzendoorn, 1987; MacTurk, Meadow-Orlans, Sanford, & Spencer, 1993).

This chapter considers the conceptual and empirical support for the notion that adult social responsiveness to children's behavior and communication acts facilitates their journey through preintentional communication up to the point at which they are using multiword combinations. What difference does contingent, social responsiveness make in terms of a child's early communication and language development? To answer this question we first define responsiveness and classify the varied types of adult responsiveness that occur early in child development. This sets the stage for review of relevant literature, which is followed by a summation of this literature in terms of its clinical and research implications. We also consider how cultural variation may influence the effect that social responsiveness has on communicative development.

This chapter was written while the research of the first and second authors was supported by National Institute of Child Health and Human Development Grant No. RO1HD27594 and Office of Special Education Programs Grant No. HO23C20152.

DEFINITION AND FUNCTIONAL
CLASSIFICATION OF ADULT SOCIAL RESPONSIVITY

The behaviors of infants and toddlers that mothers tend to consider communicative are the opportunities for adult contingent responses (Harding, 1983; Yoder & Feagans, 1988). The form and function of these behaviors undoubtedly change with development (Harding, 1984). At earlier periods of development, mothers respond to behaviors that they consider communicative but that many researchers do not necessarily consider to be intentionally communicative (e.g., Yoder, 1986). These include actions involving toys (Dawson & Galpert, 1990), vocalizations (Poulson, Kymissis, Reeve, Andreatos, & Reeve, 1991), facial expressions (Malatesta, Culver, Tesman, & Shepard, 1989), crying (Hubbard & van Ijzendoorn, 1987), or gazes toward adults or objects (Beckwith & Cohen, 1989). As the child develops, the behaviors to which mothers respond are clearly communicative. These include verbal or symbolic behavior (e.g., Nelson, 1989), conventional gestures (e.g., Masur, 1982), or intentional communication that does not necessarily involve conventional gestures or symbols (e.g., Yoder, Warren, Kim, & Gazdag, 1994).

Adult responses to an infant's or a child's behavior occur immediately after and are semantically related to or are imitations of the behavior. The criterion of immediacy is included because reliably measuring delayed responses to children's behavior is quite difficult. In addition, there is reason to believe that immediate responses may be more facilitative of various aspects of development than are delayed responses (Roth, 1987).

Over the course of early development, three classes or types of adult responsiveness can be observed. These three types are nonlinguistic contingent responses, linguistic contingent responses to the child's or infant's focus of attention, and linguistic contingent responses to the child's or infant's communicative act. These responses are aggregated into three types because each type may facilitate communicative development for different reasons and may be important at different developmental periods.

Nonlinguistic Contingent Responses

During the preintentional prelinguistic communication development stage, adult responses to child behavior typically add little linguistic information beyond acknowledging the child's behavior. This class of responses includes imitation of facial expression (MacTurk et al., 1993), imitation of children's play (Dawson & Galpert, 1990), and exact or reduced imitation of children's vocalizations (Pelaez-Nogueras & Gewirtz, 1993). Nonimitative forms of such responses include vocal turn-taking, for example, vocalizing after infant's vocalization with a different vocalization than the infant uses (Beckwith & Cohen, 1989); turn-taking in a play episode with a complementary, not imitative, action (Beckwith & Cohen, 1989); verbally acknowledging a change in the child's focus of attention without adding linguistic information to the child's act (e.g., "Uh huh")

(Fischer, 1988); attempting to soothe a distressed infant (Beckwith & Cohen, 1989); and complying with the presumed meaning of the infant's behavior (van den Boom, 1994).

Nonlinguistic contingent responses may influence communication development by enhancing other abilities that may enhance communication (i.e., mediating variables). These mediating variables include contingency or cause-and-effect learning, that is, the child learning in a general way that his or her behavior has an effect on the world (Riksen-Walraven, 1978); generalized exploration of the social and object environment; joint attentional focus, that is, adult and child attending to the object or event; and secure attachment to mother (Ainsworth, 1973). The rest of this section reviews the theory for why responsivity should influence these mediating variables and why the mediating variables should influence later communication or language development.

White (1959) suggested that parental responses to children's behavior helped the children to acquire a generalized expectation that their behavior has an effect on the world. Such a realization may motivate exploration of the environment in search of more environmental responses (White, 1959), with children eventually learning that adults can produce some of these desired effects (Golinkoff, 1983). The latter realization may lay part of the groundwork for intentional communication because intentional communication behaviors are directed toward the listener (Golinkoff, 1983).

Following the child's lead (i.e., doing what the child wants) may facilitate joint attentional focus. Joint attentional focus to an object the child selects is important because the child is more likely to communicate about an object or event that he or she is interested in than with objects in which there is no interest. It is also probably easier for the child to maintain attention to an object or event than to switch to the adult's focus of attention (Bruner, 1981; Tomasello & Farrar, 1986; see also Chapter 2). The child may be better able to understand and analyze an adult utterance in joint attentional episodes than outside of such episodes because the referents for some of the words in the former utterances match the child's focus of attention (Bruner, 1981; Tomasello & Farrar, 1986).

Ainsworth (1973) and Stern (1985) suggested that maternal responsiveness encourages babies to be securely attached to their mothers because the babies learn that their needs will be taken care of and that their interaction is valued. Secure attachment is believed to provide a secure base from which to explore the environment. Exploration of the environment may influence communication development because it may enhance learning about objects and relations between objects (i.e., the early content of communication and language) (Bloom, 1993).

Contingency learning, exploratory behavior, object play, joint attentional focus of mother and infant to the same object, and secure attachment are each empirically related to some aspect of later communication or language level. Ohr and Fagen (1994) found that contingency learning in 3-month-old children with

Down syndrome predicted their Bayley Mental Development Index 6 months later. In typically developing infants, exploratory behavior has been shown to be empirically related to later intelligence (Messer et al., 1986), part of which is verbal. Combinatorial and symbolic play have been found to be associated with several measures of communication and language in children with and without disabilities (see Bates, Benigni, Bretherton, Camaioni, & Volterra, 1979; Bloom, 1993; Yoder, Warren, & Hull, 1995). Babies who are securely attached to their mothers tend to have more exploratory behavior and more sophisticated play skills (Belsky, Garduque, & Hrncir, 1984) and more frequent intentional prelinguistic communication later in their development (Bates et al., 1979).

Linguistic Contingent Responses

The second class of adult responses—linguistic contingent responses to the child's or infant's focus of attention—includes comments (Tomasello, 1988) and directives (McCathren, Yoder, & Warren, 1995) about the child's focus of attention. The syntactic form of the utterance is probably not important. What is important is that the content of the utterance be about the child's focus of attention and/or communicative message. It can be argued that this type of input may be most important for children who are developmentally ready for early receptive vocabulary acquisition. Children begin to understand words and to communicate intentionally as evidenced by showing and giving adults objects at about the same period in development—about 9–10 months of age in typically developing infants (Bates et al., 1979). Talking about the child's focus of attention may provide the child with labels for the objects and actions to which he or she is attending (MacDonald, 1989; Tomasello, 1988). This facilitates the association between a referent class and the label (Tomasello, 1988).

The third class of adult responses—linguistic contingent responses to the child's or infant's communicative act—is contingent on child communication and adds linguistic information to the child's act. These responses include saying what the child might be trying to communicate, also known as linguistic mapping (Yoder, Warren, et al., 1994), contingent labeling (Tannock & Girolametto, 1992), and labeling responses (Masur, 1982). Expansions and recasts, also known as adult utterances that retain the central relations and topic of the child's utterance and add semantic or syntactic information to the utterance (Nelson, 1989), also are included in this class of responses. Also included are other topic continuations that do not necessarily repeat any of the words of the child's utterance but maintain the topic (Barnes, Gutfreund, Satterly, & Wells, 1983). All of these types of linguistic responses may facilitate linguistic development by helping the child to process the linguistic information that the responses contain. The temporal proximity and semantic overlap of the adult response and the child utterance may help the child understand the adult utterance and make comparisons between his or her communication act and the adult's act. This may, in turn, make the differences between the two acts salient, thereby facilitating parsing and analysis of the different elements of the adult's utterance (Nelson, 1989).

In this chapter, our definition of responsivity excludes concerns about leaving pauses that allow children to respond to questions, attempting to match how often the child speaks (i.e., turn-balancing), and matching the mood and pace of the child (see MacDonald, 1989; Mahoney & Powell, 1988). Although these excluded classes of behaviors also may facilitate development, we have excluded them because the mechanism by which they may facilitate interaction and linguistic development is different from the classes of behavior on which this chapter focuses.

SCOPE OF THE REVIEW

The published literature on responsiveness is extensive; therefore, we have set a number of parameters for this review. First, due to the focus of this volume, the review is limited to studies of children in the prelinguistic or early linguistic stages of development (i.e., birth through 24 months of age in typically developing children). Second, we limited the review to studies in which the child outcome variable was related to or was an aspect of early communication development. Third, to improve the probability that the findings indicated an effect of adult social responsivity, we excluded experiments or correlational studies in which the investigators "lumped" responsivity with other aspects of adult–child interaction while manipulating the independent variable or while measuring the predictor variable. Fourth, to reduce the probability that the associations between responsivity and child communication were a function of child effects on the adult, we excluded studies that were exclusively concurrent correlational and nonequivalent group comparisons. Finally, because we were interested in enduring effects of adult social responsivity on communication development, we excluded experimental studies (i.e., those in which responsivity was trained or manipulated) in which the responsivity treatment resulted in only temporary changes in child behavior. These excluded studies were those in which the responsivity treatment affected changes in child behavior in a single session or in which the withdrawal of the responsivity treatment covaried with the child's behavior returning to baseline levels.

Both experimental and longitudinal correlational studies are valuable in investigating a possible enduring causal link between responsivity and later communication. The advantage of well-conducted experiments is the confidence that the changes in the mothers' behavior caused the changes in the children. When one aspect of an interaction style changes, however, other aspects also usually change. In addition, more than one type of responsivity is frequently manipulated in experiments. Therefore, it is difficult to isolate the effect of responsivity on child development by only using evidence from experiments.

The inclusion of longitudinal correlational studies can help to better specify which aspects of maternal interaction style covary with the child variable. When used in isolation from experiments, however, longitudinal correlational studies cannot be used to infer that responsivity caused the individual differences in child communication. In such correlational studies, unmeasured variables may account for the relationship between responsivity and child communication; therefore, both experimental and longitudinal correlational studies were included in the review.

Regardless of the study's design, it is not sufficient to use only mother–child interaction sessions as the context for measuring the effects of maternal responsivity on generalized communication ability. Because some mothers are very responsive, children may perform at their best with their mothers but communicate at much less sophisticated levels with others. Therefore, studies that suggest enduring effects that measure the child outcome variable only within responsive mother–child interaction sessions are less persuasive evidence for more generalized effects on the child than are studies that measure child outcomes in other, less scaffolded interactions. We refer to the former group of studies as demonstrating *limited evidence of generalization*. These include studies with dependent measures taken only from mother–child interaction sessions and from mothers' reports of vocabulary size. We refer to the latter group of studies as *stronger evidence of generalization*. These include measures derived from standard protocol tests or interaction sessions with people other than the primary caregivers.

Nonlinguistic Contingent Responses

This section reviews the literature on responsivity specific to the first class of adult responsiveness, nonlinguistic contingent responses.

Limited Evidence of Generalization In typically developing infants and infants who are at risk, nonlinguistic responsivity has been shown to facilitate or predict several positive changes when the babies are with their responsive mothers. In a study with preterm 1-month-olds with unknown developmental status, Beckwith and Cohen (1989) found that maternal responsiveness to infant crying and fussing was positively related to receptive vocabulary as reported by the mothers 23 months later. In a randomized group experiment, van den Boom (1994) trained mothers to imitate the behavior of their 6-month-olds, to maintain silence when infants averted their gaze, to immediately soothe in response to infant distress signals, and to read and respond to the meaning of nondistress social cues. The babies were from Caucasian, low socioeconomic status (SES), and mostly intact families in the Netherlands. In interactions with the mothers after the intervention, van den Boom found that the intervention caused the babies to have more positive social behavior, to fuss and cry less often, to be much more securely attached to their mothers, and to show more exploration. In another study of typically developing 9-month-olds, maternal imitation of the facial expressions and actions of their babies was positively associated with the frequency of the infants' spoken utterances in mother–child sessions recorded 9 months later (MacTurk et al., 1993).

Stronger Evidence of Generalization Similar findings are apparent in studies in which the child communication or outcome measure is derived from testing or observation sessions in which the mother is not involved. In a study with typically developing 5-month-olds, maternal response to nondistress infant vocalizations was positively associated with symbolic play and language comprehension on a discrimination task 7 months later (Bornstein & Tamis-LeMonda, 1989). Bornstein and Tamis-LeMonda (1989) also reported that Japanese mothers' responsiveness to nondistress vocalizations of their 5-month-olds was positively associated with intelligence 13 months later. In two well-conducted randomized group experiments with low-SES or blue-collar families in the Netherlands, training mothers to use a variety of nonlinguistic responses to infant behaviors increased the babies' exploratory behavior in sessions in which the mother was not present (Riksen-Walraven, 1978; van den Boom, 1994). In addition, Riksen-Walraven (1978) found that increased maternal responsivity to infant communication acts increased the extent to which the typically developing 9-month-olds solved contingency learning tasks. Again, it is not specified which type of nonlinguistic responsivity was most frequently used by the mothers in the Riksen-Walraven (1978) study, but the impression is given that mothers were instructed to comply with the presumed meaning of the infant's behavior and to imitate or take a vocal turn.

Summary These studies were conducted exclusively with typically developing babies, most of whom were in the first half of their first year of life. In studies measuring the outcomes in mother–child interaction sessions, babies of mothers who used relatively high levels of nonlinguistic responding tend to be highly social, securely attached, loquacious, and less distressed than mothers who used relatively low levels of nonlinguistic responding. In studies measuring the outcomes in more controlled circumstances, nonlinguistic maternal responsivity has been shown to facilitate exploratory behavior and contingency learning. It also predicts later levels of language comprehension and production and other aspects of cognition. However, no work on the enduring effects of nonlinguistic responsivity has been done with children with disabilities.

Linguistic Contingent Responses to the Child's Focus of Attention

This section presents findings from the responsivity literature specific to linguistic contingent responses to the child's focus of attention.

Limited Evidence of Generalization It is clear that the form of the maternal utterance is not nearly as important as whether it is about the child's focus of attention (McCathren et al., 1995). In typically developing children who are in the early part of their second year, early maternal labeling of objects predicts later maternal reports of noun vocabulary. Akhtar, Dunham, and Dunham (1991) conducted a study with typically developing 13-month-olds. They found that the proportion of maternal utterances that were directives about the child's actions with an object to which the child was attending was positively related to total vocabulary and number of nouns mothers reported the children using 9 months later. In a study of typically developing 15-month-olds, Tomasello and Farrar (1986 [Study I]) found that labeling the child's object of attention inside joint attentional episodes was related to later maternal reports of total productive vocabulary and of the proportion of words said that were nouns. When used outside of joint attentional episodes, directives (Akhtar et al., 1991) and noun reference (Tomasello & Farrar, 1986) were not related to later vocabulary.

Stronger Evidence of Generalization Linguistic contingent responses to children's focus of attention also predict or affect child language as assessed by language tests. In typically developing children, Harris (1994) found that the number of times mothers labeled objects to which 14-month-olds were attending was positively associated with the children's expressive language as assessed by the Reynell Developmental Language Scales (Reynell, 1985) 13 months later. In addition, the use of commands for actions during joint attentional episodes was positively associated with both receptive and expressive Reynell scores 13 months later. Again, when using outside joint attentional episodes, these same behaviors did not predict later language scores. In an experimental study with typically developing children in the single-word stage of language learning, children learned to understand more novel words (e.g., "clip") if they were modeled when the children were looking at the object rather than when the novel words were modeled after the experimenter asked the children to shift their attention to the referent (Tomasello & Farrar, 1986 [Study II]). This result was maintained 2 weeks after the intervention ended.

Similar findings have been reported with children with Down syndrome in the single-word stage of language learning (mean chronological age [CA] 23 months, $SD = 8$ months; average mental, expressive, and receptive age-equivalent scores of about 16 months). Harris (1994) found that the number of *wh-* questions mothers used in joint attentional episodes was positively associated with expressive Reynell scores 13 months later. In addition, the number of yes/no questions mothers used in joint attentional episodes also was positively associated with receptive Reynell scores 13 months later. When used outside of joint attentional episodes, however, these same behaviors did not predict later language scores.

Summary In both typically developing children and children with Down syndrome who are developmentally in the first half of their second year of life, maternal labeling of the objects to which they are attending predicts later language scores. It should be noted that the developmental period in which there is evidence of facilitative effects of linguistic input in joint attentional episodes is later than we predicted. We have evidence of facilitation after children begin to speak, not when they first begin to intentionally communicate. In typically developing children, the evidence suggests that verbal modeling of the label of objects to which children are attending facilitates noun learning. Mentioning the action before it occurs, however, has been shown to facilitate action-verb acquisition better than mentioning the action while it is occurring (Tomasello & Kruger, 1992). Given this finding, it is probably most prudent to assume that linguistic input in joint attentional focus facilitates noun acquisition. More research is needed to determine whether linguistic input in joint attentional episodes facilitates aspects of language development other than nouns.

Linguistic Contingent Responses to the Child's Communicative Act

This section presents the review of literature specific to the third type of adult responsivity, linguistic contingent responses to the child's or infant's communicative act.

Limited Evidence of Generalization   In the second half of the second year, maternal recasts predict later aspects of grammar in typically developing children. Nelson, Denninger, Bonvillian, Kaplan, and Baker (1984) found that frequency of simple maternal recasts (i.e., a type of recast that changes or adds only one major element) when the children were 22 months old positively related to individual differences in mean length of utterance (MLU) and verb complexity 5 months later. Farrar (1990) found that the frequency of maternal recasts with the plurals and verbs ending with "ing" when children were 22 months old positively related to the children's use of plurals and verbs ending with "ing" in mother–child sessions 6 months later.

At about the same developmental period, use of topic-continuing utterances also predicts later use of various aspects of grammar in typically developing children. In a study with typically developing children in the single-word stage (MLU = 1.68; range 1.0–2.21; mean CA = 24 months), Barnes et al. (1983) found that the number of maternal utterances that continued the established topic of conversation was positively associated with children's MLU 3 months later. Farrar (1990) investigated maternal utterances that continued the topic but did not repeat any part of the child's utterance and contained the unfronted copula verbs (e.g., "This *is* a book") or regular past-tense verbs (e.g., call*ed*). He found that frequency of these types of utterances, used when the children were 22 months old, positively related to the children's use of unfronted copula verbs and regular past-tense verbs 6 months later. In contrast, frequency of maternal utterances that changed the topic with unfronted auxiliary verbs (e.g., "He *has* been here") negatively related to the children's use of unfronted auxiliary verbs 6 months later.

Stronger Evidence of Generalization   In studies using measures from tests or observation sessions that did not include the mother, there is evidence of a relationship between linguistic responsivity to children's communication in the first half of the second year and in later language. In a study with typically developing 14-month-olds, Harris (1994) found that mothers' uses of utterances that maintained the established topic of conversation were positively related to receptive Reynell scores 13 months later; however, redirecting the conversation was unrelated to later language.

In samples of children with disabilities, the evidence is even stronger. In a study of children with Down syndrome in the first stage of language development, mothers maintaining the child's topic of conversation positively predicted receptive Reynell scores 13 months later. Redirecting the topic was negatively related to receptive Reynell scores (Harris, 1994). In a study of preschoolers with autism who were in the first stage of language learning, Scherer and Olswang (1989) found that expanding (i.e., repeating the child's word and adding one semantic role to it) the children's object labels facilitated their spontaneous imitation of and eventual spontaneous production of targeted early word combinations (e.g., possession, location, attribution). Yoder, Spruytenburg, Edwards, and Davies (1995) used a similar procedure with children with developmental disabilities in the single-word stage. With no particular semantic relation being targeted, they found that expanding the children's utterances in the context of a very familiar activity facilitated the children's MLU. The measurement context for MLU was generalization sessions in which nontrainers used a different interaction style and different objects than were used in training sessions.

Summary Adults' uses of expansions when children are in the single-word stage of productive language development have been shown to facilitate the development of early multiword combinations in children with autism and developmental disabilities. In children with Down syndrome in the single-word stage, maternal use of topic-continuing utterances predicts later general language scores. In typically developing toddlers in the second half of their second year, recasts and topic-continuing utterances predict later grammatical level in sessions with their mothers.

Studies that Do Not Allow Specification of Type of Responsivity

Because of the way responsivity was manipulated or measured in the following studies, it was impossible to separate the effects of different types of responsivity. The findings of these studies contribute, however, to the understanding of the general effect of responsivity on communication development.

Limited Evidence of Generalization Girolametto and colleagues (Girolametto, 1988; Girolametto, Verbey, & Tannock, 1994) conducted two experiments that indicate that increasing the use of a variety of types of responsivity influences the context of communication and the children's vocal participation in mother–child exchanges. In both studies, the children had developmental delays and were at about the 16-month developmental level. In both studies, the Hanen curriculum (Manolson, 1985) was used to train parents to respond to the child's focus of attention, follow the child's attentional lead, comment on activities of both the child and self, and use linguistic contingent responses to the child's communicative attempts.

In the Girolametto et al. (1994) study, a randomized group experiment, the authors found that increasing the use of Hanen program components increased sustained joint attentional episodes. Although tested, the increased joint attentional focus did not transfer to semistructured sessions with an experimenter.

In his 1988 study, Girolametto used another internally valid experiment with children with developmental delays to show that the increased use of Hanen program components increased the proportion of child turns that were verbal and the diversity of vocabulary children used in sessions with the mothers. The increase in the measure of vocabulary diversity (i.e., number of different words) used with mothers could be due to increases in the amount of talking to mothers and not to a true increase in vocabulary. Generalization to sessions without mothers was not measured.

Studies by Wilcox and colleagues (Wilcox, 1992; Wilcox, Shannon, & Bacon, 1992) indicated that using a variety of types of responsivity may influence children with developmental disabilities to use more frequent intentional and symbolic communication with their mothers. In both studies, toddlers with developmental delays who were just beginning to use intentional communication participated. In both studies, the parents and professionals working with the children were trained to consistently interpret, comply with, or ask clarification of the meaning of their children's prelinguistic communication attempts. An important part of this intervention was that, near the end of the program, communicative partners of the children were taught to require increasingly clear and conventional cues from the children before they responded. That is, when the children consistently communicated by using a target cluster of behaviors (e.g., eye contact, vocalizations), parents were taught to briefly delay complying with the meaning of the behavior and ask for clarification.

It should be noted that both of these studies were matched-group studies and, therefore, constitute an exception to the types of studies we reviewed (all other experimental studies were randomized group experiments). These studies were included because they constitute strong evidence that responsivity may aid children with disabilities in developing intentional and linguistic communication abilities.

In the first of these two studies, Wilcox (1992) found that children who experienced the intervention used more intentional communication with their mothers than did children who did not experience the responsivity intervention. The method of implementation (i.e., through all caregivers including classroom teachers) made random assignment to intervention or control groups impossible. The groups were matched on Batelle Developmental Inventory (BDI) (Newborg, Stock, Wrek, Guidubaldi, & Svinicki, 1988) age-equivalency scores. If matching was inadequate, however, preintervention group differences could explain the results.

In the second of these studies, Wilcox et al. (1992) reported that children who experienced the responsivity intervention used more symbolic communication with their mothers 12 months after the end of the intervention than did children who did not experience the responsivity intervention. Again, random assignment was not possible in this study. Groups were matched before intervention on Battelle communication age-equivalency scores.

Stronger Evidence of Generalization In addition to the previously mentioned effects on interaction with responsive mothers, Wilcox and colleagues (1992) found that children of mothers whom the experimenters had taught to be more responsive had higher scores on global language tests (i.e., Sequenced Inventory of Communication Development [SICD]; Hedrick, Prather, & Tobin, 1975) and on a global test of developmental level (i.e., Battelle) than did children in the control group 12 months after the intervention ended. Even though these children were not randomly assigned to control and experimental groups, this finding is important because it suggests that responsivity training may have affected not just increased performance of preexisting skills in a very responsive interaction but also affected the acquisition of new language skills. Most of the items at the low end of the SICD are vocabulary items. The SICD and BDI were administered not by the parents but by staff not involved in the responsivity training.

Summary All of these findings were with children who have disabilities. It is clear that a variety of types of responsivity, when organized into an intervention program, facilitates joint attentional episodes and vocal turn-taking. Such an intervention may increase frequency of intentional communication and frequency of symbolic communication in sessions with responsive mothers and vocabulary acquisition.

CLINICAL IMPLICATIONS

This review generally supports the notion that social responsivity can influence later child communication and language development. The studies reviewed support an intervention model that specifies types of responsivity that most appropriately fit different developmental periods. In this model, high levels of nonlinguistic responsivity to a variety of infant preintentional communication behaviors (i.e., vocal, nonvocal, distress related, nondistress related) are most appropriate during the preintentional communication stage (i.e., developmentally ages birth to 6 months). The expected results of such responsivity are increased exploratory behavior, contingency learning, secure attachment with the mother, and more frequent preintentional and intentional communication with responsive partners. The more enduring effects of maternal nonlinguistic responsivity on communication or language may be indirect. Once children have begun to use language to communicate (i.e., developmentally ages 12–18 months), talking about their focus of attention is likely to facilitate noun vocabulary. Finally, once children are talking more frequently (i.e., developmentally ages 16–22 months), continuing the topic with recasts and expansions is likely to facilitate early multiword combinations. Therefore, as children develop, different types of responsivity are probably most likely to benefit children's language systems.

This developmentally sensitive model is similar to the ones tested by Wilcox and colleagues (Wilcox, 1992; Wilcox et al., 1992) and Girolametto and colleagues (Girolametto, 1988; Girolametto et al., 1994). The Hanen (Manolson, 1985) and Ecological Communication Organization (MacDonald, 1989) programs are two commercially available descriptions of such a model. The empirical support for the efficacy of these models would be strengthened by looking for effects on child intentional and symbolic communication in interactions with less familiar and less responsive adults than with parents who implement these intervention approaches. When conducting such studies, it is important that preexisting differences in control and experimental groups be controlled through the use of random assignment.

Limitations of Social Responsivity in Facilitating Early Language Development

There is evidence that social responsivity is not the most efficient method of facilitating early linguistic development (Kaiser et al., 1997; Yoder, Kaiser, et al., 1995). When children are just beginning to talk, another method, Milieu Language Teaching, may be more effective in facilitating early vocabulary and semantic relation development.

In Kaiser et al. (1997) and Yoder, Kaiser, et al. (1995), a Responsive Interaction intervention similar to the Hanen program used by Girolametto (1988) was compared with another naturalistic language intervention, Milieu Language Teaching, to facilitate generalized language development. The Responsive Interaction intervention used was an adaptation of one used by Rogers, Herbison, Lewis, Pantone, and Reis (1986) and Weiss (1981), which emphasizes imitating the child's actions and vocalizations, topic continuations, and expansions as primary facilitating techniques. Milieu Language Teaching emphasizes prompts for general or specific language use in the context of child-initiated play episodes and topic continuations and expansions of child responses to teaching prompts (Kaiser, 1993). The children in both studies had developmental disabilities and varied widely in their developmental levels. Both studies used group experiments to investigate the research question.

In both studies, Milieu Language Teaching was more efficient than Responsive Interaction in increasing receptive and expressive language scores in children who began the intervention in the single-word stage of language learning. In contrast, the children in the simple-sentence stage and beyond made greater gains in the Responsive Interaction group than in the Milieu Language Teaching group (Kaiser et al., 1997; Yoder, Kaiser, et al., 1995). Therefore, although responsive interaction probably does facilitate some aspects of communication and language development, it may not be the most efficient method of facilitating the early linguistic transitions in children with developmental disabilities.

There are two probable explanations for these results. First, the focus of milieu teaching on eliciting use of language may increase the child's attention to the linguistic information in the adult's model or intended child response more often than the methods of responsive interaction, which provide contingent linguistic responses to the child's focus of attention or communication.

Second, the methods of milieu teaching may be more effective than those of responsive interaction in getting a child in the single-word stage of language development to linguistically communicate. This is important to both interventions because both employ teaching techniques immediately after child communication. These child-contingent teaching techniques may be the most effective methods in either intervention model (e.g., incidental teaching, expansions). If the children do not talk very often, then the number of opportunities for using teaching methods that are contingent on child communication is minimal. Milieu Language Teaching explicitly prompts linguistic communication with topic-continuing questions and elicits imitation prompts about the child's focus of attention. Responsive Interaction methods of getting the child to communicate linguistically include continuing the child's topic with comments about the child's and the adult's activities (Tannock & Girolametto, 1992). In support of the hypothesis that the methods of milieu teaching in eliciting linguistic communication are more effective than the methods of responsive interaction, Yoder, Davies, Bishop, and Munson (1994) found that topic-continuing questions were more effective than topic-continuing comments in getting children with disabilities to use their existing language.

Cross-Cultural Similarities and Differences

In Western culture (particularly the mainland of the United States), there is stronger evidence that linguistic responses, more than nonlinguistic responses, facilitate later communication development. Adults in all the cultures reviewed responded to infant vocalizations, gazing, and crying with linguistic responses at least some of the time (Bornstein, Tal, & Tamis-LeMonda, 1991; Fogel, Toda, & Kawai, 1988; Keller, Scholmerich, & Eibl-Eibesfeldt, 1988; Richman, Miller, & LeVine, 1992). The extent to which the adults' responses are linguistic, however, covaries with the age of the child. When the infant is birth to 6 months old, adults from a variety of cultures tend to respond to infant vocalizing, gazing, and crying with similar types and frequencies of nonlinguistic responses (Richman et al., 1992). In older infants (i.e., 6–12 months old), adults tend to use increasingly more linguistic responses to vocalizations, gazing, and crying but only if the adults are from a technologically advanced culture (Richman et al., 1992).

In looking at maternal responsivity to the behavior of older infants (i.e., older than 6 months), the extent to which mothers' responses are linguistic varies as a function of how developed the nation is or how highly educated the mothers are. Adults with more formal education or from technologically advanced cultures (e.g., Japan, Germany, United States) tend to respond linguistically to older infants' behavior more often than adults who have less formal education or who are from agrarian or hunting/gathering cultures (e.g., Trobriand, Yanomani, Gusii cultures) (Bornstein et al., 1991; Fogel et al., 1988; Keller et al., 1988; Richman et al., 1992).

It is highly unlikely that the agrarian/industrial classification of a nation by itself influences frequency or type of responsivity. Instead, it is assumed that this distinction covaries with other variables that influence responsivity. For example, the agrarian/industrial distinction may covary with the frequency and type of maternal responsivity because maternal education level may be higher in industrial nations, which may influence the mothers' views of their roles in raising their children. Their views of their roles may, in turn, influence how and when they respond to their children. For example, if mothers read that responding to their infants may reduce the frequency of child crying, then they may come to believe that they are helping their children, not spoiling them by responding.

The most important question is whether cultural differences in the type and extent of maternal responsiveness affect relative rates of any important developmental indices across cultures (e.g., vocabulary size). We do not know the answer to this question; we can only clarify the question. The most important cultures to compare would be those that differ dramatically in their view of the mothers' roles in raising the child or in their view of the goal of child rearing. These views may covary with each nation's level of development. Therefore, the studies from Japan (Bornstein & Tamis-LeMonda, 1989) or from the Netherlands (Riksen-Walraven, 1978; van den Boom, 1994) do not constitute the most important comparisons with findings on U.S. families. We need contrasts to identify what elements of the agrarian/industrial distinction covaries with responsivity; for example, a four-way comparison of maternal responsivity in literate and illiterate mothers from industrialized and agrarian countries would be a possible study. Once the mothers were selected, it should be determined whether there is a significant difference across cultures and subsamples within cultures in the degree to which social responsiveness predicted later communication development.

Even if responsivity has an effect on child development in cultures that do not value responsivity, there is still the possibility that more serious, negative side effects could result from training an interaction style that conflicts with dominant cultural values. An example is the case of a mother who lives in a culture that believes that children develop optimally on their own without direct responsive interaction. If we taught this mother to be more responsive when her baby cried, the husband, grandmother, and friends may criticize the mother for "spoiling" her child.

We can take comfort in the notion that children learn and develop in varying cultural milieus, despite cultural differences in responsivity. Rogoff, Mistry,

Goncu, and Mosier (1993) convincingly showed that children in agrarian cultures can become acculturated through observation just as well as children in industrialized cultures, who are often directly taught cultural information.

CONCLUSION AND DIRECTIONS FOR FUTURE RESEARCH

Although a substantial body of research exists on the effects of responsiveness on communication and language development, many important questions remain unanswered or in need of additional investigation. The review in this chapter suggests that the effect of adult responsiveness may be important, yet limited. Responsiveness seems to play an important role in the acquisition of nouns and early multiword utterances and in indirectly enhancing other abilities that may facilitate communication development (e.g., joint attentional focus, exploration). However, it appears that interventions based solely on responsive interaction principles are not the most efficient means of facilitating early linguistic development in children with developmental delays (Kaiser et al., 1997; Yoder, Kaiser, et al., 1995). As the effects of adult social responsiveness become clearer, other research questions will move to the forefront.

In addition to the cultural issues that were previously mentioned, one issue that has occasionally engendered some debate is the extent to which adult responsivity is responsible for the naturally occurring wide variation in children's early language development. Some researchers argue that its effects are likely to be quite modest (e.g., Pinker, 1994; Rosenburg & Abbeduto, 1993); others suggest that it could play a central role in the overall process (e.g., Hart & Risley, 1995). Those who think responsivity plays a minimal role consider most differences between mothers to be inconsequential (Pinker, 1994). Those who think it might play a more important role in explaining individual differences argue that, over several years, small differences in responsivity become huge cumulative differences in the number of facilitative interactions children experience (Hart & Risley, 1995). The short responsive interactions that are used to measure responsivity are not sufficient to influence development. Instead, these brief samples are assumed to index relative responsivity levels that the children experience over time. Along these lines, the number of responsive interactions (i.e., high, medium, low, control) children were exposed to could be manipulated to determine whether such manipulations covaried with differences in language or communication. Such manipulations would be a more explicit test of the hypothesis that varying amount of exposure to responsive interactions influences individual differences in language development.

Those interested in intervention are concerned with identifying optimally facilitative environments. The generalized effects of responsivity-based interventions outside the mother–child context are unclear and require additional study. Further research also needs to be conducted on the effects of responsivity-based interventions relative to other intervention approaches in unstudied populations (e.g., children with specific language impairments, late talkers, children with autism). If we are to develop optimally effective interventions, it is important that we determine the relative effects and limitations of each type of intervention (Warren & Yoder, 1994).

REFERENCES

Ainsworth, M.D.S. (1973). The development of infant–mother attachment. In B.M. Caldwell & H.M. Ricciuti (Eds.), *Review of child development research 3* (pp. 1–94). New York: Russell Sage Foundation.

Akhtar, N., Dunham, F., & Dunham, J. (1991). Directive interactions and early vocabulary development: The role of joint attentional focus. *Journal of Child Language, 18,* 41–50.

Barnes, S., Gutfreund, M., Satterly, D., & Wells, G. (1983). Characteristics of adult speech which predict children's language development. *Journal of Child Language, 10,* 65–84.

Bates, E., Benigni, L., Bretherton, I., Camaioni, L., & Volterra, V. (1979). *The emergence of symbols: Cognition and communication in infancy.* New York: Academic Press.

Beckwith, L., & Cohen, S.E. (1989). Maternal responsiveness with preterm infants and later competency. In M.H. Bornstein (Ed.), *Maternal responsiveness: Characteristics and consequences* (pp. 75–87). San Francisco: Jossey-Bass.

Belsky, J., Garduque, L., & Hrncir, E. (1984). Assessing performance, competence, and executive capacity in infant play: Relations to home environment and security of attachment. *Developmental Psychology, 20,* 406–417.

Belsky, J., Rovine, M., & Taylor, D.G. (1984). The Pennsylvanian Infant and Family Development Project, III: The origins of individual differences in infant–mother attachment: Maternal and infant contribution. *Child Development, 55,* 718–728.

Bloom, L. (1993). *The transition from infancy to language.* New York: Cambridge University Press.

Bornstein, M.H., Tal, J., & Tamis-LeMonda, C. (1991). Parenting in cross-cultural perspective: The U.S., France, and Japan. In M.H. Bornstein (Ed.), *Cultural approaches to parenting* (pp. 69–90). Hillsdale, NJ: Lawrence Erlbaum Associates.

Bornstein, M.H., & Tamis-LeMonda, C.S. (1989). Maternal responsiveness and cognitive development. In M. Bornstein (Ed.), *Maternal responsiveness: Characteristics and consequences* (pp. 49–62). San Francisco: Jossey-Bass.

Bruner, J. (1981). The social context of language acquisition. *Language and Communication, 1,* 155–178.

Dawson, G., & Galpert, L. (1990). Mothers' use of imitative play for facilitating social responsiveness and toy play in young autistic children. *Development and Psychopathology, 2,* 151–162.

Farrar, M.J. (1990). Discourse and the acquisition of grammatical morphemes. *Journal of Child Language, 17,* 607–624.

Fischer, M.A. (1988). The relationship between child initiations and maternal responses in preschool-age children with Down syndrome. In K. Marfo (Ed.), *Parent–child interaction and developmental disabilities* (pp. 126–144). New York: Praeger.

Fogel, A., Toda, S., & Kawai, M. (1988). Mother–infant interaction in Japan and the U.S.: A laboratory comparison using 3-month-old infants. *Developmental Psychology, 24*(3), 398–406.

Girolametto, L.E. (1988). Improving the social-conversational skills of developmentally delayed children: An intervention study. *Journal of Speech and Hearing Disorders, 53,* 156–167.

Girolametto, L.E., Verbey, M., & Tannock, R. (1994). Improving joint engagement in parent–child interaction: An intervention study. *Journal of Early Intervention, 18,* 155–167.

Golinkoff, R.M. (1983). Infant social cognition: Self, people, and objects. In L. Liben (Ed.), *Piaget and the foundations of knowledge* (pp. 179–196). Hillsdale, NJ: Lawrence Erlbaum Associates.

Harding, C.G. (1983). Setting the stage for language acquisition: Communication development in the first year. In R.M. Golinkoff (Ed.), *The transition from prelinguistic to linguistic communication: Issues and implications* (pp. 93–111). Hillsdale, NJ: Lawrence Erlbaum Associates.

Harding, C.G. (1984). Acting with intention: A framework for examining the development of the intention to communicate. In L. Feagans, C. Garvey, & R. Golinkoff (Eds.), *The origins and growth of communication* (pp. 123–135). New York: Ablex.

Harris, S. (1994). *The relation of maternal style to the language development of children with Down syndrome.* Unpublished doctoral dissertation, University of California at Los Angeles.

Hart, B., & Risley, T.R. (1995). *Meaningful differences in the everyday experience of young American children.* Baltimore: Paul H. Brookes Publishing Co.

Hedrick, D.L., Prather, E.M., & Tobin, A.R. (1975). *Sequenced Inventory of Communication Development (SICD).* Seattle: University of Washington Press.

Hubbard, F.O.A., & van Ijzendoorn, M.H. (1987). Maternal unresponsiveness and infant crying. A critical replication of the Bell & Ainsworth study. In L.W.C. Tavecchio & M.H. van Ijzendoorn (Eds.), *Attachment in social networks: Contributions to the Bowlby-Ainsworth attachment theory* (pp. 339–375). New York: North-Holland.

Kaiser, A.P. (1993). Functional language. In M.E. Snell (Ed.), *Instruction of students with severe disabilities* (4th ed., pp. 347–379). New York: Macmillan.

Kaiser, A.P., Yoder, P.J., Fischer, R., Keefer, M., Hemmeter, M.L., & Ostrosky, M.M. (1997). *A comparison of milieu teaching and responsive interaction implemented by parents.* Manuscript in preparation. [Available from Ann Kaiser, GPC Box 328, Vanderbilt University, Nashville, TN 37203]

Keller, H., Scholmerich, A., & Eibl-Eibesfeldt, I. (1988). Communication patterns in adult–child interactions in Western and non-Western cultures. *Journal of Cross-Cultural Psychology, 19*(4), 427–445.

MacDonald, J.D. (1989). *Becoming partners with children: From play to conversation.* San Antonio, TX: Special Press, Inc.

MacTurk, R.H., Meadow-Orlans, K.P., Sanford, L., & Spencer, P.E. (1993). Social support, motivation, language, and interaction. *American Annals of the Deaf, 138,* 19–25.

Mahoney, G., & Powell, A. (1988). Modifying parent–child interaction: Enhancing the development of handicapped children. *Journal of Special Education, 22*(1), 82–96.

Malatesta, C., Culver, C., Tesman, J.R., & Shepard, B. (1989). The development of emotion expression during the first two years of life. *Monographs of the Society for Research in Child Development, 54*(1–2, Serial no. 219).

Manolson, H.A. (1985). *It takes two to talk: A Hanen early language parent guide-book.* [Available from the Hanen Early Language Resource Centre, 4-126, 252 Bloor St. West, Toronto, Ontario, Canada]

Martin, J.A. (1989). Personal and interpersonal components of responsiveness. In M.H. Bornstein (Ed.), *Maternal responsiveness: Characteristics and consequences* (pp. 5–14). San Francisco: Jossey-Bass.

Masur, E.F. (1982). Mothers' responses to infants' object-related gestures: Influences on lexical development. *Journal of Child Language, 9,* 23–30.

McCathren, R., Yoder, P.J., & Warren, S.F. (1995). The role of directives in early language intervention. *Journal of Early Intervention, 19,* 91–101.

Messer, D.J., McCarthy, M.E., McQuiston, S., MacTurk, R.H., Yarrow, L., & Vietze, P. (1986). Relation between mastery behavior in infancy and competence in early childhood. *Child Development, 22,* 366–372.

Nelson, K. (1989). Strategies for first language teaching. In M.L. Rice & R.L. Schiefelbusch (Eds.), *The teachability of language* (pp. 263–310). Baltimore: Paul H. Brookes Publishing Co.

Nelson, K.E., Denninger, M.M., Bonvillian, J.D., Kaplan, B.J., & Baker, N. (1984). Maternal input adjustments and nonadjustments as related to children's linguistic advances and to language acquisition theories. In A.D. Pellegrini & T.D. Yawkey (Eds.), *The development of oral and written languages: Readings in developmental and applied linguistics* (pp. 31–56). New York: Ablex.

Newborg, J., Stock, J.R., Wrek, L., Guidubaldi, J., & Svinicki, J.S. (1988). *Battelle Developmental Inventory (BDI).* Chicago: Riverside.

Ohr, P., & Fagen, J.W. (1994). Contingency learning in 9-month-old infants with Down syndrome. *American Journal of Mental Retardation, 99,* 74–84.

Pelaez-Nogueras, M., & Gewirtz, J. (1993, March). *Mother's contingent imitation increases infant vocalizations.* Poster presented at the biennial meeting of the Society for Research in Child Development, New Orleans, LA.

Pinker, S. (1994). *The language instinct.* New York: William Morrow.

Poulson, C.L., Kymissis, E., Reeve, K., Andreatos, M., & Reeve, L. (1991). Generalized vocal imitation in infants. *Journal of Experimental Child Psychology, 51,* 267–279.

Reynell, J. (1985). *Reynell Developmental Language Scales.* Los Angeles: Webster Psychological Services.

Richman, A.L., Miller, P.M., & LeVine, R.A. (1992). Cultural and educational variations in maternal responsiveness. *Developmental Psychology, 28*(4), 614–621.

Riksen-Walraven, J.M. (1978). Effects of caregiver behavior on habituation and self-efficacy in infants. *International Journal of Behavioral Development, 1,* 105–130.

Rogers, S., Herbison, J.M., Lewis, H.C., Pantone, J., & Reis, K. (1986). An approach for enhancing the symbolic, communicative, and interpersonal functioning of young children with autism or severe emotional handicaps. *Journal of the Division for Early Childhood, 10,* 135–148.

Rogoff, B., Mistry, J., Goncu, A., & Mosier, C. (1993). Guided participation in cultural activity by toddlers and caregivers. *Monographs of the Society for Research in Child Development,* Serial no. 236.

Rosenburg, S., & Abbeduto, L. (1993). *Language and communication in mental retardation.* Hillsdale, NJ: Lawrence Erlbaum Associates.

Roth, P.L. (1987). Temporal characteristics of maternal verbal styles. In K.E. Nelson & A. vanKleeck (Eds.), *Children's language* (Vol. 6, pp. 137–159). Hillsdale, NJ: Lawrence Erlbaum Associates.

Scherer, N.J., & Olswang, L.B. (1989). Using structured discourse as a language intervention technique with autistic children. *Journal of Speech and Hearing Disorders, 54,* 383–394.

Stern, D. (1985). *The interpersonal world of the infant.* New York: Basic Books.

Tannock, R., & Girolametto, L. (1992). Reassessing parent-focused language intervention programs. In S.F. Warren & J. Reichle (Eds.), *Communication and language intervention series: Vol. 1. Causes and effects in communication and language intervention* (pp. 49–79). Baltimore: Paul H. Brookes Publishing Co.

Tomasello, M. (1988). The role of joint attention in early language development. *Language Sciences, 11*, 69–88.

Tomasello, M., & Farrar, M.J. (1986). Joint attention and early language. *Child Development, 57*, 1454–1463.

Tomasello, M., & Kruger, A.C. (1992). Joint attention on actions: Acquiring verbs in ostensive and non-ostensive contexts. *Journal of Child Language, 19*, 311–333.

van den Boom, D.C. (1994). The influence of temperament and mothering on attachment and exploration: An experimental manipulation of sensitive responsiveness among lower-class mothers with irritable infants. *Child Development, 65*, 1457–1477.

Warren, S.F., & Yoder, P.J. (1994). Communication and language intervention: Why a constructivist approach is insufficient. *Journal of Special Education, 28*, 248–258.

Weiss, R.S. (1981). INREAL intervention for language handicapped and bilingual children. *Journal of the Division for Early Childhood, 4*, 40–52.

White, R.W. (1959). Motivation reconsidered: The concept of competence. *Psychological Review, 66*, 297–323.

Wilcox, M.J. (1992). Enhancing initial communication skills in young children with developmental disabilities through partner programming. *Seminars in Speech and Hearing, 13*, 194–212.

Wilcox, M.J., Shannon, M.S., & Bacon, C.K. (1992, December). *Longer term outcomes of prelinguistic intervention.* Paper presented at the Division for Early Childhood meeting, Washington, DC.

Yoder, P.J. (1986). Clarifying the relation between the degree of infant handicap and maternal responsivity to infant cues: Measurement issues. *Infant Mental Health Journal, 7*(4), 281–293.

Yoder, P.J., Davies, B., Bishop, K., & Munson, L. (1994). The effect of adult continuing wh-questions on conversational participation in children with developmental disabilities. *Journal of Speech and Hearing Research, 37*(1), 193–204.

Yoder, P.J., & Feagans, L. (1988). Mothers' attributions of communication to prelinguistic behavior of infants with developmental delays and mental retardation. *American Journal on Mental Retardation, 93*(1), 36–43.

Yoder, P.J., Kaiser, A.P., Goldstein, H., Alpert, C., Mousetis, L., Kaczmarek, L., & Fischer, R. (1995). An exploratory comparison of milieu teaching and responsive interaction in classroom applications. *Journal of Early Intervention, 19*, 218–242.

Yoder, P.J., Spruytenburg, H., Edwards A., & Davies, B. (1995). Effect of verbal routine contexts and expansions on gains in the mean length of utterance in children with developmental delays. *Language, Speech, Hearing Services in the Schools, 26*, 21–32.

Yoder, P.J., Warren, S.F., & Hull, L. (1995). Predicting children's responses to prelinguistic communication intervention. *Journal of Early Intervention, 19*, 74–84.

Yoder, P.J., Warren, S.F., Kim, K., & Gazdag, G. (1994). Facilitating prelinguistic communication in very young children with developmental disabilities II: Systematic replication and extension. *Journal of Speech and Hearing Research, 37*, 841–851.

4

Communicative Transitions

There's More to the
Hand than Meets the Eye

Jana M. Iverson and Donna J. Thal

A 10-MONTH-OLD IS PLAYING WITH toys while his mother looks on. Reaching for a car, he holds it up for her to see and looks intently into her face. When his mother comments, he puts the car down and resumes playing with his toys. As they stroll in the park, a 13-month-old and her father come upon a dog. Vocalizing excitedly, the child points to the dog and turns to her father for his response. A 15-month-old walks into the kitchen, looks first at the water faucet, then at his father, and produces a DRINKING[1] gesture (i.e., bringing a curved hand to the mouth). The father responds by giving the child a drink of water. A 17-month-old who is seated at the breakfast table with his mother points at a coffee cup and says "Daddy." His mother responds, "That's right, that's Daddy's coffee cup."

These examples illustrate an important developmental phenomenon. Even before young children have begun to talk and throughout the initial phases of language acquisition, early gesture serves an important communicative function. This chapter describes the forms and functions of early gesture, outlines developmental patterns in the emergence and production of gesture, and discusses the relevance of gesture research for clinical intervention.

THE NATURE OF GESTURE

Although the gestures just described differ in form (e.g., pointing with the finger extended versus curving the hand in a drinking gesture) and in function (e.g., commenting on the presence of the dog versus requesting a drink), they share two defining characteristics: They are actions, and they are produced with the

This chapter was supported by a National Science Foundation Graduate Fellowship to the first author and by National Institutes of Health (NIH) Grant No. DC00089 and NIH Grant No. DC00482 to the second author. The authors thank Linda Acredolo and Robert Wozniak for their comments on earlier versions of the chapter.

[1]Throughout this chapter, gesture glosses are indicated in small capital letters.

intention to communicate. Gestural actions typically involve fingers, hands, and arms (e.g., in POINTING or SHOWING) and also may employ facial features (e.g., lip smacking for COOKIES) or even the entire body (e.g., bouncing up and down for HORSE).

The intentional and communicative nature of gestures is evident in the way in which children use them to convey meaning. Gestures are often accompanied by eye contact with the adult (or gaze alternation from the adult to the object of interest and back), and they may be accompanied by vocalization. When children produce a gesture, they frequently pause and wait for the adult to acknowledge the communication. If the adult fails to respond, the gesture may be repeated. If a gesture is not understood, the child may supplement it with additional cues to ensure that the gesture is acknowledged as a communicative signal (Bates, O'Connell, & Shore, 1987).

Types and Functions of Gesture

This chapter focuses primarily on young children's use of two types of gestures: *deictic* and *representational* gestures. Deictic gestures are those whose sole function is to establish reference—to indicate or call attention to an object or event (Bates, 1976; Bates, Benigni, Bretherton, Camaioni, & Volterra, 1979). They include SHOWING (i.e., holding up an object into another's line of sight), POINTING (i.e., extending the index finger toward an object of interest), GIVING (i.e., transferring an object to another person), and REACHING (i.e., extending the arm toward a desired object, frequently accompanied by opening and closing of the fingers). Because deictic gestures only establish reference, they can be used with regard to a potentially infinite number of objects or events (e.g., POINTING can refer to a pencil, a car, or a person; REACHING can be used to indicate a toy, a cup, or a book) and can be interpreted only in relation to the context in which they occur.

Bates, Camaioni, and Volterra (1975) demonstrated that young children use deictic gestures in two functionally different ways. The researchers term these functions *proto-imperative* and *proto-declarative,* respectively. Proto-imperatives, which appear early in development (at around 9 months of age), are gestures that function to engage the adult as a tool for obtaining a desired object. In one proto-imperative sequence observed by Bates and colleagues (1975), for example, the infant Carlotta, seated on the floor in a hallway in front of the kitchen, looked toward her mother and called, using the sound "ha." When her mother came to her, Carlotta looked toward the kitchen. Her mother carried her into the kitchen, and Carlotta pointed toward the sink. When her mother gave the child a glass of water, she drank eagerly.

Proto-declaratives, which appear after proto-imperatives, are gestures that function to indicate an object with the goal of gaining the adult's attention. Thus, for example, Carlotta was frequently observed to point to objects while looking back at the adult for confirmation. Rather than using pointing (or other deictic gestures) to obtain a desired object, in other words, Carlotta had now begun to use pointing to initiate interactions with an adult.

Unlike deictic gestures, representational gestures both establish reference and carry some fixed semantic content. Representational gestures are of two types: object-related gestures and culturally defined conventional gestures. Variously termed *symbolic* gestures (Acredolo & Goodwyn, 1985, 1988, 1990; Nokony, 1977) or *characterizing* gestures (Goldin-Meadow & Morford, 1985, 1990), object-related gestures represent some aspect of a referent (e.g., flapping the hands for BIRD, twisting closed fists toward the body for MOTORCYCLE).

Object-related gestures can in principle be produced either with or without the referent object in hand (e.g., DRINKING can be produced either with a cup in hand or empty-handed), and children produce both varieties. Although empty-handed gestures are infrequent (Goldin-Meadow & Morford, 1985, 1990; Iverson, Capirci, & Caselli, 1994; Petitto, 1992), they tend to be used for communicative purposes and are closely related to linguistic development (Acredolo & Goodwyn, 1988). Referent-in-hand gestures do not appear to be primarily communicative (Bates, Bretherton, Shore, & McNew, 1983), and they tend to occur in the context of private cognition, especially when children are confronted with new instances of a known category of objects (e.g., when given a novel cup, a very young child may produce a drinking gesture, bringing the cup to the lips). Although their view is somewhat controversial, Bates and colleagues interpreted these findings as indicating that such gestural conventions (e.g., "drinking" with a cup) are a kind of naming because they are used by children to recognize, identify, or categorize objects as members of a known class.[2]

Culturally defined conventional gestures are used as social markers (e.g., nodding the head YES, shaking the head NO, and waving the hand BYE-BYE). Although some researchers explicitly exclude conventional gestures from their analyses (e.g., Acredolo & Goodwyn, 1988; Goldin-Meadow & Morford, 1985, 1990; Petitto, 1988, 1992), we believe that the effect of excluding these gestures may be to underestimate the size of the child's gestural repertoire. Our decision to include them within the representational gesture category is based on the fact that both object-related and conventional gestures are used referentially and contain fixed semantic content that generally does not vary across contexts.

---

[2]In making this argument, Bates et al. (1983) pointed out that gestural names closely resemble early verbal names in that they are derived imitatively, refer to external objects and events, point to specific objects and events, emerge at around the same time, and are strongly correlated across children with respect to frequency of use and rate of emergence. In addition, similar patterns of correlation exist between vocal and gestural names and other cognitive measures (particularly items related to means–ends relations and tool use). Based on these findings, Bates and colleagues concluded that verbal and gestural names reflect the same underlying cognitive symbolic process. Petitto (1988, 1992), however, argued that if children's gestures are to be thought of as names, they should meet the same criteria for naming (e.g., the form of a name must be physically independent of that to which it refers; names must be used consistently to refer to members of specific classes of referents; names must be used for multiple, communicative functions) as verbal names. Because they do not, Petitto (1988) argued against thinking of referent-in-hand gestures as names.

Before beginning the discussion of children's early gestural development, we would like to emphasize that early gesture as discussed in this chapter differs from the signs of signed languages such as American Sign Language. Early gestures appear before the emergence of speech in speaking children or the first signs in signing children and continue to develop during the earliest stages of language acquisition. The developmental patterns outlined in this chapter are believed to be typical of children exposed either to spoken or signed language (see Volterra & Iverson, 1995, for a review).

With these issues in mind, we now turn to the main focus of this chapter: the emergence of communicative gesture and its relationship to intentional, symbolic, and linguistic communication in very young children. As with linguistic communication, communicative gesture can be studied with regard to both comprehension and production. The first section of this chapter reviews what little is known about the development of gesture comprehension. The remainder of the chapter is organized into four sections. First, we review a set of methods used to assess children's gesture production. Next, we describe the development of gesture with respect to the emergence of first gestures, the acquisition of lexical items, and the transition to multiword speech. Some applications of these findings in research on gesture use by toddlers with language delays and gesture training with typically developing infants are then highlighted. Finally, we discuss potential educational and clinical implications of gesture research and conclude by suggesting some directions for future work.

COMPREHENSION OF GESTURE

Gesture appears to be one aspect of communicative development in which comprehension may not precede production. Young children tend to produce gestures slightly before they give evidence of comprehending them. In some cases, the gap between production and comprehension onset may even be several months or years. In addition, when gesture is comprehended, children may sometimes be able to use it as an aid to the comprehension of concomitant speech.

The majority of studies that have examined receptive aspects of gesture have focused on comprehension of deictic gestures, especially POINTING. This work has revealed that despite the fact that the average 12-month-old has already been pointing for a month or so, he or she is generally unable to follow points until after the first birthday (Butterworth & Grover, 1990; Murphy & Messer, 1977).[3] When confronted with a pointing gesture, young infants show a strong tendency to fixate only on the hand. When they do manage to look at both the hand and the target, they are likely to look first at the hand and then at the target in a two-step movement.

Young infants also experience difficulty in following POINTING across the mid-line when hand and referent are in different visual fields (Murphy &

---

[3]Infants of this age, however, can be readily conditioned to follow pointing gestures (e.g., Moore & Corkum, 1994).

Messer, 1977). Early in the second year, however, evidence of pointing comprehension begins to emerge. When 14-month-olds are presented with a pointing gesture, they not only can look swiftly and smoothly from hand to target but also can successfully follow the POINT even when the two are in different visual fields (Butterworth & Grover, 1990; Murphy & Messer, 1977).

Additional research on gesture comprehension has focused on children's ability to distinguish GIVING from POINTING. In a classic study, Macnamara (1977) found that children between 13 and 20 months of age responded differentially to GIVING and POINTING. When presented with a giving gesture, children displayed a strong tendency to take the object from the experimenter. In contrast, children tended either to look at the referent object or do nothing at all when the experimenter's gesture was a POINT.

With respect to representational gestures, comprehension studies have found that children give little evidence of understanding. Morford and Goldin-Meadow (1992), for example, noted that almost none of their 15- to 28-month-old subjects understood the representational gestures THROW and SHAKE, either when presented alone or accompanied by speech. Along similar lines, Petitto (1988) reported that her subjects demonstrated almost no comprehension of representational gestures until near the beginning of their third year. This was true even for gestures that were produced by the children themselves before comprehension testing.

Several studies have looked at children's use of gesture to guide their understanding of speech. When Allen and Shatz (1983) asked 16- to 18-month-old children a series of "what" questions, some of which were accompanied by SHOWING, they found that these children were more likely to respond to questions accompanied by gesture than to those asked without gesture. In an earlier study, Macnamara (1977) observed that when information conveyed in gesture and in speech was conflicting (i.e., the referent of the gesture was different from that conveyed in speech) or when speech was uninterpretable (i.e., in a foreign language), children up to 20 months of age tended to ignore speech entirely and focused exclusively on the object referred to by the gesture.

Morford and Goldin-Meadow (1992) conducted a study in which 1- to 2-year-old children were asked to follow a series of simple verbal commands accompanied by no gesture, by a redundant gesture (i.e., one that communicated the same content as one of the content words in the command), or by a replacement gesture (i.e., one that provided information that would have been communicated by an omitted content word). The third condition was of particular interest because children had to understand the gesture to respond correctly to the command. The authors reported that relative to the no-gesture condition, children's performance was better in the two conditions including gesture. Children also produced a greater proportion of correct responses in the replacement condition than in the no-gesture condition, suggesting that they treated the replacement gesture as a word substitute. These results, however, held only when the gestures involved were POINT and REACH/REQUEST. When the gestures were representational (e.g., THROW, SHAKE), children performed no better in the redundant gesture condition and worse in the replacement condition than in the no-gesture condition. These findings suggest that gestures can be interpreted along with speech and that information from gestures can be integrated with that from speech (see also Bates, Thal, Fenson, Whitesell, & Oakes, 1989).

ASSESSMENT OF GESTURE

Studies of young children's gesture use differ with respect to whether they employ nonexperimental observational methods or experimental tasks specifically designed to evaluate gesture production. Researchers have employed two different nonexperimental methods in studies of early gesture production. The first is the parental diary, a tool that has long been used by researchers in the field of language development. The diary method is used in gesture studies in much the same way as in studies of early speech (e.g., Acredolo & Goodwyn, 1988; Caselli, 1990). Parents are asked to record occurrences of gestures produced by their children in the course of daily routines, along with notes on the context in which the gestures were produced, the forms of the gestures, and whether they were accompanied by vocalizations or speech.

Parental diaries have two main advantages as methods for assessing gesture. First, they can provide a wealth of information about children's gesture use, revealing patterns of emergence and disappearance of individual gestures in ways that other methods cannot. Second, because this information is gathered by those who are most familiar with the child's communicative repertoire and style, parental diaries provide a valid measure of spontaneous gesture production in everyday settings.

There are also several disadvantages to this technique. Although parents respond to their children's gestures, they often do not recognize that gestures function as communicative signals in the same way as words. In addition, parents generally do not understand the distinction between gestures and other types of manual and play behaviors. This problem may be eliminated in part by providing parents with training designed to heighten sensitivity to gestural communication (e.g., Goodwyn & Acredolo, 1993) or by use of parent questionnaires, such as the Macarthur Communicative Development Inventory (Fenson et al., 1993), which lists commonly produced gestures, actions, and play behaviors. Lists of this sort may help parents by providing descriptions of what children's gestures look like and examples of how and when they might be used.

The second nonexperimental method is naturalistic observation. This method generally involves in-home videotaping of a parent in typical interaction with the child (e.g., Butcher & Goldin-Meadow, in press; Capirci, Iverson, Pizzuto, & Volterra, 1996; Iverson et al., 1994). Variation can be introduced into the setting by having the child interact with the experimenter for a brief time, by observing the child in different contexts (e.g., playing, at snacktime, going for a walk), and by introducing different sets of toys (e.g., varying play with experimenter-provided toys and the child's own toys; providing books, toys that make interesting movements, or toys specifically chosen to elicit naming behaviors).

Several experimental tasks have also been designed to assess gesture production in young children (e.g., Thal & Bates, 1988). Two of these tasks examine production of single gestures, and a third evaluates the production of gesture sequences embedded in the context of a culturally familiar script. The first of the single-gesture tasks measures children's spontaneous production of recognitory gestures. A series of familiar objects (e.g., a small car, an airplane, a doll, a cup) is presented to the child, one at a time, and the child is asked, "What's that?" Children's responses are coded according to whether they spontaneously label the object and whether the label they produce is verbal or gestural.

The second single-gesture task is an imitation task in which the child is asked to imitate recognitory gestures with objects produced by an experimenter. These gestures vary along two dimensions: whether they are accompanied by supportive (e.g., "Look at the car") or by neutral (e.g., "Look at this") language and whether they are performed with the correct object or with a placeholder (a block). Thus, each gesture can be performed in one of four possible conditions: supportive language with real object, supportive language with placeholder, neutral language with real object, and neutral language with placeholder. Examples of gestures included in this task are presented in Table 1. Children are given credit for a correct response if they imitate the gesture produced by the experimenter.

In the gesture sequences task, children are asked to imitate a series of scripted actions performed on a teddy bear by the experimenter (e.g., putting the

Table 1. Examples of gestures,[a] objects, and language used in the single-gesture imitation task

Gesture	Object	Language
drink	cup	"Look at this." (N)
fly	plane	"Look at this." (N)
brush teeth	toothbrush	"Look at this." (N)
put on head	hat	"Look at this." (N)
push	car	"Look at the car." (S)
eat	spoon	"Look at the spoon." (S)
hug	baby	"Look at the baby." (S)
sniff	flower	"Look at this." (N)
walk	dog	"Look at the dog." (S)
receiver to ear	phone	"Look at this." (N)

From Thal, D., & Tobias, S. (1994). Relationships between language and gesture in normally developing and late-talking toddlers. *Journal of Speech and Hearing Research, 37,* 169; adapted by permission.

[a]Each gesture is presented twice, once with a real object and once with a placeholder. S = supportive language, N = neutral language.

bear to bed, feeding the bear an apple, giving the bear a bath). Children are first given the objects with no model to establish a baseline rate of sequence play. When the child begins to tire of spontaneous play with the objects, the experimenter models the actions once in canonical order and once in reverse order, with the child being invited to imitate at the end of each presentation. Performance is scored on the basis of number of gestures imitated and number of gestures imitated in the modeled order.

In sum, observational and experimental methods tap different aspects of children's gestural performance. Experimental tasks provide a measure of the child's ability, on demand, to label objects gesturally, to imitate gestures and actions produced by other people, and to sequence gestures. Naturalistic observation and parent diaries, which sample the child's use of gesture in everyday interactions, provide assessment of the child's communicative repertoire.

DEVELOPMENT OF GESTURE: FIRST GESTURES

Deictic Gestures

The body of research conducted on deictic gestures and the development of referential skills since the 1970s has reinforced Werner and Kaplan's (1963) idea that referential behavior emerges through the sharing of contemplated objects in an interpersonal context. Along these lines, Bruner (1977) suggested that "the objective of early reference ... is to indicate to another by some reliable means which among an alternative set of things or states or actions is relevant to the child's and mother's shared line of endeavour" (p. 275). He further argued that the behavioral basis for referential skills is present from early in the first year of life in the form of eye gaze and other motor activities. Over time, however, the child begins to employ more efficient methods (e.g., deictic gestures) for singling out objects that are less tied to the specific situation or action pattern in which they are embedded. In other words, deictic gestures emerge out of motor skills that appear early in development and are refined to meet the demands of effective referential communication.

An initial form of reference—eye gaze and gaze following—is employed as a means of inferring attentional focus by mothers and infants early in the first year of life, long before the emergence of deictic gestures. For instance, Collis and Schaffer (1975) observed that mothers followed their infants' line of regard as a means of monitoring the infants' focus of attention. With respect to infants' gaze-following abilities, Scaife and Bruner (1975) reported that babies as young as 2 months old were able to follow an adult's line of regard when it was turned toward a locus removed from the child. Taken together, these results suggest that very young infants and their caregivers both employ gaze to monitor attentional focus.

Although young infants' gaze-following abilities are quite impressive, they are by no means fully developed. Developmental changes have been documented in a series of laboratory interaction studies carried out by Butterworth and colleagues (see Butterworth & Grover, 1990, for a review). In these studies, mothers were asked to play with their infants as they typically would. At a signal, mothers turned to look at a designated member of a set of targets placed at various positions around the room. Butterworth's findings were striking. Six-month-olds looked to the correct side of the room but stopped at the first target that fell within their scan path. In cases where there were multiple targets placed along the same wall, infants often failed to distinguish the correct target from others if it was not the first one encountered in their scan path. By 9 months of age, infants were able to localize targets regardless of their position along the scan path by extrapolating information from the orientation of their mother's head and gaze. For infants of both ages, however, gaze-following skills were restricted to objects within the visual field. When mothers looked at targets placed behind the infants, for example, babies either fixated on a target in front of them or within the visual field or failed to respond entirely. By the age of 18 months, gaze-following skills had generalized beyond the infant's own visual field. Babies now looked correctly at targets in any location, even when they did not fall in the immediate line of sight.

Despite young infants' skill at following adult eye gaze, they do not appear to use gaze as a means of actively engaging adults' attention until the beginning of the second year. At around 12 months of age, children begin to employ gaze alternation to draw an adult's attention to an interesting object or toy. Children will follow the gaze of an adult to an object and then immediately look back at the adult, seemingly to check that the adult is continuing to attend to the object. The simultaneous, active coordination of the child's attention to both the adult and to an object is a hallmark of joint attention situations that begin to occur with some frequency at 12 months of age (see Tomasello, 1995; see also Chapter 2).

Since the early part of the 20th century, numerous investigators have pointed out the close relationship between early eye-gaze behaviors and the development of deictic gestures (e.g., Stern & Stern, 1928). In early gaze-following situations, infants gain at least two important pieces of information that are essential to the development of reference. First, they begin to understand that looking where someone else is looking is a valuable clue to the current focus of the other person's attention. Second, they discover that their own line of regard can be used by others to obtain similar information. Understanding that attentional states are identifiable and can be redirected by such cues plays an important role in the emergence of deictic gestures.

Between the ages of 8 and 14 months, the cues that infants use to establish reference become more explicit. They begin to produce deictic gestures (e.g., GIVING, SHOWING, POINTING, REACHING) to mark the current focus of their attention and to draw the adult's attention to it. Among these gestures, GIVING, SHOWING, and REACHING are the first to emerge (Bates, 1976; Bates et al., 1979; Masur, 1990), with POINTING appearing slightly later (i.e., between 12 and 14 months of age; e.g., Bates, 1976; Bates et al., 1979; Lock, Young, Service, & Chandler, 1990; Masur, 1990). GIVING, SHOWING, and REACHING appear to function as primitive devices for establishing reference, and their emergence signals an important moment of transition in communicative development. As children begin to use these gestures to seek an adult's acknowledgment of an interesting toy or object, they reveal their emerging ability to be an active partner in establishing a shared object world (Bates et al., 1987).

Initially, GIVING, SHOWING, and REACHING tend to occur as responses to adult behavior (e.g., giving a requested object to an adult, reaching for an object that is being manipulated or extended by an adult). Gradually, they become less tied to the specific situations and action patterns in which they occur. For example, an initial form of REACHING might consist of exaggerated reaching toward an object accompanied by fussing. Over time, the child begins to produce a more peremptory reach while looking toward the caregiver's face (Bruner, 1977). Rather than being simply a signal of difficulty in reaching toward and obtaining a desired object, REACHING now serves as a signal for indicating interest in a particular object.

Some authors (e.g., Bates et al., 1987; see also Werner & Kaplan, 1963) interpret infants' use of GIVING, SHOWING, and REACHING as evidence that they are coming to terms with the idea of referential communication. These authors have suggested that these gestures are necessary precursors to POINTING because they allow the child to work out the principles of referential communication on a simpler level, with objects that are close at hand. Evidence for this claim comes from reports of robust correlations between the appearance of GIVING, SHOWING, and REACHING and later onset of communicative POINTING (Bates et al., 1979). The emergence of POINTING, which involves establishing reference to distant objects, occurs once children have had some practice with referential communication.

Like gaze following, the pointing form has a long developmental history before its emergence as a communicative signal (e.g., Leung & Rheingold, 1981; Murphy & Messer, 1977). For instance, index finger extension occurs reliably during mother–child interaction with infants as young as 2 months. The finger does not single out specific objects, nor is it correlated with gaze or arm extension, but it is reliably preceded and followed by vocalization or mouth movements and occurs in an interpersonal context (Fogel & Hannan, 1985).

Use of the pointing form has also been observed with some regularity among older infants. For example, 6-month-old infants will spontaneously point when an object attracts their attention in a social context, but the form lacks the full arm extension characteristic of communicative pointing. Instances of pointing-for-self are found in older infants, in which the child points at an object while exploring it closely. In a series of detailed observations, Bates (1976) noted that at the age of 9 months, the infant Carlotta frequently oriented toward new objects or unexpected sounds and pointed while staring fixedly in the direction of the novelty. She also pointed for long periods at details in storybook drawings. During this time, however, she never looked up from the object being explored to see if an adult was watching her. The use of communicative POINT-ING emerged only after Carlotta had been pointing for several weeks in such contexts and had begun to use other gestures (e.g., GIVING) in a communicative fashion.

Observations such as these have led to the idea that although the pointing form may be available early in development, its function is not fully established until after the first birthday. The process by which pointing becomes a communicative signal involves at least two changes. First, pointing becomes distanced from its referent. Early instances of pointing generally occur in the context of exploring an object that is either in the child's hand or nearby. Gradually, pointing is used to refer to proximal objects and finally to indicate objects that are removed from the child (Bates, 1976; Lock et al., 1990; Werner & Kaplan, 1963).

Second, pointing acquires a social function. Early points seem to function as self-directing attentional gestures that allow children to highlight the current focus of their attention for themselves (Bates, 1976; Masur, 1990). With growth in the domain of referential communication, pointing becomes a social gesture used to direct the attention of others to an object of interest. A striking demonstration of this shift occurs once infants begin to coordinate pointing with gaze alternation: Infants will point to an object while looking back at the adult, seeming to check that the referent of the gesture has been located and is now the focus of the adult's attention (e.g., Bates, 1976; Butterworth & Grover, 1990; Masur, 1990). In these instances, pointing is used to attract the attention of another person to an object for purposes of communication and interaction.

Representational Gestures

One of the earliest discussions of the emergence of representational gestures is in Werner and Kaplan's (1963) classic account of symbol formation. Beginning with the view that "a novel emerging function becomes actualized at first through the use of a means articulated and structured in the service of genetically earlier ends…" (p. 66), Werner and Kaplan argued that when children begin to employ symbols in communication, they do so first by making use of skills acquired earlier in development and employing them in a novel way.

Specifically, Werner and Kaplan (1963) suggested that very young children employ sensorimotor action schemas initially developed within the context of "action on the world" in their earliest communications. In effect, early sensorimotor schemes serve as the basis for first gestures. For Werner and Kaplan, the most important feature of these early gestures is that they can eventually become symbols. Children's initial representational gestures are highly context bound, presumably because children lack the understanding that symbols "stand for" their referents. Gestures are associated with specific contexts and activities and are produced only within those settings. As children begin to understand that symbols are used to represent referents, there is a shift toward the distancing of a symbol from its referent, a process Werner and Kaplan referred to as *decontextualization*. In other words, over development and with increasing experience in the symbolic domain, children begin to produce symbols across a wide variety of contexts and in the absence of referents.

In Werner and Kaplan's account of the transition to symbolic communication, representational gestures serve an important function for the child who is beginning to learn about symbols and the concept of representation. These authors argued that because the relationship between action-based gestures and their referents becomes highly practiced and is often iconic, representational gestures become increasingly distanced from their referents over time, leading to a gradual understanding of the type of arbitrary symbol–referent relation that characterizes most words. Once the child recognizes the underlying relationship between referents and symbols, such gestures function much like words and thus mark an intermediate phase in the shift toward increasingly abstract symbol–referent relationships that are typical of words and their referents.

Although Werner and Kaplan (1963) did not have longitudinal data of their own available to support their arguments, they cited examples from numerous case studies that substantiated their views. With respect to the transition from action to gesture, for example, they cited an anecdotal report from observations carried out by Perez (1878). Perez noted that one child's NO gesture emerged in the following way: At the age of 11 months, the child indicated his dislike for certain objects by pushing them away. By the age of 13 months, this pushing away gesture had become a NO gesture, consisting of waving the hand back and forth. In their discussion of the decontextualization process, Werner and Kaplan (1963) cited a classic observation by Piaget (1951), who noted that his daughter produced a DRINKING gesture initially with a full glass, then with an empty glass, and finally with no object in her hand.

Findings from longitudinal studies of early representational gestures are consistent with Werner and Kaplan's (1963) claims. With respect to their views on the transition from action to gesture, a number of authors (e.g., Acredolo & Goodwyn, 1988; Caselli, 1990) have reported that children's first representational gestures emerge out of familiar games and routines and tend to be actions that children perform with their own bodies. For example, Caselli (1990) observed that her son's first representational gestures consisted of actions extracted from favorite routines that were employed for communicative purposes. One gesture, DANCING, originated as part of a routine in which the child was asked to dance to music. At the age of 11 months, the child used the same dancing action in the absence of music to request that his mother turn on the radio.

In addition, Werner and Kaplan's (1963) description of the transition from context-bound to decontextualized symbols is supported by longitudinal data indicating strong links between context and early representational gesture production. For instance, Caselli's (1990) son initially produced the gesture BYE-BYE only when other people left the house, suggesting that, for him, production of BYE-BYE was tightly linked to this particular situation. This gesture gradually began to appear in other contexts, first as a request to go out, and then as a comment about objects (e.g., cars) moving away from the child. A similar pattern of decontextualization has also been observed in children's early word production (Volterra, Bates, Benigni, Bretherton, & Camaioni, 1979). Taken as a whole, these findings suggest that, as the symbolic function develops, children's representational gestures gradually become more context flexible, are available to refer to absent objects and events, and can be used for a variety of communicative functions (Caselli, 1990; Caselli & Volterra, 1990; Zinober & Martlew, 1985).

THE EARLY LEXICON

During the earliest stages of lexical development, gesture provides young children with an additional modality in which to acquire new vocabulary items. At first, gestures and words develop in parallel and tend to be equally represented in the child's emerging lexicon. Eventually, however, the relationship between gesture and speech is reorganized, and the role of gesture becomes subordinate to that of speech.

Emergence of Words and Gestures

Children's gestural and vocal lexicons begin to develop at roughly the same time (Acredolo & Goodwyn, 1985, 1988; Caselli, 1990; Caselli & Volterra, 1990). In a longitudinal diary study that followed one Italian child from 10 to 20 months of age, for example, Caselli (1990) observed that the child's first words ("bau bau" <dog> and "cl cl" <horse>) appeared only a few days before his first representational gestures (clapping the hands for GOOD BOY and waving BYE-BYE), a parallelism noted by other investigators in studies of larger groups of infants (e.g., Acredolo & Goodwyn, 1988). In a parent report study of early vocal and gestural vocabularies in 20 children at the age of 14 months, Casadio and Caselli (1989) found that the children's lexicons consisted of both words and gestures. That representational gestures and words begin to emerge within the same time frame means that both gesture and speech are potentially available to the young child as modalities in which new lexical items can be acquired. This combined availability may make it easier for young children who are cognitively capable of producing words but still grappling with the problems of production in the oral modality to acquire new lexical items.

Although the gestural modality is potentially available to all children acquiring their first lexical items, children vary widely in the extent to which they add verbal or gestural items to their vocabularies. Some children may have many symbolic gestures referring to a variety of referents, whereas others may produce only a few such gestures (Acredolo & Goodwyn, 1988). Analyzing the spontaneous verbal and gestural productions of a group of Italian children at ages 16 and 20 months, Iverson et al. (1994) found that the 16-month-olds could be classified into three subgroups according to the relative sizes of their speech and gestural vocabularies. In one group of children, gestures outnumbered words; in a second group, gestures and words appeared in equal numbers; and in a third group, children had many more words than gestures.

Just as there are individual differences in the relative numbers of words and gestures in the child's first vocabulary, so too is there variability in the extent to which children make use of words and gestures as they interact. Iverson et al. (1994) examined the relationship between the size of children's vocabularies (word and gesture types) and their use of these words and gestures (tokens) during a 45-minute videotaped observation. At 16 months of age, 8 of their 12 children, including 3 who actually had as many or more words than gestures in their vocabularies, showed a clear preference for communication in the gestural modality. Four children (all of whom had relatively large speech vocabularies) produced many more word than gesture tokens during the course of the session.

These findings indicate that the gestural and vocal modalities are equally available to young children who are just beginning to acquire their first lexical items and that during this time, at least for some children, new lexical items may be added as gestures more readily than as speech. Children who regularly add and use new lexical items in the gestural modality may, in effect, possess a large communicative repertoire (as measured by the number of different words and gestures produced), even when their spoken vocabularies are still quite limited.

Development of the Early Lexicon

As the child's early lexicon grows, speech and gesture develop in tandem: New lexical items are added in both modalities, and children make use of both gestures and words when interacting with others. This section presents evidence suggesting that, at this stage of development, gesture and speech function as a single communicative system.

Several observations provide support for this claim. First, early gestures and words appear to share the same communicative functions. Young children use lexical items in both modalities to refer to objects, to request objects and events, to comment on the attributes of a referent, and to reply to an interlocutor's communication (Acredolo & Goodwyn, 1988). Second, children use words and gestures in similar contexts to refer to the same general semantic domains, such as eating, drinking, and the appearance or disappearance of objects and people (e.g., Bates et al., 1979). Third, although children's early words and gestures tend to refer to a common set of referents, lexical overlap between individual verbal and gestural items is minimal (Acredolo & Goodwyn, 1988, 1990;

Caselli & Volterra, 1990; Iverson et al., 1994). Children's gestural lexicons serve to complement rather than duplicate their verbal lexicons. If a child produces a gesture for a given referent such as "fish," for example, it is very likely that he or she does not yet have a word for "fish." Similarly, if a child can produce the word "fish," then it is likely that he or she will not have a corresponding gesture.

In short, evidence from the functional use and content of children's early vocabularies suggests that the initial relationship between gesture and speech is one of reciprocity. Gestures and words exhibit little semantic redundancy and are used interchangeably in similar contexts to refer to the same broad set of referents. By functioning as a single communicative system at a stage when the child's oral production is limited, gesture and speech augment the child's communicative and referential potential.

Reorganization of the Gesture–Speech System

Within a few months, however, the relative relationship of gesture to speech begins to change. Exposed to a communicative environment that consists primarily of speech, hearing children move rapidly toward spoken language as their primary means of communication. The gesture–speech system undergoes a radical reorganization. As children begin to focus on speech and to acquire words in earnest, gesture becomes subordinated to speech. Gesture–speech reorganization is reflected in a number of developmental changes that take place at this time. First, children ultimately abandon any early preference for gestural communication that they may have shown and begin to favor speech as their primary means of communication. Iverson et al. (1994), for example, noted that as children's production of words increased between ages 16 and 20 months, overall production of gesture underwent a proportionate decline, and the relative prevalence of deictic and representational gestures also changed. Although production of deictic gestures (especially POINTING) increased significantly over time, representational gestures declined radically, suggesting that the change in gesture production was due to changes in the way gesture was used and its function relative to speech. Second, as speech becomes children's preferred channel of communication and new words are rapidly added to their vocabularies (Acredolo & Goodwyn, 1985; Caselli, 1990; Iverson et al., 1994), the acquisition of new gestures "freezes," and very few new gestures are added to the lexicon (Caselli & Volterra, 1990).

The nature of this change has been clarified by Acredolo and Goodwyn (1988), who noted that as children's speech vocabularies expand, gestures become redundant with items present in their verbal lexicons. When this redundancy occurs, it is resolved through the eventual disappearance of the gesture. Apparently, gestures serve as transitional forms that ease the child into symbolic communication and substitute until the production of specific words can be worked out (Acredolo & Goodwyn, 1988). Although gesture production does not disappear and gestures continue to be used frequently by one-word speakers (e.g., Acredolo & Goodwyn, 1988; Bates et al., 1979; Butcher & Goldin-Meadow, in press; Capirci et al., 1996; Goldin-Meadow & Morford, 1985; Greenfield & Smith, 1976; Morford & Goldin-Meadow, 1992), the gestural system shifts from a position of relative communicative equivalence with respect to speech to a new role as a secondary support system integrated with speech.

DEVELOPMENT OF GESTURE: GESTURE–SPEECH COMBINATIONS

Just as gesture appears to ease the child into the production of words, it also plays an important role in the transition from one- to two-word speech. Several months before the transition to two-word speech, children begin to combine gestures with single-word utterances. The emergence of gesture–word combinations is an important step in language acquisition. The child who was previously able to use only one word or gesture at a time can now produce and combine two communicative elements within the framework of a single utterance.

Once children begin to combine gestures and single words, they do so in two different ways. The first type of gesture–word combination, which we call *complementary*, generally appears between the ages of 14 and 16 months (e.g., Bates et al., 1979; de Laguna, 1927; Goldin-Meadow & Morford, 1985; Greenfield & Smith, 1976; Guillaume, 1927). In these complementary combinations, gestures and words convey similar, often redundant information. A child producing complementary combinations might POINT to a cup while saying the word "cup" or shake his head NO while saying "no."

The second type of gesture–word combination, which we call *supplementary*, emerges somewhat later, between the ages of 16 and 18 months, and only after children have begun to produce some complementary combinations (Butcher & Goldin-Meadow, in press; Goldin-Meadow & Morford, 1985; Greenfield & Smith, 1976; Morford & Goldin-Meadow, 1992). In supplementary combinations, gestures contain information that is different from but related to that conveyed by words. A child producing supplementary combinations might POINT to a cup while saying "Mommy" to indicate that this is Mommy's cup or wave BYE-BYE while saying "car" to indicate that a car is driving away. Supplementary combinations are similar to two-word utterances in the amount of information they convey. In a supplementary combination, however, one element is expressed in speech and the other is expressed in gesture.

On the basis of the available evidence, it appears that two-word utterances begin to emerge only after children have been producing both complementary and supplementary gesture–word combinations (Butcher & Goldin-Meadow, in press). This progression appears to be a robust feature of communicative development, even across potentially significant variations in language and culture. Thus, for example, Capirci and colleagues (1996) reported that children learning

Italian, like children learning English, move from complementary to supplementary gesture–word combinations and finally to two-word utterances.

Gesture–Word Combinations and the Transition to Two-Word Speech

Although the appearance of both complementary and supplementary combinations seems to mark an important intermediate stage in the progression from one- to two-word speech, research suggests that production of supplementary combinations may also be a particularly good indicator of the imminence of the transition to two-word speech. For example, Iverson, Volterra, Pizzuto, and Capirci (1994) observed that, relative to children who have not yet produced supplementary gesture–word combinations, children who produced such combinations by age 16 months were more likely to produce two-word combinations at age 20 months. Along similar lines, Butcher and Goldin-Meadow (in press) found a strong ($r = .90$) and significant correlation between the age at which children produced supplementary gesture–word combinations and the age at which they began to use two-word combinations. Thus, children who were among the first to produce supplementary gesture–word combinations also tended to be among the first to produce two-word utterances.

It might also be noted that children who gesture about one referent while talking about another are not showing signs of a gap in productive speech vocabulary. Capirci et al. (1996) pointed out that several of the children in their study produced gesture–speech combinations in which the children referred to two elements that they could say. In the most compelling of these observations, a child pointed to his shoe while saying "shoe" at one point in the observation. Then, 5 minutes later, he again pointed to his shoe, but this time he said "untied." Capirci and colleagues suggested that the limitation on production of a word combination such as "shoe untied" was not simply a lexical one but rather one of producing the two words together within the frame of a communicative combination.

This observation also provides a striking example of the fact that early gesture–word combinations serve two different functions for young children as they attempt to communicate. The redundancy in a complementary combination (e.g., POINTING to a shoe while saying "shoe") functions to reinforce and disambiguate the child's intended message. This added reinforcement seems to help the child, who is both vocally uncertain and still moderately unintelligible, to ensure that the message is understood. Supplementary combinations (e.g., POINTING to a shoe while saying "untied") extend the child's intended message. Combinations of this sort, in which vocal and gestural elements provide different pieces of information, contain a more complex informational content, make greater demands on the child's cognitive capacities, and appear only after children are already producing complementary combinations.

To understand the order of emergence of complementary and supplementary combinations, it is important to realize that there are two general cognitive processes that play important roles in the transition to two-word speech. The first such process involves the general ability to combine two elements, and this seems to be evidenced by production of complementary gesture–word combinations. The second process involves the general capacity to coordinate two different pieces of information within a single, integrated message, and this appears to be in place in children who produce supplementary combinations. Supplementary combinations, in other words, appear to be indicative of a child's transitional status in the language-learning process and to reflect a compromise between readiness to produce word combinations and constraints (e.g., phonological and articulatory skills; Johnson, Lewis, & Hogan, 1995) on the ability to produce two words in succession. The production of supplementary combinations seems to indicate that a child is cognitively equipped to produce two-word utterances but has not yet reached the moment of full transition into two-word speech (Morford & Goldin-Meadow, 1992).

Gesture–Speech Integration

Another index of the changing relationship between gesture and speech involves alteration in the temporal parameters constraining the co-occurrence of gesture with speech. In adults, it has been suggested that gesture and speech form a single, integrated system (McNeill, 1992). One piece of evidence for this claim comes from observed temporal links between gestures and semantically related speech. When an individual says, "I carried the box to the basement," for example, the word "box" may be produced on the stroke of a gesture conveying information about box size or weight. Thus, gesture is very tightly timed with respect to speech in adults and even in children as young as 2½ years (McNeill, 1992).

Butcher and Goldin-Meadow (in press) reported that for children who have not yet achieved the transition to two-word speech, gesture and speech are *not* timed according to the adult pattern. Words are not produced on the stroke of the gesture; rather, gestures tend to be produced either just before (e.g., POINT at duck [pause] "duck") or just after (e.g., "duck" [pause] POINT at duck) related speech. During the transition period before the onset of two-word speech, the proportion of correctly timed utterances increases, and by the time children begin to produce two-word utterances, the majority of their gesture–word combinations are timed in the adult fashion. Based on these findings, Butcher and Goldin-Meadow concluded that for very young children, gesture and speech begin to function as a single, unified system before the transition to two-word speech.

GESTURE AND LANGUAGE DELAY

In a series of studies, Thal and colleagues examined gesture use in late talkers, young children who are identified by delayed acquisition of productive vocabulary in the absence of hearing loss, mental retardation, behavioral disturbances, or known forms of neurological impairment. The researchers reported that gesture production can distinguish between children who are late bloomers (i.e., children who "recover" and begin to produce language in a typical manner) and those who are truly delayed.

In an initial study, Thal and Bates (1988) presented 18- to 32-month-old late talkers in the one-word stage and two groups of control children with two tasks: 1) a single-gesture imitation task, in which children were asked to imitate object-related gestures produced by an experimenter; and 2) a gesture-sequencing task, in which the child was asked to reproduce a familiar series of actions first modeled by the experimenter (cf. Table 1). In addition, each late talker was individually matched to two typically developing control children: one on the basis of productive vocabulary level (language-matched controls) and one for age and gender (age-matched controls).

Results indicated that late talkers performed like their younger language-matched controls on the single-gesture imitation task and like their age-matched controls on the gesture-sequencing task. That is, late talkers behaved like younger children with similarly limited productive vocabularies, whereas their ability to reproduce a sequence of gestures was similar to that of their typically developing age-mates. Based on these findings, Thal and Bates (1988) concluded that there appears to be a dissociation between language and gesture for late talkers, with gesture falling somewhat ahead of language. They suggest that late talkers' relatively poor performance on the single-gesture imitation task may reflect problems related to the retrieval of individual symbols, but that sequencing skills may develop "underground" as long as the child has a minimal set of retrievable symbols and is acting in a context that facilitates retrieval. Thal and Bates further hypothesized that if these skills are first manifested in gesture, then it may be the case that a "catch-up" will soon follow in speech.

Thal, Tobias, and Morrison (1991) tested this hypothesis by looking at the same cohort of children at a 1-year follow-up visit. The authors looked at data from the children's initial visit to determine whether any measure reliably predicted outcome at the follow-up visit. At this visit, 6 of the 10 late talkers had apparently "caught up" in their speech skills (the *late bloomers*), while the other 4 children remained delayed (the *truly delayed* children). Two measures from the initial visit appeared to distinguish between the late bloomers and the truly delayed children. The first was language comprehension: Truly delayed children were delayed in language comprehension as measured by both parent inventory and an experimental two-way, forced-choice picture identification task, while late bloomers fell within the normal range on both comprehension tasks. The second measure was performance on the set of gesture tasks: Truly delayed children did much worse on all gesture task measures than did late bloomers.

These findings provide some support for the "catch-up" hypothesis. Sequencing skills, as measured by performance on the gesture-sequencing task at the initial visit, did predict whether children were identified as late bloomers or truly delayed at the follow-up visit. However, language comprehension was also an important mediating factor in predicting recovery from delay. In addition to their good performance on the gesture-sequencing task at the initial visit, children who were later identified as late bloomers also demonstrated high levels of comprehension at the initial visit. Taken together, these results suggest that vocabulary comprehension measures and the production of conventional gestures embedded within familiar scripts may provide valuable prognostic information about recovery from early language delay.

Although gesture production in the context of imitation paradigms provides a valuable means of distinguishing among late talkers, such measures provide little information about the extent to which late talkers might employ communicative gestures to compensate for poor verbal production skills. To address this question, Thal and Tobias (1992) looked at communicative production of gestures by 18- to 28-month-old late talkers in the one-word stage and their language-matched controls across a series of structured play sessions. They reported that late talkers used significantly more communicative gestures and produced more gestures spontaneously than their language-matched controls. Late talkers also used gestures as answers to adult questions whereas language-matched controls did not. When Thal and Tobias (1992) compared production of communicative gestures at the initial visit by the subgroups of late talkers later identified as late bloomers and truly delayed, they found a striking difference between the groups: Late bloomers produced significantly more communicative gestures at the initial visit than truly delayed children, who used gestures about as often as their language-matched controls.

This result suggests that late bloomers may have made use of gesture as a way to compensate for oral language delay while truly delayed children did not. The authors speculated that the low frequency of communicative gesture use in truly delayed children may reflect delays in the development of symbolic representational abilities or in recognition that symbols can be used for communication. The finding that late bloomers do use gesture as a compensatory device, however, suggests that, for these children, an understanding of the vehicle–referent relationship and of the communicative value of symbols is in place. In this case, delayed language production may be an indication of difficulties with symbol retrieval (especially in the oral modality), articulatory problems, or other temporary obstacles to language production.

GESTURE INTERVENTION: TEACHING GESTURES TO CHILDREN

Although much of the knowledge about children's production of gestures and the relationship between gesture and spoken language acquisition comes from work on spontaneous or elicited production of gestures, some work has begun to explore these issues from a different perspective: by training parents to teach and encourage gesturing in their children. In a series of studies of typically developing children, Acredolo and Goodwyn (1988, 1989, 1995) and Goodwyn and

Acredolo (1993) observed that gesture training has a positive effect on verbal development, that children tend to use these gestural symbols earlier than verbal symbols, and that they add symbolic gestures to their vocabularies at a significantly faster rate than words.

In their initial pilot study, Acredolo and Goodwyn (1989) followed six infants longitudinally from the age of 11 months until they reached the 100-word milestone. The phenomenon of symbolic gesturing was explained to parents, and they were instructed to encourage gesture production in their infants. Specifically, families were provided with a set of five toys, each of which was the focus of a specific target gesture. The set of gestures included the following: lip smacking for "fish," hand waving (as if pushing) for "ball," sniffing for "flower," hand flapping for "chickie," and a Peekaboo gesture for Mickey Mouse. Parents were instructed to embed each toy into at least one daily routine (e.g., bathtime, diaper changing) and to model *both* the gesture and the verbal label (e.g., "See the fishie? [smack smack] Fishie, fishie!"). Parents were also told to provide the gesture and the label outside of these routines whenever an example of the object was encountered.

Based on data from weekly parent interviews, Acredolo and Goodwyn (1989) reported two main findings. First, and most important, the experimenters' efforts to train parents and parents' efforts to teach gestures to their infants were successful. On average, children in the study produced 20 gestures, considerably more than the typical mean of about 5 gestures reported in studies of spontaneous gesturing (e.g., Acredolo & Goodwyn, 1988). Second, infants in the study achieved a number of language development milestones at earlier ages than children not exposed to gesture training. In comparison to untrained children, who achieved the 50-word milestone anywhere from 17.3 (Rescorla, 1980) to 19.6 (Nelson, 1973) months on average, infants in Acredolo and Goodwyn's study reached this milestone at an average age of 16.5 months. Achievement of two-word combinations was also reached at an earlier age (16.5 months on average) in children trained to gesture than is typical for untrained children (18 to 24 months on average). Early experience with gesture training, in short, appeared to have a positive effect on syntactic as well as lexical development.

In a subsequent study, Goodwyn and Acredolo (1993) asked whether the effects of gesture training might be manifested even earlier at the onset of symbolic communication. They hypothesized that the emergence of symbolic communication may be facilitated when the articulatory demands imposed by the verbal modality are removed. In other words, production of gestural symbols may be easier for infants, and if they are cognitively equipped for symbolic communication but lack control over the articulatory apparatus required for verbal symbol production, then symbolic communication may begin earlier in the gestural modality than in the vocal modality.

To explore this possibility, Goodwyn and Acredolo (1993) carried out a within-subject comparison of the ages of onset of verbal and gestural symbols in a group of 22 hearing infants exposed to symbolic gestures from the age of 11 months. The training procedure was identical to that described previously, with the exception that the set of target gestures was expanded to include eight symbolic gestures. Parents were interviewed biweekly about their children's production of gestures and words and the contexts in which these items were employed. The data revealed a small but reliable tendency for symbol use to begin earlier in the gestural modality. The average age for symbol onset in the gestural modality was 11.94 months compared with a mean age of 12.64 months for word onset. Similarly, children reached the five-symbol milestone slightly earlier in the gestural than in the vocal modality. Based on these results, the authors concluded that although emergence of gestural symbols does tend to precede the appearance of verbal symbols, the size of the gestural advantage is small and varies widely from infant to infant.

Acredolo and Goodwyn (1995) followed up these findings by asking whether, after the onset of symbolic communication, new symbols are added more readily in the gestural modality than in the vocal modality. To address this issue, they followed two groups of children longitudinally beginning at the age of 11 months. As in previous studies, one group of children (the sign training group) was exposed to a set of eight target symbolic gestures. A second comparison group was added to test the question of whether infants add symbolic gestures to their vocabularies at a significantly faster rate than words. Children in this group (the verbal training group) were exposed to a set of target words, with parents instructed to model and use these words in the same way as parents of infants in the sign training group. The sets of words and gestures were not identical, with the exception of two overlapping items (*more* and *all gone*).

Again using parent interview data, Acredolo and Goodwyn (1995) looked at the number of target symbols acquired by the two groups at the ages of 12, 13, 14, and 15 months. They reported that the number of target gestures acquired by the sign training group was significantly greater than the number of target words learned by the verbal training group at all age points beyond 12 months. They also noted that although infants in the sign training group had target items available to them in both their gestural and verbal forms, children tended either to acquire the gesture first or to learn neither the gesture nor the word by the end of the study. The two items included in the target sets for both the sign training and the verbal training groups (*more* and *all gone*) were acquired by more children in the sign training than in the verbal training group. These findings suggest that when the phonological requirements for symbol production are eliminated, concept naming proceeds at a faster pace.

Taken together, these studies indicate that although infants may be cognitively and communicatively ready to produce symbols, they may be prevented from doing so initially by difficulties with articulation and speech production. When infants are encouraged to use the gestural modality, these limitations can be circumvented, and the onset of symbolic communication may be earlier and lexical acquisition may proceed at a more rapid pace, a finding consonant with results on the emergence and development of spontaneous gesturing in children not exposed to specific gestural input.

EDUCATIONAL AND CLINICAL IMPLICATIONS

Patterns of gesture use reported for typically developing children and late talkers validate early interventionists' incorporation of gesture assessment into evaluation procedures. The studies reviewed indicate that gesture is intimately connected with language in the earliest stages of language development. Children begin to communicate intentionally by using deictic gestures before they produce their first words. Representational gestures emerge at about the same time as first words and undergo a similar process of decontextualization, progressing from initial highly context-bound production to use in a variety of situations and for different communicative functions. These milestones are easily identifiable in children referred for communication assessment, and their presence, in combination with other developmental achievement, may be a positive prognostic indicator.

Assessment

Because gesture and speech seem to function as a single communicative system in the early stages of vocabulary development, assessing gesture use can help to determine whether language delay is related to a symbolic deficit or is more likely to be the result of other peripheral factors. Speech-language pathologists should look for gestures that carry out the communicative functions and refer to the same basic set of meanings as typical first words. If the child is using symbolic gestures where typically developing children use words, then the language delay is not likely to be due to problems with symbolic representation, and a different course of intervention would be appropriate.

For children who have acquired a substantial number of words but are not yet combining them, information from typically developing children may help to determine whether and how to proceed. Before the transition to two-word speech, typically developing children appear to circumvent limitations on the production of two-word utterances by making use of gesture–word combinations. Such combinations permit the production of two-element utterances that convey the same amount of information as a two-word combination but place less demand on limited symbolic and articulatory skills. The presence of gesture–word combinations may support a decision to focus on two-word utterances in language intervention; their absence suggests that a focus on teaching two-unit communicative acts with simpler gesture–word forms may be more appropriate.

Intervention

It is clear that gestures can be powerful communicative tools for children experiencing temporary obstacles to the acquisition of verbal language. Although it would be logical to extend this finding into clinical intervention—except for some work with populations with severe cognitive impairments—this is rarely done. Parents, and even some clinicians, often do not recognize that children's gestural abilities are closely and supportively linked to the development of verbal language. Some even explicitly discourage use of gesture, arguing that it is in competition with expressive language and, as a result, will inhibit language (e.g., Whitehurst et al., 1991). We believe that this notion is mistaken. Encouraging gesture use does not seem to impair later language development. On the contrary, the work of Acredolo and Goodwyn (1989, 1993, 1995; Goodwyn & Acredolo, 1993) suggests that explicitly teaching children a small repertoire of communicative gestures accompanied by the appropriate verbal referent and encouraging their use enhances later language development.

In light of these findings, we believe that gesture training may be highly effective in intervention, particularly for children who already appear to be compensating for lack of oral language through use of gestures. If clinicians temporarily set aside communicative emphasis on speech and related demands imposed by verbal communication, such children may be able to practice and refine newly acquired cognitive and communicative skills, become more effective and skilled communicators, and ultimately apply these abilities within the domain of vocal production. However, demands for speech before children are ready or capable of using their oral mechanism may set up a situation in which children experience more failure and, as a result, lose motivation. Take, for example, a child who produces a number of homophones but who understands the names for the different objects when spoken by someone else. This child may say "ba" for ball, bottle, banana, book, and so forth. Parents and clinicians have a great deal of difficulty understanding such a child unless the context is clear. However, if the child is taught a gesture for each object, he or she can use "ba" plus the appropriate gesture to disambiguate the communicative situation. This approach may have a number of benefits, not the least of which is reducing the frustration of both parent and child. It also creates a situation in which the parent can consistently provide an accurate model for the child (e.g., "Yes, that's the ball!") each time the child communicates, rather than guessing what the child intends to say and often providing an incorrect label.

DIRECTIONS FOR FUTURE RESEARCH

Although the evidence for a strong relationship between language and gesture in typically developing children is strong, studies focused on children with delayed language are few and have small numbers of subjects. One of the most important needs is to replicate and extend these studies by using larger numbers of participants. An important question is whether gesture production can differentiate between subgroups of children with language impairment resulting from different etiologies. Future studies also need to explore differences in the use of symbolic and nonsymbolic communicative gestures by toddlers with language delays and to examine the function of gesture–word combinations in the transition to multiword speech.

Finally, whether gesture training is an effective means of helping children with language delays learn language or whether it interferes with language learning is an empirical question of great significance. Acredolo and Goodwyn's work with typically developing toddlers (Acredolo & Goodwyn, 1989, 1993, 1995; Goodwyn & Acredolo, 1993) suggests that gesture training should have a positive outcome. However, experimental evidence is necessary to demonstrate whether the same approach will work with children who have delayed language.

CONCLUSION

We believe that the field of gesture research holds great promise for both researchers and clinicians. Because early gesture production seems to provide children with a means of producing progressively more complex communicative forms while reducing the demand on developing productive and cognitive skills, young children's gestural abilities may reveal more about their current status in the process of language learning than does their speech. Children's early gestures may thus provide clinicians and researchers with a unique window into processes underlying communicative development and the acquisition of language (McNeill, 1992) and may serve as valuable tools for assessment and intervention.

REFERENCES

Acredolo, L.P., & Goodwyn, S.W. (1985). Symbolic gesturing in language development: A case study. *Human Development, 28,* 40–49.

Acredolo, L.P., & Goodwyn, S.W. (1988). Symbolic gesturing in normal infants. *Child Development, 59,* 450–466.

Acredolo, L.P., & Goodwyn, S.W. (1989, April). *Symbolic gesturing in normal infants: A training study.* Paper presented at the biennial meetings of the Society for Research in Child Development, Kansas City, MO.

Acredolo, L.P., & Goodwyn, S.W. (1990). Sign language in babies: The significance of symbolic gesturing for understanding language development. In R. Vasta (Ed.), *Annals of child development* (pp. 1–42). London: Jessica Kingsley Publishers, Ltd.

Acredolo, L.P., & Goodwyn, S.W. (1993, April). *Symbolic gestures and vocal development: Patterns of interaction.* Paper presented at the biennial meetings of the Society for Research in Child Development, New Orleans, LA.

Acredolo, L.P., & Goodwyn, S.W. (1995). *Symbolic gestures versus words in early vocabulary acquisition.* Manuscript under review.

Allen, R., & Shatz, M. (1983). "What says meow?" The role of context and linguistic experience in very young children's responses to *what*-questions. *Journal of Child Language, 10,* 14–23.

Bates, E. (1976). *Language and context.* New York: Academic Press.

Bates, E., Benigni, L., Bretherton, I., Camaioni, L., & Volterra, V. (1979). *The emergence of symbols: Cognition and communication in infancy.* New York: Academic Press.

Bates, E., Bretherton, I., Shore, C., & McNew, S. (1983). Names, gestures, and objects: The role of context in the emergence of symbols. In K.E. Nelson (Ed.), *Children's language* (Vol. IV, pp. 59–123). Hillsdale, NJ: Lawrence Erlbaum Associates.

Bates, E., Camaioni, L., & Volterra, V. (1975). The acquisition of performatives prior to speech. *Merrill-Palmer Quarterly, 21,* 205–226.

Bates, E., O'Connell, B., & Shore, C. (1987). Language and communication in infancy. In J. Osofsky (Ed.), *Handbook of infant development* (pp. 149–203). New York: John Wiley & Sons.

Bates, E., Thal, D., Fenson, L., Whitesell, K., & Oakes, L. (1989). Integrating language and gesture in infancy. *Developmental Psychology, 25,* 1004–1019.

Bruner, J. (1977). Early social interaction and language acquisition. In H.R. Schaffer (Ed.), *Studies in mother–infant interaction* (pp. 271–289). New York: Academic Press.

Butcher, C.M., & Goldin-Meadow, S. (in press). Gesture and the transition from one- to two-word speech: When hand and mouth come together. In A. Kendon, D. McNeill, & S. Wilcox (Eds.), *Gesture: An emerging field.* New York: Cambridge University Press.

Butterworth, G., & Grover, L. (1990). Joint visual attention, manual pointing, and preverbal communication in human infancy. In M. Jeannerod (Ed.), *Attention and performance XIII* (pp. 605–624). Hillsdale, NJ: Lawrence Erlbaum Associates.

Capirci, O., Iverson, J., Pizzuto, E., & Volterra, V. (1996). Communicative gestures and the transition to two-word speech. *Journal of Child Language, 23,* 645–673.

Casadio, P., & Caselli, M.C. (1989). Il primo vocabolario del bambino [The child's first vocabulary]. *Età Evolutiva, 36,* 32–42.

Caselli, M.C. (1990). Communicative gestures and first words. In V. Volterra & C.J. Erting (Eds.), *From gesture to language in hearing and deaf children* (pp. 56–67). New York: Springer-Verlag.

Caselli, M.C., & Volterra, V. (1990). From communication to language in hearing and deaf children. In V. Volterra & C.J. Erting (Eds.), *From gesture to language in hearing and deaf children* (pp. 263–277). New York: Springer-Verlag.

Collis, G.M., & Schaffer, H.R. (1975). Synchronization of visual attention in mother–infant pairs. *Journal of Child Psychology and Psychiatry, 16,* 315–320.

de Laguna, G.A. (1927). *Speech: Its function and development.* New Haven, CT: Yale University Press.

Fenson, L., Dale, P., Reznick, J.S., Thal, D., Bates, E., Hartung, J., Pethick, S., & Reilly, J. (1993). *The MacArthur Communicative Development Inventories: User's guide and technical manual.* San Diego, CA: Singular Publishing Group.

Fogel, A., & Hannan, T.E. (1985). Manual actions of nine to fifteen week-old human infants during face-to-face interactions with their mothers. *Child Development, 56,* 1271–1279.

Goldin-Meadow, S., & Morford, M. (1985). Gesture in early child language: Studies of hearing and deaf children. *Merrill-Palmer Quarterly, 31,* 145–176.

Goldin-Meadow, S., & Morford, M. (1990). Gesture in early child language. In V. Volterra & C.J. Erting (Eds.), *From gesture to language in hearing and deaf children* (pp. 249–262). New York: Springer-Verlag.

Goodwyn, S.W., & Acredolo, L.P. (1993). Symbolic gesture versus word: Is there a modality advantage for the onset of symbol use? *Child Development, 64,* 688–701.

Greenfield, P.M., & Smith, J.H. (1976). *The structure of communication in early language development.* New York: Academic Press.

Guillaume, P. (1927). Les débuts de la phrase dans le langage de l'enfant [The emergence of the sentence in the child's language]. *Journal de Psychologie, 24,* 1–25.

Iverson, J.M., Capirci, O., & Caselli, M.C. (1994). From communication to language in two modalities. *Cognitive Development, 9,* 23–43.

Iverson, J.M., Volterra, V., Pizzuto, E., & Capirci, O. (1994, June). *Gesture-speech combinations as predictive of the emergence of two-word speech.* Poster presented at the Ninth International Conference on Infant Studies, Paris, France.

Johnson, J.S., Lewis, L.B., & Hogan, J.C. (1995, April). *A production limitation in the syllable length of one child's early vocabulary: A longitudinal case study.* Poster presented at the biennial meetings of the Society for Research in Child Development, Indianapolis, IN.

Leung, E., & Rheingold, H. (1981). Development of pointing as a social gesture. *Developmental Psychology, 17,* 215–220.

Lock, A., Young, A., Service, V., & Chandler, P. (1990). Some observations on the origin of the pointing gesture. In V. Volterra & C.J. Erting (Eds.), *From gesture to language in hearing and deaf children* (pp. 42–55). New York: Springer-Verlag.

Macnamara, J. (1977). From sign to language. In J. Macnamara (Ed.), *Language learning and thought* (pp. 11–35). New York: Academic Press.

Masur, E.F. (1990). Gestural development, dual-directional signaling, and the transition to words. In V. Volterra & C.J. Erting (Eds.), *From gesture to language in hearing and deaf children* (pp. 18–30). New York: Springer-Verlag.

McNeill, D. (1992). *Hand and mind: What gesture reveals about thought.* Chicago: University of Chicago Press.

Moore, C., & Corkum, V. (1994). Social understanding at the end of the first year of life. *Developmental Review, 14,* 349–372.

Morford, M., & Goldin-Meadow, S. (1992). Comprehension and production of gesture in combination with speech in one-word speakers. *Journal of Child Language, 19,* 559–580.

Murphy, C.M., & Messer, D.J. (1977). Mothers, infants, and pointing: A study of a gesture. In H.R. Schaffer (Ed.), *Studies in mother–infant interaction* (pp. 325–354). New York: Academic Press.

Nelson, K. (1973). Structure and strategy in learning to talk. *Monographs of the Society for Research in Child Development, 38,* Whole No. 149.

Nokony, A. (1977). Word and gesture usage by an Indian child. In A. Lock (Ed.), *Action, symbol, and gesture* (pp. 291–308). New York: Academic Press.

Perez, B. (1878). *Les trois premières anneés de l'enfant* [The child's first three years]. Paris: Alcan.

Petitto, L.A. (1988). "Language" in the prelinguistic child. In F. Kessel (Ed.), *The development of language and language research: Essays in honor of Roger Brown* (pp. 187–221). Hillsdale, NJ: Lawrence Erlbaum Associates.

Petitto, L.A. (1992). Modularity and constraints in early lexical acquisition: Evidence from children's early language and gesture. In M.R. Gunnar & M. Maratsos (Eds.), *Modularity and constraints in language and cognition: The Minnesota Symposia on Child Psychology* (Vol. 25, pp. 25–58). Hillsdale, NJ: Lawrence Erlbaum Associates.

Piaget, J. (1951). *Play, dreams, and imitation in childhood.* New York: Norton.

Rescorla, L. (1980). Overextension in early language development. *Journal of Child Language, 7,* 321–335.

Scaife, M., & Bruner, J. (1975). The capacity for joint visual attention in the human infant. *Nature, 253,* 265–266.

Stern, W., & Stern, C. (1928). *Die kindersprache* [Children's speech]. Leipzig, Germany: Barth.

Thal, D., & Bates, E. (1988). Language and gesture in late talkers. *Journal of Speech and Hearing Research, 31,* 115–123.

Thal, D., & Tobias, S. (1992). Communicative gestures in children with delayed onset of oral expressive vocabulary. *Journal of Speech and Hearing Research, 35,* 1281–1289.

Thal, D., & Tobias, S. (1994). Relationships between language and gesture in normally-developing and late-talking toddlers. *Journal of Speech and Hearing Research, 37,* 157–170.

Thal, D., Tobias, S., & Morrison, D. (1991). Language and gesture in late talkers: A one year follow-up. *Journal of Speech and Hearing Research, 34,* 604–612.

Tomasello, M. (1995). Joint attention as social cognition. In C. Moore & P. Dunham (Eds.), *Joint attention: Its origins and role in development* (pp. 103–130). Hillsdale, NJ: Lawrence Erlbaum Associates.

Volterra, V., Bates, E., Benigni, L., Bretherton, I., & Camaioni, L. (1979). First words in language and action: A qualitative look. In E. Bates, L. Benigni, I. Bretherton, L. Camaioni, & V. Volterra (Eds.), *The emergence of symbols: Cognition and communication in infancy* (pp. 141–222). New York: Academic Press.

Volterra, V., & Iverson, J.M. (1995). When do modality factors affect the course of language acquisition? In K. Emmorey & J. Reilly (Eds.), *Gesture, sign, and space* (pp. 371–390). Hillsdale, NJ: Lawrence Erlbaum Associates.

Werner, H., & Kaplan, B. (1963). *Symbol formation.* New York: John Wiley & Sons.

Whitehurst, G., Fishel, J., Lonigan, C., Valdez-Menchaca, M., Arnold, D., & Smith, M. (1991). Treatment of early expressive language delay: If, when, and how. *Topics in Language Disorders, 11,* 55–68.

Zinober, B., & Martlew, M. (1985). The development of communicative gestures. In M.D. Barrett (Ed.), *Children's single-word speech* (pp. 183–215). New York: John Wiley & Sons.

5

Role of Babbling and Phonology in Early Linguistic Development

Carol Stoel-Gammon

LEARNING TO TALK IS ONE of the major accomplishments in the first years of life. Infants enter the world with the biological capacity for understanding and producing speech; social interactions create a world in which language becomes the primary means of communication. By the end of the first year, typically developing babies are able to say a few words. By 2 years of age, they are speaking in short sentences and have a vocabulary of about 300 words. Communication begins before words are spoken, however, with cries, gestures, and vocalizations that occur in the prespeech period. Even in the first few months, infant vocal behaviors often are interpreted by caregivers as having meaning, although it is unlikely that the infant has a conscious intention to communicate. Gradually, infants become aware that such behaviors can be used to regulate the behavior of others, and their vocal and gestural behaviors move from being preintentional to intentional. With the appearance of words, babbled vocalizations become verbalizations, and symbolic communication takes on the functions of presymbolic signals.

This chapter focuses on vocal and verbal development in the first 2 years of life, with emphasis on the role of phonology. The chapter begins with a comparison of the form and function of vocalizations in the prespeech period; it is shown that both form and function appear to proceed through a regular sequence of developmental stages, relatively independent of one another. The second half of the chapter focuses on phonological acquisition during the period of meaningful speech, that is, the period during which the child produces adult-based words. Particular attention is paid to the role of babble in early speech development and to the relationship between phonological and lexical acquisition in three populations of children: 1) those who are developing in a typical fashion, 2) those who have delays in the onset of speech and/or the development of a lexicon, and 3) those with a cognitive impairment resulting from Down syndrome. The chap-

Preparation of this chapter was supported in part by Grant No. 1-R01-HD32065 from the National Institute of Child Health and Human Development.

ter concludes with a brief discussion of the clinical implications of research on early phonological development and suggestions for future areas of research.

Although this chapter focuses on the nature and use of vocal and verbal communication in young children, it should be noted that cries and gestures also play important roles as means of communication (see Chapter 4). In the beginning, infants learn to influence the behavior and attitudes of others by signaling in any modality. Cries and gestures often represent the most successful means in the first few months. Before the emergence of words, however, infants learn to produce vocal signals that communicate a broad range of intentions. As more sophisticated and conventional methods of communicating are acquired, reliance on cries and gestures diminishes. The preverbal period during which vocal and gestural behaviors coincide provides a foundation for the acquisition of communicative competence that follows and is seen as a necessary precursor to the subsequent development of the intentional use of language.

INFANT VOCAL DEVELOPMENT:
FROM PREINTENTIONAL TO INTENTIONAL

Although the intentions underlying infant communication are not always transparent, parents attribute intention to their infants' gestures and vocalizations almost from birth. To be successful, preintentional infant communication depends on two complementary types of behavior: the ability of the infant to signal intent, coupled with the ability of the parent or caregiver to interpret these signals. Initially, the burden of successful communicative exchanges lies primarily with the adult. Infants vocalize from their first days through cries and vegetative noises (also called reflexive vocalizations [e.g., fussing, coughing, sneezing, burping]); if these "signals" are ignored, no communication occurs. If, however, an adult responds by attending to the infant's physical needs and/or emotional state, a rudimentary form of communication has taken place. Around the second month, infants produce more varied signals as they begin to smile and coo, eliciting smiles and vocalizations from the parent. Thereafter, vocal exchanges, along with gaze and gesture, form an integral part of social interactions (Snow, 1977).

Even though parents consider the vocal behaviors of infants as young as 3 months to be communicative (C.Y. Miller, 1988), it is doubtful that infants of this age consciously intend to communicate. During the first year, there is a gradual shift from nonintentional to intentional use of gesture and sound as infants come to realize that they can influence those around them through their vocal and gestural signals. By 9–10 months of age, gestures and vocalizations are produced in a consistent and persistent manner, allowing infants to achieve their goals. From a Piagetian perspective, it would be said that the infant has become aware of the means–end relation (Bates, 1979). During this period, infant communication begins to take on discrete functions, such as regulating the behavior of others or engaging in social interactions (Coggins & Carpenter, 1981). As communication moves from preintentional to intentional, the form and functions of infant vocal signals become more varied. The developmental stages of form and function are described in the following sections.

The Form of Infant Vocalizations

During the first year, the infant produces a wide variety of sounds. Some are speech-like in that they resemble speech sounds of an adult language; others, such as coughs or burps, are clearly non–speech-like. Among the speech-like vocalizations are forms such as [mama] or [dædæ], which are sometimes interpreted as being attempts at the words "mommy" and "daddy." Such forms are considered to be prelinguistic unless it can be shown that they have the stable sound–meaning relationships of conventional adult-based words. Around 9 months of age, infants begin to demonstrate limited comprehension of words and simple phrases in particular contexts (see Chapter 9); by 12 months of age, the average receptive vocabulary is around 50 words, according to parental reports (Fenson et al., 1993).

Infant vocal productions can be divided into two general categories: 1) *reflexive* vocalizations (e.g., cries, coughs, hiccups), which seem to be automatic responses reflecting the physical state of the infant; and 2) *nonreflexive* vocalizations (e.g., cooing, babbling, playful yelling and screaming), which are productions containing some of the phonetic features found in adult languages (Oller, 1980; Stark, 1980). Nonreflexive vocalizations pass through a sequence of developmental stages, beginning with vowel-like utterances at 2 months of age and progressing through a period of vocal play to productions of sequences of consonant–vowel strings toward the end of the first year. Although the terms *consonant* and *vowel* appear in this discussion of prelinguistic vocalizations, early infant vocalizations are most accurately characterized as consonant- or vowel-like because they do not have all the features associated with mature productions of consonant and vowel sounds. Researchers such as Kent and Bauer (1985) prefer to use the terms *closant* and *vocant* for consonantal and vocalic elements, respectively.

Developmental Stages All infants, regardless of the linguistic community in which they are being raised, pass through the same stages of vocal development. These stages, with the approximate ages for each, are briefly characterized in this section. Although called stages, the periods are not discrete, and vocalizations from previous stages continue to be used in the subsequent ones. The onset of a new stage is marked by the appearance of vocal behaviors not observed (or observed only rarely) in the preceding period; the new behaviors do not necessarily constitute the most frequent vocalization type during that stage.

Stage 1 The first stage, phonation, begins at birth and is characterized by productions that bear little resemblance to speech (Oller, 1980). The vocal behaviors of this stage consist primarily of reflexive (sometimes called vegetative) vocalizations such as crying, fussing, coughing, sneezing, and burping.

Stage 2 At 2–3 months of age, a new type of vocal production appears as infants begin smiling and interacting with adults in their environment. These vocalizations are characterized by nasal resonance and are generally perceived as back vowels (i.e., vowels articulated at the back of the mouth) or as syllables consisting of back consonants (i.e., velars, uvulars) and back vowels. The term used to describe these infant utterances in this stage is cooing or gooing, because it seems as though the infant is saying [ku] or [gu]. Consonant–vowel (CV) syllables produced at this stage are considered primitive because the timing of opening and closure of the consonantal and vocalic elements is far less regular than that which occurs in adult speech (Oller, 1980).

Stage 3 The cooing stage is followed by a period during which infants seem to be intentionally exploring the capabilities of their vocal tract. From 4 to 6 months of age, productions range from repetitions of vowel-like elements to squeals, growls, yells, raspberries (bilabial or labiolingual trills), and friction noises. The predominant type of vocalization can vary from week to week or even from day to day, making it difficult to characterize an infant's productions without an extensive sample. During this stage the infant produces some sequences of CV syllables. As in the previous stage, the timing of the opening and closure of these CV syllables is not yet adult-like.

Stage 4 This stage begins when infants are 6–7 months of age and is characterized by the appearance of canonical syllables, composed of alternating consonants and vowels. The timing of these syllables approximates that of adult speech; consequently, the productions sound very speech-like. A striking characteristic of the productions in the canonical babbling stage is the presence of repeated syllables that may resemble words of the language (e.g., [mamama], [dididi]). Upon hearing a sequence such as [mama] or [dada], parents often report with delight that their 7-month-old has begun to call them by name. At this stage, however, there is no evidence of a sound–meaning correspondence in the infant's productions, and thus [mama] should not be considered a word. During this stage the repertoire of phones (i.e., speech sounds) is relatively limited, with stops, nasals, and glides the most common consonantal sounds, and lax vowels (e.g., [ɛ, æ, ʌ]) the most frequent vocalic types. The place of articulation of the consonantal phones shifts dramatically at about this stage, as the frequency of velars declines sharply, and front consonants, both alveolars and labials, become predominant. Multisyllabic utterances in this period are often categorized as *reduplicated* babbles (i.e., strings of identical syllables like [bababa]) or *variegated* babbles (i.e., syllable strings with varying consonants and vowels like [bagu]). Although both types of utterances occur in the canonical babbling stage, reduplicated babble predominates initially, and variegated babble increases after 9–10 months (Smith, Brown-Sweeney, & Stoel-Gammon, 1989).

Stage 5   This next stage of babbling, jargon babble (also called intonated babble) begins around 12 months of age; it co-occurs with both the canonical babbling stage and the use of early words. It is characterized by strings of sounds and syllables uttered with a variety of stress and intonational patterns. To many adults, it seems as though children are speaking in whole sentences, that is, they are making statements and asking questions, but are using their "own" language rather than the standard language spoken by older children and adults around them.

In spite of the developmental trend toward the use of consonants, more than half of infant babbled utterances are short (monosyllabic) and formed exclusively of vocalic elements, even in later stages. Findings from research on vocal development show that canonical babbles, produced either as single CV syllables or as repetitive strings, account for between 25% and 40% of the total utterances at 9–12 months (Menyuk, Liebergott, & Schultz, 1995; Stoel-Gammon, 1989; Vihman, Macken, Miller, Simmons, & Miller, 1985).

The Sounds of Babble   The speech-like sounds used by infants change dramatically during the first year of life. In the first 6 months, vowel articulations tend to predominate; most consonantal sounds are produced in the back of the mouth, that is, sounds like [k] or [g]. With the onset of the canonical babbling stage, there is a marked shift toward front consonants with frequent occurrences of [m], [b], and [d] in particular. Between 6 and 12 months, the sound repertoire expands considerably, but claims that babies produce all the sounds of all languages of the world (Jakobson, 1968) during this period have not been substantiated. Studies have shown that a relatively small set of consonants accounts for the great majority of consonantal sounds produced. Locke (1993) stated that the consonants [p, b, m, w, t, d, n, j, k, g, h] comprise about 90% of the consonants produced by infants raised in American-English–speaking environments. In terms of articulatory features, these consonants represent particular manner classes, namely the stops [p, b, t, d, k, g], the nasals [m, n], and glides [w, j]. Cross-linguistic research has shown that these same manner classes predominate in the babble of infants raised in all linguistic environments (Locke, 1983).

The Effects of Audition

For many years, it was believed that deaf infants vocalize during the first year in the same way that hearing infants do and that differences become apparent only when hearing babies begin to produce words and their peers with hearing impairments do not. It is now known that this view is not true. Although deaf babies do vocalize in the months after birth, their productions do not conform to the sequence of stages observed for hearing infants. Most notably, babies with a moderate to severe loss of hearing fail to enter the canonical babbling stage when expected (Oller & Eilers, 1988). Moreover, after 8 months, the variety of consonants in their vocalizations decreases with age, in contrast to the increase documented for hearing babies (Stoel-Gammon & Otomo, 1986). In terms of consonantal types, infants with hearing loss tend to produce an unusually high proportion of labial consonants, such as [b] and [m], presumably because of the visual movements associated with the production of these speech sounds (Stoel-Gammon, 1988).

In summary, prelinguistic vocal development follows a regular sequence of stages from birth through the onset of speech. At around 6–7 months of age, typically developing infants begin to produce utterances that have phonological characteristics similar to those found in word productions: CV syllables with adult-like timing. Consonants occurring frequently in these canonical syllables are generally stops, nasals, or glides; most vowels are mid to front in terms of tongue and jaw placement and are lax. Although canonical syllables represent a key stage in vocal development, they do not represent the most frequently occurring type of vocalization. More than half the vocalizations are vowels only, and monosyllabic utterances occur with greater frequency than multisyllabic ones.

The Functions of Infant Vocalizations

As with the form of early vocal productions, the functions of infant vocalizations follow a regular sequence of stages, beginning with the preintentional cries and vegetative noises that are present at birth and continuing to the stage of intentional production of adult-based words. This section presents a description of the vocalizations associated with the different functions of vocal communication.

Stage 1 The first functional stage is referred to as a period of reflexive sound making (Stark, Bernstein, & Demorest, 1993). The vocal behaviors of this stage (the phonation stage in the form of infant vocalizations) consist primarily of reflexive vocalizations, including crying, fussing, coughing, sneezing, and burping. Although the infant is not aware of the intentional function at this stage, these productions are interpreted by adults as indications of hunger, pain, or discomfort requiring attention to the infant's physical state. Whereas vegetative noises show little change from infancy through adulthood, cry patterns take on distinctive features with age. D'Odorico (1984) found that "call" cries of infants 4–5 months old had different duration and nonsegmental patterns than their "discomfort" cries. Some nonreflexive sounds usually perceived as vowels or syllabic consonants also occur during this stage. In the Stark et al. (1993) study, reflexive vocal behaviors accounted for 93% of the vocalizations at 2 weeks, dropping to 54% at 8 weeks.

Stage 2 The next functional stage, termed reactive sound making (Stark et al., 1993), appears at 2–3 months of age; reactive vocalizations occur frequently until approximately 10 months of age, accounting on average for more than 40% of the vocal behaviors during this 8-month period. Reactive sound making typically occurs in face-to-face interactions between the infant and caregiver, and gaze may be as important as sound. Of particular importance during this period is the development of turn taking, that is, vocal exchanges that adhere to the temporal characteristics of mature conversational interactions. During these proto-conversations, participants alternate between speaking and listening; adults pause after producing an utterance, thereby providing an opportunity for the infant to respond. Initially, caregivers accept almost any vocal behavior, including vegetative noises, as constituting an infant's turn in the conversation. Later, the adults become more selective, responding to speech-like babbles but not to burps or coughs (Snow, 1977).

Bloom (1988) and Bloom, Russell, and Wassenberg (1987) reported that the timing and phonetic form of adult productions affect the frequency and quality of reactive sound making. Three-month-old infants produced a greater proportion of syllabic speech-like utterances in two conditions: 1) when adult utterances were temporally contingent (i.e., maintaining a turn-taking pattern), and 2) when adult vocalizations were verbal rather than nonverbal and gestural. Syllabic utterances were described as sounding as though "the baby was really talking." They were characterized by greater oral resonance, more varied pitch contour, articulations formed in the front of the mouth, and more "relaxed" affect. Vocalic utterances, in contrast, were those that were classified as non–speech-like. They were characterized by greater nasal resonance, articulated more in the back of the mouth, had more uniform pitch contours, and seemed "more effortful" than syllabic utterances. Overall, infants produced a higher proportion of vocalic utterances, but the ratio of syllabic to vocalic vocalizations increased when infants were engaged in turn-taking exchanges with an adult partner.

Stage 3 The stage of reactive sound making is followed by a stage referred to as activity sound making, which begins at about 4–5 months of age. The key feature of activity sound-making vocalizations is that they are produced while the infant is engaged in behaviors directed toward the environment and *do not* involve interaction with an adult, although an adult may be present. In the Stark et al. (1993) study, this type of vocal activity constituted about 25% of all vocalizations from 6 to 12 months of age. Using a slightly different classification scheme, Delack (1976) compared the quantity of vocalizations produced by infants in various settings: alone, with their mother, and with a stranger. He found that, from 18 to 53 weeks of age, more than half of the vocalizations occurred when the infant was alone; at 38 weeks of age, about 70% of the vocalizations were produced in this context. Such vocalizations would presumably conform to Stark et al.'s category of activity sound making.

Stage 4 The last stage in the Stark et al.'s (1993) model is communicative sound making, which begins around 9 months of age and includes words as well as babbled utterances. Using Halliday's (1973) classifications, Stark et al. (1993) noted that this stage is characterized by four communicative intentions frequently expressed by young children: 1) instrumental/regulatory, 2) personal, 3) interactional, and 4) heuristic/imaginative. Communicative sound-making behaviors accounted for 20% of all vocalizations at 40 weeks of age and 31% at 55 weeks of age; these behaviors represented the predominant type of vocal communication from 71 to 88 weeks of age (65% at 71 weeks; 82% at 88 weeks).

As noted previously, infant communication involves both gesture and sound. Wetherby, Cain, Yonclas, and Walker (1988) reported that among prelinguistic infants ages 11–14 months, gestures accompanied by vocalization accounted for 40% of the communicative acts observed in a 30-minute recorded sample; gestures alone accounted for 35% of the acts, and vocalizations alone accounted for 24%. Similar findings were reported by Carpenter, Mastergeorge, and Coggins (1983).

Form and Function of Prelinguistic Vocalizations

Both the form and function of infant vocalizations follow a regular sequence of stages, beginning with relatively primitive utterance types and evolving toward speech. Comparison of the stages in the two domains reveals similarities in terms of onset. For example, the cooing stage begins at about the same time as the reactive sound-making stage, and the onset of the canonical babbling stage occurs at about the same time as the emergence of activity sound making. The presence of these parallels does not necessarily mean that there is a one-to-one link between form and function. A single communicative function can be signaled by a variety of types of vocalizations (and gestures), and the same vocalization type can serve various communicative functions (Stark et al., 1993). Thus, Vihman and Miller (1988) reported finding no differences in the phonological characteristics of babbles used in interactional and noninteractional contexts. In both cases, vocalizations lacking consonants occurred most frequently. They did find a difference between the phonetic form of interactional babbles and of words, which were assumed to be interactional: Roughly 50% of the babbles had no consonantal elements whereas only 25% of words lacked consonants. Vihman and Miller concluded that it is not the function of an utterance that determines its phonological form but whether the utterance is an attempt at a word of the ambient language.

As children make the transition from prespeech to speech, they continue to use their vocal output for the same communicative functions as in the prespeech period. The change comes not in the nature of their communicative intents but in the transition from vocal to verbal behaviors. Phonologically, the babble of infancy, particularly the production of canonical syllables, serves as the basis for the formation of early words.

FROM PRESYMBOLIC TO SYMBOLIC COMMUNICATION

Perhaps the most heralded linguistic milestone for a child is the appearance of words. When the infant produces his or her first "bye-bye," "daddy," or "all-gone," he or she is technically no longer an infant (i.e., no longer without speech). Although parents view this step as a quantal leap, it in fact represents the marriage of aspects of communication that were already present. To be considered a word, a vocal production must have both sound and meaning; specifically, a sequence of speech sounds must be linked to a specific meaning. As shown previously, infant communication is linked to intention from around age 9 months; both gesture and vocal output can be linked to particular functions, such as requesting, showing, protesting, and commenting. Sound also is present in the speech-like productions of canonical syllables and jargon babble. What distinguishes words from babble is the use of speech sounds as they are used in the target language. To become a word of English, prelinguistic forms like [mama] and [ba] must be linked to conventional words like "mommy" and "ball," respectively. As this linking is accomplished, children begin to acquire a core vocabulary of adult-based words. There are cases in which children invent their own words, producing vocalizations with consistent sound–meaning relationships but with no identifiable adult models. These proto-words (also referred to as phonetically consistent forms or vocables) are generally understood only by the immediate family and are gradually replaced by conventional forms.

Babble as the Basis for Speech

The first words typically appear during the period of canonical babble, and for a period of 7–10 months, babble and speech coexist. When children are around 18 months of age, the proportion of babbled utterances declines markedly as words and short phrases begin to predominate. The relationship of babbling to speech has been debated at length. Roman Jakobson, the linguist who greatly influenced the study of child phonology, argued strongly that infants' vocalizations before the first words were not related to subsequent phonological development. According to his view, babbling is a purely biologically based phenomenon characterized by "an astonishing quantity and diversity of sound productions…consonants of any play of articulation, palatalized and rounded consonants, sibilants, affricates, clicks, complex vowels, diphthongs…." (Jakobson, 1968, p. 21). With the onset of speech, Jakobson claimed that the child suddenly loses the ability to produce a diverse set of speech sounds and, in effect, begins all over with a limited repertoire of consonants and vowels in first words. Although many of Jakobson's predictions regarding phonological acquisition have subsequently been supported, his views on the relationship between babbling and speech have not.

Infants may indeed produce a wide array of sound types during the prelinguistic period, but only a subset of these appears regularly. The consonant classes that occur most frequently in late babbling, namely, the manner classes of stops, nasals, and glides, are the same classes that predominate in early word productions. The manner classes that are infrequent in babble (liquids, fricatives, and affricates) are precisely those that appear later in the acquisition of speech (Stoel-Gammon, 1985). Moreover, the CV syllable structure, characteristic of the canonical babbling period, is also the most frequent syllabic type in early

word productions. Thus, babbling and early speech share the same basic phonetic properties in terms of sound types and syllable shapes. Developmentally,
the sounds of babble serve as the building blocks for the subsequent production
of words.

Support for the notion of continuity from babble to speech comes from longitudinal investigations showing that individual production patterns in place and
manner of articulation, syllable shape, and vocalization length in the prelinguistic period often are "carried forward" to a child's first words (Stoel-Gammon &
Cooper, 1984; Vihman, Ferguson, & Elbert, 1987; Vihman et al., 1985). Additional evidence comes from an experimental study of the acquisition of nonsense
words. Messick (1984) examined children's phonetic inventories in babbling,
and then taught them nonsense words that were either phonetically similar or
dissimilar to their own babbled forms. After 10 sessions of exposure to the two
types of words, the children produced a significantly greater number of phonetically similar words, although they showed no differences in their ability to
understand the two types of nonsense forms.

In addition to the studies showing continuity in the phonetic patterns of
babble and speech, there is a growing body of evidence linking prelinguistic
vocal development with general speech and language skills throughout early
childhood. Longitudinal studies (summarized in Stoel-Gammon, 1992) have
shown correlations among the age of onset of canonical babble and the age of
onset of speech; the amount of vocalization at age 3 months and vocabulary size
at age 27 months; the number of CV syllables at age 12 months and age at use of
first words; use of consonants at age 12 months and phonological skills at age 3
years; and diversity of syllable and sound types at 6–14 months of age and performance on speech and language tests at 5 years of age. In each case, more in
the prelinguistic period (i.e., more vocalizations at age 3 months; more CV syllables at age 12 months) was linked to better performance on speech and language
measures. These correlations provide further support for the view that babbling
serves as a foundation for subsequent acquisition of speech and language.
Infants who produce a greater number of prelinguistic vocalizations, particularly
a greater number of canonical utterances with a variety of consonants and vowels, have amassed a greater arsenal of building blocks that can be recruited for
the production of words.

The Role of Practice and Feedback

The link between babble and speech can be attributed, at least in part, to practice
and feedback in the prelinguistic period. Speech has a skill component and, as
with any skilled activity, practice increases the control and precision with which a
movement is performed. Thus, the more often a baby produces the movements
that shape the vocal tract to produce particular sounds and sound sequences, the
more automatic those movements become and ultimately the easier it is to exe-
cute them in producing words. Vihman (1992) identified a set of frequently

occurring CV syllables ("practiced" syllables) for each subject and reported that for most children the syllables used in early words were "primarily drawn from the repertoire of practiced syllables" (p. 406). Given this finding, it would seem that babies who have a large stock of practiced CV syllables in babbling will have an advantage in early word acquisition because they will have a larger repertoire of forms to which meaning can be attached. Vihman noted that subjects who evidenced slower vocabulary acquisition were those who failed to use their practiced syllables in speech production. In a similar vein, Stoel-Gammon (1989) reported that one of the two late talkers studied produced many CV syllables in his babbled utterances but did not use these forms in his attempts at real words.

Practice in the production of speech-like vocalizations is important for another domain: feedback. Infants are exposed to two types of vocal input, the speech of others and their own productions. Both are crucial for the acquisition of adult language, and studies of prelinguistic vocalizations of deaf babies demonstrate that the effects of a lack of auditory input can be detected at 7–8 months of age. In addition to improving the skill component of speech production, practice is important because it provides infants the opportunity to hear their own vocalizations.

The nature of the feedback loop was described by Fry (1966) in the following way: "As sound producing movements are repeated and repeated, a strong link is forged between tactual and kinesthetic impressions and auditory sensations that the child receives from his own utterances" (p. 189). Awareness of the links between one's own oral-motor movements and the acoustic signal that results is a prerequisite to auditory-vocal matching that underlies word production. It seems logical that the more a baby babbles, the greater the opportunity to establish the feedback loops necessary for producing and monitoring his or her own speech. Moreover, the feedback loop may make infants pay attention to words in the adult language that resemble their own babbled forms. Thus, for example, a baby who frequently produces [ba] or [baba] might be likely to acquire the word "ball" or "bottle" because these words are similar to forms for which auditory and kinesthetic feedback patterns have been established.

Practice and feedback are not independent aspects of early vocal development; practice involves the repeated production of sounds, and feedback involves hearing and monitoring these practiced productions. It is possible to have practice without auditory feedback, but feedback cannot occur in the absence of practice. Babies with hearing impairments, for example, have a typically developing vocal apparatus that would allow them to practice the movements associated with the production of CV syllables. They would have tactile and kinesthetic feedback from oral movements, but their hearing loss prevents them from forming an auditory feedback loop like that of hearing babies. Although they have the capability of producing canonical syllables at the same developmental stage as other babies, babies with hearing impairments are significantly delayed in the onset of the canonical babbling stage and in the frequency and diversity of supraglottal consonants in their vocalizations, as noted previously. Presumably, this failure is linked to the lack of auditory input from others and from their own output.

At the same time, it appears that lack of practice also affects the timetable of development. Locke and Pearson (1990) examined the linguistic development of a young, cognitively typical girl who was tracheostomized and "generally aphonic" from 5 to 20 months. During this period, she vocalized infrequently, producing utterances that usually consisted of "a single vocalic sound of approximately syllable length" (p. 7). Thus, although exposed to speech from the adults around her, she was unable to produce canonical babbles and had little opportunity to form auditory or tactile feedback loops based on her own vocalizations. Following decannulation (i.e., removal of the tube that prevented normal respiration) just before 21 months of age, the girl evidenced a marked increase in the frequency of vocal output. Of the 909 utterances produced in the weeks following decannulation, however, only 6 met the criteria for canonical syllables. In addition to the lack of well-formed syllables, the girl's speech samples were characterized by a limited repertoire of consonantal types. The authors noted that her speech was similar to that of deaf infants studied by Oller and Eilers (1988) and Stoel-Gammon and Otomo (1986). Thus, the findings of this investigation, though limited to a case study of a single child, suggest that the ability to practice and to hear one's own vocalizations plays a critical role in typical vocal development.

Acquiring a Vocabulary

The first word period is characterized by the appearance of adult-based words and the growth of productive vocabulary to 50 words or more. There is considerable variation in both the age of onset of speech and rate of lexical acquisition. The MacArthur Communication Development Inventories, referred to hereafter as the CDI, present data from 86 infants at 12–13 months of age, showing a range of 0–67 words across their subjects at this age period (Fenson et al., 1993). The data are based on parent report, with parents using a checklist to indicate which words their children understand and which words they can produce. Within this format, it is not possible to determine the situational contexts for comprehension and production of words; as noted in Chapter 9, production and comprehension often are limited to particular settings in the early stages and then are decontextualized with age. At age 18–19 months, the productive vocabularies of 80 infants on the CDI ranged from 13 to 471 words with a mean of about 100. The wide ranges in these data show the extent of variability in early lexical acquisition.

In terms of phonology, the first word period is characterized by productions of simple syllabic structure, typically CV, CVC, or CVCV. The repertoire of speech sounds is limited, consisting primarily of stops, nasals, and glides. The child's words seem to be learned and produced as whole units rather than as sequences of segments; thus, the first contrasts of the child's system are in terms of words. Only later does the child show convincing evidence of contrasts in terms of syllables or phonemic oppositions. Because of this whole-word approach to word production and the concomitant lack of one-to-one correspondence between the adult target and the child's form, the first words often are understood only by immediate family members who are familiar with the child's productive vocabulary. The end of the first word stage, at about 18 months of age, is signaled by a rapid increase in vocabulary size, an expansion of phonetic repertoire, and the onset of two-word utterances.

By age 24 months, the typically developing child has acquired a productive vocabulary of 300–350 words and can produce multiword sentences. Although children's phonological systems are far from complete, the basic syllable shapes and sound classes are present; about 50% of what they say can be understood by a stranger (Coplan & Gleason, 1988). The intelligibility level of any speaker is influenced by a variety of factors, and the relationship between intelligibility and speech production is not straightforward (Kent, 1993); as a consequence, estimates of intelligibility may vary widely. For young children, the most important factor for intelligibility is the interaction between accuracy of pronunciation and general language ability. If a 2-year-old's productions are relatively accurate in terms of phonology and length of utterance is short, the child will be producing a high proportion of one-word utterances that are easy to understand. In this case, intelligibility would be high even though language level might be low. In contrast, if a child's speech is characterized by long, syntactically complex utterances, but a limited inventory of speech sounds and syllable types, intelligibility is likely to be low.

In terms of segments and sound classes, the typical 2-year-old's phonetic inventory contains labial, alveolar, and velar stop consonants, both voiced and voiceless; labial and alveolar nasals; glides [w], [j], and [h]; and some fricatives, usually [f] and/or [s] (Paynter & Petty, 1974; Prather, Hedrick, & Kern, 1975; Stoel-Gammon, 1985, 1987). In terms of syllable and word shapes, the child's repertoire has expanded to include open and closed syllables that can combine to form disyllabic words. In addition, the average 2-year-old can produce some words with consonant clusters in initial and final positions (Stoel-Gammon, 1987). Compared with consonants, the vowel repertoire at age 2 years is relatively complete, and accuracy levels average about 75%. Most errors occur on the lax vowels /ɪ, ɛ, æ/ and the r-colored vowels (Hare, 1983; Stoel-Gammon & Herrington, 1990).

The Phonology–Lexicon Interface

For many years it was assumed that the particular words that appeared in children's productive vocabularies were the result of semantic and pragmatic pressures, that is, that children learned to say words that would be the most useful in communicating their needs and in talking about actions and objects that were important to them. In a longitudinal study of three children's first 50 words, however, Ferguson and Farwell (1975) noted patterns of lexical acquisition that were apparently related primarily to the phonological composition of the target words rather than to the semantic or pragmatic features. For example, one child produced an unusually high number of words with the sibilant consonants [s, z, ʃ, tʃ, dʒ], such as "cereal, shoes, cheese, juice, see, eyes, ice, sit"; in contrast, the other two children had relatively few words with sibilants. A second child acquired a large number of words beginning with the voiced bilabial stop /b/ but few with its voiceless cognate /p/. Noting the high degree of accuracy of pronunciation across the subjects, Ferguson and Farwell argued that children attempt to say words, sounds, and syllable structures that they can accurately produce, while avoiding words that are difficult for them phonologically. They hypothesized that individual patterns of lexical selection and avoidance reflect the production capabilities of the child. The phonologically based selection and avoidance patterns observed by Ferguson and Farwell were subsequently documented by other researchers (see, e.g., Menn, 1976; Stoel-Gammon & Cooper, 1984; Vihman, 1981).

Although the notion that children actively select or reject words on the basis of the words' phonological features was viewed as intriguing, some researchers were not fully convinced, noting that the findings of apparent phonologically based lexical selection could be attributed to other factors. An alternative explanation is that the child who acquires a large number of words with sibilant consonants is simply exposed to more words of this type, thus implicating input frequency as the critical feature. The only way to determine whether input frequency or phonological composition is the crucial variable is to trace lexical acquisition when both variables are strictly controlled. Using an experimental paradigm involving the teaching of nonsense words, Schwartz and Leonard (1982) did just that. They analyzed spontaneous productions to determine the inventory of consonants and syllable structures used by each child and then created individualized sets of nonsense words, half of which were characterized by consonants and syllable structures that were "in" a child's repertoire (IN words), and half of which contained consonants "outside" the child's productive repertoire (OUT words). The words in each set then were presented to the child an equal number of times in a play-like format. Analysis of production and comprehension patterns yielded two consistent findings: 1) Children produced more IN words than OUT words, and 2) there were no differences in the comprehension of IN words and OUT words. Thus, Schwartz and Leonard confirmed a phonological basis in early lexical acquisition.

As the productive vocabulary grows toward 100 words, the influences exerted by lexical selection patterns decline, and children attempt to produce words with a wider range of target phonemes and syllable structures. At this stage, a different type of relationship between phonological and lexical systems becomes apparent. Children with large lexicons tend to have large inventories of speech sounds and syllable structures; conversely, children with smaller vocabularies have limited phonetic inventories. In her longitudinal study of 34 children, Stoel-Gammon (1991b) reported a strong statistical correlation between the size of children's initial and final consonantal inventories and the size of their productive lexicon at 24 months of age. In a companion study, Stoel-Gammon and Dale (1988) compared the phonological systems of typically developing children with those of "precocious" talkers who had extraordinarily large lexicons for 18 months of age (400–600 words compared with an average lexicon of 50–60 words). At age 20 months, the phonetic inventories of subjects in the precocious group were much larger than those of the typically developing group at 21 or even 24 months of age. Among the precocious children, affricates, fricatives, and liquids were common, in addition to the stops, nasals, and glides that would be expected.

Children with Delayed Language: The Relationship of Babble to Speech

There are only a few studies that have examined the relationship of babble and speech among children who are late to acquire words. Reporting the findings of a longitudinal study of 34 children followed from age 9 months to 24 months, Stoel-Gammon (1989) noted that one child's prespeech vocalizations from age 9 to 21 months differed from those of her peers in that she produced almost no utterances with CV syllables. The child was also the slowest of the group to enter the stage of meaningful speech (defined as the production of 10 identifiable words in a 60-minute speech sample). This finding supports the view of a strong link between phonological patterns of babble and the onset of speech.

In a study focusing exclusively on children with specific expressive language delay, Whitehurst, Smith, Fischel, Arnold, and Lonigan (1991) analyzed speech samples from 37 children at two points in time. The first session occurred when children were, on average, age 28 months; the second session took place 5 months later. Because the purpose of the study was to determine which variables from the first session were the best predictors of expressive language abilities at the second session, a range of variables was analyzed, including rate of word use, amount of vowel babble versus consonantal babble, amount of interactive versus noninteractive babble (i.e., babble with and without communicative intent), and vowel babble length in syllables. At age 28 months, the children's speech samples displayed characteristics usually associated with younger typically developing children. Uninterpretable utterances (either babbles or unintelligible productions) occurred more than twice as often as utterances with identifiable words, and 63% of the uninterpretable utterances were categorized as vowel babble. Two variables from the samples at age 28 months were strongly related to expressive language scores 5 months later: a positive correlation with rate of word use and a negative correlation with rate of vowel babble. The authors concluded that for children with language delay, "vowel babble competes with expressive language, consonantal babble facilitates expressive language, and the length and social responsiveness of babble are independent of expressive language" (p. 121).

Phonological and Lexical Development of Late Talkers

Studies of children with delayed onset of speech also provide evidence of a link between phonological and lexical acquisition. In terms of phonology, typically developing 2-year-olds have a phonetic inventory of 9–10 different consonants in word-initial position and 5–6 different consonants in word-final position; all three major classes of place of articulation (i.e., labial, alveolar, velar) are present as well as a variety of manner classes. The typical 2-year-old produces both open and closed syllables and can combine them to form disyllabic words (Stoel-Gammon, 1987). At this age, the average number of words in the productive vocabulary is about 320 (Fenson et al., 1993).

By comparison, 24- to 30-month-old children with smaller vocabularies (often called "late talkers") exhibit a different set of phonological patterns, characterized by smaller consonantal inventories and more limited syllable structures (Stoel-Gammon, 1991a). It cannot, however, be concluded that these children have atypical phonological systems. In view of their small lexicon, expectations regarding their phonologies should be different from the expectations for children with vocabularies within the typical range. For the late talkers, the phonological system should include at least CV syllables with supraglottal consonants, at least one nasal and one oral consonant, at least one labial and one lingual consonant, and a vowel system with a distinction between high and low vowels and front and back vowels (Stoel-Gammon & Stone, 1991). From this perspective, the relationship between phonology and the lexicon is more important than the size of the phonetic inventory in determining whether a child's phonological system is typical.

Studies examining the relationship between lexical and phonological acquisition among late talkers suggest that a limited phonological system generally goes hand in hand with a small productive vocabulary, even if the phonological measures include nonmeaningful (i.e., uninterpretable) utterances as well as words. Paul and Jennings (1992), for example, compared the phonologies of late talkers and controls matched for age, sex, and socioeconomic status. The late talkers were divided into two groups, a younger group (ages 18–23 months) with productive vocabularies under 10 words, and an older group (ages 24–34 months) with productive vocabularies under 50 words and no use of two-word combinations. The children's phonological systems were analyzed in three ways: 1) number of different consonants produced in words and uninterpretable utterances, 2) complexity of syllable structures in words and uninterpretable utterances, and 3) accuracy of consonants in word productions.

Findings showed that late talkers in both groups were phonologically less advanced than their age-matched peers on all three measures. In addition, the older group of late talkers was more advanced than the younger group on measures of size of consonantal inventory and accuracy of consonants in word productions; the two groups did not differ with respect to syllable structure. Examination of the sound classes and syllable structures used by the typically developing children and the late talkers revealed commonalties across all children, leading the authors to conclude that the late talkers were delayed, but not deviant, in their phonological development.

Rescorla and Ratner (1996) examined the speech patterns of 30 late talkers, ages 24–31 months (mean 26 months) and compared them with 30 controls matched for age, sex, and socioeconomic status. The two groups differed in receptive and expressive language abilities and particularly on productive vocabularies: a mean of 22.8 words for the late talkers compared with a mean of 224.9 for the controls. Phonological analysis of the children's speech was based on a naturalistic 10-minute sample gathered as each child interacted with his or her mother. The findings showed that the late talkers vocalized less frequently than the controls (a mean of 51.4 versus 118.2 vocalizations in the sample). In addition, the late talkers displayed significantly smaller inventories of consonants and vowels and greater proportional use of open syllables (vowel only or consonant–vowel). The authors argued that the phonological systems of the group of late talkers are best characterized as delayed rather than deviant in that they resemble the systems of younger typically developing children. They hypothesized that the low rate of vocalization and phonological delay are interdependent: "children with some underlying phonemic inadequacy may elect to vocalize less, thus diminishing opportunities for the kind of vocal practice that fosters phonemic development" (p. 163).

Finally, Thal, Oroz, and McCaw (1995) examined the phonological patterns of late talkers who scored below the 10th percentile on the CDI (Fenson et al., 1993) and compared the findings with two groups of control children, one matched for age, the other for language level. The late talkers were divided into two subgroups on the basis of their performance on a 30-minute spontaneous language sample. Children who produced fewer than 10 different words in the sample were placed in the premeaningful speech group (7 children ranging in age from 18 to 33 months, with an average age of 22.5 months); children who produced more than 10 words formed the meaningful speech group (10 children ages 19–28 months, with an average age of 23.5 months). Each subject in the late-talker groups was paired with two typically developing children, an age-matched control and a language-matched control who had the same size productive vocabulary (as determined by the CDI). The spontaneous language sample served as the basis for seven phonological measures: 1) complexity of syllable structure in babble, 2) complexity of syllable structure in intelligible speech, 3) number of different consonants produced in babbled utterances, 4) number of different consonants produced in word-initial position, 5) number of different consonants produced in word-final position, 6) number of babbled utterances containing true consonants, and 7) number of intelligible utterances containing true consonants.

The strongest and most straightforward support for a clear link between phonological and lexical acquisition in these children was the finding that the late talkers performed like their lexicon-matched peers on measures of phonology and functioned at a lower level than their age-matched controls. This type of evidence was clearest for the seven children in the premeaningful speech group. There were no significant differences between the performance of these children and their language-matched controls on any of the phonological measures. Furthermore, they were significantly lower than their age-matched controls on all measures except two: number of different consonants in babbled utterances and proportion of true consonants in babble. These findings suggest a close tie between phonological and lexical development. For this group of children with substantial delays in the acquisition of a productive vocabulary, performance on phonological measures was similar to that of children with the same size productive vocabulary who were, on average, 8 months younger.

For the second group of late talkers, the meaningful speech group, the relationship between phonology and lexicon was somewhat more complex. The performance of late talkers in this group did not differ statistically from their language-matched controls on any of the seven phonological measures. At the same time, these late talkers differed from their age-matched controls on only one of the seven measures, number of different consonants produced in word-final position. These findings suggest that the phonological abilities of children in the meaningful speech group fell between the two control groups. Thus, the link between lexicon size and phonological behaviors in this group is present but is not as strong as for late talkers in the premeaningful speech group.

Phonological Development in Children with Down Syndrome

Delays in the onset of speech are also apparent in children with cognitive delays. A population that has been of interest to researchers in prelinguistic and early linguistic development is children with Down syndrome; these children can be identified early, thus making it possible to track development from birth. Studies show that, for the most part, prelinguistic development of babies with Down syndrome differs very little from that of their cognitively typical peers (Dodd, 1972; Smith & Oller, 1981; Smith & Stoel-Gammon, 1996; Steffens, Oller, Lynch, & Urbano, 1992; Stoel-Gammon, 1981). Unlike infants with hearing impairments who display clear delays in the onset of canonical babbling, infants with Down syndrome follow the same general stages of prespeech vocal development and approximately the same timetable.

The major difference between early speech patterns of typically developing children and those with Down syndrome is in the onset of meaningful speech and subsequent linguistic development. In a longitudinal study with data collected at 3-month intervals, Smith (1984) reported that, although the babbling patterns of 10 typically developing infants and 10 infants with Down syndrome were comparable, the appearance of words was delayed by approximately 6 months in the group with Down syndrome. Furthermore, after the onset of speech, the proportion of interpretable utterances increased rapidly in the output of typically developing children, reaching an average of 50% at 18 months. In contrast, the proportion of utterances judged to contain words for the group with Down syndrome at 30 months of age, 9 months after the first use of words, was approximately 5%. These findings indicate that the association between pre-speech and early speech development documented for children with typical cognitive abilities does not hold for children with Down syndrome. There seems to be a dissociation in the abilities of infants with Down syndrome, with babbling patterns being typical, at least in terms of sound classes and onset of canonical babble, but lexical acquisition showing a clear delay.

Subsequent studies of lexical development among children with Down syndrome have revealed that the number of different words produced in language samples from these children is significantly less than the number produced by control children matched for mental age. Thus, even when cognitive level is controlled, children with Down syndrome seem to have difficulties acquiring and using words. However, when groups of typically developing children and children with Down syndrome are matched on mean length of utterance (MLU) rather than mental age, the performance of the children with Down syndrome is superior to that of the controls in terms of number of different words produced in a language sample (J.F. Miller, 1988). A full discussion of these findings is beyond the scope of this chapter; it is clear, however, that the interrelationships among prespeech, lexical, and syntactic development (as measured by MLU) in children with Down syndrome are qualitatively different from those in typically developing subjects. Research with populations of children with other types of disorders, such as fragile X or Prader Willi syndrome, may reveal other relationships among these aspects of early linguistic development.

CLINICAL IMPLICATIONS

What are the clinical implications of the findings presented in this chapter? The most obvious is that prespeech vocal patterns should be considered an integral part of any clinical assessment and diagnosis. Oller, Basinger, and Eilers (1996) noted that parents are good observers of their children's vocal development and can reliably determine whether their child has entered the stage of canonical babbling. Thus, parent report coupled with a clinical assessment could serve as an early identifier of atypical development (Eilers, Neal, & Oller, 1996). When faced with a child who is delayed in acquiring words, a clinician should determine whether the quantity and quality of prespeech vocalizations are within typical limits. If they are, it could be assumed that the child's difficulties do not result from limited proficiency in the area of phonology. If the quantity and quality of vocalizations are below expectation, then prespeech vocal development may be considered as one of the underlying problems. It should be noted that there are exceptions to the link between prelinguistic vocal development and the acquisition of speech. Some children with atypical babbling patterns develop language in a typical fashion, just as some children with typical babble do not adhere to typical patterns of language acquisition. It appears that babble, particularly the onset of use of canonical babble, is one of the most reliable markers for early identification of speech and language disorders in children.

The relationship between phonological and lexical acquisition should also be considered in the assessment of children with delayed speech. Given that a limited lexicon is typically associated with small inventories of sound types and syllable structures, the late talker would not be expected to exhibit a phonological system comparable to that of his or her age-matched peers. Stoel-Gammon and Stone (1991) suggested that one focus of assessment would be to determine if phonology and lexicon are commensurate (i.e., developing at equal rates). These authors suggested that if lexical acquisition and phonology are delayed to the same extent (i.e., are commensurate, but delayed), intervention should first focus on language while phonology is monitored. The rationale for this view is that if the basic problem lies with language, the phonological system will expand to accommodate the newly acquired words as the child acquires a larger lexicon. However, if both phonological and lexical development are delayed, but a child's phonological system shows greater delay, then intervention should focus first on phonology because the phonological system may be a prime factor in the delay in lexical acquisition. In either case, information regarding both phonology and the lexicon would be important for designing an appropriate program of intervention.

FUTURE RESEARCH DIRECTIONS

The research summarized in this chapter supports the view that the phonetics of babble are linked to early phonological development and to the acquisition of words. Many questions remain, however, about the nature of this association:

1. The link between babble and speech has been documented for typically developing children and for late talkers but not for children with Down syndrome. What about other populations, such as children with cerebral palsy, apraxia of speech, autism, otitis media, or delayed motor development?
2. Research has reported correlations between babble and speech. The presence of correlations between two phenomena, however, does not necessarily mean the two are causally related. Can it be shown that atypical prespeech development causes speech and language delays? What kinds of evidence would be construed as causal rather than correlational?
3. In what way(s) is babbling related to language development beyond acquisition of the lexicon? Are there links to syntax, semantics, and/or pragmatics?

4. To what extent is babbling influenced by input? Does the amount of input create differences in output? Does the nature of input (e.g., motherese) exert strong influences on babble and speech? Can input be directly linked to delay or deviancy in early speech and language development?

CONCLUSION

This chapter has focused on the link between prespeech and early speech development in typically developing children, with brief discussion of the effects of hearing loss and cognitive deficit. Numerous studies of children with typical cognitive functioning have shown that prelinguistic vocal development is linked to subsequent acquisition of speech and language, particularly acquisition of the lexicon. Delays in the onset of canonical babble and the infrequent use of consonants in babble are associated with delays in the onset of speech, a slow rate of lexical acquisition, and a phonological system that is limited in terms of sound types and syllable structures. In children with Down syndrome, the relationship between babble and speech appears to be different; despite almost typical babbling patterns, the onset and development of speech are markedly delayed. Future research should be directed toward examining the nature of the link between prespeech and early speech across populations of children with atypical development and across linguistic domains.

REFERENCES

Bates, E. (1979). *The emergence of symbols: Cognition and communication in infancy.* New York: Academic Press.

Bloom, K. (1988). Quality of adult vocalizations affects the quality of infant vocalizations. *Journal of Child Language, 15,* 469–480.

Bloom, K., Russell, A., & Wassenberg, K. (1987). Turn taking affects the quality of infant vocalizations. *Journal of Child Language, 14,* 211–247.

Carpenter, R., Mastergeorge, A., & Coggins, T. (1983). The acquisition of communicative intentions in infants eight to fifteen months of age. *Language and Speech, 26,* 101–116.

Coggins, T.E., & Carpenter, R.L. (1981). The communicative intention inventory: A system for observing and coding children's early intentional communication. *Applied Psycholinguistics, 2,* 235–251.

Coplan, J., & Gleason, J. (1988). Unclear speech: Recognition and significance of unintelligible speech in preschool children. *Pediatrics, 82,* 447–452.

Delack, J.B. (1976). Aspects of infant speech development in the first year of life. *Canadian Journal of Linguistics, 21,* 17–37.

Dodd, B.J. (1972). Comparison of babbling patterns in normal and Down's syndrome infants. *Journal of Mental Deficiency Research, 16,* 35–40.

D'Odorico, L. (1984). Non-segmental features in prelinguistic communications: An analysis of some types of infant cry and non-cry vocalizations. *Journal of Child Language, 2,* 17–27.

Eilers, R., Neal, R., & Oller, D.K. (1996, April). *Late onset babbling as an early marker of abnormal development.* Poster presented at the 10th International Conference on Infant Studies, Providence, RI.

Fenson, L., Dale, P., Reznick, J.S., Thal, D., Bates, E., Hartung, J., Pethick, S., & Reilly, J. (1993). *MacArthur Communicative Development Inventories (CDI)*. San Diego, CA: Singular Publishing Group.

Ferguson, C.A., & Farwell, C. (1975). Words and sounds in early language acquisition: Initial consonants in the first fifty words. *Language, 51,* 419–439.

Fry, D.B. (1966). The development of the phonological system in the normal and deaf child. In F. Smith & G.A. Miller (Eds.), *The genesis of language* (pp. 187–216). Cambridge, MA: MIT Press.

Halliday, M.A.K. (1973). *Explorations in the function of language.* London: Edward Arnold.

Hare, G. (1983). Development at 2 years. In J.V. Irwin & S.P. Wong (Eds.), *Phonological development in children: 18 to 27 months* (pp. 55–88). Carbondale: Southern Illinois University Press.

Jakobson, R. (1968). *Child language, aphasia, and phonological universals.* The Hague, The Netherlands: Mouton. (First published in 1941)

Kent, R.D. (1993). Speech intelligibility and communicative competence in children. In A.P. Kaiser & D.B. Gray (Eds.), *Communication and language intervention series: Vol. 2. Enhancing children's communication: Research foundations for intervention* (pp. 223–239). Baltimore: Paul H. Brookes Publishing Co.

Kent, R.D., & Bauer, H.R. (1985). Vocalizations of one year olds. *Journal of Child Language, 12,* 491–526.

Locke, J.L. (1983). *Phonological acquisition and change.* New York: Academic Press.

Locke, J.L. (1993). *The child's path to spoken language.* Cambridge, MA: Harvard University Press.

Locke, J.L., & Pearson, D. (1990). The linguistic significance of babbling. *Journal of Child Language, 17,* 1–16.

Menn, L. (1976). *Pattern, control and contrast in beginning speech: A case study in the development of word form and word function.* Unpublished doctoral dissertation, University of Illinois, Champaign-Urbana.

Menyuk, P., Liebergott, J.W., & Schultz, M.C. (1995). *Early language development in full-term and premature infants.* Hillsdale, NJ: Lawrence Erlbaum Associates.

Messick, C. (1984). *Phonetic and contextual aspects of the transition to early words.* Unpublished doctoral dissertation, Purdue University, West Lafayette, IN.

Miller, C.Y. (1988). Parents' perceptions and attributions of infant vocal behaviour and development. *First Language, 8,* 125–142.

Miller, J.F. (1988). The developmental asynchrony of language development in children with Down syndrome. In L. Nadel (Ed.), *The psychobiology of Down syndrome* (pp. 167–198). Cambridge, MA: The MIT Press.

Oller, D.K. (1980). The emergence of speech sounds in infancy. In G.H. Yeni-Komshian, C.A. Ferguson, & J. Kavanagh (Eds.), *Child phonology: Production* (Vol. 1, pp. 93–112). New York: Academic Press.

Oller, D.K., Basinger, D., & Eilers, R. (1996, April). *Intuitive identification of infant vocalizations by parents.* Poster presented at the 10th International Conference on Infant Studies, Providence, RI.

Oller, D.K., & Eilers, R. (1988). The role of audition in infant babbling. *Child Development, 59,* 441–449.

Paul, R., & Jennings, P. (1992). Phonological behavior in toddlers with specific expressive language delay. *Journal of Speech and Hearing Research, 35,* 99–107.

Paynter, E., & Petty, N. (1974). Articulatory sound: Acquisition of two-year-old children. *Perceptual and Motor Skills, 39,* 1079–1085.

Prather, E., Hedrick, D., & Kern, D. (1975). Articulation development in children aged two to four years. *Journal of Speech and Hearing Disorders, 53,* 179–191.

Rescorla, L., & Ratner, N.B. (1996). Phonetic profiles of toddlers with specific expressive language impairment. *Journal of Speech and Hearing Research, 39,* 153–165.

Schwartz, R., & Leonard L. (1982). Do children pick and choose? An examination of phonological selection and avoidance in early lexical acquisition. *Journal of Child Language, 9,* 319–336.

Smith, B.L. (1984). Implications of infant vocalizations for assessing phonological disorders. In N. Lass (Ed.), *Speech and language: Advances in basic research and practice* (Vol. 11, pp. 169–194). New York: Academic Press.

Smith, B.L., Brown-Sweeney, S., & Stoel-Gammon, C. (1989). A quantitative analysis of reduplicated and variegated babbling. *First Language, 9,* 175–190.

Smith, B.L., & Oller, D.K. (1981). A comparative study of pre-meaningful vocalizations produced by normally developing and Down's syndrome infants. *Journal of Speech and Hearing Disorders, 46,* 46–51.

Smith, B.L., & Stoel-Gammon, C. (1996). A quantitative analysis of reduplicated and variegated babbling in vocalizations by Down syndrome infants. *Clinical Linguistics and Phonetics, 10,* 119–129.

Snow, C. (1977). The development of conversation between mothers and babies. *Journal of Child Language, 4,* 1–22.

Stark, R.E. (1980). Stages of speech development in the first year of life. In G.H. Yeni-Komshian, C.A. Ferguson, & J. Kavanagh (Eds.), *Child phonology: Vol. 1. Production* (pp. 73–92). New York: Academic Press.

Stark, R.E., Bernstein, L.E., & Demorest, M.E. (1993). Vocal communication in the first 18 months of life. *Journal of Speech and Hearing Research, 36,* 548–558.

Steffens, M.L., Oller, D.K., Lynch, M., & Urbano, R.C. (1992). Vocal development in infants with Down syndrome and infants who are developing normally. *American Journal on Mental Retardation, 97,* 235–246.

Stoel-Gammon, C. (1981). Speech development of infants and children with Down's syndrome. In J.K. Darby (Ed.), *Speech evaluation in medicine* (pp. 341–360). New York: Grune & Stratton.

Stoel-Gammon, C. (1985). Phonetic inventories, 15–24 months: A longitudinal study. *Journal of Speech and Hearing Research, 28,* 505–512.

Stoel-Gammon, C. (1987). The phonological skills of two-year-old children. *Language, Speech, and Hearing Services in Schools, 18,* 323–329.

Stoel-Gammon, C. (1988). Prelinguistic vocalizations of hearing-impaired and normally hearing subjects: A comparison of consonantal inventories. *Journal of Speech and Hearing Disorders, 53,* 302–315.

Stoel-Gammon, C. (1989). Prespeech and early speech development of two late talkers. *First Language, 9,* 207–224.

Stoel-Gammon, C. (1991a). Issues in phonological development and disorders. In J. Miller (Ed.), *Research on child language disorders* (pp. 255–265). Austin TX: PRO-ED.

Stoel-Gammon, C. (1991b). Normal and disordered phonology in two-year-olds. *Topics in Language Disorders, 11,* 21–32.

Stoel-Gammon, C. (1992). Prelinguistic vocal development: Measurement and predictions. In C.A. Ferguson, L. Menn, & C. Stoel-Gammon (Eds.), *Phonological development: Models, research, implications* (pp. 439–456). Timonium, MD: York Press.

Stoel-Gammon, C., & Cooper, J. (1984). Patterns of early lexical and phonological development. *Journal of Child Language, 11,* 247–271.

Stoel-Gammon, C., & Dale, P. (1988, May). *Aspects of phonological development of linguistically precocious children.* Paper presented at the Child Phonology Conference, University of Illinois, Champaign.

Stoel-Gammon, C., & Herrington, P. (1990). Vowel systems of normally developing and phonologically disordered children. *Clinical Linguistics and Phonetics, 4,* 145–160.

Stoel-Gammon, C., & Otomo, K. (1986). Babbling development of hearing-impaired and normally-hearing subjects. *Journal of Speech and Hearing Disorders, 51,* 33–41.

Stoel-Gammon, C., & Stone, J. (1991). Assessing phonology in young children. *Clinics in Communication Disorders, 1,* 25–39.

Thal, D., Oroz, M., & McCaw, V. (1995). Phonological and lexical development in normal and late-talking toddlers. *Applied Psycholinguistics, 16,* 407–424.

Vihman, M. (1981). Phonology and development of the lexicon. *Journal of Child Language, 8,* 239–265.

Vihman, M. (1992). Early syllables and the construction of phonology. In C.A. Ferguson, L. Menn, & C. Stoel-Gammon (Eds.), *Phonological development: Models, research, implications* (pp. 393–422). Timonium, MD: York Press.

Vihman, M., Ferguson, C.A., & Elbert, M. (1987). Phonological development from babbling to speech: Common tendencies and individual differences. *Applied Psycholinguistics, 7,* 3–40.

Vihman, M., Macken, M., Miller, R., Simmons, H., & Miller, J. (1985). From babbling to speech: A reassessment of the continuity issue. *Language, 61,* 397–445.

Vihman, M., & Miller, R. (1988). Words and babble at the threshold of language acquisition. In M.D. Smith & J.L. Locke (Eds.), *The emergent lexicon: The child's development of a linguistic vocabulary* (pp. 151–183). New York: Academic Press.

Wetherby, A., Cain, D., Yonclas, D., & Walker, G. (1988). Analysis of intentional communication of normal children from prelinguistic to the multi-word stage. *Journal of Speech and Hearing Research, 31,* 240–252.

Whitehurst, G., Smith, M., Fischel, J., Arnold, D., & Lonigan, C. (1991). The continuity of babble and speech in children with specific expressive language delay. *Journal of Speech and Hearing Research, 34,* 1121–1129.

6

Nonverbal Communication, Affect, and Social-Emotional Development

Peter Mundy and Jennifer Willoughby

GESTURAL NONVERBAL COMMUNICATION SKILLS, SUCH as pointing or giving to achieve goals in social interactions, emerge in the behavioral repertoires of most children after approximately 6 months of age. The study of the development of these skills most often has been associated with research on early social-cognitive development and the precursors of language development (e.g., Bates, Benigni, Bretherton, Camaioni, & Volterra, 1979; Bretherton, McNew, & Beeghly-Smith, 1981; Bruner, 1975; Butterworth & Jarrett, 1991; Golinkoff, 1983; Sugarman, 1984; Tomasello, 1988, 1995). However, research on the development of different types of nonverbal communication skills in the second year of life also may hold considerable promise for understanding social-emotional development in young children. An exploration of this hypothesis constitutes the central theme of this chapter.

Perhaps the most obvious rationale for this hypothesis is based on possible links between communication development and behavior disorder. Children who evidence delays in language development are at risk for the development of emotional and behavior disorders (Baker & Cantwell, 1987; Beitchman, Hood, & Inglis, 1990). Furthermore, individual differences in the development of nonverbal referential and social-communication skills appear to be related to the individual differences in language development (Bates et al., 1979; Dunham, Dunham, & Curwin, 1993; Mundy, Kasari, Sigman, & Ruskin, 1995; Olson, Bates, & Bales, 1984; Tomasello, 1988). If observations of nonverbal communication skills can provide predictive information about the language development of preschoolers (e.g., Bates et al., 1979; Mundy et al., 1995; Olson et al., 1984), then the early observation of these skills also may help to identify children who are likely to develop emotional and behavior disorders secondary to language delays.

Alternatively, it may be that nonverbal communication development in the second year reflects both constitutional and environmental factors that contribute

Preparation of this chapter was supported by National Institute on Deafness and Other Communication Disorders Grant No. 00484.

directly to the social-emotional development of the child, rather than only indirectly through association with language development. This possibility is inherent in three related strands of theory and research.

Research and theory has suggested that an impairment of nonverbal communication skills may be an important marker of interactional processes that play a role in subsequent social-emotional difficulties in young children. For example, it has been argued that infants' or toddlers' displays of difficult-to-read nonverbal signals or unresponsiveness to the communicative bids of others may potentiate child–caregiver relationship disturbance (Howlin & Rutter, 1987; Mundy, Seibert, & Hogan, 1985; Wetherby & Prizant, 1993b). Alternatively, others have suggested that a disturbance in the child–caregiver attachment system may negatively affect the early nonverbal communication development of children (Bretherton, Bates, Benigni, Camaioni, & Volterra, 1979; Papoušek, Papoušek, Suomi, & Rahn, 1991; Stern, 1985).

A second strand of theory suggests that the development of nonverbal communication skills may be indicative of developments in distinct, albeit rudimentary, aspects of social cognition (Bretherton et al., 1981; Bruner, 1975; Mundy & Hogan, 1994; Tomasello, 1995; Wellman, 1993). Impairments or differences among children in social cognition may play a role in emotional and behavior regulation in social interactions (Dodge, 1986; Stern, 1985). Therefore, it may be that measures of nonverbal communication skills provide an index of individual differences in early social-cognitive development that in turn may be related to the emotional and behavior regulation of young children in social interactions.

Finally, an even more direct connection between nonverbal communication and social-emotional development has been suggested. Certain types of nonverbal communication skills, especially declarative or joint attention skills (see Chapter 2), may reflect developments in the capacity of the child to initiate shared, positive, affective states with others in reference to a third object or event (Adamson & Bakeman, 1985, 1991; Bates, Camaioni, & Volterra, 1975; Jones, Collins, & Hong, 1991; Mundy, Kasari, & Sigman, 1992; Rheingold, Hay, & West, 1976). Thus, the development of joint attention skills may mark an important aspect of the development of individual differences in the tendency to engage in what may be called affective intersubjectivity (Mundy et al., 1992; Stern, 1985). Hypothetically, individual differences in this characteristic may have important ramifications for emotional outcomes for young children (Stern, 1985).

Each of these related possibilities is deserving of extended consideration; however, that is beyond the scope of this chapter. Instead, this chapter focuses on the last hypothesis, which suggests the possibility of a direct connection between early communication and social-emotional development. First, the chapter discusses research and theory on the features that distinguish different nonverbal communication skills that emerge in this period. As part of this presentation, evidence is marshaled to support the assumption that different types of nonverbal communication skills reflect distinct aspects of early development. In particular, the discussion argues that measures of joint attention skill development reflect the tendency to share positive emotional experiences with others vis-à-vis objects or events. Two models of how individual differences in this tendency may affect emotional outcome in children are discussed. In one model, the potential effect of the caregiver on the development of affective sharing is described (Stern, 1985); in another model, the possibility that individual differences in affective sharing in joint attention reflect constitutional or innate factors as well as environmental effects is considered.

DEVELOPMENT AND ASSESSMENT
OF NONVERBAL COMMUNICATION SKILLS

The development of nonverbal, gestural social-communication skills is marked by an important shift from dyadic to triadic, or referential communicative interactions, in the first year of life (Bakeman & Adamson, 1984; see also Chapter 2). From birth to about 6 months of age, infants and caregivers primarily engage in face-to-face or dyadic interactions. However, after the fourth or fifth month, infants become increasingly attentive to objects. With this increased interest in objects, the interactions of the child and caregiver gradually expand to incorporate attention to both the social partner and objects. This expansion continues through the second year of life, so that by 18 months of age, a significant portion of infant–caregiver interactions may be characterized as triadic (Bakeman & Adamson, 1984). The term *triadic* refers to the apparent capacity of the toddler to deploy attention between self, other, and a referent in social-communicative interactions. For example, a toddler may point to a toy (i.e., the referent) while looking at his or her mother (i.e., the other) to communicate his or her desire for toys (i.e., the self).

In seminal theory and research concerning infants' abilities to manage these triadic interactions, Bruner and colleagues distinguished between different types of social-communication skills that emerged in the latter part of the first year of life (Bruner, 1975; Bruner & Sherwood, 1983; Scaife & Bruner, 1975). These included the ability to engage in object-oriented offering and turn-taking routines and the ability to use or respond to visual line of regard to coordinate attention to events or objects with another person (Bruner, 1975; Scaife & Bruner, 1975). The latter capacity to engage in joint attention routines was not clearly manifest in most infants until about 9–12 months of age, at which point infants began to visually orient themselves in directions consistent with the line of regard of others (Scaife & Bruner, 1975).

In independent but equally fundamental efforts, Bates et al. (1979) emphasized that infants' capacities to direct the line of regard of a social partner to objects appeared to bifurcate with regard to function in the 9- to 12-month-old period. Late in the first year of life, gestural acts were used by infants for imperative functions, such as pointing to elicit aid in obtaining an object that is out of reach. However, the functionally distinct use of gestures and eye contact for declarative purposes, such as showing an object to another person, also could be distinguished (Bates et al., 1979). Thus, by the end of the 1970s, research and theory had culminated in a taxonomy of different forms of nonverbal social-communication skills that emerged in the later part of the first year of life and were consolidated throughout the second year of life.

Applied researchers often have called on elements of this taxonomy in their attempts to devise measures of individual differences in the development of communication skills (Seibert, Hogan, & Mundy, 1982, 1987; Snyder, 1978; Wetherby & Prizant, 1993b; Wetherby & Prutting, 1984). These efforts have made it possible for different researchers to use similar methods in explorations of early nonverbal communication development. Versions of these methods include the abridged version of Seibert and Hogan's Early Social-Communication Scales (ESCS; Mundy, Sigman, & Kasari, 1990; Mundy, Sigman, Kasari, & Yirmiya, 1988) and the Communication and Symbolic Behavior Scales (CSBS; Wetherby & Prizant, 1993a). These very similar instruments use a structured, videotaped child–tester interaction designed to elicit nonverbal communicative bids. Child–tester interactions are used to minimize the possible variability that care-givers may contribute to the display of communicative skills among young children. Both instruments yield frequency scores for the number of bids within a taxonomy of three categories of nonverbal communication. Bruner and Sher-wood's (1983) terminology for this taxonomy is used in both assessment systems.

In this terminology, social-interaction skills refer to the use of eye contact, gestures, and affective signals to elicit and maintain episodes of turn taking, such as when infants repeatedly give and take objects from a caregiver. According to Bruner and Sherwood (1983), turn taking was considered to be a social skill that was fundamental to most communicative interactions that often involve a send-reply, turn-taking sequence of information exchange. Behavior regulation skills refer to the capacity to use gestures and eye contact to direct attention and elicit aid in obtaining an object or event (e.g., requesting). An example would be the act of giving a jar while making eye contact with an adult to elicit aid in opening the jar. Finally, joint attention skills involve communicative bids that appear to be used to share the experience of an object or an event with someone (e.g., commenting). This function is less instrumental but perhaps inherently more social than with behavior regulation bids. An example here might be a child who holds a novel toy up to a caregiver to show the toy. Both joint attention and behavior regulation presumably reflect the child's developing awareness of the rules of reference within social interaction and, as such, were considered to be fundamental to the development of verbal communication skills (Bruner & Sherwood, 1983).

Nonverbal Communication and Social Cognition

Researchers are interested in nonverbal communication skills because of their relation to social-cognitive development (Bretherton et al., 1981; Moore &

Corkum, 1994; Tomasello, 1995). To some degree, this perceived relationship hinges on the judgment that the intentionality of the communicative bids of the child becomes more apparent with the emergence of triadic/referential communication bids (Bates et al., 1979; Golinkoff, 1983). This judgment, in turn, is based on several observations. Infants and young children increasingly combine gestures, such as reaching or pointing to objects, with eye contact, suggesting that they are monitoring the potential reception of their signal by a social partner. Infants and young children also increasingly use conventional signals, such as pointing, suggesting that they understand something of the signal value of specific types of gestures. Finally, and perhaps most important, with the emergence of triadic skills, infants and young children begin to display communicative repair when their initial gestural bids do not yield desired responses, suggesting that they recognize when the intent or goal of their signal has not been realized (Golinkoff, 1983; see also Chapter 7).

To be intentional with regard to communicative acts suggests that the child has some awareness of self and others as capable of sending and receiving signals (Bruner, 1975). Extending this notion, Bretherton et al. (1981) suggested that referential nonverbal communication skills reflect rudimentary aspects of a developing "theory of mind" in infants and young children. That is, triadic nonverbal communicative acts indicate that the child can appreciate that others have perceptions and intentions relative to objects or events and that these perceptions or intentions can be affected by the child's behaviors. Numerous researchers have attempted to expand on the notion that referential nonverbal communication skills reflect an awareness that self and others can experience common covert psychological phenomenon relative to objects and events (Baron-Cohen, 1989; Bretherton et al., 1981; Hobson, 1993; Moore & Corkum, 1994; Mundy, Sigman, & Kasari, 1993; Stern, 1985; Tomasello, 1995; Wellman, 1993).

Several of these elaborations converge on a similar perspective. For example, in an attempt to understand interpersonal development, Stern (1985) proposed that between 7 and 12 months of age, infants develop the capacity to share three aspects of mental states with others. Accordingly, infants in this period can share intentions or a common goal orientation with regard to objects or events, engage in joint attention and share a common visual perspective on objects or events, and share affective states or a common emotional response to objects and events. Similarly, Wellman (1993), theorizing about early cognitive development, proposed that in the last quarter of the first year of life, infants understand people in terms of three aspects of behavior: 1) desire or that people can seek to attain the same objects or experiences; 2) perception or that people can see, hear, or feel the same object or event; and 3) emotion or that people can have the same affective reactions to objects or events.

The aspects of social cognition described by Stern (1985) and Wellman (1993) may be directly related to the three categories of nonverbal communication skills described by Bates et al. (1975) and Bruner and Sherwood (1983).

The ability to recognize that self and others can experience intentions, or goal orientations, may be reflected by the capacity of the child to initiate and respond to nonverbal requests. The capacity to understand that both self and others can share a common visual perspective of an event or object may be involved in both joint attention and behavior regulation, as these both involve coordinating attention between self and another person vis-à-vis an object or event. Finally, and most pertinent to this discussion, is the possibility that both social-interaction and joint attention skills may involve affective sharing. In the former, affective sharing occurs in the face-to-face enterprise of turn taking. In the latter, the tendency to share affective states may have a more sophisticated expression as the child initiates shared affective states in a triadic context, that is, in reference to an object or event (Mundy et al., 1992).

This line of thinking would suggest that different types of nonverbal communication skills may reflect distinct aspects of social-cognitive and social-emotional development in young children. However, this hypothesis presupposes that the distinctions made among nonverbal communication skills, such as joint attention skills versus behavior regulation skills, reflect truly distinct domains of early development. This important issue has received almost no attention in research on typical development. Nevertheless, direct support for the importance of the distinctions among nonverbal communication skills made by Bruner, Bates, and others is apparent in applied research on children with developmental disorders. A brief examination of this literature may be useful before considering how measures of different nonverbal communication skills may reflect social-emotional development.

Psychological Distinctions Among Nonverbal Communication Skills

One piece of evidence that suggests that nonverbal communication skills reflect distinct domains in early development is the observation that young children with distinct forms of biologically based disorders display different profiles of strengths and limitations in nonverbal communication skill acquisition (Mundy, Sigman, Ungerer, & Sherman, 1986; Mundy et al., 1995; Wetherby & Prutting, 1984; Wetherby, Yonclas, & Bryan, 1989). Young children with autism display a profound disturbance of joint attention skill development but display relatively better development of other nonverbal communication skills. Alternatively, children with Down syndrome display a disturbance of behavior regulation skills but display less disturbance of gestural joint attention or social-interaction skills (Loveland & Landry, 1986; McEvoy, Rogers, & Pennington, 1993; Mundy, Sigman, & Kasari, 1994; Mundy et al., 1986; Mundy et al., 1988; Mundy et al., 1995; Wetherby & Prutting, 1984; Wetherby et al., 1989). The contrasting pattern of nonverbal communication skill development observed across these groups cannot be understood simply in terms of caregiver or other environmental effects (Kasari, Sigman, Mundy, & Yirmiya, 1988; Mundy et al., 1988). This alignment of particular types of nonverbal communication skill impairment within groups of children with specific types of developmental disorders suggests that different nonverbal communication skills may reflect distinct and, to some degree, constitutional aspects of early psychological development in young children.

Studies on the cognitive and neurological correlates of nonverbal communication skills are consistent with this hypothesis. McEvoy et al. (1993) observed a significant relation between joint attention and social-interaction skills, as assessed on the ESCS, and a putative measure of executive functions in children with autism and typical development. A comparable relation was not observed for behavior regulation skills.

Executive functions refer to the regulatory processes that enable planned and flexible problem solving. In McEvoy et al. (1993), the critical executive function task was one in which children had to repeatedly find a hidden object under one of two screens and then periodically shift their problem-solving set to find the object under the alternative screen. McEvoy et al. interpreted their results to suggest that deficient joint attention and better behavior regulation skill development in children with autism could be explained by the different degree to which these two types of skills may reflect cognitive executive function processes. Furthermore, because executive functions may be mediated by neurological processes associated with the frontal lobes, McEvoy et al. suggested that joint attention development, and the lack thereof in children with autism, was related to neurological processes involving the frontal lobes.

Data consistent with this conclusion have been reported in an intervention study with young children with intractable seizure disorders (Caplan et al., 1993). The data in this study indicated that positron emission tomography (PET) indices of individual differences in metabolism in the frontal hemispheres of this sample of 13 children with seizure disorders predicted joint attention development months after surgical intervention for these children but did not predict behavior regulation or social-interaction skill development. These results suggested that individual differences in the functioning of the frontal lobes, as indexed by a measure of metabolic rate, were associated with joint attention skill development measured with the ESCS. Although consistent with the results of the McEvoy et al. (1993) study, this research goes beyond that study by providing a direct empirical link between neurological functioning and nonverbal communication development.

These studies begin to suggest that different types of nonverbal communication skills reflect different types of cognitive and neurological processes. Data indicate that measures of joint attention skills may be particularly sensitive indices of both cognitive problem-solving and frontal-neurological processes as applied to the domain of early social-communication development. This observation, in combination with the segregation of different types of nonverbal communication skill deficiencies with different developmental disorders, provides a basis for the assumption that different types of nonverbal communication skills may reflect different aspects of early psychological development. This assumption is critical to the remainder of this chapter, which explores the possibility that some types of nonverbal communication skills reflect critical components of early social-emotional development.

THE AFFECTIVE CORRELATES
OF NONVERBAL COMMUNICATION SKILLS

In attempting to understand the nature of nonverbal communication skill development, Bates and colleagues emphasized the cognitive, representational processes that may be involved in these skills (Bates et al., 1979). Initially, however, they also observed that joint attention acts serve not only to direct the attention of the adult to an object but also are used for social-affective sharing purposes. Bates et al. (1979) stated, "Long before he can understand the utilitarian value of sharing information, the child will engage in declaring for primarily social purposes" (p. 115). Accordingly, children's declaring or joint attention acts involve the "use of an object (through pointing, showing, giving, etc.) as a means to attain adult attention" (p. 115). Furthermore, the attention-getting component, as described by Bates et al. (1979), appeared to involve the conveyance or exchange of affective signals. They suggested that the development of joint attention acts marks the emergence of attempts to "seek a more subtle kind of adult response—laughter, comment, smiles and eye contact" (p. 121) in reference to an object and event.

It is difficult to observe a young child engaged in a joint attention bid and not be struck by the social, affect-sharing quality of the communicative bid. Other researchers have expressed similar views of joint attention development. Rheingold et al. (1976) interpreted joint attention acts as a means to share experience with others. They described this experience-sharing function as distinct from the function of imperative, requesting gestures. Bruner (1981) also perceived that there may be "some primitive mood marking procedure to distinguish indicating from commanding or requesting" (p. 67) among preverbal acts of communication. These observations suggest that joint attention acts may involve the attempts of young children to convey or share their affective experience of an object with others. Alternatively, affective sharing may play a lesser role in behavior regulation acts. Thus, theoretically, nonverbal joint attention may involve affective sharing to a greater extent than does nonverbal requesting.

The empirical literature supports and expands on this view of joint attention behaviors. Bates et al. (1975) suggested that joint attention bids may involve seeking an affective response from adults; however, research suggests that by 10 months of age infants may initiate positive affective exchanges in a joint attention context. In play with objects, infants often first express positive affect to objects and then turn to display this affect to a social partner (Jones et al., 1991). Jones and Raag (1989) also presented data that suggest that by 18 months the tendency of young children to share positive affect vis-à-vis an object is as strong with strangers as it is with familiar caregivers. In addition, Adamson and Bakeman (1985) reported that higher proportions of all affective displays occur within joint attention episodes than in face-to-face interaction in caregiver–child interaction observations conducted with infants at the ages of 6, 9, 12, 15, and 18 months (Adamson & Bakeman, 1985). Thus, their data suggest that joint attention episodes may be a prepotent context for the conveyance of affect in mother–infant interaction.

Although important and informative, these studies did not attempt to directly distinguish among nonverbal communication skills in terms of their affective correlates. However, a direct comparison of the affective components of nonverbal joint attention and requesting was presented by Kasari, Sigman, Mundy, and Yirmiya (1990) who examined facial affect and nonverbal communication in an attempt to understand the disassociation between joint attention and behavior regulation skill development in children with autism. The results of this study indicated that children with typical development displayed much more positive affect in conjunction with joint attention bids compared with behavior regulation bids. The children with autism displayed equivalent levels of affect in conjunction with both types of communicative behavior and displayed significantly less positive affect in conjunction with joint attention bids than did the comparison children.

A related study was conducted with a sample of 32 typically developing young children who were approximately 20 months old (Mundy et al., 1992). This study indicated that the young children displayed more positive affect in conjunction with each of the four types of joint attention acts relative to four types of requesting acts. The results of this study were interpreted to suggest that the assessment of joint attention bids on the ESCS reflects a tendency to initiate states of affective intersubjectivity or states of shared positive affect vis-à-vis objects or events (Mundy et al., 1992).

Data also indicate that infants and young children display considerable individual differences in affective intersubjectivity in structured measures of gestural communication development. Wetherby and Prizant (1993a) assessed 282 children who were either prelinguistic or used holophrastic speech with the CSBS. One measure on the CSBS is an index of shared positive affect. It is not clear to what degree this CSBS measure is derived from observations of joint attention bids or other nonverbal communication bids. Nevertheless, their data suggested that considerable individual differences in the tendency to display positive affect to the tester in a structured nonverbal communication measure may be displayed by young children. The potential importance of these individual differences is discussed in the next section.

Joint Attention and Social-Emotional Development

Much more research is needed before a definitive perspective on the nature of nonverbal communication skills will exist. However, the foregoing review provides the basis for some interesting, if tentative, conclusions. Research and theory suggest that the types of nonverbal communication skills that develop in the second year of life may reflect partially independent domains of early psychological development. Data on the correlates of nonverbal communication skills suggest that the domain assessed under the rubric of joint attention may reflect higher order self-regulatory behavior organization mechanisms associated with frontal lobe neurological processes to a greater degree than behavior regulation and, perhaps, social-interaction skills. In addition, and perhaps most important, joint attention skills may provide a window to individual differences in the tendency of infants and young children to initiate states of positive affective sharing with others that are referenced to objects or events.

Although the empirical links between joint attention and social-emotional behavior development in children are few, the theoretical links are readily observed, especially when joint attention is viewed as involving affective sharing. Stern (1985) suggested that the "capacity to share affective states is the most pervasive and clinically germane feature of intersubjective relatedness" (p. 138) that arises in infants and young children.

Intersubjectivity refers to a phenomenon in which social partners perceive that they share the experience of similar thoughts or feelings, and consequently a sense of connectedness, during social interaction (cf., Ickes, Tooke, Stinson, Baker, & Bissonette, 1988). As noted previously, nonverbal communication skills theoretically reflect the development of processes involved in the capacity to experience episodes of intersubjectivity. That is, they reflect a developing awareness in infants and young children that the self and others can have similar goals, perceptions, or feelings regarding objects or events. Moreover, joint attention behaviors may be especially important in the development of the intersubjective experience of affect (Mundy et al., 1992). For Stern, the development of this capacity, or the capacity for "interaffectivity" (1985, p. 132), constitutes a critical step in the social-emotional development of the child.

In Stern's (1985) view, it was most important to consider how caregivers respond when infants and young children initiate a potential state of shared affect in reference to objects or events. Caregiver responsiveness was referred to as "affective attunement," or the degree to which a parent aligned his or her response appropriately to the affect expressed by the child. For example, a parent might smile and laugh along with a child's positive affect but also display concern and comfort in response to a child's expression of negative affect expressed vis-à-vis an object or event. Parental attunement was viewed as critical to emotional development because it enabled young children to begin to understand what was and what was not within the realm of shareable personal, emotional experience. Furthermore, the effects of attunement were thought to become increasingly robust as triadic nonverbal communications emerged and the child became more capable of processing intersubjective information, or shareable experiences, that were anchored to a greater variety of reference points in the world.

Stern referred to the potentially pathogenic expression of affective attunement as "selective attunement" (1985, p. 207). *Selective attunement* refers to the tendency of a caregiver to more consistently or tolerantly respond with respect to a particular style or valence of their child's affect (e.g., positive or negative affective expressions). Selective attunement occurs in all caregiver–child dyads to some degree, at some times. However, problems arise in dyads where selective attunement occurs chronically and there is a systematic, long-term bias toward responsiveness to one affective valence or another. For example, a parent may be responsive to positive affective expressions but intolerant of negative expressions, or vice versa. In Stern's view, selective attunement is fundamental to the development of emotional disturbance because the child comes to emphasize "the portion of inner experience that can achieve intersubjective acceptance with the inner experience of other, at the expense of the remaining, equally legitimate portion of inner experience" (1985, p. 210). Thus, selective attunement to affective states in infants is thought to precipitate the early disavowal of segments of the child's affective experience. For example, some children have difficulty expressing pleasure in their achievements, whereas others may claim that they never experience negative feelings. Thus, an emotional disturbance is created, with certain aspects of the child's emotional internal life split off or invalidated. This process, in Stern's view, is a primary contributor to the development of behavior disorders in children as well as in adults.

According to this interactional view, the degree to which children express positive affect in the context of joint attention could largely be an effect of caregiver affective attunement or selective attunement. Accordingly, joint attention skills may be one marker of the mental health of a caregiver–child dyad. For example, stressed, ambivalent, or inadequate caregivers might not be well attuned to the expression of positive affect in their children. Consequently, a decrease in joint attention bids might be observed among children exposed to this type of caregiving.

One study reported data consistent with this hypothesis (Flanagan, Coppa, Riggs, & Alaro, 1994). In this study, a group of 13 teenage mothers and their infants was assessed with a measure of quality of parent–child interaction and a measure of nonverbal communication skill development, the CSBS. The results indicated that the infants displayed typical levels of social-interaction behavior but less joint attention behavior and more requesting behavior than expected based on comparisons with the CSBS normative data. It was not clear to what degree this reflected differences between this sample and the CSBS normative sample on potentially critical factors such as socioeconomic status of the mothers. However, correlation analyses did indicate that infants in more positively interacting dyads, based on direct observations of social interactions, displayed relatively more joint attention and social-interaction behaviors and relatively fewer requesting behaviors.

Interpretation of this one study must be cautious because of a variety of methodological issues. Nevertheless, the results of this study appear to be consistent with the caregiver interaction perspective noted previously. However, the results do not speak to specific mechanisms. It is not clear from this study whether selective attunement or some other process was responsible for the relations observed between caregiver interactions and nonverbal communication. At the very least, though, Flanagan et al.'s (1994) study suggested that further research on nonverbal communication skills as markers of the social-emotional outcome in at-risk caregiving environments may be useful.

Stern's (1985) model of selective attunement and Flanagan et al.'s (1994) data emphasize the possible effects of caregiver behavior on nonverbal communication and consequent social-emotional outcome. However, a complementary but more nativistic view of the meaning of nonverbal communication and social-emotional development also should be considered. In a nativistic model, it is assumed that joint attention and affective sharing are influenced not only by environmental caregiver effects but also by inherent qualities of the child. This view emerges from applied research on nonverbal communication in children with autism (Mundy, 1995) but may have implications for research on nonverbal communication and social-emotional development in all children.

Joint Attention and Social-Emotional Approach Behavior

Why do young children initiate joint attention bids? It is tempting to address this question solely in terms of the cognitive processes that are involved in coordinated attention and reference to objects (e.g., Butterworth & Jarrett, 1991; Tomasello, 1995). However, such an approach may be more appropriate for understanding how a child is able to initiate a joint attention bid but not necessarily why a child initiates joint attention bids. To understand why young children initiate joint attention bids, it may be important to consider motivational processes, as Bates et al. (1979) did when observing that joint attention bids mark the emergence of attempts to "seek a more subtle kind of adult response—laughter, comment, smiles and eye contact" in episodes involving reference to an object or event (p. 121). Research also suggests that joint attention bids may reflect the tendency of young children to share their own positive affect with others relative to objects or events (Kasari et al., 1990; Mundy et al., 1992). If these observations are valid, then individual differences in joint attention bids may reflect differences in the degree to which children are motivated by the reinforcement value of a social partner's positive regard, the experience of establishing shared positive affect with others, or both (Mundy, 1995).

The tendency of a child to initiate episodes of shared positive affect through joint attention bids may be referred to as a social and emotional approach tendency (Fox, 1991; Mundy, 1995). This tendency may have a positive effect on the potential for developing a relationship between children and potential caregivers. The degree to which the child is disposed to positive affective sharing in communication with others may be expected to play a role in the degree to which the child is able to establish a positive sense of relatedness with caregivers and other less familiar people. If this sequence of assumptions and hypotheses is correct, then observations of joint attention behaviors may provide an index of a behavior domain (i.e., social-emotional approach) that is related to children's capacity to elicit positive attachment relations with potential caregivers.

It may be argued that individual differences in joint attention development and the related disposition toward positive social-emotional approach behaviors may be explained in terms of learning processes (e.g., Moore & Corkum, 1994). For example, Stern's (1985) model of affective attunement illustrates how it might be expected that caregiver influences would lead to more or less joint attention and positive social-emotional approach behavior in young children. However, several lines of reasoning may be marshaled to suggest that neurobiological variability among children also contributes to individual differences in the disposition toward joint attention bids and social-emotional approach behaviors.

First, observations of the profound disturbance in joint attention development among children with autism lead to considering the development of joint attention, and positive affective sharing, from a biological perspective. Much research on autism suggests that the primary causal path in its etiology is neurobiological (see Schopler & Mesibov, 1987). Several models are available that depict biological mechanisms that may specifically support the capacity for social-emotional approach behaviors, and positive affective intersubjectivity may be disturbed in children with autism (Fotheringham, 1991; Mundy, 1995; Panksepp & Sahley, 1987). One of the lessons of research on autism for the field of typical development may be that there is a very large degree of variability in the degree to which people tend to establish states of positive affective intersubjectivity with others and that some portion of this variance may be due to neurobiological differences among people.

Second, the observation that individual differences in joint attention development could be predicted from individual differences in frontal lobe functioning among young children with histories of intractable seizure disorders (Caplan et al., 1993) provides some support for the notion that joint attention development reflects individual differences in neurobiological processes. Furthermore, this finding provides a bridge to a finding in developmental psychobiological research. Before the end of the first year of life, neurological subsystems may be organized and lateralized to regulate social approach behaviors as opposed to social withdrawal behaviors (Fox, 1991). In particular, left frontal lobe processes appear to play a role in behaviors that are child initiated, involve a focus on a person, and include the display of positive affect to the social partner (Davidson, Ekman, Saron, Senulis, & Friesen, 1990; Dawson, 1994; Fox, 1991). In the first year of life, reaching to a caregiver while smiling would be prototypical of a social approach behavior. Hypothetically, positive affective sharing in joint attention bids in the second year of life reflects an elaboration of this frontally mediated, social-emotional approach tendency. This speculation is bolstered by the finding that left rather than right lobe frontal functioning was most powerfully related to joint attention development in the study of children with seizure disorders (Caplan et al., 1993). This possible lateralization of neurological processes also would be consistent with the notion that some component of individual differences in positive social-emotional approach disposition (as measured by frequency of joint attention bids) is associated with differences innate to neurobiological propensities.

The previous hypotheses and assumptions constitute a model that is on the speculative side of research and theory on joint attention skill development. However, it is not beyond the reach of empirical verification or refutation. For example, one prediction that may be derived from this model is that higher rates of joint attention bids or social-emotional approach behavior would be associated with more positive perceptions of the child's social or affiliative behavior by caregivers. There are at least two studies that provide some support for this possibility.

Paul (1991) reported on a study in which thirty 2-year-olds with specific expressive language delays were compared with 30 children displaying a more typical pattern of expressive language development. The results indicated that parents of late talkers reported observing more evidence of disruptive and hyperactive behavior than did the parents of children with more typical language. The reports of parents of late talkers also yielded lower scores on the socialization index of the Vineland Adaptive Behavior Scales, even when items associated with language development, such as saying "please," were excluded (Paul, 1991). The critical items on this measure include items that assess the degree to which the parent confirms that the child shows interest in children or peers; plays simple interactive games, shows a desire to please his or her caregiver, and imitates complex tasks displayed by others. Paul also reported that the late talkers produced significantly fewer overall communicative acts with their mothers and that this difference was primarily due to an attenuated tendency of the late talkers to initiate joint attention acts. Indeed, late talkers displayed a higher mean for behavior regulation acts (6.3, $SD = 5.1$) than did the comparison children (4.2, $SD = 3.1$) but a much lower mean for joint attention acts (23.27, $SD = 12.3$ versus 40.7, $SD = 15.2$, respectively) (Paul & Shiffer, 1991).

The interpretation of these data is not straightforward. On the one hand, it may be that processes specific to delayed language development account for the links observed in this study among socialization, behavior disorder, and joint attention behaviors in 2-year-olds. On the other hand, the uneven profile of communicative functions displayed by the late talkers leaves open an alternative. Paul (1991) suggested that this profile was indicative of a child who may engage in social interactions for instrumental purposes but who was limited in tendency to engage in communicative interaction for the more social purposes inherent to joint attention bids. Thus, a tentative hypothesis raised in this study was that an attenuation of joint attention bids reflected a reduced drive to initiate communicative bids that involve social experience sharing. This reduced drive may be linked both to language delays and behavior disorder in some children (Paul, 1991).

A serendipitous but related finding was reported in a study of 30 preschool children with autism and comparison children, including a sample of 30 typically developing children (Mundy et al., 1994). The children in this study had developmental mental ages of about 20 months. They were presented with the ESCS, and parents provided a report of their children's symptoms on the Autism Behavior Checklist (ABC; Krug, Arick, & Almond, 1979). The ABC yields measures of impairment in five areas: 1) a relating scale that assesses the tendency to use and respond to touching, eye contact, facial affect, and imitation and to establish friendships; 2) a language scale that measures the frequency of language use and atypical vocal behavior; 3) a social/self-help scale that assesses temperament and adaptive behavior; 4) a sensory scale measuring hypersensitivity and hyposensitivity to stimulation; and 5) a body/object use scale that measures stereotypes and repetitive actions.

The results indicated that observations of nonverbal joint attention bids in interactions with a tester were correlated with the parents' reports on the relating scale of the ABC for both the children with autism ($r = -.37, p < .05$), and for the children with typical development ($r = -.40, p = <.05$). Higher scores on the ABC relating scale indicated that parents confirmed more negative observations about the social behavior of their children, such as not responding to others' affect, resisting being touched or held, not imitating others in play, and not developing friendships. Thus, in both the samples of children with autism and with typical development, children who reportedly had fewer positive social behaviors by parental report also had lower ESCS joint attention scores. These data suggest that the frequency of joint attention behaviors, as assessed in interaction with a tester, may be related to parent's perception of the display of positive social behaviors among typically developing young children as well as among children displaying atypical social development. Although tentative, these results are consistent with the notion that joint attention behavior, via effects associated with caregiver perceptions of and responsivity to the social behavior of young children, could have an effect on the development of caregiver–child relationships. The next section extends this notion to the consideration of how joint attention skill development and social approach behaviors may relate to the development of attachment.

Joint Attention and Attachment

The social approach model leads to a premise regarding a possible interaction between joint attention skill development and attachment. This model assumes that joint attention bids, at least those associated with the expression of positive affect, reflect a disposition toward social-emotional approach behavior in children. Furthermore, it is assumed that social-emotional approach behaviors play a facilitating role in establishing bonds or a positive sense of relatedness between the child and others. Finally, it is also assumed that individual differences in joint attention development are affected by both environmental, especially caregiver effects, and innate neurobiological characteristics of the child. This suggests the possibility that different types of environmental and biological combinations may affect joint attention and, more important, social-emotional approach tendencies in children.

If the focus is on caregiver effects, the tendency is to suggest that a child's joint attention skill development may be augmented by positive caregiving and attenuated by negative caregiving. However, if it also is assumed that a child has an innate reaction range with regard to the development of joint attention skills, then more of a transactional perspective may be adopted. From this perspective, one potential combination is the child with a biological disposition toward higher frequencies of joint attention, or social approach behavior, who is growing up in an environment that presents a risk for less-than-optimal caregiving. A less optimal caregiver environment may have a negative effect on the social-emotional development of a child. However, a possible hypothesis is that a child with a higher predisposition toward joint attention and social-emotional approach behavior may be less vulnerable to the negative effects of a poor caregiver environment. Although poor caregiving may decrease social-emotional approach tendencies, children with higher biological predispositions toward joint attention skill development may have a sufficiently broad reaction range so that they express an adaptive level of social-emotional approach behaviors with the primary caregiver and with other potential caregivers. This, in turn, may allow the child to elicit whatever positive social interactions are possible in the poor caregiving environment. More important, it also may increase the likelihood that the child will establish bonds with others that mitigate the negative effects of the primary caregiver interactions. Thus, the display of good joint attention skills by a toddler with a tester may be one significant indicator of the degree to which this child may be more, or less, vulnerable to negative caregiving effects.

This hypothesis of the social-emotional approach model leads to a testable prediction about the relationships among joint attention development, attachment, and behavioral outcome in children. The assessment of early attachment is often undertaken with a paradigm called the "strange situation" (Ainsworth & Bell, 1970). The strange situation involves observations of infants or young children in a sequence of separations and reunions with a caregiver. Observations of the child's behavior during separation and particularly during reunion episodes are scored to yield a categorical index of the degree to which a child and caregiver appear to have a secure or insecure attachment relationship. This provides a measure of the quality of the caregiving environment with insecure attachment ratings associated with less optimal caregiving (Main, Tomasini, & Tolon,

1979). This model leads to the expectation that ratings of attachment in the strange situation and ratings of joint attention bids to a tester may yield partially independent predictors of early behavioral development in preschool children. In particular, it might be expected that data from attachment measures and joint attention measures would interact in their prediction of behavioral outcome with positive joint attention development mitigating the negative effects associated with indices of disturbed attachment. However, the toddler with both poor attachment and poor joint attention development may be at higher risk than other children for the development of behavior disorders.

These predictions presuppose that measures of attachment and the tendency to display joint attention bids reflect at least partially independent processes in early development. In this regard it should be noted that the electroencephalogram correlates of infants' responses to separation situations and social approach situations appear to be different (Fox, 1991). Furthermore, research on autism suggests that, although children with autism display profound joint attention disturbance, the behavior they display in strange situations is not so disturbed relative to control children with mental retardation (Sigman & Mundy, 1989). Similarly, individual differences in joint attention behavior do not appear to be correlated with attachment ratings of children with autism, although behavior regulation does appear to correlate with attachment in these children (Capps, Sigman, & Mundy, 1994). Thus, although little research may be applied to this important issue, the data that exist are not inconsistent with the hypothesis that joint attention and attachment measures may provide independent, but complimentary indices of risk for social-emotional disturbance in preschool children. The authors of this chapter are examining this hypothesis in a longitudinal study of infants and young children who are at risk for the development of behavior disorders.

EDUCATIONAL AND CLINICAL IMPLICATIONS

The clinical and educational implications of the theory outlined in this chapter may be most apparent to those involved in the national movement toward attempting to provide early educational opportunities for children in need by the age of 3 years, or earlier when possible. One impediment in the effective provision of such services is that the ability to identify all children who may benefit from early intervention, or recognize and address individual differences among children that may affect their responsiveness to early intervention efforts, is limited. One limiting factor is that there are few tools in the clinical armamentarium of assessments that focus on individual differences evident among children in the second year of life, even though the second year of life is a period that is rich with significant developments in cognitive, communication, social, and emotional skills.

In this regard, one of the more useful applications would be the development of assessment instruments that could contribute to the identification of future language delays in children before the age of 2 years. It is still not clear to what degree measures of nonverbal communication skills provide important and unique information about language development in young children. Nevertheless, findings are encouraging (e.g., Dunham et al., 1993; Mundy et al., 1995; Tomasello, 1988). For example, two studies suggest that simple measures of individual differences in the tendency of children in the middle of the second year of life to follow the gaze and pointing of others may be very strong predictors of expressive language development (Mundy & Gomes, 1996; Mundy et al., 1995). Thus, these studies alone suggest there may be optimism about the clinical utility of measures such as the ESCS or CSBS in screening for early educational interventions.

In addition to possible language development prediction, however, the observational platform used in measures of nonverbal communication skills, such as the CSBS or ESCS, is rich with information about other important domains of development. These measures have the potential for providing a standardized view of the child that may be informative about emotional and temperamental factors as well as about cognitive or social-cognitive components of early development. If this potential can be realized, then these types of measures may make a very real contribution to the clinical assessment of the mental and behavioral health of young children and to the assessment of early factors associated with language development. Although often not considered to be primary, these factors may be critically important to consider in the design and implementation of early intervention programs for very young children.

DIRECTIONS FOR FUTURE RESEARCH

According to the theory reviewed and developed in this chapter, the pursuit of at least three areas of nonverbal communication skills research may be edifying. Understanding the connection between nonverbal communication and language development may be essential to understanding the putative links between nonverbal communication and subsequent emotional or behavioral development. Several of the most important issues in this realm of inquiry have been considered at length (Mundy & Gomes, 1997). This section offers the chapter authors' views on some of the essential issues.

It is not yet clear to what degree measures of nonverbal communication simply predict individual differences in initial aspects of language acquisition or predict stable individual differences in language development that are manifest beyond the preschool period. This would appear to be an essential issue to resolve. It is also not clear whether measures of nonverbal communication skills provide information about language development that goes beyond the information provided by more object-oriented measures of early cognitive development. If they do not provide additional information, the incremental utility or validity of measures of nonverbal communication may be called into question. As always, nature versus nurture is an important issue. In this regard, it will be useful to determine the contribution of both environmental and inherent factors to individual differences in nonverbal communication development among young children.

Above and beyond language, there may be direct linkages between nonverbal communication and emotional and behavioral outcome. One important possibility noted previously in this chapter is the connection to emotional and behavioral outcome by way of social-cognitive development. Thus, a second line of inquiry may be to explore the hypothetical connection between nonverbal communication and social-cognitive development. The importance of this line of research in studies is increasingly well recognized in the literature (e.g., Moore & Corkum, 1994; Mundy, 1995; Tomasello, 1995).

A third important line of inquiry also exists. Measures of nonverbal communication may reflect important and stable aspects of children's early emotional and temperamental status and, therefore, may be directly predictive of emotional and behavioral outcome. The single most important study for future research in this regard involves a direct test of this hypothesis that individual differences on nonverbal measures of joint attention, behavior regulation, or social-interaction skills obtained in the second year of life contribute to the prediction of behavioral outcome in the third, fourth, or fifth year of life. Other hypotheses, such as those previously enumerated about the relationships among nonverbal communication, attachment, and behavioral outcome, may be useful to pursue as well. However, the first and most important step is to determine if the link between nonverbal communication and behavioral outcome can be established. We are working toward this goal in a longitudinal study of 120 infants with prenatal exposure to cocaine who are being followed from birth through the preschool period. Thus, we will soon see whether the theory espoused in this chapter can stand up to the rigors of empirical scrutiny.

CONCLUSION

This chapter has argued that the study and assessment of nonverbal communication skill development, especially in the second year of life, may be of considerable value for research on early social-emotional development. Several systems of assessment of nonverbal communication skills have been developed. However, these assessments often are considered only in conjunction with research on language development. Nevertheless, research and theory strongly suggest that nonverbal communication development may reflect processes that are critical to adaptive and maladaptive social-cognitive and social-emotional development in preschool children.

To illustrate this point, Stern's (1985) theory on early intersubjectivity and affective attunement between caregivers and young children was described as possibly being related to the development of nonverbal communication skills. A social motivational model of joint attention development was described, and extrapolated from this model was the hypothesis that joint attention and attachment measures may be complementary but independent predictors of behavior development in preschool children. At the outset, though, it was noted that the model presented in this chapter did not do justice to the numerous possible connections between early nonverbal communication and subsequent social-emotional development in children. The authors hope this chapter serves to encourage others to begin to examine these potentially important linkages in early development.

REFERENCES

Adamson, L., & Bakeman, R. (1985). Affect and attention: Infants observed with mothers and peers. *Child Development, 56,* 582–593.

Adamson, L., & Bakeman, R. (1991). The development of shared attention during infancy. In R. Vasta (Ed.), *Annals of child development,* (Vol. 8, pp. 1–41). London, UK: Jessica Kingsley Publishers, Ltd.

Ainsworth, M., & Bell, S. (1970). Attachment, exploration and separation: Illustrated by behavior of one-year-olds in a strange situation. *Child Development, 56,* 582–593.

Bakeman, R., & Adamson, L. (1984). Coordinating attention to people and objects in mother–infant and peer–infant interactions. *Child Development, 55,* 1278–1289.

Baker, L., & Cantwell, D. (1987). A prospective psychiatric follow-up of children with speech/language disorders. *Journal of the American Academy of Child and Adolescent Psychiatry, 26,* 546–553.

Baron-Cohen, S. (1989). Joint-attention deficits in autism: Towards a cognitive analysis. *Development and Psychopathology, 3,* 185–191.

Bates, E., Benigni, L., Bretherton, I., Camaioni, L., & Volterra, V. (1979). *The emergence of symbols: Cognition and communication in infancy.* New York: Academic Press.

Bates, E., Camaioni, L., & Volterra, V. (1975). The acquisition of performative prior to speech. *Merrill-Palmer Quarterly, 21,* 205–224.

Beitchman, J.H., Hood, J., & Inglis, A. (1990). Psychiatric risk in children with speech and language disorders. *Journal of Abnormal Child Psychology, 18,* 283–296.

Bretherton, I., Bates, E., Benigni, L., Camaioni, L., & Volterra, V. (1979). Relationship between cognition, communication and quality of attachment. In E. Bates, L. Benigni, I. Bretherton, L. Camaioni, & V. Volterra, *The emergence of symbols: Cognition and communication in infancy* (pp. 223–269). New York: Academic Press.

Bretherton, I., McNew, S., & Beeghly-Smith, M. (1981). Early person knowledge as expressed in verbal and gestural communication: When do infants acquire a theory of mind? In M. Lamb & L. Sherrod (Eds.), *Infant social cognition* (pp. 333–373). Hillsdale, NJ: Lawrence Erlbaum Associates.

Bruner, J. (1975). From communication to language: A psychological perspective. *Cognition, 3,* 255–287.

Bruner, J. (1981). Learning how to do things with words. In J. Bruner & A. Garton (Eds.), *Human growth and development* (pp. 62–84). London: Oxford University Press.

Bruner, J., & Sherwood, V. (1983). Thought, language and interaction in infancy. In J. Call, E. Galenson, & R. Tyson (Eds.), *Frontiers of infant psychiatry* (pp. 38–55). New York: Basic Books.

Butterworth, G., & Jarrett, N. (1991). What minds have in common is space: Spatial mechanisms serving joint visual attention in infancy. *British Journal of Developmental Psychology, 9,* 55–72.

Caplan, R., Chugani, H., Messa, C., Guthrie, D., Sigman, M., Traversay, J., & Mundy, P. (1993). Hemispherectomy for early onset intractable seizures: Presurgical cerebral glucose metabolism and postsurgical nonverbal communication patterns. *Developmental Medicine and Child Neurology, 35,* 582–592.

Capps, L., Sigman, M., & Mundy, P. (1994). Attachment security in children with autism. *Development and Psychopathology, 6,* 249–261.

Davidson, R., Ekman, P., Saron, C., Senulis, J., & Friesen, W. (1990). Approach-withdrawal and cerebral asymmetry: Emotion expression and brain physiology. *Journal of Personality and Social Psychology, 58,* 330–341.

Dawson, G. (1994). Development of emotional expression and emotion regulation in infancy: Contribution of the frontal lobe. In G. Dawson & K. Fischer (Eds.), *Human behavior and the developing brain* (pp. 518–536). New York: Guilford Press.

Dodge, K. (1986). A social information processing model of social competence in children. In M. Perlmutter (Ed.), *Minnesota symposium on child psychology* (Vol. 18, pp. 72–125). Hillsdale, NJ: Lawrence Erlbaum Associates.

Dunham, P., Dunham, F., & Curwin, A. (1993). Joint-attentional states and lexical acquisition at 18 months. *Developmental Psychology, 29,* 827–831.

Flanagan, P., Coppa, D., Riggs, S., & Alaro, A. (1994). Communication behaviors of teen mothers. *Journal of Adolescent Health, 15,* 169–175.

Fotheringham, J. (1991). Autism: Its primary psychological and neurological deficit. *Canadian Journal of Psychiatry, 36,* 686–692.

Fox, N. (1991). It's not left, it's right: Electroencephalograph asymmetry and the development of emotion. *American Psychologist, 46,* 863–872.

Golinkoff, R. (1983). The preverbal negotiation of failed messages: Insights into the transition period. In R. Golinkoff (Ed.), *The transition from prelinguistic to linguistic communication* (pp. 57–78). Hillsdale, NJ: Lawrence Erlbaum Associates.

Hobson, P. (1993). *Autism and the development of mind.* Hillsdale, NJ: Lawrence Erlbaum Associates.

Howlin, P., & Rutter, M. (1987). The consequences of language delay for other aspects of development. In W. Yule & M. Rutter (Eds.), *Language development and language disorders* (pp. 103–131). Philadelphia: J.B. Lippincott.

Ickes, W., Tooke, W., Stinson, L., Baker, V., & Bissonette, V. (1988). Social cognition: Intersubjectivity in same sex dyads. *Journal of Nonverbal Behavior, 12,* 58–84.

Jones, S., Collins, K., & Hong, H. (1991). An audience effect on smile production in 10-month-old infants. *Psychological Science, 2,* 45–49.

Jones, S., & Raag, R. (1989). Smile production in older infants: The importance of a social recipient for the facial signal. *Child Development, 60,* 811–818.

Kasari, C., Sigman, M., Mundy, P., & Yirmiya, N. (1988). Caregiver interactions with autistic children. *Journal of Abnormal Child Psychology, 16,* 45–56.

Kasari, C., Sigman, M., Mundy, P., & Yirmiya, N. (1990). Affective sharing in the context of joint attention interactions of normal, autistic and mentally retarded children. *Journal of Autism and Developmental Disorders, 20,* 87–100.

Krug, D., Arick, J., & Almond, P. (1979). Autism screening instrument for educational planning: Background and development. In J. Gilliam (Ed.), *Autism: Diagnosis, instruction, management and research* (pp. 117–126). Austin: Texas University Press.

Loveland, K., & Landry, S. (1986). Joint attention and language in autism and developmental language delay. *Journal of Autism and Developmental Disorders, 16,* 335–349.

Main, M., Tomasini, L., & Tolon, W. (1979). Differences among mothers of infants judged to differ in security. *Developmental Psychology, 15,* 472–473.

McEvoy, R., Rogers, S., & Pennington, R. (1993). Executive function and social communication deficits in young, autistic children. *Journal of Child Psychology and Psychiatry, 34,* 563–578.

Moore, C., & Corkum, V. (1994). Social understanding at the end of the first year of life. *Developmental Review, 14,* 349–372.

Mundy, P. (1995). Joint attention and social emotional approach behavior in children with autism. *Development and Psychopathology, 7,* 63–82.

Mundy, P., & Gomes, A. (1996, April). *Responding to joint attention bids and language development.* Paper presented at the 10th Biennial International Conference on Infant Studies, Providence, RI.

Mundy, P., & Gomes, A. (1997). A skills approach to early language development: Lessons from research on developmental disabilities. In L. Adamson & M. Romski (Eds.), *Research on communication and language disorders: Contributions to theories of language development* (pp. 107–132). Baltimore: Paul H. Brookes Publishing Co.

Mundy, P., & Hogan, A. (1994). Joint attention, intersubjectivity and autistic psychopathology. In D. Cicchetti & S. Toth (Eds.), *Rochester symposium on developmental psychopathology: Disorder and dysfunction of the self* (pp. 1–31). Rochester, NY: University of Rochester Press.

Mundy, P., Kasari, C., & Sigman, M. (1992). Nonverbal communication, affective sharing, and intersubjectivity. *Infant Behavior and Development, 15,* 377–381.

Mundy, P., Kasari, C., Sigman, M., & Ruskin, E. (1995). Nonverbal communication and early language acquisition in children with Down syndrome or normal development. *Journal of Speech and Hearing Research, 38,* 157–167.

Mundy, P., Seibert, J., & Hogan, A. (1985). Communication skills in mentally retarded children. In M. Sigman (Ed.), *Children with emotional disorders and developmental disabilities* (pp. 45–70). New York: Grune & Stratton.

Mundy, P., Sigman, M., & Kasari, C. (1990). A longitudinal study of joint attention and language development in autistic children. *Journal of Autism and Developmental Disorders, 20,* 115–123.

Mundy, P., Sigman, M., & Kasari, C. (1993). The theory of mind and joint attention deficits in autism. In S. Baron-Cohen, H. Tager-Flusberg, & D. Cohen (Eds.), *Understanding other minds: Perspectives from autism* (pp. 181–203). Oxford, England: Oxford University Press.

Mundy, P., Sigman, M., & Kasari, C. (1994). Joint attention, developmental level, and symptom presentation in young children with autism. *Development and Psychopathology, 6,* 389–401.

Mundy, P., Sigman, M., Kasari, C., & Yirmiya, N. (1988). Nonverbal communication skills in Down syndrome children. *Child Development, 59,* 235–249.

Mundy, P., Sigman, M., Ungerer, J.A., & Sherman, T. (1986). Defining the social deficits in autism: The contribution of non-verbal communication measures. *Journal of Child Psychology and Psychiatry, 27,* 657–669.

Olson, S., Bates, J., & Bales, K. (1984). Mother–infant interaction and the development of individual differences in children's cognitive competence. *Developmental Psychology, 20,* 166–179.

Panksepp, J., & Sahley, T. (1987). Possible brain opioid involvement in disrupted social intent and language development of autism. In E. Schopler & G. Mesibov (Eds.), *Neurobiological issues in autism* (pp. 357–372). New York: Plenum.

Papoušek, H., Papoušek, M., Suomi, S., & Rahn, C. (1991). Preverbal communication and attachment: Comparative views. In J. Gerwitz & W. Kurtines (Eds.), *Intersections with attachment* (pp. 97–122). Hillsdale, NJ: Lawrence Erlbaum Associates.

Paul, R. (1991). Profiles of toddlers with slow expressive language development. *Topics in Language Disorder, 11,* 1–13.

Paul, R., & Shiffer, M. (1991). Communicative initiations in normal and late-talking toddlers. *Applied Psycholinguistics, 12,* 419–431.

Rheingold, H., Hay, D., & West, M. (1976). Sharing in the second year of life. *Child Development, 83,* 898–913.

Scaife, M., & Bruner, J. (1975). The capacity for joint visual attention in the infant. *Nature, 253,* 265–266.

Schopler, E., & Mesibov, G. (Eds.). (1987). *Neurobiological issues in autism.* New York: Plenum.

Seibert, J.M., Hogan, A.E., & Mundy, P. (1982). Assessing interactional competencies: The Early Social-Communication Scales. *Infant Mental Health Journal, 3,* 244–245.

Seibert, J.M., Hogan, A.E., & Mundy, P. (1987). Assessing social and communication skills in infancy. *Topics in Early Childhood Education, 7*(2), 38–48.

Sigman, M., & Mundy, P. (1989). Social attachments in autistic children. *Journal of the American Academy of Child and Adolescent Psychiatry, 28,* 74–81.

Snyder, L. (1978). Communicative and cognitive abilities in the sensorimotor period. *Merrill-Palmer Quarterly, 24,* 161–180.

Stern, D. (1985). *The interpersonal world of the infant.* New York: Basic Books.

Sugarman, S. (1984). The development of proverbial communication. In R.L. Schiefelbusch & J. Pickar (Eds.), *The acquisition of communicative competence* (pp. 23–67). Baltimore: University Park Press.

Tomasello, M. (1988). The role of joint attention in early language development. *Language Sciences, 11,* 69–88.

Tomasello, M. (1995). Joint attention as social cognition. In C. Moore & P. Dunham (Eds.), *Joint attention: Its origins and role in development* (pp. 103–131). Hillsdale, NJ: Lawrence Erlbaum Associates.

Tomasello, M., & Farrar, J. (1986). Joint attention and early language. *Child Development, 57,* 1454–1463.

Wellman, H. (1993). Early understanding of the mind: The normal case. In S. Baron-Cohen, H. Tager-Flusberg, & D. Cohen (Eds.), *Understanding other minds: Perspectives from autism* (pp. 40–58). Oxford, England: Oxford University Press.

Wetherby, A.M., & Prizant, B.M. (1993a). *Communication and Symbolic Behavior Scales: Normed ed.* Chicago: Applied Symbolix.

Wetherby, A.M., & Prizant, B. (1993b). Profiling communication and symbolic abilities in young children. *Journal of Childhood Communication Disorders, 15,* 23–32.

Wetherby, A.M., & Prutting, C.A. (1984). Profiles of communicative and cognitive-social abilities in autistic children. *Journal of Speech and Hearing Research, 27,* 367–377.

Wetherby, A.M., Yonclas, D., & Bryan, A. (1989). Communicative profiles of handicapped preschool children: Implications for early identification. *Journal of Speech and Hearing Disorders, 54,* 148–158.

7

The Ontogeny and
Role of Repair Strategies

Amy M. Wetherby,
Dianne G. Alexander, and Barry M. Prizant

REBECCA WAS RIDING IN THE car with her mother in downtown Tallahassee. Rebecca, who was 20 months old, pointed out the window and excitedly exclaimed, "/fag, fag/" to direct her mother's attention to a spectacle in the distance. Her mother could not figure out what Rebecca was referring to and said, "What?" Rebecca repeated her vocalization "/fag, fag/" and continued pointing. Her mother still could not determine what she was referring to and again asked "What?" Rebecca continued pointing but then said, "/tag, tag/." Finally realizing what Rebecca was pointing to, her mother then said, "Oh, pretty flag! Look at all the flags," as they drove by the capitol building. Her mother was able to identify the referent once Rebecca reverted to her previous form of /tag/ for the word "flag." Her new approximation of /fag/ was not clear enough for her mother to recognize. Rebecca's ability to persist in her communicative goal and to modify the form of her communicative signal ensured that her intention was understood.

The example of Rebecca modifying her utterance to clarify her intention is a sophisticated repair strategy used by a competent young communicator. A repair can be defined as the ability to persist in communication and to modify or revise a signal when faced with a breakdown in communication (Wetherby & Prizant, 1993). A communicative breakdown can occur if the speaker's intended goal is not achieved either because the message is not responded to or is not understood. The ability to repair communicative breakdowns develops very early. It is dependent on at least two significant developmental achievements: 1) a child's repertoire of communicative means to express intentions; and 2) the child's awareness of the need to persist and, if necessary, to modify or revise the signal if the communicative partner does not respond as desired. With the acquisition of words, the child has access to an ever-growing variety of verbal means to clarify intentions.

This chapter examines the ontogeny of repair strategies of young children from early gestural stages of communication beginning at the transition to intentional communication through early linguistic stages of communication development. Explanatory theories on the ontogeny of repairs are considered and developmental patterns of repair strategies are described by reviewing research on preverbal as well as verbal children at more advanced linguistic stages. The chapter then presents developmental findings on the use of repair strategies in young children ranging from the prelinguistic to early stages of verbal development, based on the research of the authors of this chapter. Research on repair strategies of individuals with communication disabilities is examined. The chapter closes with a discussion of clinical and research implications.

DEVELOPMENT OF INTENTIONALITY
AND ROLE OF COMMUNICATIVE REPAIRS

Communicative repair is a behavior that reflects and is dependent on a child's social awareness and emotional regulation and is an index of the degree of intentionality or goal directedness in communication. Consequently, it is an important measure of the interrelationship of a child's developing socioemotional and communicative systems. Children begin to repair at the same time they begin to produce intentional communication. This supports the concept that children are "active and creative participants" (Bates, Bretherton, & Snyder, 1988, p. 3) in the process of acquiring language.

Bates's (1979) work identified behavioral indices from which communicative intent may be inferred. Infant communicative behaviors initially are produced in reaction to internal physiological states and are interpreted by the listener without the infant's awareness or intent. A child is considered to be an intentional communicator when he or she develops an awareness "*a priori* of the effect that a signal will have on [the] listener, and [develops persistence] in that behavior until the effect is obtained or failure is clearly indicated" (Bates, 1979, p. 36). Bates's description of intentional communication mentions two important indices: 1) the child's awareness of the communicative signal's effect and 2) the child's ability to persist in signaling the communicative behavior.

The ability to use repair signals may emerge in the same manner as other communicative behaviors, from preintentional to intentional. Brazelton (1982) described infant behaviors that are probably not intentional but that are potent in their ability to "fix" interactions. As early as 4–6 weeks after a baby is born, the parent–child dyad functions in such a way that the infant's behavior communicates a need for alterations in parental input. Using the "still face" situation, Tronick, Als, Adamson, Wise, and Brazelton (1978) described infants' use of affect displays to alter their mother's inappropriate and unexpected response (Conn & Tronick, 1982). Mothers were directed to sit in front of their infants, expressionless and unresponsive. Their 1- to 4-month-old babies exhibited an intense reaction that demonstrated not only the importance of interactional reciprocity but also demonstrated the infants' abilities to regulate their affect to achieve the social goals of the interaction.

As the communicative development of children emerges in the context of regulation of emotion and social interactions with others, it also develops in relation to the child's emergence as an intentional being (see Chapters 2 and 6). Wetherby and Prizant (1989) suggested that rather than considering intentionality as an all-or-none achievement, it may be viewed along a continuum in the following manner: 1) absence of awareness of a goal; 2) awareness of the goal; 3) simple plan to achieve the goal; 4) coordinated plan to achieve the goal; 5) alternative plan to achieve the goal; and 6) metapragmatic awareness of the plan to achieve the goal. Several of the indices that account for increasing intentionality involve Bates's (1979) concepts of increasing awareness and persistence and are reflected in the child's repair behaviors. The emergence of alternative plans to achieve the goal requires that the child be able to repeat or modify his or her failed communicative signal, that is, to repair his or her communication.

It appears, then, that the emergence of communicative repairs is a direct result of a process that involves socioemotional, communicative, and cognitive development and is a significant achievement closely related to the transition to intentional communication. However, determining the presence or absence of intentionality is a continuing problem. A dilemma exists over identifying a boundary between the perlocutionary (i.e., preintentional) and illocutionary (i.e., intentional) stages of communication development. The presence of at least rudimentary efforts to repair may provide the hallmark for the transition to intentional communication.

Thus, the ability to repair communicative breakdowns clearly reflects the intention to communicate. Bretherton (1992) described gestural communicative exchanges between preverbal children and their mothers to illustrate the child's communicative intentionality. Bretherton found that it was the children's persistence and communicative repairs that provided striking support for the intentionality of their messages. Bretherton further argued that the infant's ability to produce and understand intentional gestures provides evidence for the emergence of "intersubjective understanding" (1992, p. 63). This development is important for the understanding of communicative repairs.

When communicative partners interact to intentionally exchange messages about a common topic, they exhibit intersubjectivity or the interfacing of minds through conventional signals (Bretherton, 1992; Trevarthen & Hubley, 1978). This achievement implies that the infant possesses two important capacities: 1) the ability to understand others as psychological beings and 2) the knowledge that others can be deliberately influenced through intentional signals (Bretherton & Bates, 1979). These capacities reflect the acquisition of a "theory of mind," which means that along with the emergence of intentionality (including the ability to persist and repair), the infant is able to impute mental states to self and others (Bretherton, 1992). A child's ability to clarify messages for the listener is evidence of a theory of mind. An example of preverbal negotiation provided by Golinkoff (1986) illustrates the emergence of a theory of mind. At age 14 months, Jordan vocalizes to get his mother's attention and then points to request a toy out of reach. His mother offers him the wrong toy, and he shakes his head NO and continues pointing. His mother then offers him another toy, and he rejects it. Finally, his mother offers him the requested toy, and he is content. Jordan's preverbal negotiation suggests that he is aware that his mother is trying to discover his communicative goal. The presence of a theory of mind presupposes the ability and social motivation to use repair behaviors, which provide support for intentionality, and an awareness of the mental states of others, which is necessary for the application of repairs.

The communicative repair is acquired as an ability that reflects emerging intentionality. It provides a window into the child's socioemotional as well as communicative, linguistic, and cognitive development. The child's competence as a communicator is both a result of and an indicator of developing social, emotional, and communicative systems. This competence is first noted as the child develops communicative intentionality and awareness of his or her listener and continues to develop as efforts to achieve communicative goals are made through persistence and modification of signaling.

DEVELOPMENTAL PATTERNS OF REPAIR STRATEGIES

Young children rely on preverbal communication to clarify intentions and to repair breakdowns; that is, children have a variety of gestures, vocalizations, or both, which may be used to achieve communicative goals. The following two examples of preverbal repairs illustrate how young typically developing children with limited communicative repertoires negotiate meaning.

At 14 months of age, Michelle, in the early one-word stage, communicated with a large repertoire of preverbal gestures and vocalizations and a small number of word approximations. Michelle was seated at a table between her mother and an unfamiliar adult. The adult engaged Michelle with a kangaroo windup toy, and together they shared the spectacle of the kangaroo jumping until it stopped. Michelle held up the kangaroo and showed it to her mother while smiling. Then she gave the kangaroo to the adult and vocalized "uh uh" with a rising intonation to request the adult to wind it up. The adult then showed the kangaroo to Michelle, commented by saying, "kangaroo jump," and set the kangaroo on the table without winding it up. Michelle shifted her gaze between the adult and the kangaroo, then with great determination waved her arms up and down depicting the movement of the kangaroo in an attempt to clarify her request for the adult to wind up the toy. Michelle's use of a depictive gesture at 14 months of age was an impressive repair strategy that reflected her persistence in pursuing her goal to request action as well as her ingenuity in clarifying her meaning.

At 11 months of age, Robbie was in the prelinguistic stage and communicated with a variety of conventional gestures (e.g., giving and showing objects) and some vocalizations. Like Michelle, Robbie was interacting with his mother and another adult. Robbie's mother engaged him with a kangaroo windup toy, and they watched it together. When the kangaroo stopped jumping, Robbie gave the kangaroo to his mother. She wound it up and, subsequently, the kangaroo jumped again. They both laughed heartily. When the kangaroo stopped, Robbie again gave it to his mother, clearly requesting recurrence of this activity. This time his mother set the kangaroo on the table without winding it up and commented, "kangaroo." Robbie looked at the kangaroo, looked at his mother, and looked back at the kangaroo. Then he picked up the kangaroo and gave it to the second adult. This repair strategy reflects Robbie's persistence in pursuing his communicative goal. Although Robbie did not change his means of communicating (i.e., he again used a giving gesture to request action), he did direct his communication to a different person when his mother did not respond. Thus, even by the end of the first year, preverbal children demonstrate abilities in repairing breakdowns in communication. These examples provide qualitative information about repairs used by prelinguistic children and suggest developmental patterns of the emergence of repair strategies.

Research on Preverbal Repair Behaviors

Although verbal repair strategies have received much attention in the literature, few studies have examined repairs used by preverbal children. Golinkoff (1986) conducted a hallmark study of the preverbal repair strategies of three typically developing children. She sampled the children's communication shortly after their first birthday and then again two more times at about 2-month intervals. Each sample was about 30 minutes during lunchtime with the child positioned in a high chair and the mother nearby. Golinkoff identified three types of communicative episodes: 1) *immediate successes,* when the mother understood the child's intention; 2) *missed attempts,* when the mother failed to respond to the child's signal; and 3) *negotiations,* when the mother failed to understand the meaning initially and helped the child to clarify his or her intention. Golinkoff found that a mean of 49% of the communicative interactions were negotiation episodes, whereas 13% were missed attempts, and 38% were immediate successes over all three samples. The relative proportion of negotiation episodes and missed attempts decreased from the first to the third sample, whereas that of immediate successes increased.

A negotiation episode commenced following the child's initial signal, when the mother failed to comprehend and respond appropriately. The children then repaired, protested, or abandoned the communicative goal. A negotiation episode terminated with an outcome of success, compromise, or failure to accomplish the goal. It is noteworthy that the negotiation episodes consisted of an average of 7.3 turns, which reflect the perseverance of these young children in spite of their limited communicative repertoire. Golinkoff (1986) found that the percentage of repairs that occurred during negotiation episodes increased from

26% in the first sample to 42% in the third sample, whereas the percentage of protests decreased from 22% to 4%.

In Golinkoff's (1986) study, a child's repair was coded as either a repetition or a modification of the previous signal. A modification consisted of either an addition to the previous signal or a change to a different signal. Golinkoff found that about 36% of the repairs were repetitions, and 32% were additions, with minimal differences in the proportions across the three samples. The use of changes to repair increased from 13% in the first sample to 32% in the third sample, which is likely associated with the child's increasing communicative repertoire.

In this study, children relied on a limited repertoire of communicative signals, including pointing, reaching, giving, showing, vocalizing, and idiosyncratic gestures. The ability to indicate the object of reference greatly enhanced the mothers' abilities to comprehend the message. The children focused the mothers' attention to objects of interest by either leaning toward the object, gesturing with the object, or naming the object. The use of words occurred in 7% of negotiation episodes and 22% of immediate successes. Thus, words occurred three times more often in immediate successes than in negotiation episodes; however, the use of words did not guarantee success.

Directed eye gaze toward the mother also assisted the mothers' comprehension of the children's intentions. Children directed gaze to their mothers most often during immediate successes, and directed gaze increased in negotiation episodes from 37% in the first sample to 53% in the third sample. In contrast, the children directed gaze toward the desired object and not at their mothers for 83% of the initial signals of negotiation episodes during the first sample, which decreased to 33% in the third sample. Thus, as they acquired more skill in obtaining and checking their mother's attention with visual regard over the three samples, children's successful communication increased.

The findings of Golinkoff (1986) indicated that as children develop during the preverbal stage of intentional communication, their repair attempts increase. She demonstrated that typically developing young children were frequently faced with failed communicative attempts, even with familiar caregivers, and more often than not tried to negotiate the failed messages by repeating the signal or adding something to the initial signal. Golinkoff found that it was less likely for prelinguistic children to change to a different signal.

Few other investigations have examined the presence of early persistence and repairs in intentional, preverbal communicators (Bretherton, 1992). A study by Ross and Kay (1980) of mother–infant play found that 12-month-olds used a variety of strategies to revive failed turn-taking games that had been stopped by an adult. The infants exhibited repair strategies including gaze alternation between the adult and the toy, retaking of their own turn and then waiting, and use of gestures (e.g., holding up their hands) to invite a turn from the adult.

Research on Repair Strategies in Verbal Children

Because of the paucity of research on preverbal repairs, this chapter examines research findings on verbal repairs in an attempt to identify developmental patterns of repair strategies at linguistic stages. Early conversational competence requires the successful use of language in communicating over multiple turns and depends on the ability to repair communicative failures. Opportunities for communicative breakdowns are pervasive in the midst of communicative attempts. Brinton and Fujiki (1989) noted that "production is sprinkled with false starts, incomplete constructions, and ill-formed utterances. Comprehension often is hampered by distraction, inattention, or misperception" (p. 63). Without communicative repairs, successful communication in conversation is unlikely.

The form and content of verbal communicative repairs vary according to the skills of the communicative partners and which partner takes responsibility for rectifying the breakdown. Schegloff, Jefferson, and Sacks (1977) provided four categories that described communicative repairs according to who initiated the repair and who provided the clarification:

1. *Other-initiated self-repairs* occur when the speaker produces an unclear message, the listener requests clarification, and the speaker provides it.
2. *Self-initiated self-repairs* occur when the speaker produces an unclear or unsuccessful communication, identifies it, and repairs it.
3. *Other-initiated other-repairs* occur when the listener identifies an unclear utterance and repairs it him- or herself.
4. *Self-initiated other-repairs* occur when the speaker identifies his or her unclear utterance but the listener provides the repair.

Most research has examined the other-initiated self-repairs of verbal children as examples of conversational monitoring in children during linguistic stages of development. Gallagher (1977) examined patterns of repairs in the speech of 18 typically developing children, 6 in each of Brown's language stages, Stages I, II, and III. Brown's (1973) stages begin at the point when children combine words and are defined by major changes in syntactic development that correlate with mean length of utterance (MLU) measured in morphemes. Children in Brown's Stage I had a mean age of 21 months and mean MLU of 1.5; children in Stage II had a mean age of 23 months and mean MLU of 2.2; and children in Stage III had a mean age of 29 months and mean MLU of 2.9. Each child was presented with the query "What?" about 20 times during a 1-hour language sample with an experimenter who pretended to misunderstand.

Gallagher (1977) found that, regardless of language stage, the children modified linguistic form to repair their misunderstood messages 77% of the time and failed to respond only 2% of the time. Patterns of modified repairs were evident across language stages. Modifications were coded as phonetic changes, additions, reductions, and substitutions in the following manner:

- Phonetic change indicated that the phonetic shape of any element in the child's original utterance differed from the phonetic shape of that element in his or her response utterance.
- Addition indicated that a morpheme not appearing in the original utterance was added.
- Reduction indicated that a morpheme appearing in the original utterance did not appear in the repair.
- Substitution indicated that a word in the child's repair replaced a word in the original utterance while maintaining the original word's major grammatical and semantic features.

Additions occurred 30% of the time across all language stages. Even at Stage I of language development, children seemed to appreciate that adding linguistic elements to an utterance was an effective strategy to repair breakdowns. Significant differences were evident across language stages in the proportion of the other three categories of modification.

The majority of modifications used by children in Stage I were either additions or phonetic changes, with the latter being the most frequent. The repair strategy used by Rebecca as described previously (i.e., replacing/fag/with/tag/) is an example of a phonetic change. Gallagher (1977) theorized that the reliance on phonetic changes at this stage of language development was due to the primitive organization of the child's language system. Other structural options for modification were simply not available to the unsophisticated users of language.

The majority of modifications used by children in Stage II were additions and reductions. The modifications produced at this stage seem to reflect the development of the language system in general. Both additions and reductions used the same linguistic elements (i.e., modifiers of the object-noun phrase and verb). If the modifier was added to the utterance as an addition, it served to clarify the message. If it had been present in the original utterance, its deletion served to focus attention on the major information-bearing elements.

Children operating in Brown's Stage III employed three major modification behaviors: additions, reductions, and substitutions. Unique to children in Stage III was the high frequency of substitutions (30%). Because substitutions occurred with markedly less frequency at Stage I (13%) and Stage II (14%), the findings indicate that substituting elements requires greater language sophistication than simply adding or deleting elements.

Gallagher's (1977) study indicated that as children's knowledge of language structure developed, any one of the modification strategies could be used. At Stage I, only one modification strategy accounted for 45% of the children's repairs; children in Stage II tended to use two strategies; and children in Stage III employed three strategies with approximately equal frequency.

The form of the request for repairs also has been found to influence the type of repairs. Wilcox and Webster (1980), using procedures similar to Gallagher's (1977), compared children's responses with different requests for clarifications and found that "What?" was more likely to elicit repetitions and commenting on the object requested, whereas "Yes, I see it" was more likely to elicit modifications. Gallagher (1981) identified three types of requests for clarification: 1) requests for confirmation (e.g., "You want this cookie?"); 2) general queries (e.g., "What?"); and 3) specific queries (e.g., "Which one do you want?"). She found that typically developing children as young as 2 years of age were able to respond differentially to different types of queries but that specific requests were more difficult.

The familiarity of the interactant also has been found to influence repairs used by young children. Tomasello, Farrar, and Dines (1984) studied repairs of ten 2-year-old children in each of Brown's Stages I and II, interacting with their mothers and with an unfamiliar adult. Both adults provided about a dozen misunderstandings of children's requests by saying, "What do you want?" Tomasello et al. found that children in both stages with both interactants repeated their original request about 35% of the time and modified their request about 65% of the time. Differences were found in the types of modifications. Children in Brown's Stage I were more likely to use reductions to modify with their mothers, which made the key word more salient, and use substitutions as well as additions with the unfamiliar adult. By Stage II, the children's modifications were more evenly distributed among reductions, substitutions, and additions. These findings indicate that very young children are able to consider the needs of the listener to modify their messages.

Some investigators have examined conversational repairs used by verbal children in relation to level of linguistic functioning (e.g., Brinton, Fujiki, Loeb, & Winkler, 1986; Brinton, Fujiki, & Sonnenberg, 1988; Gallagher & Darnton, 1978; Kahmi & Koenig, 1985; Purcell & Liles, 1992). These studies found that a developmental pattern exists both in a child's responsiveness to requests for clarification and in pragmatic abilities to appreciate and consider how to clarify the message for the listener, consistent with the findings of Gallagher (1977). Furthermore, the ability to respond to several requests for clarification in sequence (i.e., a stacked repair sequence) continues to develop in older children (Brinton et al., 1986). Investigating the effective use of linguistic structures to negotiate and achieve successful communication is an important part of the process for understanding the development of conversational competence. This line of research needs to be extended to prelinguistic development.

NORMATIVE STUDY OF REPAIR STRATEGIES

Since the 1970s, much research and theory has focused on preverbal communication; however, little is known about developmental patterns of preverbal repairs. In light of the potential importance of understanding and enhancing repairs in prelinguistic children, further research is needed in this area. Because of the limited research on preverbal repairs, Alexander (1994) conducted a cross-sectional study of the ontogeny of repair strategies using the normative samples from the Communication and Symbolic Behavior Scales (CSBS) (Wetherby & Prizant, 1993). The CSBS is a standardized assessment instrument designed to examine communicative, social/affective, and symbolic abilities of children whose functional communication abilities range from prelinguistic intentional communication to early stages of language acquisition (i.e., a developmental level of between 8 and 24 months). The CSBS uses a standard but flexible format for gathering data through a combination of a caregiver questionnaire and behavior sampling procedures. The direct child assessment involves varying degrees of relatively structured and unstructured sampling procedures that resemble natural adult–child interactions and provide opportunities for documenting a child's use of a variety of communicative and symbolic behaviors. The caregiver is present during the entire sample and is encouraged to respond naturally to the child's bids for interaction. During the CSBS sampling procedures, opportunities for repair are created when a child's communicative attempts are not responded to as intended. The child's ability to persist and repair then can be examined.

Normative data on a sample of more than 300 typically developing American-English–speaking children from 8 to 24 months of age and 30 children with developmental disabilities from 18 to 30 months of age have been published (Wetherby & Prizant, 1993). In addition to norms referenced to chronological age, the CSBS presents norms based on language stages that include the prelinguistic, early one-word, late one-word, and multiword stages. The definitions of these language stages are presented in Table 1.

Analysis of Repair Signals

Alexander (1994) selected videotaped communication samples of 120 children from the normative samples collected during the field-testing of the CSBS to study repairs in greater depth than was analyzed during the standard scoring procedures. The tapes for this study were sampled such that there were 30 children in each of the four language stages with a mean age comparable to the mean age of each group of children in the normative samples. The mean ages of the chil-

Table 1. Definitions of language stages based on the use of words and word combinations during the CSBS

Language stage	Number of different words	Number of different word combinations
Prelinguistic	0 to 1	0 to 1
Early one-word	2 to 5	0 to 1
Late one-word	6 to 9	0 to 1
Multiword	10 or more	2 or more

From Wetherby, A.M., & Prizant, B.M. (1993). *Communication and Symbolic Behavior Scales manual* (p. 56). Chicago: Applied Symbolix; reprinted by permission.

dren in the study were 12.4 months in the prelinguistic stage, 14.8 months in the early one-word stage, 18.1 months in the late one-word stage, and 20.7 months in the multiword stage.

To describe the development of repair signals in children across these language stages, only the segments of the CSBS samples designed to provide opportunities for repairs were analyzed and coded. These segments consist of four communicative temptations (i.e., the windup toy, balloon, bubbles, jar) during which the child's requests for activation of the toy, blowing up the balloon, blowing more bubbles, and opening the jar for more food were deliberately not responded to by the interactant according to the CSBS protocol in the following manner. Following the initial activation or presentation of the object to the child, the interactant responded to the child's first two communicative request signals for continuation of the activity. After the child's third communicative signal for continuation, the interactant purposely failed to comply with the child's request by commenting on the object and returning it to the child without activation or assistance. If the child persisted in his or her request, the next or fourth communicative signal was considered to be the communicative repair.

The child's third or failed communicative attempt and fourth or persistent communicative signal for each of the four communicative temptations were described in the following manner: The third communicative signal was coded as the referent act; the fourth signal was coded as the repair signal, a repetition or modification with reference to the preceding referent act. Failures to repair, given the opportunity to do so, were included in the analysis. If the child failed to produce two communicative request signals and/or if the interactant failed to provide an opportunity for the child to repair, those communicative temptations were not coded or included in the analysis. Thus, data were collected from most children on four repair opportunities and from other children on fewer opportunities. Therefore, the total repair opportunities were less than the total of 120 possible repair opportunities at each language stage (i.e., four communicative temptations per 30 children). It should be noted that the CSBS procedures provide a second repair opportunity after the first in each communicative temptation, if the child persists after the first repair. The response to the second repair opportunity was not included for analysis in this study.

Data were analyzed to determine whether repair attempts were repetitions or modifications along the parameters of form (i.e., gestures and vocalizations), content (i.e., words and phrases), and use (i.e., interactant and prosodic changes). Modified repair components were further described as additions, reductions, and changes (i.e., substitutions).

Developmental Patterns of Repair Strategies

One major finding was that 98% (118 of the 120 children) across all stages who communicated to request an action or object also produced at least one communicative repair when their request failed. Only two 8-month-old infants failed to persevere following their failed communicative requests. This important finding indicates that the ability to repair communicative breakdowns emerges essentially simultaneously with the emergence of intentional communicative functions.

This study also provided information about the types and patterns of repair behaviors used by children in the prelinguistic, early one-word, late one-word, and multiword stages of language development. The number and percentage of occurrence of no repair, repetition, modification, and total repair opportunities for all children in each language stage are presented in Table 2. The percentage of repair attempts ranged from 88% (81 of 92) in the prelinguistic stage to 93% (95 of 102) in the multiword stage. Consistent with the findings of Golinkoff (1986), these children attempted to repair the vast majority of their failed communicative attempts.

The use of repetition as a repair strategy increased from the prelinguistic to the early one-word stage and then decreased. The use of modifications was predominant in the prelinguistic stage and increased in frequency through the multiword stage. Repetition, as an overall repair strategy, was only used by 6% of the total participants as their only method of repair; however, exclusive use of repetitions to repair was more likely to occur with the developmentally younger children. Modification as a child's only repair strategy was used by 49% of the total participants. Thus, repetition only as the primary repair strategy appeared to decrease with development; exclusive use of modification to repair increased with development.

The use of gestural, vocal, word, and phrase repairs out of total repairs is summarized in Table 3. Developmental patterns are described in this section for form, content, and use variables.

Form Variables of Repair

Gestural Repairs   The overwhelming reliance by all of these children on gestural forms to repair was remarkable. Of the 118 children who exhibited communicative repairs, 100% of them used gestures as a component in one or more repairs. When the individual repair acts were summed across children in each language stage, it was found that about 95% of the repairs of children in prelinguistic, early one-word, and late one-word stages contained a gestural

Table 2.   Frequency and percentage of occurrence of no repairs, repetitions, modifications, and total repairs out of total repair opportunities for each language stage

	Prelinguistic	Early one-word	Late one-word	Multiword
No repairs	11 (12%)	4 (4%)	13 (12%)	7 (7%)
Repetitions	27 (29%)	42 (40%)	25 (19%)	17 (14%)
Modifications	54 (59%)	60 (57%)	69 (64%)	78 (76%)
Total repairs	81 (88%)	102 (96%)	94 (88%)	95 (93%)
Total repair opportunities	92	106	107	102

Table 3. Frequency and percentage of occurrence of gestural, vocal, word, and phrase repairs out of total repairs for each language stage

	Prelinguistic	Early one-word	Late one-word	Multiword
Form				
Gestural repairs	77 (95%)	96 (94%)	93 (99%)	90 (88%)
Vocal repairs	42 (52%)	64 (63%)	58 (54%)	70 (74%)
Content				
Word repairs	0 (0%)	3 (3%)	22 (23%)	16 (17%)
Phrase repairs	0 (0%)	0 (0%)	4 (4%)	37 (39%)
Total repairs	81	102	94	95

form; 88% of the repairs of multiword-stage children contained a gesture. Furthermore, gestures were used in the referent act and then abandoned in the repair less than 4% of the time across all stages.

Bates's (1979) research on the development of intentionality emphasized the importance of intentional gestures for prelinguistic communication. The gestural components of preconversational repairs appear to be equally important. The use of a depictive gesture, as described previously in the repair strategy of Michelle, is an example of a modified gestural repair and illustrates how explicit a child can be with the use of gestures before the emergence of words. This study demonstrated that gestural repairs are a critical component during the transition to intentional communication as well as the transition to symbolic communication.

At all stages of development, children repeated their gestures more often than they modified them. When gestures were modified at all stages of communicative development, the forms of the gestures were most likely to be changed. That is, rather than clarifying by adding or reducing gestural components, all of the children who did modify their gestures tended simply to try a different gesture.

Vocal Repairs In general, the use of vocal forms to repair increased developmentally as the spoken language skills of children emerged and became established. The percentage of children who used one or more vocal repairs increased from 83% of the prelinguistic children to almost 87% of the early and late one-word–stage children to more than 93% of the multiword-stage children. When the individual repair acts were summed across children in each language stage, it was found that the percentage of repairs that did not contain a vocal component decreased from 48% in the prelinguistic stage and 38% in the early and late one-word stage to 26% in the multiword stage. Furthermore, vocalizations were used in the referent act and then abandoned in the repair about 15% of the time in the prelinguistic stage, which decreased to 10% by the multiword stage. When comparing these findings with those of gestural repairs, it can be seen that the majority of repairs consisted of a gesture plus a vocalization and that the coordination of gesture and vocalization to repair increased with advancing language stage.

At all stages of development, children used vocal modifications more often than vocal repetitions to repair. The general trend was that at least twice as many vocal repairs were modified than were repeated across all language stages. Many of the children in this study lacked a reliably established phonological system. The vocal repair modifications of the developmentally younger participants consisted primarily of the addition of consonants, vowels, or both, which is likely related to the simplicity of the referent act. Children in the late one-word stage were about as likely to add phonemes as they were to simply change phonemes. The vocalizations of participants in the multiword stage usually contained a variety of different consonants in the referent act and, thus, were more likely to use vocal changes than additions or reductions.

Content Variables   Developmental patterns in the use of words to repair were identified. Word and phrase repairs rarely were used by the developmentally youngest children but were observed increasingly as a function of increasing vocabularies in more advanced stages of language development. However, even with increasing sophistication, 63% of the participants in the late one-word stage and 75% of the participants in the multiword stage failed to use words to repair; 84% of the late one-word–stage and 54% of the multiword-stage participants failed to use phrases to repair.

Children in the late one-word and multiword stages used at least twice as many word modifications as repetitions and three times as many phrase modifications as repetitions to repair. The two developmentally older groups used word modifications that were widely dispersed among the possibilities of word changes, additions, and reductions. The lack of a discernible pattern of word repair strategies may be an indication that the availability of a variety of repair strategies has emerged. Phrase modifications of the late one-word–stage children were rare but did occur when the children added or removed words. The multiword-stage children frequently used phrases to repair and were able to clarify their requests by changing their phrases or adding words to them.

Use Variables of Repair   Whether children's abilities to direct communicative acts to a different interactant to repair increased with development also was examined. The repair strategy used by Robbie, as described previously, which consisted of redirecting a request for action from his mother to another adult, is an example of an interactant change. A trend did emerge suggesting that communicating to another person "for help" may increase with development and concomitant experience. Proportions of participants who used interactant changes increased from 13% in the prelinguistic stage, to 17% in the early one-word stage, to 27% in the late one-word stage, and to 33% in the multiword stage. Changes in the use of prosodic features for repair were also examined. No developmental trends appeared; instead, approximately 20% of all the participants, regardless of language stage, used changes in prosody to repair. Thus, changes in interactant and prosody appear to be repair strategies used by some, but not all, children in the early stages of communication development and language acquisition.

Comparisons with Gallagher's (1977) Study In general, the results of Alexander's (1994) study are consistent with those of Gallagher (1977). Gallagher's study revealed three important patterns with regard to children who were all verbal communicators: 1) The majority of children modified rather than repeated their utterances to repair breakdowns; 2) with increasing development, children used increasing numbers of strategies to repair; and 3) children in Brown's Stage I tended to modify their vocalizations *or* add words or phrases to repair; children in Stage II tended to add *and* reduce words and phrases to repair; and children in Stage III tended to add, reduce, *and* change words and phrases to repair.

As a result of the communication levels of the participants and the organizational structure of Alexander's (1994) study, exact comparisons are not possible. The following patterns from Alexander's study, however, are consistent with those of Gallagher (1977): 1) The majority of children in this study modified rather than repeated their communication to repair breakdowns; however, these children were more likely to repeat gestures; 2) with increasing development, children have at their disposal increasing numbers of strategies for repair; and 3) children increase in the coordination of gestural plus vocal and then verbal repairs with advancing language skills. Both Gallagher's (1977) study and Alexander's study agreed that children's communicative repairs are more likely to contain modifications than repetitions and that there is an increase in the number of repair strategies employed by children as they develop. Finally, there appear to be patterns associated with the elements of repair used by children as they acquire communicative skills and linguistic abilities.

Because children in Alexander's (1994) study were in the early stages of language acquisition, this necessitated investigation of repair elements not included in Gallagher's study. Alexander's study examined nonverbal components of communicative repairs, whereas Gallagher's study investigated semantic and grammatical components of conversational repairs. Despite these contrasts, the two studies had similarities in outcomes. Repair behaviors of typically developing children, whether preverbal or linguistic, tend to consist more of modifications than repetitions. Repair behaviors of children in either prelinguistic or language stages demonstrate developmental progressions in the variety of repair strategies used.

Comparisons with Golinkoff's (1986) Study Alexander's (1994) study and Golinkoff's (1986) study examined the use of repairs during the transition from presymbolic to symbolic communication. The age range of the participants in this study is broader than Golinkoff's participants, both at the lower and upper limit. Also, Golinkoff examined repairs that occurred naturally in a familiar setting while this study examined simulated repairs in a natural communicative interaction with both a familiar and an unfamiliar adult present in a clinical setting. This study was cross-sectional and sampled up to 4 repairs from 120 participants, whereas Golinkoff's study was longitudinal and sampled about 60 repairs from 3 participants over about 6 months.

One finding common to both studies is that among typically developing children, preverbal communicators attempted to repair many failed communicative messages. Golinkoff found a lower percentage of repairs, which is likely due to the methods of sampling repairs. Golinkoff documented many stacked repairs, as indicated by the mean number of turns-per-negotiation episodes, which were not analyzed in the CSBS study. Responding to stacked repairs is expected to be more challenging than responding to a single repair opportunity, particularly for young children.

Another common finding is that the majority of young children have access to a variety of combinations of repair strategies that include repetitions and modifications of gestural and vocal signals. The children in Golinkoff's study were more likely to repeat a signal or to add a component to the initial signal. During the CSBS, the children were more likely to repeat gestures, but they did modify gestures more frequently than Golinkoff found, and they were more likely to modify vocalizations to repair across language stages. The greater use of modified repairs found with the CSBS may be due to the presence of an unfamiliar adult as well as the nature of the repair opportunity. Both studies documented the persistence and creativity of very young preverbal communicators and demonstrated the effectiveness of verbal repairs as children became verbal communicators.

RESEARCH ON COMMUNICATIVE
REPAIRS IN CHILDREN WITH DISABILITIES

It is likely that children with communication disabilities will be faced with the need to repair communication breakdowns even more often than typically developing children because, by definition, their messages usually are less sophisticated and may be more difficult to understand. Therefore, it is important to consider how children with disabilities develop and use repair strategies. There is a substantial amount of research on repairs in verbal children with language-learning disabilities (LLD) and with mental retardation but limited information on preverbal children with communication disabilities. This section reviews briefly the research on verbal children and examines more carefully the few studies available on preverbal children or individuals with severe disabilities.

Research on Verbal Communicators

Research investigating the conversational competence of school-age children with LLD has identified several aspects of conversational ability that are deficient. Children with LLD have been found to be impaired in their ability to formulate useful descriptions, to repair communicative breakdowns, to take an assertive position in conversation, to use advanced syntactic and morphological structures, to retrieve words, and to exhibit fluent speech commensurate with that of typically developing children (Bryan, Donahue, & Pearl, 1981; MacLachlan & Chapman, 1988). Donahue (1983) suggested that children with LLD are more competent participants in conversation when their conversational partner takes responsibility for maintaining the conversation but that they will have a more difficult time when they are required to direct the conversational interchange.

MacLachlan and Chapman (1988) compared the breakdowns of typically developing children and children with LLD and found that the group with LLD exhibited higher rates of communication breakdown in narration than conversation. The researchers hypothesized that, in the narration task, the requirements for more complex syntax, the lack of discourse support, and the more difficult organization problems were problematic for the children with LLD. In a study of responses to stacked repairs, Brinton and colleagues (1986) found that 5- to 9-year-old children with LLD produced more inappropriate responses or failed attempts to the second and third clarification requests in a sequence than typically developing peers. They suggested that children with LLD lacked not the ability to repair but the persistence necessary to negotiate a stacked communicative repair.

Preschool children with specific language impairments have been found to be deficient in repair strategies compared with typically developing children at the same language stage. Using procedures similar to Gallagher (1977), Gallagher and Darnton (1978) found that children with language impairments in Brown's Stages I, II, and III modified repairs more often than repeated; however, their use of modifications did not follow the developmental patterns of typically developing children. The children with language impairments used an equal proportion of phonetic changes, additions, and reductions across all three stages. They rarely used substitutions, which would be expected to increase across these stages. Gallagher and Darnton concluded that the selection and execution of repair strategies of these children with language impairments were unsystematic and not commensurate with their linguistic stage compared with children without disabilities.

In addition to research on children with specific language disabilities, several studies have examined repairs used by individuals with mental disabilities. Responses to requests for clarification used by individuals with mental retardation highlight the social underpinnings of repair strategies. Paul and Cohen (1984) compared repairs of adults with pervasive developmental disorders (PDD) to a control group of adults with mental retardation matched for nonverbal IQ. The participants had an average performance IQ of 63 and were functioning at or near Brown's Stage III. Using three different types of requests for clarifications, Paul and Cohen found that both groups confirmed requests for confirmation and repeated or modified in response to general and specific queries. Both groups used more modifications than repetitions for all three types of queries. However, the participants with PDD were deficient in providing the specific piece of information solicited in the specific queries, reflecting the social-pragmatic difficulties associated with PDD.

The ability to repair may be related to the social experiences of the individual. Brinton and Fujiki (1991) compared responses to triple-stacked repair sequences (i.e., three requests for clarification in sequence) in two groups of adults with mental retardation, one residing in community-based programs and the other in institutions. All of these participants were functioning in or beyond Brown's Stage III. Both groups of participants were less responsive than typically developing children previously studied at comparable developmental levels, particularly as the sequence progressed. However, both groups did use an equal distribution of repetitions and modifications to repair. Both groups of participants also used gestural and suprasegmental responses to supplement verbal repairs. Differences were identified in the types of modifications. Participants who lived in the community were more likely to add information to their modifications than were the individuals who lived in institutions. The use of addition repairs suggests an awareness that additional information is needed by the listener to interpret the message and may be enhanced by experiences with a greater variety of interactants, as would be the case with those living in a community-based setting.

Calculator and Delaney (1986) compared the use of repairs by five nonspeaking and five speaking individuals with moderate to severe mental retardation. All of these individuals constructed syntactic forms and had an MLU that corresponded to Brown's Stages II and III with communication boards; therefore, they could be compared with verbal communicators. The nonspeaking participants used repair strategies similar to a matched group of speaking participants in regard to the responsiveness to requests for clarification and proportion of repetitions and modifications. However, compared with typically developing children at comparable stages of linguistic development, these individuals relied more on repetitions. Both the nonspeaking and speaking participants demonstrated the following patterns: 1) They failed to respond to requests for clarification in about 18% of the opportunities; 2) they used repetitions slightly more frequently than modifications to repair; and 3) the most common type of modification was additions, with substitutions and reductions being infrequent and phonetic changes rare.

The nonspeaking individuals used communication boards, which are characterized by a slow rate of transmission and frequent breakdowns in communication. Calculator and Delaney (1986) found that all five nonspeaking individuals changed modality only 14% of the time and were just as likely to go from board to nonboard communication as from nonboard to board. For these individuals, motor demands may be an important variable affecting repair. The speaking individuals rarely changed modality; thus, these participants tended to persevere within the same modality most of the time.

These findings for verbal communicators who have disabilities indicate that repair strategies are deficient compared with typically developing children, both in frequency and sophistication. These findings also highlight the importance of developing the active use of repair strategies along with targeting and expanding vocabulary and grammatical forms and enhancing other conversational skills.

Research on Nonverbal Communicators

As with typically developing children, there is a paucity of research on repairs of nonverbal communicators with disabilities. Brady, McLean, McLean, and Johnston (1995) studied repairs of 28 individuals with severe to profound mental retardation who resided in an institution. Each individual was provided with five opportunities to repair when requests for help were not responded to or were misunderstood in a variety of ways and was provided with five opportunities to repair when requests for attention to an object or event were similarly not responded to or were misunderstood. Brady et al. (1995) found that 25 of the 28 participants initiated at least one repair. Significantly more participants repaired when requests for help were misunderstood. The individuals who did repair tended to either repeat the same signal or change to a different signal; additions were used rarely by these individuals.

Preliminary Study of Repairs with
Preverbal Children with Communication Impairments

Alexander (1994) conducted a preliminary study of repair behaviors of a small group of children with hearing impairment (HI) and a small group with PDD using the CSBS protocol described previously. These two populations were selected because of the contrast in social abilities. Videotaped samples of six children with HI and six with PDD were analyzed. Each group consisted of four children in the prelinguistic stage and two in the early one-word stage. The mean age of the group with HI was 24 months and of the group with PDD, 48 months.

The methods used by Alexander (1994) for analysis of the repair behaviors of typically developing children appeared to be effective for analysis of the repair behaviors of this small sample of children with HI and PDD. As with the typically developing children, all 12 of these children used gestures when they repaired. Prelinguistic children with HI, like the typically developing children in the study, used repetition of gestures to a greater extent than modifications. Prelinguistic children with PDD, who were older than the children with HI, tended to modify their gestures more than they repeated them. It is noteworthy that the gestural repairs of children with HI frequently contained gestures that were obviously more forceful or energetic than the gesture in the referent act. This was also true for the children with PDD. Therefore, the changes in gestural prosody should be considered in addition to vocal prosody change.

None of the children with HI used vocal repetition to repair. The prelinguistic children with HI had noticeably low proportions of vocal modification repairs: 83% of their repairs had no vocal components. However, the children with PDD had higher proportions of vocal repair: 63% of their prelinguistic repairs and 75% of their early one-word–stage repairs contained a vocal component. Only one participant with HI out of six children demonstrated the use of consonants in the referent act or repair; the remainder relied solely on vowel sounds. Two out of six children with PDD produced consonants in vocal repairs; the remainder vocalized using only vowel sounds or nontranscribable utterances. Because these participants were in the prelinguistic and early one-word stages of language development, their limited use of words to repair was not unexpected. Only one child with HI who was in the early one-word stage used word repairs. This child added a vocal approximation of "eat" in conjunction with the sign for eat to repair his failed communication. No children with PDD used words during communicative or repair acts.

Use of interactant and prosody changes were noted. Only one prelinguistic child with HI changed interactant to repair; no instances occurred with the children with PDD. No changes of prosody occurred with the group with HI; however, 25% of repairs of children with PDD contained a change in prosody. The prosodic changes employed by the children with PDD were applied primarily to vowel sounds and nontranscribable sounds and consisted primarily of increased loudness.

In general, the protocol used in the CSBS for sampling opportunities for communicative acts and communicative breakdowns seemed to be appropriate for children who appear to be developing typically and also for those who are known to have communicative impairments. Problems of preference for activities; attentional requirements; and differences in personality, culture, and experience that affect a child's inclination to persevere occur with all children, regardless of ability level. The difference in the chronological ages between the typically developing children and those with HI and PDD must be considered in comparing results. The children with PDD were considerably older than all of the typically developing children and were older than most of those with HI. Children with PDD may have had increased opportunities for communicative experiences but also an increased likelihood of frustrating experiences associated with failed communicative attempts.

The apparent reliance of prelinguistic children with PDD on the use of modification as a strategy for repair was surprising. It may be that the behavioral inconsistency associated with the disorder makes it difficult for the child to "recover" a recent behavior to repeat it. The finding also may indicate that children with PDD have the same lack of awareness for their own behaviors as they appear to have for the behaviors of others. The apparent dependence on modification may be the result of catching the child in the midst of a sequence of behaviors. Children with PDD tend to learn by memorizing chunks or sequences of information (Prizant, 1983). If a child has a repertoire of behaviors that he or she cycles through to repair, the identified modification repair may be a component of a larger sequence of behaviors that is repeated. Furthermore, the abundant use of prosodic feature change appeared to be the result of negative emotion that is frequently displayed by children with PDD.

IMPLICATIONS FOR RESEARCH AND CLINICAL PRACTICE

Further research on repair strategies is needed with children in the prelinguistic stage, both for children who are typically developing and for children with communication disabilities. Research is particularly needed to document further the use of repair strategies during the transitions to intentional communication and to symbolic communication. Of particular importance for preverbal individuals is to document the relationship vis-à-vis the rate of communicating, the repertoire of communicative means, and the use of repair strategies. For individuals with communication disabilities who display challenging behavior as a means of communicating, the ability to repair with appropriate behaviors may lead to reductions in challenging behaviors.

The issue of changing the modality of the communicative signal to repair needs to be investigated with individuals with a range of communication disabilities. The developmental findings with the CSBS suggest that children from the prelinguistic through the multiword stage persist with a gestural repair and abandon the vocalization a small portion of the time; it is rare that they abandon the gestural component. These findings are consistent with the modality changes reported by Calculator and Delaney (1986). Further research is needed to examine patterns of changing modality and to consider whether the use of vocal repairs by preverbal children with communication delays has predictive value for later language development.

Research emphasizing the interrelationships among communication, language, and socioemotional development (Prizant & Meyer, 1993) supports the idea that communicative repairs may be an early index of social and communicative development. Failure to exhibit communicative repairs early in development may indicate an impairment in the ability to engage successfully in social and/or communicative interactions. Children with language impairments have deficits in repair strategies that are evident from preschool through school age.

Differences in patterns of preverbal repair strategies may be an early indicator of a problem in communication and/or language development. Therefore, a child should be considered at risk for a communicative delay if he or she exhibits a lack of communicative repair behaviors at any stage beyond the transition to intentional communication. The following are high-risk indicators: 1) diminished ability to repair due to a limited repertoire of repair strategies (e.g., reliance on a single, repetitive strategy); 2) limited use of conventional gestural components to repair, especially in conjunction with a substantial display of frustration; 3) lack of awareness of the listener's needs or failure to recognize that the communicative partner can be used as a means to achieve goals; and 4) failure to develop an array of multimodal communicative repair strategies that include gestural, vocal, and, ultimately, verbal repetitions and modifications.

The findings of the research reviewed in this chapter suggest several implications that should be considered for clinical practice. Communicative repairs are an integral aspect of typical communicative development. Their absence should be considered as a significant limitation, and development of repairs should be targeted in intervention. Because children with language impairments are likely to encounter frequent communicative breakdowns, the need for communicative repairs is critical. The acquisition of communicative repairs follows a developmental progression; therefore, intervention techniques should reflect appropriate developmental trends as they apply to the child, to communication acquisition, and to the patterns of repair behaviors. Communicative repairs emerge in conjunction with other aspects of development. Intervention to support the development and use of repairs also should address the child's socioemotional, cognitive, and communicative functioning.

An important intervention goal for prelinguistic children is to develop more sophisticated and successful repairs to use when a child's intent is misunderstood or is unclear to the listener. The development of repairs can be easily targeted within intervention contexts by holding out for an extra turn. For example, prelinguistic milieu intervention described by Warren, Yoder, Gazdag, Kim, and Jones (1993; see also Chapter 15) incorporates repair opportunities by teaching prelinguistic children to request the continuation of a turn-taking interaction. Once children begin to initiate requests or comments, they need to be able to persist until the listener understands their intended meaning. The preverbal negotiation of meaning is a critical step in developing communicative competence.

Typical development indicates that gestural repetitions are an important means for repair during both the transition to intentional and to symbolic communication. Therefore, initial intervention should target the use of gestural repairs. Subtle or idiosyncratic repairs may be used by children with disabilities and should be responded to as repairs. Gestural prosody or the increased forcefulness of gestures should be recognized as repair attempts by children with language impairments. As children begin to use vocalizations with communicative intent, the use of vocal repairs and the coordination of gestural and vocal repair components should be enhanced. Increasing numbers of strategies for repair should be encouraged as the child develops.

The interaction between repair strategies and challenging behaviors should be considered for individuals who display challenging behaviors as a means to communicate. Individuals with limited communicative repertoires may display challenging behaviors after one or more attempts to communicate with an appropriate behavior. Patterns in the number of failed communicative attempts that an individual can tolerate before the display of challenging behavior should be identified and increased, which can be done by setting up stacked repair opportunities and prompting an appropriate behavior to repair before the point at which the individual is likely to display challenging behavior.

CONCLUSION

The ability to repair communicative breakdowns emerges in synchrony with and is a significant component of the development of the ability to communicate intentionally. Communicative repair may represent the outcome of socioemotional, communicative, and cognitive development, strongly influenced by psychosocial and constitutional factors. As such, its importance is considerable. Also meaningful are the findings that gestural components are integral to early communicative repairs and that the inclusion of vocalizations and verbalizations to repair increases with development. The number and type of repair components that a child is able to use increases with development. Although further research on preverbal repairs is needed, the findings reviewed in this chapter suggest an ontogeny of repair strategies and indicate that the quality of a child's preverbal repairs has important implications for early identification. Finally, the use of repair strategies is an important intervention target for children at prelinguistic stages of development.

REFERENCES

Alexander, D. (1994). *The emergence of repair strategies in chronologically and developmentally young children.* Unpublished dissertation, Florida State University, Tallahassee.

Bates, E. (1979). Intentions, conventions, and symbols. In E. Bates, L. Benigni, I. Bretherton, L. Camaioni, & V. Volterra (Eds.), *The emergence of symbols* (pp. 33–42). New York: Academic Press.

Bates, E., Bretherton, I., & Snyder, L. (1988). *From first words to grammar.* New York: Cambridge University Press.

Brady, N.C., McLean, J.E., McLean, L.K., & Johnston, S. (1995). Initiation and repair of intentional communication acts by adults with severe to profound cognitive disabilities. *Journal of Speech and Hearing Research, 38,* 1334–1348.

Brazelton, T.B. (1982). Joint regulation of neonate–parent behavior. In E.Z. Tronick (Ed.), *Social interchange in infancy* (pp. 7–35). Baltimore: University Park Press.

Bretherton, I. (1992). The interfacing of minds. In S. Feinman (Ed.), *Social referencing and the social construction of reality in infancy* (pp. 57–77). New York: Plenum.

Bretherton, I., & Bates, E. (1979). The emergence of intentional communication. In I. Uzgiris (Ed.), *New directions for child development* (Vol. 4, pp. 81–100). San Francisco: Jossey-Bass.

Brinton, B., & Fujiki, M. (1989). *Conversational management with language-impaired children.* Rockville, MD: Aspen Publishers.

Brinton, B., & Fujiki, M. (1991). Responses to requests for conversational repair by adults with mental retardation. *Journal of Speech and Hearing Research, 34,* 1087–1095.

Brinton, B., Fujiki, M., Loeb, D.F., & Winkler, E. (1986). Development of conversational repair strategies in response to requests for clarification. *Journal of Speech and Hearing Research, 29,* 75–81.

Brinton, B., Fujiki, M., & Sonnenberg, E. (1988). Responses to requests for clarification by linguistically normal and language impaired children in conversation. *Journal of Speech and Hearing Disorders, 53,* 383–391.

Brown, R. (1973). *A first language: The early stages.* Cambridge, MA: Harvard University Press.

Bryan, T., Donahue, M., & Pearl, R. (1981). Learning disabled children's communicative competence on referential communication tasks. *Journal of Pediatric Psychology, 6,* 383–393.

Calculator, S., & Delaney, D. (1986). Comparison of nonspeaking and speaking mentally retarded adults' clarification strategies. *Journal of Speech and Hearing Disorders, 51,* 252–259.

Conn, J.F., & Tronick, E.Z. (1982). Communicative rules and the sequential structure of infant behavior during normal and depressed interaction. In E.Z. Tronick (Ed.), *Social interchange in infancy* (pp. 59–77). Baltimore: University Park Press.

Donahue, M. (1983). Learning-disabled children as conversational partners. *Topics in Language Disorders, 4,* 15–27.

Gallagher, T. (1977). Revision behaviors in the speech of normal children developing language. *Journal of Speech and Hearing Research, 20,* 303–318.

Gallagher, T. (1981). Contingent query sentences with adult–child discourse. *Journal of Child Language, 8,* 51–62.

Gallagher, T., & Darnton, B.A. (1978). Conversational aspects of the speech of language-disordered children: Revision behaviors. *Journal of Speech and Hearing Research, 21,* 118–135.

Golinkoff, R.M. (1986). "I beg your pardon?": The preverbal negotiation of failed messages. *Journal of Child Language, 13,* 455–476.

Kahmi, A., & Koenig, L. (1985). Metalinguistic awareness in normal and language disordered children. *Language, Speech, and Hearing Services in Schools, 16,* 199–210.

MacLachlan, B., & Chapman, R. (1988). Communication breakdowns in normal and language learning-disabled children's conversation and narration. *Journal of Speech and Hearing Disorders, 53,* 2–7.

Paul, R., & Cohen, D. (1984). Responses to contingent queries in adults with mental retardation and pervasive developmental disorders. *Applied Psycholinguistics, 5,* 349–357.

Prizant, B. (1983). Language acquisition and communicative behavior in autism: Toward an understanding of the "whole" of it. *Journal of Speech and Hearing Disorders, 48,* 296–307.

Prizant, B., & Meyer, E. (1993). Socioemotional aspects of language and social-communication disorders in young children. *American Journal of Speech-Language Pathology: A Journal of Clinical Practice, 2,* 56–81.

Purcell, S., & Liles, B. (1992). Cohesion repairs in the narratives of normal-language and language-disordered school-age children. *Journal of Speech and Hearing Research, 35,* 354–362.

Ross, H.S., & Kay, D.A. (1980). The origins of social games. In K. Rubin (Ed.), *Children's play* (pp. 17–32). San Francisco: Jossey-Bass.

Schegloff, E.A., Jefferson, G., & Sacks, H. (1977). The preference for self-correction in the organization of repair in conversation. *Language, 53,* 361–382.

Tomasello, M., Farrar, M., & Dines, J. (1984). Children's speech revisions for a familiar and an unfamiliar adult. *Journal of Speech and Hearing Research, 27,* 359–363.

Trevarthen, C., & Hubley, P. (1978). Secondary intersubjectivity: Confidence, confiding, and acts of meaning in the first year. In A. Lock (Ed.), *Action, gesture, and symbol* (pp. 183–229). New York: Academic Press.

Tronick, E., Als, H., Adamson, L., Wise, S., & Brazelton, T.B. (1978). The infant's response to entrapment between contradictory messages in face-to-face interaction. *Journal of the American Academy of Child Psychiatry, 17,* 74–84.

Warren, S.F., Yoder, P.J., Gazdag, G., Kim, K., & Jones, H. (1993). Facilitating prelinguistic skills in young children with developmental delay. *Journal of Speech and Hearing Research, 36,* 83–97.

Wetherby, A.M., & Prizant, B. (1989). The expression of communicative intent: Assessment guidelines. *Seminars in Speech and Language, 10,* 77–91.

Wetherby, A.M., & Prizant, B.M. (1993). *Communication and Symbolic Behavior Scales manual.* Chicago: Applied Symbolix.

Wilcox, J., & Webster, E. (1980). Early discourse behavior. Children's response to listener feedback. *Child Development, 51,* 1120–1125.

8

Intentionality and the Role of Play in the Transition to Language

Karin Lifter and Lois Bloom

PLAY IS A PERVASIVE, NATURAL activity in a child's life. Young children will take almost any opportunity, in almost any place, to play by themselves or with care-givers and peers. Play can be defined in many ways, but perhaps the most insight-ful definition was offered by Virginia Axline: "Play is the child's natural medium of self-expression" (1947, p. 9). Although researchers have differed in their views of just what it is that children express in their play, most would agree on what play behaviors are. Play is an infant making noises and laughing at their effects, or a 9-month-old dropping spoons and watching them land, or a 1-year-old dumping beads out of a can or blocks out of a box, or a toddler putting objects together to form thematic relations among them, or a preschooler playing "Daddy" or "Baby" in a game of house. Play is also Peekaboo with a caregiver, splashing at the water table with peers, or "running the show" in a pretend family trip. Children are playing when they reenact pleasant and unpleasant events with dolls to act out and reshape experiences that they have had, and they are playing when they engage in rough-and-tumble activities on a playground. Children engage in many of these kinds of activities before and as they are learning to talk.

One purpose of this chapter is to present a definition of play to examine the role of play in the transition to language. Two major themes inform this defini-tion. The first theme is that play is expression: Actions in play are one way that children have, like language, to embody and make manifest the representations that they have in mind. The second theme is that play is interpretation: Play is a way for children to embrace and learn about objects, events, and relations in the world through interpreting the results of their own actions and by revising what they know about the world. The definition we propose expands earlier defini-

The authors are especially grateful to the teachers, staff, children, and families of the May Center for Early Education, Arlington, Massachusetts, and the May Institute, Inc., Harwich, Massa-chusetts, for their enthusiasm and support for the study of play in children who are developing more slowly than or differently from their peers. The authors also thank Krista Wilkinson for her thoughtful reading of earlier versions of the chapter.

161

tions in the literature that have focused on play only as expression. A second purpose of this chapter is to show how the definition of play can provide a framework for planning programs of assessment and intervention for children whose development is delayed and proceeding with difficulty. Play as expression provides a window on what children know, which allows for the use of play for assessment activities. Play as interpretation means that it is an activity for acquiring knowledge—allowing for the design of intervention programs to facilitate developmental progress.

This chapter begins with a brief review of earlier definitions of play and with a rationale for the definition to be presented here. The argument is made that developments in cognition contribute to the contents of the mind that are expressed in both play and language and that the children's play activities contribute to such developments as much as they are influenced by them. A brief review of cognitive development from the period of late infancy through the second year then is presented to set the stage for a review of those research studies that have examined the relationship between play and language and that have evaluated the role of play in the transition to language. Discussions of play as a context for learning and the educational and clinical implications of prior research follow. The chapter concludes with an overview of the role of culture for developments in play and some directions for future research.

DEFINITIONS OF PLAY

The developmental approach to theory and research in the study of play originated in the constructivist tradition (Piaget, 1954, 1962), with play used as a window on what children know and on the changes taking place in their knowledge over time (Lifter & Bloom, 1989; Lowe, 1975; McCune, 1995). Play was seen as an expressive activity on the part of the child so that researchers could infer developments in knowledge for exploring relationships between play and language.

Early Definitions of Play

Definitions of play were largely influenced by Piaget's description of play as "a happy display of known actions" rather than as an "effort to learn" (1962, p. 93). In a strict Piagetian interpretation, play is a form of assimilation (i.e., the child incorporates new information into existing knowledge structures about objects and events) rather than an accommodation to learn something new. In this view, children can be "playful" because they are engaged in something that they already know.

Many definitions of play described play as spontaneous, intrinsically motivated behavior, with active engagement and attention to the activity itself rather than to a goal and with freedom from externally imposed rules. Play was distinguished from exploratory behavior in the sense that play is not about learning but about having fun while engaging in known activities, with an "as if" quality that requires an element of pretense (Elkind, 1990; Rubin, Fein, & Vandenburg, 1983). Implicit in these definitions was the component of positive affect. If children were engaged in known activities of their choosing, it was assumed that these activities would be enjoyed and would co-occur with a display of positive affect; hence, positive affect was included in many definitions of play (Butterfield, 1994; Elkind, 1990; Wolery & Baley, 1989).

However, empirical studies of children's early play, although originally motivated by traditional definitions of play, were exploratory in nature. The effort was made to determine what children were doing in play rather than to confirm the factors included in one or another definition of play (e.g., Belsky & Most, 1981; Fenson, Kagan, Kearsley, & Zelazo, 1976; Lifter & Bloom, 1989; Lowe, 1975; Nicolich, 1977). Such research incorporated the assumptions that play is intrinsically motivated and requires active engagement on the part of the player, but other factors were not addressed directly. Most often, all of the object-related activities in a sample of play behaviors were analyzed rather than analyzing only those behaviors that demonstrated attention to the activity itself rather than to its goal, or that required a pretense quality, or that included a display of positive affect. Thus, the empirical research into the nature of play and the relationship between play and language departed from the traditional definitions of play that presumably first motivated the research.

A factor frequently overlooked in most definitions of play that were influenced by Piaget is the fundamental function of play: acquiring new knowledge. Play is not just a display of what the child already knows. Play is also what Montessori (1967) called "the child's work" (p. 180), and children are in the process of learning about objects and events when they play. For example, children pay more attention to activities that represent new learning than to those that are relatively well known (Bloom, Tinker, & Beckwith, in preparation; Ruff & Saltarelli, 1993; Wikstrom, 1994). Children playing with objects tend not to express emotions at the same time (Phillips & Sellito, 1990), but they are most likely to express emotions immediately after play activities that represent new learning rather than old learning (Bloom, et al., in preparation).

Thus, the view that play is reserved for the display of known actions or that play is restricted to assimilation (Elkind, 1990) is too limited. Play is too pervasive in young children's lives to not be an activity base for learning about the world. Indeed, Piaget (1954) had explained the child's construction of reality in terms of schemes that were developed through actions on objects, although these actions were not regarded as play. Consequently, a theoretical perspective is needed that also incorporates the fundamental function of play for acquiring new knowledge—play as a context for interpreting new events—and that takes into account the full range of object-related behaviors in which children engage.

Play Defined from the Intentionality Perspective

Bloom (1993) proposed a more inclusive definition of play and its role in development: Actions in play are expressions of intentional states, as the external embodiment of aspects of representations in consciousness at a particular moment in time. Intentional states are

> the contents of mind that are dynamically constructed as prior knowledge in memory informs perceptions, actions, and interactions in the world. The consequence of acting—including acts of expression and interpretation—is the construction of representations which, in turn, inform what the child learns about the world. Development originates in this transaction between thinking and acting because intentional states determine actions and are, in turn, informed by them. (Bloom et al., in preparation)

In this view, actions in play display what the child already knows but also display what the child is currently thinking about in efforts to make sense of ongoing events for advancing knowledge.

Consequently, new factors can be added to the definition of play while retaining and revising the factors in existing definitions of play in the literature to propose a more comprehensive definition. A revised definition of play would continue to describe play as spontaneous, naturally occurring behaviors that are intrinsically motivated and that require the active engagement of the child. Play, however, also requires attention to and interpretation of a wide range of object- and person-related behaviors for advancing knowledge. In addition, the requirement of positive affect displays for defining play needs to be revised because the expression of positive affect varies with the nature of play activities and the developments they show. Therefore, we propose this definition of play: Play is the expression of intentional states—the representations in consciousness constructed from what young children know about and are learning from ongoing events—and consists of spontaneous, naturally occurring activities with objects that engage attention and interest. Play may or may not involve caregivers or peers, may or may not involve a display of affect, and may or may not involve pretense.

This definition of play incorporates several key assumptions. First, the basis of the definition is the complementary transaction between play as evidence of what the child knows and play as an activity leading to developments in cognition. Play is both a window on the child's knowledge and a window on how that knowledge is constructed. Second, the definition affords a view of play that can be examined in relation to language because in the intentionality model, both language and play are expressions of the contents of mind, that is, expressions of intentional states informed by ongoing events and prior knowledge.

Third, this definition of play as a complementary process of expression and interpretation provides the theoretical basis for applications of play in assessment and intervention. If play is an expression of what children are thinking about (i.e., what children know about ongoing events), then play activities can be used for assessment purposes. At the same time, if children interpret and reinterpret what they know in relation to ongoing events through activities of play, then interventions in play can be used to facilitate progress in development. Given that both play and language are expressions of the contents of the mind, interventions that contribute to developments in play also may contribute to developments in language (this is discussed in more detail later in the chapter).

Distinction Between Intentional States and Intentional/Goal-Directed Behaviors

Inherent in the definition of play proposed here is a distinction between intentionality in the larger sense just discussed (Bloom, 1993) and intentional behaviors (Bates, Benigni, Bretherton, Camaioni, & Volterra, 1979; Bates, Bretherton, & Snyder, 1988; Bruner, 1983). Searle (1984) made the distinction between the larger sense of Intentionality (with a capital "I") and intention (with a lowercase "i"), which is the intention to do something, for example, to act or to communicate, and is, essentially, goal-directed activity. Intentionality with a capital "I" is what our conscious states of mind are about at any moment in time, that is, representations consisting of elements, roles, and relations under psychological attitudes of belief, desire, and feeling. An intentional state may or may not include the intention to do something, a goal, or a plan for acting. "Intentionality... doesn't just refer to our intentions (to act), but also to beliefs, desires, hopes, fears...and all of those mental states (whether conscious or unconscious) that refer to, or are about, the world apart from the mind" (Searle, 1984, p. 16).

This distinction between intentional behaviors and intentional states has different implications for interpreting both play activity and relationship of play to developments in language. Intentional behaviors are specifically purposeful and volitional. They are activities in the service of some goal, and they are observable. In describing cognition in relation to language, Bruner (1983) concluded that "much of the cognitive processing in infancy appears to operate in support of goal-directed activity" (p. 27). The development of intentional behaviors often is considered a prerequisite to the development of intentional communication, first with gestures and vocalizations and later with language (Bates, 1976; Bates et al., 1979, 1988). Thus, intentional behaviors include gestural communication with caregivers around toys, that is, to show or give something to a caregiver or to use a caregiver to obtain some desired goal. Because intentional behaviors are in the service of a social-communicative goal, they support a child's participation in the social world.

Intentional states, in contrast, are representations in conscious states of mind that are about the objects of the child's attention and engagement and that are expressed by the behaviors we observe. Intentional states are beliefs, desires, and feelings directed toward the objects of attention and engagement, and they may or may not include a goal and a plan to achieve the goal. Thus, intentional states are the products of both cognitive activity and affective engagement with a world of people, objects, and events. Because they are hidden, intentional states must be embodied and made manifest so that other people can know them, and their embodiment can be expressed by language, play, and gesture as well as by expressions of emotion (Bloom, 1993). From this perspective, play and language are always *about* something that is represented in states of mind. Caregivers and others can interpret and respond to what a child's play and language are about and thereby can contribute to the child's knowledge and promote the child's participation in a social world.

Three guiding principles govern the transaction between intentional states and the child's context for development: the principles of relevance, discrepancy, and elaboration (Bloom, 1993). The principle of *relevance* directs the child's focus of attention and determines which information from the input is worth knowing. Something in the context is relevant if it corresponds to an element or elements in the mind and is pertinent to what the child is feeling and thinking so that the child can make sense of it. "Relevance is the single property that makes information worth processing and determines the particular assumptions an individual is most likely to construct and process" (Sperber & Wilson, 1986, p. 46).

The principle of *discrepancy* has to do with the difference between contents of mind and what is perceptually available in the context. Very young infants' intentional states are constrained to what they can perceive in the immediate here and now. With developments in recall and the symbolic capacity, infants can begin to remember past events and to anticipate new events. As a result, contents of mind differ from what is immediately perceptible in the context. Learning occurs when the child acts in ways that resolve the discrepancy, such as through expression in play or in language. The principle of *elaboration* presses the child to act in increasingly more detailed and complex ways to express the increasingly intricate and elaborative intentional states that cognitive developments make possible.

These cognitive developments occur in the content, structure, and organization of knowledge as well as in the symbolic capacity, to determine what a child recalls from memory and holds in mind in intentional states. Together, the principles of relevance, discrepancy, and elaboration guide the transaction between a child's intentional states and the child's context for developments in play and language. For the child, play activities provide the contexts for expression and interpretation, for displaying prior knowledge, and for constructing new knowledge. For the researcher and teacher, play activities provide a window on the child's knowledge for planning the goals for assessment, teaching, and intervention. The next section presents a brief description of cognitive developments that have informed studies of play during the transition to language. This transition to language begins before the use of words, extends through a child's first words, and ends with the vocabulary spurt and the appearance of multiword utterances.

OVERVIEW OF COGNITIVE PREREQUISITES
AND CONTRIBUTIONS TO LANGUAGE

The descriptive studies of play, especially those in the period from late infancy through the second year of life, were centered predominantly on the cognition required for developments in play activities (e.g., Belsky & Most, 1981; Fenson et al., 1976; Lifter & Bloom, 1989; Lowe, 1975; Nicolich, 1977), whereas play as a social process was often the focus in studies of preschool-age children (e.g., Garvey, 1974; Parten, 1932; Smilansky, 1968). Studies to explore the role of social processes in children's acquisition of language (e.g., Tomasello & Farrar, 1986) have focused on episodes of joint attention between caregivers and children during object play.

Sensorimotor Stages and the Emergence of Symbolic Behavior

Researchers described cognition in terms of sensorimotor stages and the transition to symbolic behaviors, measures of play, and performance on ordinal scales of sensorimotor development. These descriptors then were related to different aspects of language.

Description of Sensorimotor Stages   Early descriptions of the cognitive structure and organization of play activities relied heavily on Piaget's work (1954, 1962), which influenced how play activities were examined as a window on cognition and, subsequently, in relation to developments in language. Piaget described cognitive developments in the first 2 years of a child's life as consisting of the evolution of conceptual thought and the emergence of symbolic behavior. The last two of these stages that he described, Stage 5 (the emergence of means–end relations) and Stage 6 (the emergence of symbolic thought and the full achievement of object permanence), coincide with the age period typically studied for the transition to language: from 8 months of age through at least the first half of the second year of life. The principal development in these last two stages is the differentiation of the self from objects and people, which allows children to break from knowing the world only in terms of their own actions. The child becomes able to keep track of objects and people, and the relationships between them in space and over time. Infants come to appreciate that objects continue to exist in space and time when the objects can no longer be seen and acted on and that objects enter into relationships with other objects and people. Similarly, infants come to consider people as independent agents who act and do things for them in events that can be thought about and planned.

Early Measures of Play in Relation to Sensorimotor Development
Because children's play behaviors often have to do with actions on objects, it was easy for researchers to describe play activities in terms of Piaget's description of the sensorimotor substages. For example, before Stage 5, the infant orients to an object or to a person, but not to both at the same time. During Stage 5, infants are able to coordinate attention to both a person and an object, for exam-

ple, by showing, giving, or pointing out an object to a caregiver (Bates et al., 1979). Stage 6 pretend play activities have been described as transitional between sensorimotor and symbolic play because the activities are self-oriented (e.g., feeds self with spoon). Differentiating self from objects and others and the beginning development of planning and control anticipate the transition to symbolic play, which is marked by two features in particular. One feature is the application of self-oriented actions to other people or objects (e.g., a shift from feeding self to also feeding a doll). The second feature of symbolic play is using one object to "stand for" another (e.g., pretending a red bead is an apple). Imitated actions also are projected onto new objects (e.g., Garwood, 1982).

The global distinction between manipulative and pretend play that has been widely used to describe children's play activities in this period followed directly from Piaget's (1962) description of practice play (Piaget's sensorimotor period) and symbolic play (Piaget's symbolic period). In manipulative play, the child's actions are determined by the objects that can be seen and handled in the here and now. In pretend play, the child's actions "symbolize" knowledge about absent objects and events. In addition to this global distinction between manipulative and symbolic play, other studies, in contrast, provided more explicit descriptions of children's play activities (e.g., Lifter & Bloom, 1989; McCune, 1995), which have then figured prominently in efforts to describe relationships between play and language.

Ordinal Scales of Development   At the time that many hypotheses about the relationships between cognition and language were being offered, ordinal scales of sensorimotor development became available and were seen as a way of objectifying Piaget's descriptions and interpretations. These scales were explicitly developed to operationalize Piaget's description of sensorimotor development and to provide an objective measure of children's progress through the period. The most widely used of these, to examine aspects of cognition in relation to other developmental domains, the Uzgiris and Hunt (1975) scales, were designed to assess six different aspects of sensorimotor development: object permanence, means–ends relations, vocal and gestural imitation, operational causality, object relations in space, and schemes for relating to objects.

Given the availability of sensorimotor scales of development, children's "scores" on task items were readily used for comparison with progress in language and with progress in play (Bates et al., 1979; Lifter & Bloom, 1989), and hypothesized relationships between cognition and language were formally tested with methods of correlation, yielding varying results. For example, Bloom's (1973) hypothesis that the development of the vocabulary spurt depended on achievements in object knowledge, in general, and object permanence, in particular. Some studies found little or no support for this hypothesis (Bates et al., 1979; Corrigan, 1978). However, as pointed out by Anisfeld (1984; see also Bloom, Lifter, and Broughton, 1985, for a review of the related studies), the lack of correlations between scale measures of object permanence and indices of language often resulted from the expectation of a

> narrow and rigid relation and did not make allowances for the complex vicissitudes of development. One should not expect two related capacities to appear in exactly the same narrow time [for a variety of reasons].... I am impressed...that the vocabulary growth-spurt and the attainment of full object permanence appeared within weeks of one another and not discouraged by findings that they did not appear in exactly the same testing sessions. (Anisfeld, 1984, p. 81)

Researchers used the scales to examine aspects of sensorimotor development other than object permanence along with measures of play to explore relationships to language. In particular, in the study by Bates et al. (1979), two general measures of play, combinatorial play and symbolic play, were correlated with progress in language at monthly intervals from 9 to 13 months of age. They also determined that specific aspects of cognition (i.e., means–ends relations) and both measures of play were related to transitions in language and concluded that other aspects of sensorimotor development were more important than object permanence in this transition.

Summary of Measures of Cognition for Examining Relationships to Language Thus, researchers examined relationships between cognition and language by operationalizing and measuring cognition in different ways. On the one hand, cognition was assessed with the ordinal scales of sensorimotor development, and scores were then correlated with progress in various aspects of language (Bates, et al., 1979; Corrigan, 1978; Lifter & Bloom, 1989). On the other hand, naturally occurring play activities were observed directly and described in terms of the distinction between their form, such as type of movement (e.g., taking apart, putting together) and content, such as construction of a familiar or new thematic relation between objects (Lifter & Bloom, 1989). Play was described in terms of the general categories of manipulative (i.e., combinatorial) and symbolic play (Bates et al., 1979) or with finer distinctions among play activities that were informed (e.g., Lifter & Bloom, 1989; McCune, 1995; Nicolich, 1977), by the kinds of activities and their outcomes.

The results of these studies have converged to reveal three developments in cognition that are important developments in both play and language in the period that begins in the last quarter of the first year and continues through the second year of life. The first development is the transition from preintentional to intentional/goal-directed behaviors. The second development is the transition from presymbolic to symbolic activities. The third contribution from cognitive development to both play and language is in the young child's intentionality, that is, developments leading to changes in the representations that are expressible by language and play. These representations are the child's intentional states—contents of mind about people, objects, and events under psychological attitudes of belief, desire, and feeling. This larger sense of intentionality embraces but is not limited to the more narrow sense of intention to act or intention to communicate. This larger sense of intentionality requires developments in the symbolic capacity, but the symbolic capacity is only one aspect of the developments in cognition, emotion, and social understanding that are required for both language and play. Intentional states are the products of both cognitive activity and affective engagement in a world of people, objects, and events. Intentional states are dynamically constructed from moment to moment in that part of the mind ordinarily referred to as consciousness (or working memory), and they are crucial to acquiring all forms of human behavior (Bloom, 1993).

EVALUATION OF THE ROLE
OF PLAY IN THE TRANSITION TO LANGUAGE

The developments shown to be important to the developmental relationship between language and play resulted from different theoretical and empirical emphases in the study of play and language, but all originated within the developmental/constructivist tradition. The three key cognitive developments—emergence of intentional behaviors, the symbolic capacity, and increasing elaboration of intentional states—led to different conclusions and the different implications that follow them about the relationship between language and play.

Transition from Preintentional to Intentional and Goal-Directed Behaviors

The development of intentional behaviors was regarded as prerequisite to the development of intentional communication, which first appears with gestures and prelinguistic vocalizations and later with language. The transition from preintentional to intentional behaviors centers specifically on developments occurring in Piaget's Stage 5 of sensorimotor development and, in particular, the relationship of means–ends behaviors to the emergence of language. Bates et al. (1979) identified three manifestations of development occurring in Stage 5 as basic to communication: 1) the noncommunicative use of tools, 2) the ability to direct an adult's attention to some object or event (e.g., pointing, giving, showing), and 3) the ability to use an adult as the means to a goal (i.e., external agency). They concluded that the emergence of single words depends on gestural communication (e.g., pointing, giving, showing), the appreciation of means–ends relations and tool use, "gestural naming" (e.g., drinking from an empty cup, putting a shoe to one's foot), and at least some limited aspects of vocal and gestural imitation (Bates et al., 1988).

Bates and colleagues (1979) also examined the relationship of play to language, but the role of play in the transition from preintentional to intentional activities was not made explicit. They compared the global measures of combinatorial play and symbolic play to the children's progress in language. They concluded that combinatorial and symbolic play were the best predictors of social-communicative development. Combinatorial play predicted both comprehension and production and social-communicative development through the period of 9–13 months of age. Symbolic play was more closely tied to production and was a stronger predictor toward the end of the period. Although the measures of play were compared with progress in language, the measures of play were not used as measures of cognition, in general, or as measures of intentional behaviors, in particular. Instead, other aspects and measures of cognition were deemed central to the development of intentional behaviors for both play and language.

The role of social interaction in the development of language was made explicit in the transition from preintentional to intentional behaviors. Because of the goal-directed focus inherent in intentional behaviors, language was conceptualized as an instrument or tool for "getting things done" in a social context by influencing other people. Intentional behaviors that are manifest in the social-interactive contexts of play activities include the proto-declarative behaviors of giving, showing, and pointing. The cognitive structure and organization underlying these play activities is centered on development of means–ends behaviors and the functions that means–ends behaviors serve for communication and joining in a social world.

In summary, Bates and colleagues (1979, 1988) provided an important advancement to the field of language development by calling attention to the transition from preintentional to intentional behaviors for the emergence of language. Recognition of this transition provided an important view of cognitive prerequisites to language in terms of children's development of means–ends relations and their ability to use objects and people in the service of various goals for participating in a social world. Bates and colleagues also opened the way for thinking about intention during the transition to language, with intention interpreted in terms of goal-directed activity (e.g., using words). However, the role of play in the transition to language was not made explicit in their work.

Transition from Presymbolic to Symbolic Activities

The transition from presymbolic to symbolic activities represents a critically important development for the relationship between cognition and language and led to the global distinction between manipulative play and symbolic play. Many studies that examined relationships between play and language described manipulative and symbolic play in the progression from self-oriented to other-oriented activities (Hill & McCune-Nicolich, 1981; Nicolich, 1977).

McCune (1995) provided detailed and explicit descriptions of the relationships between play and language, with the differentiation of self from objects and others as the prevailing cognitive task underlying play activities. McCune's descriptions have received considerable attention and are noteworthy for the differentiations within symbolic play that she provided. She described the first two play levels (Levels 1 and 2) in her categorization scheme as presymbolic play and considered them to be Stage 6 sensorimotor developments. In Level 1, called presymbolic play schemes, children showed their understanding of object use (e.g., bringing comb to hair or a cup to mouth) and their knowledge of the specific characteristics of individual objects. Other studies referred to this stage as enactive naming (Bates et al., 1979; Belsky & Most, 1981). Level 2, called self-pretend, was the child pretending in self-related activities (e.g., eating from an empty spoon, tilting head back and drinking from an empty cup). According to McCune (1995), these activities provide evidence that the child understands the link between actions in play and their counterpart in reality.

McCune's (1995) Levels 3 and higher were regarded as symbolic play. Level 3 was defined by the appearance of other-pretend activities as children extend the symbolism of an activity beyond themselves toward other people and objects (e.g., child feeding his or her mother with a spoon, giving a teddy bear a drink from a cup). Beginning to say words was associated with the onset of Levels 2 and 3 pretend behavior. Level 4 consisted of combinations of actions in play, with single action schemes (e.g., drinking) related to several actors (e.g., child taking a drink from an empty cup and then giving the doll a drink), and of different action schemes related in sequence (e.g., the child feeding the doll with a spoon, giving it a drink, then putting it to bed). The onset of combinations in language (i.e., multiword utterances) was associated with the onset of combinations in play. Level 5, the final level, was described as hierarchical pretend and consisted of actions that appear to be driven by internal mental processes and a plan for action (e.g., the child picks up a doll and then searches for the bottle to give the doll a drink), with less need to rely on the perceptual world (McCune, 1993). The beginning of rule-governed multiword utterances was associated with the onset of hierarchical pretend play.

McCune's (1995) detailed analyses of play have provided useful coding schemes for description and assessment purposes. As had Bates et al. (1979) and Lifter and Bloom (1989), McCune (1995) also (and Piaget, 1954, before them) concluded that both play and language were manifestations of the same underlying cognitive processes. However, the role of play in the transition to language was not made explicit in the studies by either Bates et al. (1979) or McCune (1995). Similar progressions from self-pretend to other-pretend were observed in other studies, but they were not explicitly related to developments in language (Lowe, 1975; Nicolich, 1977; Watson & Fischer, 1977).

Developments in Intentionality and the Transition from General to Specific Knowledge for Play and Language

Once we invoke the larger sense of intentionality, which encompasses both intentional behaviors and the symbolic capacity, we have a basis for understanding the role of developments in play for the transition to language. The major results in the Lifter and Bloom (1989) study of play and language led to the conclusion that developments from general knowledge to more specific knowledge about objects were responsible for the increasing elaboration of intentional states expressed by both play activities and language.

Evidence of Developmental Change from General to Specific Knowledge

Developments in children's play during the second year of life reveal increases in the specificity of knowledge about objects as well as their symbolic qualities. A developmental progression from general to specific activities has been observed in several studies of children's play (e.g., Beeghly, Weiss-Perry, & Cicchetti, 1990; Belsky & Most, 1981; Fenson et al., 1976; Lifter & Bloom, 1989; Lowe, 1975; Ungerer & Sigman, 1981). General object knowledge has to do with ideas about objects that apply to many different kinds of things: that they exist, that they can enter into relationships with other objects, and that they can be moved out of sight and then retrieved. These ideas are independent of the specific characteristics and functions of individual objects and appear to dominate play activities during a child's first year. Such general play activities indicate "exercise of the child's developing functions, irrespective of the materials handled" (Lowe, 1975, p. 33). Specific knowledge, in contrast, has to do with ideas about the perceptual, functional, and cultural properties of objects that permit children to enter objects into more particular relationships with themselves and with other objects.

Lifter and Bloom (1989) provided evidence of developmental change in the kinds of thematic relationships children learn to construct in their early play in the progress from general to specific knowledge, and also showed how these developments in play were related to developments in language. Their analyses focused on those activities in which children related two objects to each other and were based, originally, on the Piagetian concept of reversibility (Piaget, 1954). The ability to understand that actions on objects can be reversed is required for understanding means–ends relations, the permanence of objects, and the logic of groups that contribute to the development of higher-order thinking skills. Reversibility itself depends on the differentiation of self from objects and people and the ability to understand and plan actions apart from actions only in relation to the self.

The first evidence of the appreciation of reversibility was the distinction between separating and constructing, when children first acted on two objects in relation to each other in their spontaneous play. Separations and constructions were reversible actions. Acts of separation consisted of taking apart a configuration of objects (e.g., taking beads from a container, taking a peg person out of the seesaw); acts of construction consisted of moving two objects together to form a thematic relationship (e.g., putting the peg person into the seesaw, putting beads on a string). The separating and constructing activities of 14 children were examined, longitudinally, during three 3-month intervals defined by a continuum of developments in language: a prespeech window, that is, a baseline at 9–11 months before words were learned; the first words window, that is, the month in which the first use of words occurred in the playroom along with the months immediately before and after (mean age 13.8 months); and the vocabulary spurt window, that is, the month the vocabulary spurt was identified along with the immediately preceding and succeeding months (mean age 19.2 months).

The children's earliest prespeech activities consisted of separations—taking things apart—and constructions were reliably observed around first words. Following the initial distinction between separating and constructing activities, the remaining analyses focused on the progressive differentiation in constructing activities (as schematized in Figure 1). At first, children either put objects back into the original configurations that had been presented to them in the playroom (i.e., given relations [e.g., putting a peg person back into the see-saw or nesting the nesting cups into one another]), or they created a relationship that was different from the original presentation (i.e., imposed relations [e.g., putting a bead onto or into a nesting cup]). This development from given to imposed relationships in the children's constructing activities was evidence of

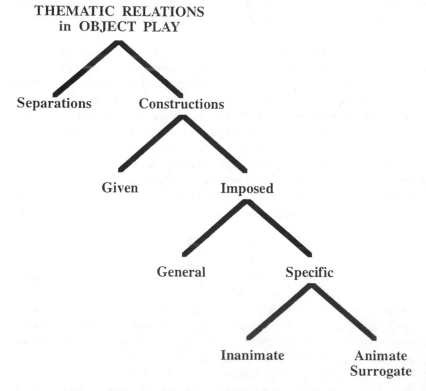

Figure 1. Categories of thematic relations in object play. (From Lifter, K., & Bloom, L. [1989]. Object knowledge and the emergence of language. *Infant Behavior and Development, 12,* 395–423; adapted by permission.)

the principle of discrepancy (Bloom, 1993) and the developments required for acting to resolve a discrepancy between what the child has in mind and what is evident from the context. For a given construction, the child needed to recall how the objects were assembled when they were first seen. However, imposed constructions required that the child have in mind a possible configuration for the objects that was different (discrepant) from how the objects originally were presented to them in the playroom.

In turn, imposed relations were either general or specific. General relationships were those that could be created with a variety of objects simply according to whether one object could serve as a support or a container for another object. Thus, family figures, beads, and miniature spoons and forks often ended up being transferred from one container or support to another. For specific relations, in contrast, the children constructed configurations in which they took account of the particular physical, functional, and/or conventional properties of objects in relation to one another (e.g., putting beads on a string, extending a spoon to feed a doll). Finally, specific constructions were subdivided into inanimate constructions and animate surrogate constructions. Inanimate constructions made use of the particular physical properties of inanimate objects (e.g., stringing beads, stacking a set of nesting cups, rolling a truck down a ramp). Animate surrogate constructions, in contrast, used a replica person or animal in the construction (e.g., feeding a doll with a spoon, putting a person figure on a horse).

Evidence of Relationships Between Play and Language In the prespeech period, when most of the children's actions consisted of separating activities, a child would take hold of an object (e.g., a peg in the seesaw, a cup in a nest of cups), perhaps explore it or mouth it, and then drop it, put it down, or cast it aside. In activities like these, the child did not need to appreciate the relationship in the configuration to take it apart; just reaching and grasping one of the objects caused the separation. Even though their mothers provided models for constructing relationships between objects, by putting them back together again in various configurations, the children's activities consisted primarily of separating. Thus, their actions were expressions of intentional states that were largely determined by what was immediately available and perceptible to them in the context.

The early predominance of separating activities also suggested that the children's organization of object knowledge consisted of unidirectional actions in which objects were moved in relation to the child; that is, the infants were basically acting on one object at a time. These activities did not provide evidence that the children appreciated the concept of reversibility (i.e., that objects are independent entities that can be moved in reciprocal relationships to other objects). However, these actions provided *opportunities* for analyzing and learning about the objects, that is, that objects can be moved from place to place and moved apart from another object in a configuration. The children evidently learned about the possible relationships between objects by first learning to take those relationships apart, and this development preceded the emergence of words.

By the time of their first words in the playroom (mean age 13.8 months), all the children were constructing relationships between objects—taking one object and putting it together in a relationship with another object—reaching the criteria used to establish "achievement" in constructions (Lifter & Bloom, 1989). Actions in play in which a child constructs a relationship between objects are expressions of intentional states that are constructed out of the data from perception *in relation to information recalled from memory:* The children had to have recalled the configuration to mind from experience and then acted to embody or make that representation manifest in the situation. The developmental progression from separating to constructing also revealed an appreciation for the reversibility of action patterns—evidence that the child now knew that a relationship that is taken apart can be put back together again. These developments provided evidence of a reorganization of object knowledge that included knowing about objects as separate entities that could enter into relationships with other objects. To create these configurations, the children needed to have a representation of that configuration in mind along with a plan for acting, which depended on developments in both the symbolic capacity and intentional behaviors. Thus, developments in intentional states embraced these two aspects of development that were the focus of much research during the late 1970s (e.g., Bates et al., 1979; Nicolich, 1977). However, the children's intentional states also depended on their affective engagement and selective attention to the relevance of objects in the situation according to what they already knew about the objects. Thus, both prior knowledge and affect contributed to these developments as well.

Initially, most of the children's constructions either reproduced a relationship given in the original presentation of the objects or, when imposed rather than given, were general relationships of containment and support. However, gradual change was observed in the kinds of imposed relationships constructed in the period from first words to the vocabulary spurt. The children increasingly constructed thematic relations in which they took account of the particular physical, functional, and/or conventional properties of objects in relation to one another. A comparison of these two categories revealed a steady increase in specific constructions, which required knowledge of the functional and conventional properties of objects, along with a steady decrease in general constructions. The general constructions depended primarily on the physical properties of objects that afforded either containment or support for other objects. Finally, inanimate constructions predominated among the earliest specific relations, and animate surrogate constructions gained in frequency later in the period. Thus, a progression from physical specificity to conventional specificity was observed in the imposed thematic relationships that the children constructed.

By the time of the vocabulary spurt, all the children were constructing imposed, specific relationships with the objects in the playroom. The foundation for these developments, however, was the child's expanding physical knowledge of objects in general. The Developments in general object knowledge included a fuller understanding of the constructs of reversibility, means–ends relations, and the permanence of an object's identity in time and space, regardless of the different physical, functional, and conventional relationships of which it might be part. Thus, development in expressing more specific intentional state representations in play followed a long period in development, spanning several months in the second year, in which the children's general knowledge about objects gradually expanded to include particular properties of objects and the different relationships in which they can enter.

Achievements in constructing specific thematic relations between objects coincided with the vocabulary spurt that, similarly, represented a period of consolidation in the acquisition of a vocabulary of words. In addition to the increase in numbers of words, which is what is captured by a vocabulary spurt, the intentional states that could be attributed to the children's words also showed developmental change (Bloom, 1994; Bloom, Beckwith, Capatides, & Hafitz, 1988). When compared with similar attributions made at the time of first words, the children were more likely to be expressing intentional states about anticipated objects and events rather than objects and events that were already evident in the situation; this development was consistent with the principle of discrepancy. The children's words at vocabulary spurt were also more likely to express meaning that was about imminent actions, that is, things they would do or wanted their mothers to do, than about what could simply be seen, shown, or presented. Thus, development was evident in the intentional state representations expressed both by words, which were about anticipated actions, and play, which was about specific relations having to do with more elements and more roles and relations between them, consistent with the principle of elaboration. Both the advance in language represented by the vocabulary spurt and the developments in play reflected in specific constructions depended on particular knowledge about objects that was physical, functional, and conventional and developments in mental representation for intentional states that enabled the children to hold more entities in mind along with increasingly elaborative, specific relationships between the entities.

Relationships Between Play and Language to Sensorimotor Development and Scale Performance   The major developments in constructing activities in play were bracketed by the beginning and end of Stage 6 object permanence behaviors, as measured with the Uzgiris and Hunt (1975) scales, which is consistent with what has been reported in other studies (Bates et al., 1979; Corrigan, 1978). Before Stage 6, the children's object-related behaviors were predominantly separations, with constructing behaviors beginning to emerge. Although Stage 5 is often regarded as presymbolic (e.g., by McCune, 1995), critically important developments in conceptual organization are already taking place, namely, the development of reversibility and notions about objects as separate entities that can be entered into relationships with other objects and people. Other studies with infants in the first year of life have revealed complementary evidence of developments in memory and conceptual understanding (Mandler, 1988, 1992). Stage 5 also has been marked as important for development in intentional behaviors, particularly with respect to means–ends behaviors as measured by scale performance (Bates et al., 1979). Taken together, the studies by Bates et al. and by Lifter and Bloom (1989) indicate that understanding objects as separate entities is required for the use of an object or person in the service of some goal.

What has ordinarily been termed Stage 6 is actually a long period in which developments in representation are gradual and cumulative; it is a period that is, nevertheless, transitional. At the time of entry to Stage 6, which coincided with the first words window, the children in Lifter and Bloom's (1989) study were already constructing relations between objects. The long period (5 months on average) that was bracketed by the beginning and end of Stage 6 performance on the scales encompassed both the gradual progressions in play, from given to imposed and from general to specific activities to the emergence of animate surrogate relations, and development in language, from expressing evident meanings to anticipated action meanings.

Inferences of Developmental Change in Intentional States The advantages of evaluating developments in play along a continuum from given to imposed and from general to specific activities are in the inferences that can be made, first, about developments in mental representation in intentional states and object knowledge, and, second, the observed developmental progressions allowed the examination of changes in play in relation to other simultaneous developments, such as language. The development from given to imposed constructions was evidence that the children could recall relationships between objects they had experienced before from memory, and this recall did not depend on seeing the configuration again each time the toys were introduced in the playroom. The development from given to imposed constructions was consistent with the principle of discrepancy, which captures the difference between acting on the information available in the context (given relationships) and prior knowledge about different possibilities (imposed relationships). The development from general to specific constructions was evidence that the children could recall more of the particular characteristics of objects that afforded more elaborative and specific physical, functional, and conventional relationships with other objects and the ability to hold such representations in mind in a plan for action, consistent with the principle of elaboration. These were the developments in cognition responsible for the developments observed in children's play activities. Developments in mental representation were not required for children's early separating activities but were required to explain the emergence and development of their increasingly elaborative constructing activities. The children had to recall a configuration and hold that representation in mind for plans for action. Increasingly complex representations, with different roles and relations between roles, were the basis for developments both in specific constructions and in the vocabulary spurt as the children learned more words and talked more about anticipated actions. Both of these developments in play and language were consistent with the principle of elaboration in the intentionality model.

In summary, different kinds of knowledge in memory and different capacities for recall and representation were required for the imposed specific constructions than for the given general constructions and for the meanings expressed by the children's words by the time of the vocabulary spurt. Thus, the continuum from given and general relations between objects to imposed, specific thematic relations allowed for explanation of developments in play and language that go beyond the global categories of manipulative and symbolic play. All the children's construction activities involved both manipulations and the symbolic capacity, but the Lifter and Bloom (1989) analysis revealed the finer distinctions within the more global categories and their development over time and also revealed the developmental relationship in progress from manipulative to increasingly symbolic actions. The sequence of developments from separating to constructing; from given to imposed constructions; and, among imposed constructions, from general to specific to animate surrogate constructions; augments the description of infant intelligence in terms of the development of object and action concepts proposed by Mandler (1992, in press). Examining play in terms of a progression from separating activities in the prespeech period to the specific animate surrogate constructing activities at the time of the vocabulary spurt resulted in a more powerful explanation of developments during the single-word period in relation to language.

Conclusions from the Three Perspectives
to the Study of Play in the Transition to Language

We have seen how the role of play during the transition to language has been framed in different ways within the constructivist tradition. The three dominant emphases in studies of relationships among language, play, and cognition—the intentionality perspective; the focus on intentional, goal-directed behaviors; and the focus on symbolic behaviors—share the view that language and play are related to each other in development by virtue of the relationship of each to developments in cognition, as predicted originally by Piaget (1962). Furthermore, the intentionality perspective embraces and subsumes developments in both the symbolic capacity and intentional behaviors. However, the three research emphases differ on how play can be used as a window on early developments in cognition and the level of differentiation used to describe play and language behaviors for the purposes of examining relationships between them. The three perspectives also differ in the part played by the role of social interaction in the development of play and the role of play in the transition to language.

First, explicit descriptions of different aspects of play were used as a window on cognition in the studies reported by Lifter and Bloom (1989) and by McCune (1995). McCune used differentiated categories of symbolic play to describe specific changes in the differentiation of self from objects and people. Categories of social and event knowledge identified by others (e.g., Bretherton, 1984; Lucariello, 1987) are subsumed in McCune's subcategories of symbolic play. Lifter and Bloom's analysis captured detailed developmental changes in the aspects of knowledge that were expressed in play and revealed differentiated subcategories of manipulative play that set the stage for the emerging developments in specific object knowledge and its relationship to symbolic play. Bates et al. (1979), in contrast, relied on the global categories of combinatorial and symbolic play to describe progress in play, and they also assessed developments in cognition with other measures of sensorimotor scale performance. Although each study employed measures of language form and, in some cases (e.g., Bates et al., 1979), measured language in terms of both comprehension and production, Bloom et al. (1988) contributed an analysis of early words that revealed developmental change in the meanings these words expressed (from evidential states to anticipated actions) and the cognition these meanings required. Thus, the qualitative differences in the different categorization schemes that have been used influence the conclusions that can be drawn about the role of play in the transition to language. A summary of measures is presented in Table 1.

Second, although the bulk of the descriptive studies focused on individual children with a caregiver, the analyses centered on what the children did. As a result, the studies differed regarding the role of social interaction in the transition. Bates et al.'s (1979) view of the cognitive and social bases for language centered on the importance of means–ends relationships and the instrumental function of language and play. They concluded that the transition to intentional,

Table 1. Measures used to examine relationships between play and language

Studies	Play analyses	Language analyses
Bates et al. (1979, 1988)	Global distinction • Manipulative (combinatorial) play • Symbolic play	Language uses • Proto-declaratives • Proto-imperatives Language forms • Early words (comprehension and production)
McCune (1995), Nicolich (1977)	Categories of symbolic (pretend) play	Language forms • Early words • Word combinations • Rule-governed combinations
Bloom (1993), Bloom et al. (1988), Lifter & Bloom (1989)	Categories of thematic relationships between objects (traditionally characterized as manipulative or symbolic play)	Language forms • Early words • Vocabulary spurt Language meanings • Presentational and action • Evident and anticipated

goal-directed behaviors provided the cognitive basis for language and resulted in the ability first to use objects and people in the service of various goals and then, soon after, to use language as a tool, enabling the child to join in a social world. (See Bloom, 1993, for a critique of the "tool use" metaphor as an explanation of language acquisition.)

McCune (1993) used the transition from presymbolic to symbolic activities in play to explain how the ability to think about the self and others develops in the context of play with a caregiver. Progress in self–other understanding was used to support developments in children's theory of mind, in particular, the ability to consciously and deliberately infer something about others' intentions, which is not fully developed until well after the transition to language.

From the intentionality perspective, play is an expression of contents of mind, which means that play is about something to which caregivers and others can respond for supporting the child's participation in a social world (Bloom, 1993; Lifter & Bloom, 1989). The consequence of developments in cognition and affect is that intentional states become both increasingly discrepant from the data of perception and increasingly elaborated. Children must learn more intricate and complex forms of expression, in play and language, to express discrepant and elaborative meanings to be able to share intentional states with others and thereby sustain the intersubjectivity that has determined emotional well-being since early infancy. A child's need to make the hidden contents of mind manifest so that other people can know them and share them is what drives development and, especially, developments in language (Bloom, 1993). The comparisons between play and language identified by Lifter and Bloom (1989) are presented in Table 2.

Finally, the three research emphases have resulted in different conclusions regarding the role of play in the transition to language. For Bates et al. (1979),

Table 2.   Correspondences between play and language from the intentionality perspective

Language analyses	Play analyses
Prespeech (9–11 months)	Separating activities • Moving objects apart: perceptually based, unidirectional actions
Early words: primarily expressing evident, presentational meanings (mean age: 13.8 months)	Reversible actions relating one object thematically to another in *general* ways • Re-creating given relationships • Creating general relationships based on simple physical properties (for containment and support)
Vocabulary spurt: primarily expressing anticipated action meanings (mean age: 19.2 months)	Reversible actions relating one object thematically to another in *specific* ways • Creating thematic relationships based on physical, functional, and conventional object roles and properties

Note: See Lifter and Bloom (1989) for empirical report.

the development of intentional behaviors in general, not play in particular, is central for the development of language. Although play behaviors may reflect developments in intentional behaviors, these researchers did not describe how play serves the development of intentional behaviors. McCune (1995; also Nicolich, 1977) provided detailed descriptions of relationships between language and play, with both language and play presented as manifestations of developments in cognition. As a result, cognition was considered the basis for the developments expressed in play, but McCune did not make explicit how play activities contribute to developments in cognition or to developments in language.

The role of play in the transition to language was made explicit within the intentionality model, where play is considered an activity base for both expression and interpretation. Acts of expressing and interpreting contents of mind, in turn, cause revision and change in the experiences that inform developments in cognition. Thus, play provides the child with a context for constructing the representations in intentional states and knowledge. At the same time, play activities provide the researcher with a window on both the representations that are the contents of the child's intentional states and the emergence and developments in knowledge that they require. The developments reported by Lifter and Bloom (1989) in language, from prespeech to first words to the vocabulary spurt, correspond to developments in play beginning with the transitions from separating to constructing activities, and within the constructing activities, from given to imposed constructions and from general to specific thematic relations. These developments in language and play provided evidence of the increasingly discrepant and elaborative intentional states that the children expressed in the single-word period in the second year of life. The developments in mental representation and object knowledge that both play and language require resulted in the close relationship between play and language that was observed.

PLAY AS A CONTEXT FOR LEARNING

Before we can consider the clinical and educational implications of play, we need to consider how play activities provide a context for learning through expression. Play provides a context for revision and change in the contents of mind that inform developments in cognition. When an infant or a very young child plays with an object, the child typically looks at an object and then acts on it, and what the child does with the object at first is based on what the child might already know about it. However, looking at and then acting on an object are opportunities for learning something more about the object and about the child's own abilities for acting. Thus, a child comes to learn about an object's properties—such as how it feels, whether soft or rigid, with edges or without, graspable or not—and other such physical properties. At first, actions are very simple: The child must pick up an object, possibly explore it by mouthing it, and then cast it aside or put it down somewhere else. This sequence might be repeated with other, different objects, and sometimes the child might turn back to retrieve an object previously discarded. Thus, the child learns that the same objects can be found in different places and that the same action can be repeated with different objects.

Certain objects will already be attached or in close proximity to other objects, such as when graduated cups are nested in each other. If the object is already part of a configuration of things that go together (e.g., nested cups, a wooden "driver" in a car, a fork and spoon in a cup), the act of separating the objects provides new information, first about the individual objects but also about the relationship between them. The new information the child gains might consist only of learning that things in relation to each other can be separated. But, eventually, the child will realize that if the objects can be taken apart, they can also be put back into their original configurations. Through separating and constructing activities, children come to realize that objects are individual entities and that such individual entities can relate to each other according to their physical properties (e.g., when one object provides a container or a support for holding another object). The early separating activities described by Lifter and Bloom (1989) provided the children with just such opportunities for learning. When a child took hold of an object that formed part of a configuration with another object and pulled the two objects apart, the groundwork was laid for appreciating the general relational properties that the objects can have to one another. The act of separating allowed the child to see the relationship between the two objects they had taken apart, and also, how they might go back together to restore the relationship. Indeed, children's earliest constructing activities consisted of reversals of their separating activities. The act of separating provided perceptual support for the experience needed to learn how things go together and for learning about the relational properties of individual objects.

At first, children "see-then-act": They look at objects and move them from place to place, in and out of containers, back and forth from cup to truck, and they do these things over and over again. Thus, acting on objects provided opportunities to learn the relationship properties of objects that were, at first, fairly general in nature; however, repeated encounters with new and different objects and applying knowledge about the physical general relationship properties of objects to new objects, expanded the possibilities for the kinds of relationships that different objects afford. These relationships become increasingly specific. Putting a toy "person" into a car takes advantage of the "container" properties of the car and the "containable" properties of the "person," just as putting one nesting cup into another uses one object as a container for another. However, something else is also involved in the relationship that is formed between the toy person and the car, because this configuration also has conventional, cultural properties that go beyond the general physical properties of the objects and the relationships the physical properties afford.

Thus, by acting on objects to join them together in general ways, children come to learn that particular objects can be related to each other in more conventionally specific ways. These early constructing activities allowed children to "play out" the increasingly elaborate events of their lives. Such conventional properties are not inherent in the objects themselves but are derived from how children participate in social and cultural exchanges in their activities of daily living. Learning to eat with a spoon, for example, is augmented when a child uses a spoon to "feed" a doll in play, creating a specific relationship between two objects, the spoon and the doll. Similarly, understanding the relationships between people and vehicles is augmented when a child puts a toy figure into a toy car and pushes it along a "roadway." By constructing increasingly specific and elaborate relationships with objects, not only are children expressing what they are learning about the world, but they are also enhancing that learning at the same time.

An important source of evidence that children are actively learning from their play with objects comes from research in children's attention and engagement. Children pay more attention to play activities that represent new learning than to those activities that are already relatively well known (e.g., Ruff & Saltarelli, 1993; Wikstrom, 1994). A related research finding is that children are more engaged and express more emotionally toned affect in the context of constructing recently learned specific thematic relationships between objects than the earlier learned given and general relationships (Bloom et al., 1997). If children are more engaged and are also paying more attention to activities that represent new learning for them, we can take their interest and engagement in the action as an indication that learning is taking place.

Finally, as children come to appreciate the many different relationships that are possible among objects by constructing increasingly elaborate and specific thematic relationships among them, they have more options to choose from when acting on objects. Their play becomes more planful and loses the "see-then-act" quality it had when they were dependent on the perceptual properties of objects for their actions. Although a child's play continues to be intrinsically motivated, behavior becomes more planful because it is guided by the new knowledge that the child is gaining, not only in activities of daily living but also by recreating those activities in play.

In summary, what children do with objects in their play has to do with what they know about objects, which is regulated by the structure and organization of knowledge. This knowledge comes from their experiences with objects in the context of their own activities and participation in everyday events with caregivers. Children's intrinsic motivation to act in play ensures the process of learning, which is often not the case for children developing more slowly than or differently from their peers. The educational and clinical implications of play as a context for learning are described in the next section.

EDUCATIONAL AND CLINICAL IMPLICATIONS

The central point of this chapter is that children engage in interpretive activities as well as expressive activities when they play, and these activities cause revision and change in the experiences that inform developments in cognition. Although for most children play activities may appear effortless, children with developmental disabilities have difficulty using play to learn about the world (Fewell & Kaminski, 1988) and are often not intrinsically motivated to learn. These same children are often those who have difficulty learning language (Lahey, 1988). It is for these children that the educational and clinical implications from the role of play in the transition to language could be and should be especially useful for assessment *and* intervention activities designed to enhance their development.

Because the traditional constructivist perspective focused on play as "the happy display of known actions" (Piaget, 1962, p. 93), connections were drawn from play to assessment activities, and a number of play assessment instruments were developed (e.g., Fewell & Rich, 1987; Lifter, Edwards, Avery, Anderson, & Sulzer-Azaroff, 1988; Linder, 1993; Wetherby & Prizant, 1992; see Lifter, 1996, for review). Play provided a window on cognition, independent of language, for assessing development in children with language delays because what children know and are thinking about can be made manifest in play activities without language.

However, the constructivist approach has been essentially silent on the usefulness of play activities for facilitating developmental change for two main reasons. First, because play was originally defined as an expression of known actions, the notion of work was antithetical to play (Elkind, 1990). The prevailing view was that when children play they use objects according to what they know; they do not adapt to objects in the sense of learning something new. Second, because development as a whole, which includes play, is ordered by the child's construction of the world, developmental change was considered outside the direct control of educators (Gratch, 1979) and not amenable to intervention. This second reason is fundamental to the procedures of developmentally appropriate practice (DAP) (Bredekamp, 1987). The procedures of DAP assume active involvement of the learner and have led to *child-directed* approaches in education. Child-directed originally meant that children will determine what they will learn because they are intrinsically motivated to learn. As a result, any kind of teacher-directed intervention was regarded as outside the guidelines of DAP.

In the intentionality perspective, however, play functions for both expression and interpretation (Bloom, 1993). This perspective provides a rationale for designing and implementing interventions in play in particular and interventions more widely to enhance development. Play is indeed "the child's work" (p. 180), as was pointed out by Montessori (1967) and confirmed by empirical findings in the 1990s that show increased allocation of children's attention and engagement in activities in their object-related play that are developmentally new (Bloom et al., in preparation; Ruff & Saltarelli, 1993; Wikstrom, 1994). Children are actively engaged in learning when they can interpret ongoing events in terms of the structure, organization, and content of their existing knowledge. Therefore, the challenge in using play activities for learning and facilitating developmental change is to identify target play activities that children can make sense of and that provide opportunities for revision and change to acquire new knowledge.

Interpretable activities are those that the child knows at least something about and is in the process of learning, not activities beyond the child's level of understanding. Interpretable activities can be determined by assessing the focus of the child's attention and the content of play relative to developmental progression. For example, researchers and teachers can determine if children relate objects to one another in thematic ways as described by Lifter and Bloom (1989), and, if so, they can determine the extent of specificity of the roles and properties of objects manifest in those thematic relations. It is possible to identify the degree of discrepancy between presented events and what has to be recalled from memory for relating objects in play, as well as the extent and kind of elaboration in the roles and properties of objects shown in play. Such analyses can provide researchers and teachers with methods for selecting play activities that are relevant to a child's learning level at a particular period in development, and this basic approach is consistent with teaching activities that are within what Vygotsky (1978) called the zone of proximal development.

The constructivist framework, and the intentionality perspective in particular, provide important insights into the role of play in development, with implications for intervention when incorporated into educational and clinical programs. For example, Lifter, Sulzer-Azaroff, Anderson, and Cowdery (1993) argued for attention to the *developmental appropriateness* of play activities, rather than activities based on the selection of appealing toys or age-appropriate behaviors (e.g., Eason, White, & Newsom, 1982), to identify play actions to teach children with developmental disabilities. Developmental appropriateness has to do with assessment of play to identify activities at the child's level of *interpretation*. Studies also have attended to the inclusion of cognitive and social-communicative prerequisites to language objectives (Warren, Yoder, Gazdag, Kim, & Jones, 1993) or have explained the success of play intervention programs in terms of relationships between play and language (Goldstein & Cisar, 1992; Stahmer, 1995). Children with higher scores in language learned symbolic play activities more easily than children with lower scores. Slade and Wolf (1994) advocated attention to the structure and organization underlying a child's play before assuming the child is able to engage in the complex play activities required for play therapy.

Descriptive categories of children's play activities are provided in the play studies reviewed in this chapter, and they form the basis for several play assessment instruments (see Lifter, 1996). For example, Lifter et al. (1988) devised the

Developmental Play Assessment (DPA) tool based on the categories of play reported in Lifter and Bloom (1989) (i.e., given and imposed, general and specific, and animate surrogate) and integrated with other reports of children's play (e.g., Belsky & Most, 1981; Nicolich, 1977; Watson & Fischer, 1977). The DPA yields an evaluation of a child's progress in play in relation to a sequence of developmentally ordered play categories, with the child's performance in each category described as "absent," emerging," and "mastered." The categories identified to be emerging are considered to tap into a child's level of interpretation and to be the relevant categories to target in an intervention program.

A preliminary validation of the DPA for use in identifying play objectives for intervention was reported in Lifter et al. (1993). They selected play activities from two different categories in the play sequence and taught the play activities to preschoolers with developmental disabilities. The particular categories were identified as developmentally appropriate (e.g., child as agent in which doll is recipient of action) and age appropriate (e.g., doll as agent in which doll is agent of action) relative to the individual children. Developmentally appropriate categories were either emerging or those at the next step in the development sequence. Age-appropriate categories of play activities were those that were used by the children's peers who did not have disabilities. Lifter et al. (1993) reported that the children reached criterion more quickly for the developmentally appropriate activities and generalized those activities to new instances to a greater extent than they did with the age-appropriate activities.

The results of the Lifter et al. (1993) study supported the usefulness of selecting intervention targets at the child's level of interpretation, that is, activities that were determined to be emerging or at the next step for an individual child. The results also supported the teaching of play activities to children whose play was limited or developing very slowly. The children did not engage in the target activities until the intervention was under way, although they were provided with the relevant play materials during the baseline observations. Further studies are obviously needed. This method of using data from the development of children without disabilities for planning assessment and intervention with children who have disabilities follows the precedent set by Bloom and Lahey (1978; Lahey, 1988) who used the data from the language development of children without disabilities for assessment and intervention with children who have language disorders.

The intentionality perspective and the use of play for both intervention and assessment activities bring together the goals of both DAP and early childhood special education (ECSE). On the one hand, "the explicit mission of early childhood special education (ECSE) is to produce outcomes that would not occur in the absence of intervention or teaching" (Carta, Schwartz, Atwater, & McConnell, 1991, p. 4). On the other hand, DAP requires active involvement of the learner (Johnson & McChesney Johnson, 1992) with child-directed approaches that are antithetical to the teacher-directed approaches suggested by

ECSE. Many children with developmental disabilities are not intrinsically motivated to learn and so cannot be expected to "determine" what they will learn as some child-directed approaches promote. Teacher-directed approaches are needed that consist of determining activities at the child's level of interpretation and providing the push needed for children to engage in them to facilitate developmental change. Child-directed approaches then should be revised to include a determination of goals based on the structure and organization of the child's knowledge at a particular time. Selecting and teaching target activities at a child's level of interpretation enhance the child's focus of attention and afford opportunities for active involvement in learning, resulting in intervention efforts that are truly child directed (Lifter, 1995; McCathren, Yoder, & Warren, 1995).

Because play contributes to a child's knowledge of the world, interventions in which children learn more about objects, people, and events provide opportunities for development in language. Children learn to talk about what they know. Learning more about the world through play means the child has more knowledge to share with caregivers and peers, and displaying that knowledge allows caregivers and peers to respond. The expectation is that teaching children to play in activities that are finely tuned to and build on their interpretation abilities will provide them with opportunities to learn to talk about ongoing events they know something about or are learning about, thereby facilitating developmental change. The impact of learning to play on the structure and organization of knowledge and on development in language and social interaction is the promise of play interventions. How that is best accomplished awaits further study.

THE ROLE OF CULTURE FOR DEVELOPMENTS IN PLAY

The descriptions of developments in play presented in this chapter have been generated within a European American cultural perspective and by empirical studies of the play of European American children to a large extent. Therefore, the comments in this section are necessarily speculative for several reasons. For one, the role of culture in the transition to symbolic processes in play has not been addressed directly, because, in part, of the dearth of descriptive studies of the development of children from divergent cultures (see Bloom, 1992, and Graham, 1992, for discussion of this point), although this is changing (Roopnarine & Johnson, 1994). Most of the studies reviewed for this chapter were based on observations of children from a subset of American cultures with an emphasis primarily on object-related behaviors, which may be a largely European American influence. Children from African American homes evidently have less object-related and more person-related influences on their language and play (Blake, 1994; Lin & Blake, 1995). The need for more culturally relevant descriptive studies of play is clear.

More important, however, for understanding the role of culture in these transitions is a fundamental change in how culture is viewed in development.

Lucariello (1995) offered a historical analysis of how the elements of mind, culture, and person have been regarded in a cultural psychology. Early versions of a cultural psychology began with mind and culture as separate entities. Lucariello argued, instead, for an analysis of mind and culture in a "person-based" cultural psychology, in which the fundamental unit of analysis is the "culturally shared realities or frames through which persons interpret the environment" (p. 3).

Until person-based cultural analyses begin to inform studies of the relationships between play and language, only speculative conclusions about the role of culture in their development are possible. The environment provided for most children includes opportunities to act on objects and to engage in a social world with caregivers and peers, unless the family is severely impoverished or the child's capacities to actively attend to objects, people, and events are compromised in some way. The assumption is, therefore, that every child will acquire knowledge of objects, people, and events that contribute to developments in play and language, and all children will make the transitions from preintentional to intentional behaviors and from presymbolic to symbolic activities. Both of these transitions contribute to developments in intentionality, that is, to developments in the representations of conscious states of mind that are expressed by language and play. The content of the particular activities themselves, however, should be culturally specific, as would the materials used, because symbols are given meaning from sociocultural processes (Fein, 1989).

All cultures have arrangements and customs by which people interact with one another, just as they have systems of expression for communicating with one another. Although the forms of interaction and communication may differ across cultures, people from all cultures engage in caregiving activities that become highly familiar to young children and are likely to reappear in the children's play activities. In descriptions of children's symbolic activities in the literature, most early activities centered around familiar feeding and other well-known activities (Lucariello, 1987) that could reasonably be expected to be represented in all children's play.

Nevertheless, physical and social environments can vary considerably. Different social contexts and cultures provide different environments for children to learn about the world, with different kinds of opportunities for engaging with caregivers and peers. An infant's environment continuously expands from the immediate environment provided by caregivers, to the larger environment of the family, and, eventually, to the environment of the larger culture, including peers. However, not much is known about the relative contributions from culture and development on children's environments; different cultures emphasize and attend to differing aspects of needs in the environment. For example, conversations in which participants take overlapping turns, talking at the same time, are acceptable in culturally different societies and even valued by the participants in certain contexts (e.g., Cazden & Dickinson, 1981; Ervin-Tripp, 1979; Heath, 1982, 1983; Whatley, 1981).

More studies of the role of culture in the development of play are needed. The promise of future research lies in more comprehensive and culturally relevant analyses of the role of play in the transition to language and the relation of both play and language to developments in cognition. Such studies also would have important educational and clinical implications in addition to the clinical and educational implications from the studies of play that are reviewed in this chapter.

DIRECTIONS FOR FUTURE RESEARCH

Several directions for research have already been described. Chief among these, perhaps, is the need to learn more about children's play in different cultures. For an assessment and intervention procedure to be valid, it must be informed by a culturally relevant descriptive base that includes the social role of play in development. Also needed are studies to document the effectiveness of play interventions and whether they contribute to a child's knowledge of the world, in general, and to a child's development in language and social interaction, in particular. Studies also are needed that examine the usefulness and feasibility of integrating language with play in intervention programs. Given the perspective that play and language are both expressions of intentional states (Bloom, 1993), the integration of language objectives with developmentally appropriate play objectives would mean including and embedding related goals in the same activity.

Descriptive studies are needed that examine the impact of the caregiver on how children learn to play and the conditions surrounding their interactions, similar to the need for descriptive studies that inform interventions in communication and language (Warren & Reichle, 1992). The role of the caregiver has been conceptualized as a scaffolder by Bruner (1983) and, in contrast, as primarily a responder by Bloom (1997; Bloom, Margulis, Tinker, & Fujita, 1996). The nature of the caregiver's role for both learning language and learning play activities has direct implications for the role that the interventionist should take, and the extent to which children require explicit scaffolding or more careful responding is another issue for research.

In addition to the needs of children, educational programs are also needed for teachers and related services providers that focus on the importance of play in children's lives (Smilansky, 1990). Beliefs about the role of play in children's lives and whether play should be "interfered with" often are not informed by empirical research. Intervention is not interference if the selection of objectives allows for the child to be actively involved in the process of learning. How learning to play can serve an important function for children who have difficulty in development is an important content area for personnel preparation programs.

Finally, it is also important that the covariation among play, language, and social competence is examined in descriptive studies (e.g., Bloom et al., 1997). Many interventions that have centered on facilitating language and social development have used play as an activity base to support these interventions (Bricker & Cripe, 1992; Kaiser, Yoder, & Keetz, 1992; Odom & Strain, 1984; Warren & Gazdag, 1990). What is not known is the relationship between the child's level of interpretation in play and the play activities selected to support language and social goals in assessment and intervention, and information about the relationship between the child's level and play activities is necessary for improving the efficacy of interventions.

CONCLUSION

Play is defined in this chapter as an interpretive activity as well as an expressive activity, and this definition was derived from the intentionality model of development proposed by Bloom (1991, 1993, 1994, in press). Developments in cognition contribute to the contents of mind that are expressed in both play and language, and, in turn, children's play activities contribute to cognitive developments as much as they are influenced by them. This definition of play relates directly to assessment and intervention activities. The challenge in using play activities for learning and facilitating developmental change in children with developmental disabilities is to identify target play activities that children can make sense of and then to provide opportunities for revision and change in their knowledge. Selecting and teaching play activities at the child's level of interpretation enhances the child's focus of attention, affords opportunities for active involvement in learning, provides activities that the child can talk about and that caregivers and others can respond to, and should result in intervention efforts that are truly child centered.

REFERENCES

Anisfeld, M. (1984). *Language development from birth to three.* Hillsdale, NJ: Lawrence Erlbaum Associates.

Axline, V.M. (1947). *Play therapy.* Cambridge, MA: Riverside Press.

Bates, E. (1976). *Language and context: The acquisition of pragmatics.* New York: Academic Press.

Bates, E., Benigni, L., Bretherton, I., Camaioni, L., & Volterra, V. (1979). *The emergence of symbols: Communication and cognition in infancy.* New York: Academic Press.

Bates, E., Bretherton, I., & Snyder, L. (1988). *From first words to grammar: Individual differences and dissociative mechanisms.* New York: Cambridge University Press.

Beeghly, M., Weiss-Perry, B., & Cicchetti, D. (1990). Beyond sensorimotor functioning: Early social-communicative and play development of children with Down syndrome. In D. Cicchetti & M. Beeghly (Eds.), *Children with Down syndrome: A developmental perspective* (pp. 329–368). Cambridge, England: Cambridge University Press.

Belsky, J., & Most, R.K. (1981). From exploration to play: A cross-sectional study of infant free play behavior. *Developmental Psychology, 17,* 630–639.

Blake, I. (1994). Language development and socialization in young African American children. In P. Greenfield & R. Cocking (Eds.), *Cross-cultural roots of minority child development* (pp. 167–195). Hillsdale, NJ: Lawrence Erlbaum Associates.

Bloom, L. (1973). *One word at a time: The use of single-word utterances before syntax.* The Hague, The Netherlands: Mouton.

Bloom, L. (1991). Representation and expression. In N. Krasnegor, D. Rumbaugh, R. Schiefelbusch, & M. Studdert-Kennedy (Eds.), *Biological and behavioral determinants of language development* (pp. 117–140). Hillsdale, NJ: Lawrence Erlbaum Associates.

Bloom, L. (1992, Fall–Winter). Racism in developmental research. *Division 7 Newsletter.* Washington, DC: American Psychological Association.

Bloom, L. (1993). *The transition from infancy to language: Acquiring the power of expression.* New York: Cambridge University Press.

Bloom, L. (1994). Meaning and expression. In W. Overton & D. Palermo (Eds.), *The ontogenesis of meaning* (pp. 215–235). Hillsdale, NJ: Lawrence Erlbaum Associates.

Bloom, L. (1997, April). Intentionality is the basis for the social foundations of language development. In *Social foundations of language development: Theoretical issues.* Symposium conducted at the biennial convention of the Society for Research in Child Development, Washington, DC.

Bloom, L. (in press). Language acquisition in its developmental context. In D. Kuhn & R. Siegler (Eds.), *Cognition, perception, and language* (Vol. II) in W. Damon (Series Ed.), *Handbook of child psychology.* New York: John Wiley & Sons.

Bloom, L., Beckwith, R., Capatides, J., & Hafitz, J. (1988). Expression through affect and words in the transition from infancy to language. In P. Baltes, D. Featherman, & R. Lerner (Eds.), *Life-span development and behavior* (Vol. 8, pp. 99–127). Hillsdale, NJ: Lawrence Erlbaum Associates.

Bloom, L., & Lahey, M. (1978). *Language development and language disorders.* New York: John Wiley & Sons.

Bloom, L., Lifter, K., & Broughton, J. (Eds.). (1985). *The emergence of early cognition and language in the second year of life.* New York: John Wiley & Sons.

Bloom, L., Margulis, C., Tinker, E., & Fujita, N. (1996). Early conversations and word learning: Contributions from child and adult. *Child Development, 67,* 3154–3175.

Bloom, L., Tinker, E., & Beckwith, R. (1997). *Developments in expression: Language, emotion, and object play.* Manuscript in preparation.

Bredekamp, S. (1987). *Developmentally appropriate practice in early childhood programs serving children birth through age 8.* Washington, DC: National Association for the Education of Young Children.

Bretherton, I. (1984). *Symbolic play.* Orlando, FL: Academic Press.

Bricker, D., & Cripe, J.J.W. (1992). *An activity-based approach to early intervention.* Baltimore: Paul H. Brookes Publishing Co.

Bruner, J. (1983). *Child's talk.* New York: Norton.

Butterfield, N. (1994). Play as an assessment and intervention strategy for children with language and intellectual disabilities. In K. Linfoot (Ed.), *Communication strategies for people with developmental disabilities: Issues from theory and practice* (pp. 12–44). Sydney, Australia: MacLennan & Petty.

Carta, J.J., Schwartz, I.S., Atwater, J.B., & McConnell, S.R. (1991). Developmentally appropriate practice: Appraising its usefulness for young children with disabilities. *Topics in Early Childhood Special Education, 11*(1), 1–20.

Cazden, C., & Dickinson, D. (1981). Language in education: Standardization versus cultural pluralism. In C. Ferguson & S. Heath (Eds.), *Language in the USA* (pp. 446–468). Cambridge, England: Cambridge University Press.

Corrigan, R. (1978). Language development as related to Stage 6 object permanence. *Journal of Child Language, 5,* 173–189.

Eason, L.J., White, M.J., & Newsom, C. (1982). Generalized reduction of self-stimulatory behavior: An effect of teaching age-appropriate play to autistic children. *Analysis and Intervention in Developmental Disabilities, 2,* 157–169.

Elkind, D. (1990). Academic pressures—too much, too soon: The demise of play. In E. Klugman & S. Smilansky (Eds.), *Children's play and learning* (pp. 3–17). New York: Teachers College Press.

Ervin-Tripp, S. (1979). Children's verbal turn-taking. In E. Ochs & B. Schieffelin (Eds.), *Developmental pragmatics* (pp. 391–414). New York: Academic Press.

Fein, G. (1989). Mind, meaning, and affect: Proposals for a theory of pretense. *Developmental Review, 9,* 345–363.

Fenson, L., Kagan, J., Kearsley, R.B., & Zelazo, P.R. (1976). The developmental progression of manipulative play in the first two years. *Child Development, 47,* 232–236.

Fewell, R.R., & Kaminski, R. (1988). Play skills development and instruction for young children with handicaps. In S.L. Odom & M.B. Karnes (Eds.), *Early intervention for infants and children with handicaps: An empirical base* (pp. 145–158). Baltimore: Paul H. Brookes Publishing Co.

Fewell, R.R., & Rich, J.S. (1987). Play assessment as a procedure for examining cognitive, communication, and social skills in multihandicapped children. *Journal of Psychoeducational Assessment, 2,* 107–118.

Garvey, C. (1974). Some properties of social play. *Merrill-Palmer Quarterly, 20,* 163–180.

Garwood, S.G. (1982). Piaget and play: Translating theory into practice. *Topics in Early Childhood Special Education, 2*(3), 1–13.

Goldstein, H., & Cisar, C.L. (1992). Promoting interaction during sociodramatic play: Teaching scripts to preschoolers and classmates with disabilities. *Journal of Applied Behavior Analysis, 25,* 265–280.

Graham, S. (1992). "Most of the subjects were white and middle-class": Trends in published research on African-Americans in selected APA journals. *American Psychologist, 47,* 629–639.

Gratch, G. (1979). The development of thought and language in infancy. In J.D. Osofsky (Ed.), *Handbook of infant development* (pp. 439–461). New York: John Wiley & Sons.

Heath, S. (1982). What no bedtime story means: Narrative skills at home and school. *Language and Society, 11,* 49–76.

Heath, S. (1983). *Ways with words.* Cambridge, England: Cambridge University Press.

Hill, P., & McCune-Nicolich, L. (1981). Pretend play and patterns of cognition in Down's syndrome children. *Child Development, 52,* 611–617.

Johnson, J.E., & McChesney Johnson, K. (1992). Clarifying the developmental perspective in response to Carta, Schwartz, Atwater, and McConnell. *Topics in Early Childhood Special Education, 12*(4), 439–457.

Kaiser, A.P., Yoder, P.J., & Keetz, A. (1992). Evaluating milieu teaching. In S.F. Warren & J. Reichle (Eds.), *Communication and language intervention series: Vol. 1. Causes and effects in communication and language intervention* (pp. 9–47). Baltimore: Paul H. Brookes Publishing Co.

Lahey, M. (1988). *Language disorders and language development.* New York: Macmillan.

Lifter, K. (1995). Strategies that make sense. Commentary on R.B. McCathren, P.J. Yoder, and S.F. Warren, The role of directives in early language intervention. *Journal of Early Intervention, 19,* 106–107.

Lifter, K. (1996). Assessing play skills. In M. McLean, D.B. Bailey, & M. Wolery (Eds.), *Assessing infants and preschoolers with special needs.* Englewood Cliffs, NJ: Prentice-Hall.

Lifter, K., & Bloom, L. (1989). Object knowledge and the emergence of language. *Infant Behavior and Development, 12,* 395–423.

Lifter, K., Edwards, G., Avery, D., Anderson, S.R., & Sulzer-Azaroff, B. (1988, November). *Developmental assessment of children's play: Implications for intervention.*

Paper presented to the annual convention of the American Speech-Language-Hearing Association, Boston.

Lifter, K., Sulzer-Azaroff, B., Anderson, S., & Cowdery, G. (1993). Teaching play activities to preschool children with disabilities: The importance of developmental considerations. *Journal of Early Intervention, 17*(2), 139–159.

Lin, L., & Blake, I. (1995, March). *The communication of Euro-American preschool children: A factive orientation.* Paper presented at the biennial meetings of the Society for Research in Child Development, Indianapolis, IN.

Linder, T.W. (1993). *Transdisciplinary play-based assessment: A functional approach to working with young children* (Rev. ed.). Baltimore: Paul H. Brookes Publishing Co.

Lowe, M. (1975). Trends in the development of representational play in infants from one to three years: An observational study. *Journal of Child Psychology and Psychiatry and Allied Disciplines, 16,* 33–47.

Lucariello, J. (1987). Spinning fantasy: Themes, structure, and the knowledge base. *Child Development, 58,* 434–442.

Lucariello, J. (1995). Mind, culture, person: Elements in a cultural psychology. *Human Development, 38,* 2–18.

Mandler, J. (1988). How to build a baby: On the development of an accessible representational system. *Cognitive Development, 3,* 113–136.

Mandler, J. (1992). How to build a baby: II. Conceptual primitives. *Psychological Review, 4,* 587–604.

Mandler, J. (in press). Representation. In W. Damon (Series Ed.) & D. Kuhn & R. Siegler (Vol. Eds.), *Handbook of child psychology: Vol. 2. Cognition, perception, and language.* New York: John Wiley & Sons.

McCathren, R.B., Yoder, P.J., & Warren, S.F. (1995). The role of directives in early language intervention. *Journal of Early Intervention, 19,* 91–101.

McCune, L. (1993). The development of play as the development of consciousness. In M.H. Bornstein & A.W. O'Reilly (Eds.), *The role of play in the development of thought* (pp. 67–79). San Francisco: Jossey-Bass.

McCune, L. (1995). A normative study of representational play at the transition to language. *Developmental Psychology, 31*(2), 198–206.

Montessori, M. (1967). *The absorbent mind.* New York: Holt, Rinehart & Winston.

Nicolich, L.M. (1977). Beyond sensorimotor intelligence: Assessment of symbolic maturity through analysis of pretend play. *Merrill-Palmer Quarterly, 23,* 89–99.

Odom, S.L., & Strain, P.S. (1984). Classroom-based social skills instruction for severely handicapped preschool children. *Topics in Early Childhood Special Education, 4*(3), 97–116.

Parten, M. (1932). Social participation among preschool children. *Journal of Abnormal and Social Psychology, 27,* 243–269.

Phillips, R., & Sellito, V. (1990). Preliminary evidence on emotions expressed by children during solitary play. *Play and Culture, 3,* 79–90.

Piaget, J. (1954). *The construction of reality in the child.* New York: Basic Books.

Piaget, J. (1962). *Play, dreams, and imitation.* New York: Norton.

Roopnarine, J.L., & Johnson, J.E. (1994). The need to look at play in diverse settings. In J.L. Roopnarine, J.E. Johnson, & F.H. Hooper (Eds.), *Children's play in diverse cultures* (pp. 1–8). Albany: State University of New York Press.

Rubin, K., Fein, G., & Vandenberg, B. (1983). Play. In E.M. Hetherington (Ed.), *Handbook of child psychology: Socialization, personality, and social development* (pp. 693–774). New York: John Wiley & Sons.

Ruff, H.A., & Saltarelli, L.M. (1993). Exploratory play with objects: Basic cognitive processes and individual differences. In M.H. Bornstein & A.W. O'Reilly (Eds.), *The role of play in the development of thought* (pp. 5–16). San Francisco: Jossey-Bass.

Searle, J. (1984). *Minds, brains, and science.* Cambridge, MA: Harvard University Press.

Slade, A., & Wolf, D.P. (Eds.). (1994). *Children at play: Clinical and developmental approaches to meaning and representation.* New York: Oxford University Press.

Smilansky, S. (1968). *The effects of sociodramatic play on disadvantaged preschool children.* New York: John Wiley & Sons.

Smilansky, S. (1990). Sociodramatic play: Its relevance to behavior and achievement in school. In E. Klugman & S. Smilansky (Eds.), *Children's play and learning: Perspectives and policy implications* (pp. 18–42). New York: Teachers College Press.

Sperber, D., & Wilson, D. (1986). *Relevance: Communication and cognition.* Cambridge, MA: Harvard University Press.

Stahmer, A.C. (1995). Teaching symbolic play skills to children with autism using Pivotal Response Training. *Journal of Autism and Developmental Disorders, 25,* 123–141.

Tomasello, M., & Farrar, M.J. (1986). Joint attention and early language. *Child Development, 57,* 1454–1463.

Ungerer, J., & Sigman, M. (1981). Symbolic play and language comprehension in autistic children. *Journal of the American Academy of Child Psychiatry, 20,* 318–337.

Uzgiris, I., & Hunt, J. (1975). *Assessment in infancy.* Urbana: University of Illinois Press.

Vygotsky, L. (1978). *Mind in society: The development of higher psychological processes* (M. Cole, V. John-Steiner, S. Scribner, & E. Souberman, Eds.), Cambridge, MA: Harvard University Press. (Original work published in 1930)

Warren, S.F., & Gazdag, G. (1990). Facilitating early language development with milieu intervention procedures. *Journal of Early Intervention, 14,* 62–86.

Warren, S.F., & Reichle, J. (1992). The emerging field of communication and language intervention. In S.F. Warren & J. Reichle (Eds.), *Communication and language intervention series: Vol. 1. Causes and effects in communication and language intervention* (pp. 1–8). Baltimore: Paul H. Brookes Publishing Co.

Warren, S.F., Yoder, P.J., Gazdag, G.E., Kim, K., & Jones, H.A. (1993). Facilitating prelinguistic skills in young children with developmental delay. *Journal of Speech and Hearing Research, 36,* 89–97.

Watson, M.W., & Fischer, K.W. (1977). A developmental sequence of agent use in late infancy. *Child Development, 48,* 828–836.

Wetherby, A.M., & Prizant, B.M. (1992). Profiling young children's communicative competence. In S.F. Warren & J. Reichle (Eds.), *Communication and language intervention series: Vol. 1. Causes and effects in communication and language intervention* (pp. 217–254). Baltimore: Paul H. Brookes Publishing Co.

Whatley, E. (1981). Language among black Americans. In C. Ferguson & S. Heath (Eds.), *Language in the USA* (pp. 92–107). Cambridge, England: Cambridge University Press.

Wikstrom, P. (1994). *The role of attention in early cognitive development.* New York: Columbia University. Unpublished doctoral dissertation. University Microfilms International. No. 9427165: Ann Arbor, MI.

Wolery, M., & Bailey, D.B., Jr. (1989). Assessing play skills. In D.B. Bailey, Jr. & M. Wolery (Eds.), *Assessing infants and preschoolers with handicaps* (pp. 428–446). Columbus, OH: Charles E. Merrill.

9

The Transition
to Symbolic Communication

Amy M. Wetherby, Joe Reichle, and Patsy L. Pierce

B Y THE TIME OF THEIR first birthday, children usually do not produce true words but can communicate intentionally using a variety of gestures and vocalizations that have shared meanings with caregivers (Bates, O'Connell, & Shore, 1987). Social interactions between infants and caregivers revolve around the sharing of affect and attention and contribute to the infant's awareness of the effect that his or her behavior can have on others (Bruner, 1981; Dore, 1986; see also Chapter 2). One-year-olds have learned to express a variety of communicative intentions, including requesting, protesting, calling, greeting, showing off, and commenting (Bruner, 1981; Wetherby, Cain, Yonclas, & Walker, 1988; see also Chapter 2). A child's behavior becomes increasingly more goal directed and shows growing evidence of intentionality over the first year, which culminates in the capacity to symbolize, evident in the child's ability to use words to refer to objects and events and to pretend with objects in play.

Typically, by their second birthday, children can use and understand hundreds of words, construct sentences, and engage in simple conversations. Communication becomes much more readable and explicit with the accumulation of successful communicative experiences. The dramatic changes in language abilities that occur between 1 and 2 years of age are reflected in two major transitions: 1) the transition to symbolic communication and 2) the transition to linguistic communication. These two transitions in spoken language development are examined in this chapter. Although a thorough discussion of the transition to linguistic communication is beyond the scope of this chapter and book, the qualitative changes that are evident as a child acquires a symbolic communi-

This chapter was supported in part by Contract No. H133B80048 to the Research and Training Center on Community Living from the National Institute on Disability and Rehabilitation Research; Grant No. HO24D40006, A Replication and Dissemination of a Model of Inservice Training and Technical Assistance to Prevent Challenging Behaviors in Young Children, U.S. Department of Education; and Grant No. HO29D050063, Preparation of Leadership Personnel: Training Leadership Personnel to Address the Needs of Preschoolers Who Engage in Challenging Behavior, U.S. Department of Education.

cation system and progresses from symbolic to linguistic communication are considered. The developmental milestones associated with these transitional points can serve as a road map for practitioners working with learners at early stages of language development. A developmental road map can provide landmarks to help identify important achievements on the way to words and to guide decisions about where to go next.

This chapter examines the transition to symbolic communication from a constructivist perspective, which considers language learning as an active process in which children construct or build knowledge and shared meanings based on interactions with people and experiences in their environment (Bates, 1979; see also Chapter 8). A primary goal of this chapter is to describe patterns in the development of symbolic communication by first examining the emergence of an expressive lexicon and considering the transition to symbols in spoken language as well as gestural and graphic modalities, and second, by considering parallel developments in the comprehension of meaning. A second goal of this chapter is to examine the acquisition process of symbolic communication by exploring theories on how and why children learn symbolic communication. The chapter closes with clinical and research implications.

EMERGENCE OF AN EXPRESSIVE LEXICON

The transition to symbolic communication refers to a child's emerging capacity to use words as symbols that represent objects, events, or concepts. There is a large body of literature on the emergence of lexicon in young children, with the acquisition of the first 50 words having received the most attention (see Bloom, 1993). Two major achievements have been recognized since the late 1800s as milestones in early lexical development: a child's first words and a vocabulary burst that occurs after the first 20–50 words. This section examines developmental patterns associated with these two achievements during the transition to symbolic communication.

First Spoken Words

There is a very gradual transition from the use of preverbal sounds and gestures to first words. At about 9 months of age, intentionality becomes evident in children's communicative behavior by their display of alternating eye gaze between a person and an object and persistence in signaling until their communicative goal is met (Bates, 1979). Before using words, children acquire a repertoire of conventional sounds and gestures to express communicative intentions (e.g., open–close hand reach to request a desired object out of reach, pointing and vocalizing "da" to direct attention to an interesting object). The capacity to use intentional communication and to acquire conventional signals is rooted in the developing cognitive knowledge that people are causal agents of actions and that people and objects can be used as tools to solve problems (Bates, 1979; Harding & Golinkoff, 1979; Snyder, 1978; Steckol & Leonard, 1981). From a constructivist perspective, intentional, conventional communication and its cognitive-social underpinnings form the foundation for the emergence of first words (Bates, 1979; Bloom, 1993).

The discovery that things have names begins to unfold at about 12–13 months of age. Initial first word acquisition has been described as context or event bound in that initially words may not refer to objects or actions, but rather, a particular word may only be used in a highly specific context or situation (Barrett, 1986). First words often mark a predictable point in an episode (e.g., waving and saying "bye bye" when closing a book, saying "uh-oh" when a tower of blocks is knocked over). Bloom (1993) described the acquisition of words as initially based on episodic associations. A child hears and remembers a word as part of an episode, and it is the episode that cues the use of early words. Participation in ritualized, turn-taking routines with caregivers provides essential scaffolding from which the child links words to events (Barrett, 1986; Bruner, 1981; Tomasello, 1992).

First words are by nature underextensions in that they are used in extremely limited contexts. The earliest of first words are not yet considered symbolic or referential because they "seem to belong to the context as a whole rather than to the referent in the peculiar way that names can be said to 'belong to' or identify referents" (Bates, 1979, p. 39). When children begin using first words, the majority of communicative signals in their repertoire continue to be preverbal sounds and gestures, with a sprinkling of words used here and there. Some early verbalizations in a child's repertoire, called *idiomorphs*, consist of consonant–vowel combinations that are not standard adult words (e.g., when a child pushes a toy car and makes the sound "vroom" or barks like the family's pet dog). Idiomorphs probably emerge as a result of the child playing with or imitating sounds in ritualized contexts.

Early in the one-word stage, new word acquisition is very slow, averaging about one new word per week, and is highly variable across children. Vocabulary attrition is a characteristic of the early one-word stage (Bloom & Lahey, 1978). It is not unusual for old words to drop out of a child's vocabulary as new words emerge, which sometimes causes concern to parents. This attrition has been characterized as the child having a window of vocabulary growth that is only so big and the child needs to lose an old word to make room for a new one (Bloom & Lahey, 1978). Another reason is that a particular word may have multiple meanings initially and may be replaced by several different new words that convey more specific meanings (e.g., /baba/ replaced by approximations of bottle, drink, juice, cup). It also may reflect the transition from pragmatic to semantic meaning. That is, proto-words may express general meanings tied to communicative functions (e.g., /duda/ used as a general request for help and /da/ as a general comment to direct attention to objects), and old forms may no longer be used once a child acquires more specific words to express those functions. Furthermore, a change in preferred topics may influence the acquisition and use of vocabulary items (Reich, 1986). Early lexical acquisition also may be limited by sound production. Lexical selection has been found to be influenced by consonant inventory (see Chapter 5). Thus, children who produce a limited number of sounds will be limited in the different forms they can produce and would be more likely to use each form to encode several meanings.

During the one-word stage, the event-bound use of words becomes decontextualized (Barrett, 1986; Bates, 1979). Children learn to free words from the context by hearing the same word in different events and hearing different words in similar situations (Bloom, 1993). The decontextualization of word use is believed to reflect the child's increasing knowledge of situations and concepts (Barrett, 1986). New word acquisition becomes associated with conceptual representations of objects and events. With the formation of concepts, different or new experiences with objects or events can cue the use of words. Thus, it is conceptual associations that enable the flexible use of words.

The question of when is a word a word has received much attention in the literature. Two major criteria have been used to determine that a spoken word is used to refer to an object or event (Vihman & McCune, 1994): 1) a phonetic form that approximates an adult word and 2) situational consistency in use. Thus, a spoken word can be operationalized as a phonetically consistent form that is used to refer to a particular object or event and only that object or event. Although the decision of whether a word is a word has challenged researchers and theorists, it is an intuitive decision for caregivers. Caregivers do not labor over whether their child's utterance is or is not a word; rather, they respond to their child's communicative intention and richly interpret the word from the context. The responsivity of caregivers can play an important role in language development (see Chapter 3).

A word is considered a symbol when it has been decontextualized or dissociated from the occurrence of a particular event. Bates (1979) stated that

> conventional communication is not symbolic communication until we can infer that the child has objectified the vehicle–referent relationship to some extent, realizing that the vehicle (i.e., the symbol) can be substituted for its referent for certain purposes, at the same time realizing that the symbol is not the same thing as its referent. (p. 38)

The capacity to use words as symbols corresponds with the cognitive achievement of mental representation (Bates, 1979; Snyder, 1978; Steckol & Leonard, 1981). Piaget (1970) argued that the capacity for mental representation is derived from the child's actions with objects in the world. From this constructivist perspective, a symbol is the "representation or internal reenactment (representation) of the activities originally carried out with objects or events" (Bates, 1976, p. 11). Children shift from responding to internal states and external events to learning by acting on objects and being able to think about representations of objects and events.

Early Gestural Production

Early gestural productions in typically developing children develop and function much like the boosting stage of a rocket propelling early productive language. Bonvillian, Orlansky, and Folven (1990) reported that typically developing children's first gestural vocabulary tends to be produced several months before spoken word approximations. Consequently, gestures may provide an important initial strategy of gaining experience in functional communicative exchanges. The relatively early appearance of gestures has been reported by a number of investigators (see Bonvillian et al., 1990). Bonvillian et al. (1990) summarized literature examining cognitive skills that have been associated with the onset of communicative spoken vocabulary. Several differences emerge in examining correlative relationships between cognitive indices and early verbal and gestural production when comparing vocabulary acquisition using gestures compared with speech. These investigators reported that 31% of the typically developing children of deaf parents that they observed produced their first recognizable sign approximations during sensorimotor Stage 3, whereas 46% of those children observed produced their first spoken words during sensorimotor Stage 4.

The prevalence of early gestural forms before vocal and verbal approximations is well supported in literature addressing the physiology of motor and vocal behavior. Braem (1990) provided a detailed review of hand movements required in sign production that emerge as early as 1–2 months of age. Similarly, Dennis, Reichle, Williams, and Vogelsberg (1982) addressed both hand shapes and movement patterns required to produce common gestures and their mean age of emergence. Other investigators (Kent, 1993) have summarized major aspects of physiological development that make the vocal mode an increasingly efficient mechanism for producing a frequent and varied repertoire of sounds. From these sources of information, it is clear that certain physiological events significantly influence communicative mode efficiency during the first several years of life.

The majority of early gestures are deictic in that they are not associated exclusively with a single referent object or event. Among early deictic gestures, pointing appears to be the most prevalent and correspondingly has received the greatest amount of attention in the literature. There are a number of contextual features that may influence pointing. Initially, a greater proportion of children's pointing gestures are directed at proximal rather than distal objects, although frequency distributions of proximal and distal pointing tend to shadow each other. Locke, Young, Service, and Chandler (1990) examined 140 pairs of typically developing children interacting with their mothers during toy-playing and book-reading activities. The greatest percent increase in usage for proximal gestures occurred between 11 and 13 months of age, and the greatest proportional increase for distal gestures was between 13 and 15 months of age (Locke et al.,

1990). As children's frequency of pointing and accompanying gaze shifts increases, mothers appear to become increasingly responsive. At 9 months of age, mothers responded to about 70% of infants' points. By 15 months of age, they responded to almost 100% of children's pointing gestures (Locke et al., 1990) in toy-playing and book-reading activities. How mothers respond to children's pointing is particularly intriguing. Vygotsky (1934/1986) hypothesized that early pointing emerges as the result of failed attempts at reaching for desired items. However, Locke et al. (1990) provided evidence to suggest that at least some mothers appear to respond to early pointing gestures as proto-commenting (i.e., proto-declarative) rather than requesting/demanding (i.e., proto-imperative) behavior. This pattern does not explain why young children's early communicative functions are often requests for objects and actions. However, the variability in interaction patterns across typically developing children and their parents is substantial. In part, this variability may be due to cultural differences in expectations for the role of speakers and listeners (van Kleeck, 1994). For example, in a culture that places great value on the listening ability of children, a smaller proportion of child requests for goods and services might be observed.

In addition to simple pointing, a child's early gestural system includes some representational gestures. Caseli and Volterra (1990) reported that at around 11 months of age, gestures that denote a more precise referent begin to emerge in typically developing children. Referential gestures more often refer to actions that mimic the action that an object produces rather than tracing the object in space. This description seems to support evidence in vocal mode production that children are more apt to attend to and use the functional features of early referents rather than the perceptual features of early referents. Caseli and Volterra (1990) reported that between 12 and 16 months of age, representational gestures are very context bound and are often used in response to adult queries for information or as early conversational repair strategies.

The decontextualization observed in the use of spoken words also is found in the development of gestures. The first representational gestures that children use entail producing an action from a familiar social game or routine (see Chapter 4), such as covering up the eyes to request a game of Peekaboo or using the motion of bringing a rounded hand to the mouth to request a drink. The transition from action to gesture may be viewed as enactive (Bruner, 1964) or indexical (Piaget, 1970) representation rather than as symbolic representation. Although the transition to symbolic representation is relatively rapid in typically developing children, it may be very protracted in children with developmental delays. For example, children with autism and other severe communication disabilities may rely on very primitive representational gestures for extended periods, such as requesting a tickle by making a tickling motion with the hand or requesting to go outside by leading an adult by the hand and putting the adult's hand on the doorknob. These gestures have been described as reenactments in that the child is repeating an action from an event to make that event reoccur (Prizant &

Wetherby, 1987; Schuler, 1980). (Similarly, a dog getting his leash and dropping it next to his master as a request to go for a walk is enactive rather than symbolic communication in that the leash is part of the action of going for a walk.) Thus, reenactments may reflect the intention to communicate with limitations in representational capacity. The acquisition of a substantial repertoire of reenactment gestures may bolster representational skills and provide a bridge for the transition to symbolic communication as these gestures become decontextualized.

Acredolo and Goodwyn (1990) reported that, although infrequently occurring, the mean number of representational gestures in the repertoires of infants examined ranged between 0 and 16 with a mean of 3.9. Referential classes in which representational gestures were observed included objects, requests, attributes, and events. They were most often observed within interactive routines. This suggests that, although an important supplement to an initial communicative repertoire, representational gestures account for a relatively small proportion of a child's working vocabulary.

Of particular interest to those describing patterns in the acquisition of spoken language is the relationship between gestural and vocal production. Several researchers have described the emergence of gestures alone, vocalizations alone, and gestures used with vocalizations in typically developing young children (Carpenter, Mastergeorge, & Coggins, 1983; Goldin-Meadow & Morford, 1990; Wetherby et al., 1988). During the prelinguistic and one-word stage, children from 9 to 15 months of age use gestures in about 75% of their communicative signals, and about half of their gestures are accompanied by vocalizations. About one fourth of communicative signals are vocalizations alone (Carpenter et al., 1983; Wetherby et al., 1988). The use of gestures alone has been found to decrease during the second year of life, with an increase in gestures plus vocalizations and vocalizations alone. By the end of the second year, children are in the multiword stage, and gestures alone account for about 10% of communicative signals, vocalizations alone account for about 40%, and gestures with vocalizations account for about 50%. During the one-word stage, only a small proportion of vocalizations are intelligible speech, but by the multiword stage, the vast majority of vocal communication is speech (Wetherby et al., 1988). By 2.5 years of age, the use of speech alone predominates (Goldin-Meadow & Morford, 1990).

Typically developing children initially appear to use gestures to supplement rather than to duplicate their spoken communicative repertoires (see Chapter 4). It is quite likely that the child uses the symbol form that has proven to be the most efficient in a particular context. Once children gain the capability of coordinating gestures and verbalizations, however, they may somewhat systematically evaluate an audience to select the most viable mode to use (Gibson & Schmuckler, 1989). Similarly, children have been reported to switch communicative mode as part of a repair strategy for a miscommunicated original message (Wetherby & Prizant, 1989; see also Chapter 7).

Over time, it is likely that vocal utterances usually result in superior communicative efficiency for the typically developing child. Unlike gestures, spoken utterances can be produced whether or not the child has already secured a listener's visual attention. In addition, spoken utterances are more likely to be decontextualized. Furthermore, spoken utterances are more apt to be understood by communities of listeners that may be less familiar with the child's communicative repertoire.

Early Graphic Symbols

Interventionists and researchers have begun to consider graphic symbols as viable means to produce communicative messages. In part, interest in graphic symbols has resulted from an emerging literature describing the use of graphic symbols to supplement vocal and verbal production among individuals with developmental disabilities. Additional interest has been spurred by the growing literature describing graphic symbol acquisition in typically developing children as part of early literacy skills.

Children may engage initially in gestures that include pointing, offering objects, or pushing objects away as a means to express proto-imperatives and proto-declaratives (see Chapter 17 for a description of the emergence of graphic symbols). Offering and pushing away gestures that involve objects probably represent an overlap of graphic and gestural modes. These gestures tend to occur when gestures have not yet been decontextualized from their object referents. As a result of increasing decontextualization, the child may first use objects and gestures as reenactments, as described previously, and learn that objects can function as communicative symbols. For example, a child may retrieve an empty wrapper of a toaster pastry and offer it in the direction of a parent as a rudimentary request. In other cases, objects associated with a desired event may be used initially as reenactments and later become symbols. For example, a child usually may see car keys only when they emerge from Mom's purse to insert into the car ignition. However, seeing keys on the kitchen table, the child may pick them up and thrust them in the direction of a parent as an overture for a car ride. The criteria that this chapter describes for spoken symbols applies to object and graphic symbols as well. Objects must reach a level of decontextualized use before they are considered symbolic. For example, if a child hands an adult a baseball as a signal to play ball, it is difficult to argue that a representation has been used. However, when a baseball is used to represent playing other sports (e.g., basketball) or when a child pretends to take a bite out of a miniature plastic apple to indicate hunger, symbols take on a more representational quality.

At the level of object symbols, the representational play literature (see Chapter 8) is particularly relevant. Around 12 months of age, children begin to use objects functionally; for example, spoons are associated with delivering food to one's mouth, and combs are run through one's hair. Slightly later, these actions with common objects are applied to dolls or other agents. If these actions are produced for the benefit of a listener, the objects are an essential part of the communicative utterance. Children who give no evidence of using objects, miniature objects, and associated objects in play may have significantly fewer opportunities to learn to use object symbols representationally; that is, adults have fewer opportunities to enhance further development by responding to object use with modeling of either language, or play, or both.

Although it is mostly understood how objects become representational for typical children who can manipulate them, there is limited information about how two-dimensional representations can be used to represent three-dimensional objects. Two-dimensional symbols include photos (black and white and color), product logos, line drawings, and traditional orthography. Infants discriminate between simple visual patterns by 2 months of age and recognize familiar from unfamiliar patterns by 6 months of age (Rosinski, 1977). The recognition of two-dimensional representations requires a comparison between the pattern presented and a representation of that pattern stored in memory. By 4 or 5 months of age, children begin to discriminate between and recognize both photos and their associated real objects (Rosinski, 1977). Between 18 months and 2 years of age, children discriminate between and match two-dimensional symbols to their real object counterparts; further levels of decontextualized representation can be considered as two-dimensional symbols become further degraded.

Logos, sometimes referred to as trademarks, are paired print and graphic symbols representing a commercial product or its producer (Chan, 1994). Logos are designed (often after significant marketing research) to be visually pleasing with salient features that will be immediately recognizable and remembered by consumers. Traditionally, logos and trademarks have been designed to maximize visual perception and retention (Chan, 1994). Typically developing children have numerous opportunities to come in contact with trademarks and product logos that occur frequently and naturally during their daily routines. Consequently, opportunities for incidental learning and use are abundant. Children as young as 2 years of age correctly recognize environmental logos and trademarks (Boudreau, 1994). Parents of young children report logo recognition associated with requesting functions at even earlier ages (Fischer, Schwartz, Richards, Goldstein, & Rojas, 1991).

Numerous investigators have examined children's ability to use graphic symbols to represent objects and events (e.g., Daehler, Perlmutter, & Myers, 1976; Mizuko, 1987; Musselwhite & Ruscello, 1984). Daehler et al. (1976) examined the equivalence of pictures and objects among 36 typically developing boys and 36 typically developing girls at each of three age groups: 24 months, 29 months, and 44.7 months. These investigators concluded that by 24 months of age, children demonstrated an equivalence between objects and pictures. Mizuko (1987) investigated the ability to match a variety of types of line-drawn symbols to their corresponding referents among children between 29 and 44 months. He reported that children have a much easier time corresponding static graphic symbols to objects than they do corresponding graphics to actions or attributes. By the time most children reach their second birthday, graphic symbols represent a supplement to speech and have a primary role in early literacy activities.

Among people with developmental disabilities, Mirenda and Locke (1989) examined the representational quality of two-dimensional symbols among non-speaking individuals ranging from 3 to 20 years of age and with mild to severe mental retardation and/or autism. The authors suggested that their results point to a hierarchy of difficulty among two-dimensional symbol types, with color photographs being the easiest, followed by black-and-white photographs, line-drawn symbols, and then traditional orthography. In this investigation, as in many addressing the salience of graphic symbols, a matching-to-sample task was used.

Keogh and Reichle (1985) described levels of visual matching that can be used in evaluating the graphic mode representational system. At a minimum, an assessment protocol should address object to identical object matching, symbol form to identical symbol form matching, and symbol form to object matching. That is, the interventionist should determine that the learner can discriminate among referents to be communicated about, discriminate among symbols to be taught, and also match symbols to corresponding items and events. If an interventionist were considering line-drawn symbols and black-and-white photos, separate identity-matching assessments might be compared that include identity photo to photo and identity line drawing to line drawing matching. Having verified that an individual can discriminate between real items and the symbols used to represent them, the interventionist can determine whether the individual can match both line drawings and black-and-white photos to corresponding referents.

Characteristics of Early Vocabulary

The literature is replete with efforts to characterize early lexical development. In a classic study of the first 50 words used by 18 children, Nelson (1973) concluded that the words that children first learned were based on functional, dynamic features; that is, these children first learned the names of objects on which they could act (e.g., socks, shoes, ball, keys, blanket, bottle). Nelson suggested that the salient functional property of objects captures the child's attention and provides the motivation to learn the name.

The literature makes a distinction between nominals (i.e., words referring to the names of objects, animals, and people; also called substantive words) and nonnominals (i.e., words referring to actions, attributes, or other relations among nominals, such as *more, up, all gone, there, no, away, stop;* also called function or relational words). Numerous researchers have studied the relative proportions of nominals and nonnominals in children's first 50 words. Some researchers conclude that the majority of first words comprises nominals (e.g., Clark, 1973; Kuczaj, 1986), and others conclude that less than half but usually a substantial proportion of the emerging lexicon comprises nominals (e.g., Bloom, 1983; Vihman & McCune, 1994). Evidence of the predominance of nominals in first word acquisition has been reported for children learning English as well as at least five other languages (Gentner, 1982). However, a bias toward nominals may not be universal. Tardif (1996) reported that verbs are the most numerous in Mandarin-speaking children's emerging lexicon. Mandarin-speaking caregivers were found to produce higher proportions of verbs than nouns, and verbs were more often in the most salient part of the caregivers' utterances. These findings support the important influence of linguistic input and sociocultural environment on emerging lexicon.

There appear to be differences in the ways in which children acquire nouns versus verbs. Tomasello (1992) pointed out that the "conceptual packaging operation involved in verbs is different than that for nouns" (p. 214) in two important ways. First, concrete nouns usually map concepts that refer to whole objects; however, it is much more uncertain what aspects of a situation are relevant for the meaning of a concrete verb. Second, object labels usually refer to static features, but verbs usually refer to actions and changes of states that are transient. Tomasello suggested that these packaging differences between nouns and verbs require different contexts for acquisition.

Tomasello and Kruger (1992) demonstrated that 1- to 2-year-old children learn verbs better in nonostensive contexts, that is, contexts in which the adult uses verbs to regulate the child's behavior or anticipate an impending event or action (e.g., "roll it to me" while child holds ball; "uh-oh, fall down" before knocking down a tower of blocks). An ostensive naming context is one in which an adult points out and names an entity that is visible, usually one to which the child is attending. Although an ostensive naming context is commonly used by parents of young children in mainstream middle-class American culture, it is uncommon in other cultures (Tomasello, 1992; van Kleeck, 1994).

It is clear that there is much individual variation across children in the proportion of nominals and nonnominals used. Children with a *referential style* of lexical development use a predominance of nominals; children with an *expressive style* use a variety of nonnominals (Nelson, 1973; Snyder, Bates, & Bretherton, 1981). It is also clear that during early lexical development, children do not simply learn the names of things but rather acquire a variety of nominals and nonnominals. Having some nonnominal words appears necessary for the capacity to construct word combinations because nominals form the subject of sentences and nonnominals form the predicate (Tomasello, 1992).

The capacity to use nominals and nonnominals flexibly is essential to vocabulary growth. Contextually flexible words are those used spontaneously in a variety of situations and are considered qualitatively different from contextually bound words, which are used only in restricted contexts (Bates, 1979). In a longitudinal study, Vihman and McCune (1994) collected monthly lexical samples of 20 children from 9 to 18 months of age. They found that these children showed a noticeable increase in the use of flexible nominals between 13 and 14 months of age, with a corresponding doubling of nonnominals the following month and another doubling again the next month. Thus, an increase in context-flexible word use may be an indicator of the transition to symbolic communication, which was made by these children between 13 and 16 months of age.

Not all words proceed from context-bound to context-flexible use. Some words emerge as context bound and may become flexible, whereas others are used flexibly from the onset (Barrett, 1986; Barrett, Harris, & Chasin, 1991). Theories and research on lexical development suggest that the way children learn to use words flexibly is based on a prototypical organization of word meanings and concept formation (Barrett et al., 1991; Kuczaj, 1986) based on the theory of Rosch (1978). Rosch proposed that concepts are formed by a prototype or "best" exemplar. In lexical development of young children, the prototypes of word classes are formed by the first exemplars (e.g., the class of dogs begins with the child's pet dog), and additional members are added to the category on the basis of similarity to the prototype. Concepts are organized with the prototype being central to the category and new instances being assigned relatively central or peripheral positions, depending on the degree of similarity to the prototype. Over time, prototypes can be modified. The prototypical organization of word meanings better accounts for patterns of child language than traditional models of classification that rely on a critical set of attributes (e.g., the class of dog has +four legs, +fur, +barks, –meow) (Bates, 1979; Kuczaj, 1986). This theory implies that children's experiences and their ability to perceive similarities and differences among objects and events contribute to concept development and the formation of word classes.

Although children appear to have good command of the early vocabulary that they acquire, evidence suggests that for some time after the acquisition process starts, children continue to under- or overextend the meanings of words. Children's lexical development is filled with underextensions (e.g., the word "doggie" used only to refer to a particular pet) and overextensions (e.g., the word "doggie" used for all four-legged animals). The extensions of word usage in lexical development provide insight into what features a child uses to categorize concepts and words. Estimates of the proportion of object names that are under- or overextended range from about 10% to 30% (Barrett, 1986).

Extensions are not unique to speech development. Overextensions of sign location, hand shape, and movement patterns have been well documented. Extensions often appear to occur in other situations calling for the same communicative function that is most often associated with a particular vocabulary item. For example, children who have been taught the sign EAT are often reported to overextend its meaning to other situations in which they are making a request (Sigafoos, Doss, & Reichle, 1991). The more explicit the class of items or events represented by a symbol, the more likely a listener is to recognize the overextended use of the vocabulary item.

Most typically developing children encounter a sufficient range of exemplars of a particular referent that, with accumulated experience, they are able to decipher the referent's critical characteristics. However, among graphic mode symbols, common patterns of overextension include position and size bias responding. Johnston (1992), in examining young typically developing children's ability to match product logos to their referents, reported that children who were early in the acquisition process often selected graphic symbols as a result of the similarity of position to a previously selected successful symbol choice. Mustonen (1995) reported that some preschoolers with mild disabilities appeared to rely on the similarity of the length and width dimensions of a two-dimensional product logo and the fronted side of its three-dimensional counterpart to make a correct choice. There is a critical need for additional investigation of the parameters of graphic symbols that may be over- or underextended. Learning more about typical children's ability to correspond graphic symbols to their referents may be helpful in deriving more efficient strategies to teach beginning literacy and in deriving practice and effective instructional strategies to use with individuals who have developmental disabilities. (See Chapter 17 for a discussion of the problem that people with significant disabilities have with this aspect of extension and instructional strategies that can be implemented to prevent overextensions and underextensions.)

The use of gestures and graphic symbols appears to follow some of the same trends previously described. However, among early graphic symbols, representations of objects appear to predominate. There is some reason to believe that very young children may be somewhat predisposed to use two-dimensional graphic symbols to represent objects and activities involving desired objects (e.g., going to McDonald's) rather than actions associated with the activities. Mizuko (1987) found that young children more easily matched object symbols than action symbols to their respective referents. Similar to the theory proposed by Tomasello (1992) regarding children's acquisition of verbs in spoken vocabulary, Mizuko formulated a hypothesis to explain mechanisms of early vocabulary acquisition in the graphic mode. He hypothesized that objects must be depicted performing static rather than dynamic actions (unless animation software is incorporated into graphic symbol displays). Because common objects often are depicted as part of action symbols, children may be biased toward matches between action symbols and objects rather than the referent action being represented. Many of the early gestures acquired by young children represent explicit actions that are part of joint activity routines. It is possible that the ability to display movement in gestures makes representing actions somewhat easier than in a static graphic mode. A critical area of exploration is the influence that animation has on the relative acquisition of object and action symbols. This could be particularly important with children with physical disabilities who find it difficult to participate in nonostensive contexts in which adults use verbs to regulate children's behavior. There have been relatively few efforts that examine teaching opportunities to criterion in comparing different two-dimensional symbol systems.

The Vocabulary Burst in the Acquisition of Symbols

Vocabulary increases slowly and steadily until about 18–21 months, when vocabulary growth begins to accelerate at a dramatic rate. This period of sudden acceleration in the rate of new word acquisition is known as the *vocabulary burst* (Bates et al., 1987). Bloom (1993) conducted a longitudinal study of 14 children from first words to sentences. The criterion used by Bloom to operationalize a vocabulary burst was at least 3 new words per week after having learned at least 20 different words. She found that the mean age at the onset of a vocabulary burst was 19 months, and these children produced an average of about 50 different words (range of 34–75 words) at the vocabulary burst.

Fenson et al. (1994) provided the largest database on early vocabulary development. They reported cross-sectional data on 1,800 healthy children ages 8–30 months from parent report derived from the MacArthur Communicative Development Inventories (CDI) (Fenson et al., 1993). They found that by 17 months of age half of the sample produced between 50 and 100 words, indicating the point of vocabulary burst, and that by 2 years of age 90% of the sample reached this point. They concluded that vocabulary development was characterized by an accelerated but regular growth pattern between 16 and 30 months of age, with much variability at each age level, and that for 10% of the children this acceleration began at 13–14 months of age.

The rate of acquisition in gestural mode seems to proceed comparably to speech during the child's first year and a half of development (see Chapter 4). At the point of the vocabulary burst, it appears that children begin to discover the relative efficiency of vocal mode productions (Bates et al., 1987), and the rate of gestural acquisition begins to wane. At the same time, gestural symbols that had been associated exclusively with certain referents now begin to be used in combination with or replaced by spoken symbols. However, there are no comparable data to report during this time frame on typically developing children's graphic mode acquisitions.

The vocabulary burst appears to define a quantitative change in vocabulary growth curve with corresponding qualitative change in language abilities. This qualitative change associated with the vocabulary burst has been described in numerous ways in the literature, all converging on a shift in the way children learn new words to account for the rapid acceleration in word learning. Nelson (1991) described this as the entry into the acquisition of a productive language and pointed out that the vocabulary burst is accompanied by the frequent use of the question "What's that?" The drive to want to know the name for everything reflects the child's solid realization that things have names. Bloom (1993) described the vocabulary burst as a shift from episodic to conceptual associations, which is consistent with Barrett's (1986) shift from context bound to prototype. Bloom argued that it is the conceptual basis of word acquisition that is the impetus for the accelerated rate of vocabulary growth. This pattern of lexical growth snowballs and leads to a diverse lexical composition. Tomasello (1992) suggested that young children's conceptual representations are organized by event structures, which are composed of actions and conceptual roles derived from cultural activities. The child's developing capacity to understand the intentional roles of adults as agents in routine activities, such as undressing the child, filling the tub, and bathing the child, allows the child to map words onto the objects, actions, and roles of event structures, which leads to cultural learning.

Considering the pragmatic context of word learning as a sociocultural activity underscores the importance of understanding the influence of parental input on lexical acquisition. Although the emergence of first words has been found to be enhanced by the caregiver's ability to follow the child's focus of attention and label the object of coordinated attention (Tomasello & Farrar, 1986), such an ostensive naming context does not appear to be essential for later word learning. That is, once a child is using words flexibly, word learning for nominals and nonnominals can proceed in nonostensive contexts. Tomasello, Strosberg, and Akhtar (1996) found that 18-month-old children could learn the names of objects when an adult announced the intention to find an object and then selected that object. The authors concluded that children use a variety of different sources of information to actively determine the adult referential intention. Barrett et al. (1991) studied the initial and subsequent uses of the first 10 words of four children from 10 months to 2 years of age. They found that although there was a strong relationship between parental speech and their child's initial word use, a relatively high proportion of subsequent uses of words was not related to parental speech. For those words in which a relationship did exist, it consisted of the mother using the word when the child was carrying out a particular action, the mother using the word when she was carrying out an action, or the mother producing a new referential use of a word.

Beyond the Vocabulary Burst:
The Transition to Linguistic Communication

Several new achievements in language abilities follow the vocabulary burst and indicate movement to a linguistic system of communication. Although this chapter and this volume focus on prelinguistic communication, it is important to understand the major changes that occur shortly after the transition to linguistic communication. This section briefly describes the major changes that characterize this next transition.

Shortly after children go through the vocabulary burst, they begin to combine two or more words in novel combinations and, hence, truly have acquired a productive language system. The passage from the single-word to the multiword stage has been documented at about 20 months of age (Bates et al., 1987). Children often produce successive single-word utterances before constructing multiword combinations (Greenfield & Smith, 1976; Werner & Kaplan, 1963). These are utterances that appear to have the characteristics of a two-word utterance except that the pause time between the two words is too great and the intonational contour of the utterance is more in keeping with single-word productions.

Another new achievement that corresponds with the onset of the vocabulary burst and the shift to multiword combinations is the ability to predicate. Predication is the ability to describe states, qualities, and relations of objects and is the essence of constructing sentences. That is, a sentence consists of a predicate (i.e., verb phrase) that provides information about the subject (i.e., noun phrase). In addition to being able to name things, children can now tell a person something about things by describing actions, attributes, or locations. Predication may first be evident when a child combines a gesture and word, such as saying "dada" while pointing to Daddy's shoe (Dore, 1986), and later in word combinations.

In the gestural mode, Bonvillian et al. (1990) reported that children begin to combine gestures with spoken words at or just before the onset of spoken two-word utterances. Two types of gesture–spoken word combinations have been reported. In one, the gesture duplicates the spoken word's meaning. In the other, the gesture and the spoken word produce different but complementary semantic meaning. The latter construction is very similar to the phenomenon of successive single words. Combinations of gestures and spoken words appear to emerge somewhat within the same time frame at around 20 months of age (Fenson & Ramsay, 1980). However, Goldin-Meadow and Morford (1990) reported that the children they observed stopped producing two-gesture combinations before their first two-word productions. Very little is known about the combining of graphic symbols with either spoken words or gestures to create semantically more complex utterances, although anecdotally Reichle (1993) reported an example of a child vocalizing "go" as she pointed to a picture of a toy store. This same child often would open a Sears catalog and say "mine" as she pointed to desired toys.

In some respects, using graphics as part of an expanded utterance may be easier than producing an expanded utterance in either gestural or vocal mode. In these latter two modes, the child must retrieve each symbol from memory. Combinations that are apt to be used frequently have a distinct advantage of appearing in early two-word combinations. However, in graphic mode an array of symbols may be concurrently displayed. This may challenge the learner's recognition rather than recall memory.

In addition, it is possible to create what appears to be a two-word utterance that actually consists of two single symbol choices. Many electronic communication aids allow the user to select individual symbols that are held in a buffer. A visual display may be continuously presented that allows monitoring of the symbol(s) in the buffer. When all relevant symbols have been selected, the user activates the buffer, which releases all stored symbols. This strategy allows multiple-word utterances to be constructed outside of some of the "real-time" constraints imposed on vocal or gestural mode productions. Although relatively uninvestigated, features of electronic communication aids may enhance an individual's ability to begin combining communicative symbols. It is possible that the permanency of a graphic mode display offers an advantage of symbol permanency in recalling events in the past; as a consequence, a learner can prepare an utterance as he or she engages in an event. An icon pneumonic can be displayed to remind how to display (i.e., recall) the message at a later time; consequently, talking about displaced events can be thought of as relying more on recognition than recall memory.

The transactional nature of language development is evident in how parental input shifts after the vocabulary burst. Poulin-Dubois, Graham, and Sippola (1995) studied parental labeling and children's developing lexicon during picture-book reading in 16 French- and English-speaking parent–child dyads at monthly intervals from 1 to 2 years of age. They found an association between the proportion of nominals used by these children and their performance on a categorization task, suggesting a cognitive achievement associated with the vocabulary burst. This finding is consistent with research documenting an association between categorization skills and onset of the vocabulary burst (see Mervis & Bertram, 1993). Furthermore, these parents changed their manner of labeling pictures after their child had gone through the vocabulary burst by increasing the use of subordinate labels over basic labels, which had a positive association with the child's acquisition of nominals once the child's lexicon exceeded 100 words.

After the vocabulary burst, a phenomenon in the strategies that children use to acquire new vocabulary appears to emerge. Mervis and Bertram (1993) described the phenomenon of *fast mapping* in which a child has a very small number of critical learning opportunities in which he or she may have been a vicarious participant. For example, a child observing a teacher interact with another child might hear the teacher refer to a toy automobile by calling it a Ford. The reference may have been made in the presence of five or six toys. Because the child knew the names of the other five items, the child concludes that the new term applies to the toy car. Mervis and Bertram reported that at least some children's propensity to use this strategy corresponds to the onset of the vocabulary burst as well as to competence in categorization skills and suggested that this strategy is based on a cognitive insight about objects. Fast mapping represents a critical acquisition because it dramatically frees the child from the exclusive reliance of intervention strategies directed exclusively at him or her. Little is known about the extension of fast mapping to gestural and graphic modes, although the same relationship previously described for the vocal mode would be expected to exist.

The dramatic growth rate and size of lexicon that follows the vocabulary burst trigger the beginning of a semantic basis of language development. Once a significant number of words have been acquired, words themselves can cue the use of words (Bloom, 1993), contributing further to the developmental momentum. Having gone through the vocabulary burst is an indicator of the transition to linguistic communication. Bloom (1993) discussed this transition:

> Only when words begin to cue recall of other words can we speak of the child's acquisition of word meanings and the beginning of the development of semantics. This development is crucial, because semantics is specifically a linguistic system, having to do with arbitrary and conventional units and the formal and functional relations among them. (p. 98)

Semantic meanings expressed in single words and word combinations have been found to be similar across languages and to include agents, actions, attributes, location, possession, disappearance, and denial (Bates et al., 1987). With the onset of semantic development, children begin requesting information, bringing up topics about things that are remote in place and time, and maintaining a topic for several turns; thus, they are truly engaging in conversation. The process of grammaticization is then set into motion, with the acquisition of the fundamentals of syntax and morphology occurring between 20 and 30 months of age (Bates et al., 1987).

PARALLEL DEVELOPMENTS IN COMPREHENSION OF MEANING

Comprehension is the process of making sense of a message. It is "an event that takes place privately within the mind of the listener" (Miller & Paul, 1995, p. 7). Comprehension requires the listener to consider many aspects of knowledge, including the intention of the speaker; knowledge about the event, the social context, and the world; assumptions about what is already known; and the meaning based on linguistic components of the message. Comprehension and production of language develop concurrently and somewhat independently in typically developing children, even though there are similarities in the developmental patterns between the two. The transition to a symbolic level of comprehension requires the ability to understand the meanings of words without nonverbal cues and culminates in the transition to linguistic comprehension, which includes the ability to understand grammatical morphemes and word order in sentences.

Children with developmental disabilities who are at a prelinguistic stage of language production show a wide range of comprehension abilities. Some may have receptive abilities that are also at a prelinguistic level, whereas others may have the capacity for linguistic comprehension despite limited expressive abilities. It is important to determine whether a child's language comprehension is commensurate with or in advance of language production. A developmental framework of comprehension can provide the practitioner with landmarks to help identify important achievements on the way to linguistic comprehension and to guide decisions about how to foster language comprehension.

Emerging Comprehension

Young children learn to respond to others' communicative signals and words, first in highly ritualized contexts. Before children comprehend the meaning of words, they use a variety of contextual cues to determine a response strategy; thus, children may appear as if they comprehend specific linguistic information (Chapman, 1978; McLean & Snyder-McLean, 1978; see also Chapter 10 for a description of many of these strategies). With the transition to intentional communication, children begin to respond to three different types of cues to determine the meaning of messages. First, they begin to comprehend nonverbal cues provided by caregivers, including gestures, facial expressions, and directed eye gaze (e.g., an adult pointing to or looking at an object "means" the child should give or attend to that object). Second, children also may respond to situational cues by using the immediate environment and knowledge of what to do with objects to respond (e.g., observe what others do, drink from a cup, put objects in a container). Graphic cues available to the child are undoubtedly part of the situational context. For example, while riding in the car, Mom says, "Wanna go to McDonald's?" as the car passes a Golden Arches signpost. The child's affirmative response may be controlled by the business signage rather than specifically by what Mom said. Third, children also may respond to paralinguistic cues by using intonation to determine how to respond (e.g., loud voice "means" angry). It is easy to overestimate a child's comprehension of language if there is no awareness of the nonverbal, situational, or paralinguistic cues that the child may be using to determine how to respond. The use of these contextual cues should not be viewed as detrimental. Rather, the child's development of comprehension response strategies serves as a bridge to the comprehension of word meanings.

By the end of the first year, children understand the meanings of words that are very familiar, and their comprehension continues to be guided by the context. The earliest evidence of comprehension of words is reported during social-action games, such as Pat-a-Cake and Peekaboo (Bruner, 1981; Chapman, 1978; Platt & Coggins, 1990). The child's understanding of how to respond is related to the familiarity of the context and the caregiver's ability to scaffold his or her verbal message with contextual cues. Platt and Coggins (1990) studied comprehension of social-action games in 29 typically developing children from 9 to 15 months of age. They identified a hierarchy in both the children's increasing levels of participation in social-action games and in the caregivers' decreasing amounts of structure and contextual cueing. The results of this study evidenced a positive relationship between a child's emerging comprehension and adult structure.

During this early period of contextually cued situational comprehension, children's burgeoning ability to interpret simple gestures and graphic symbols may serve them well (see Chapter 4 for a detailed discussion of the emergence of children's comprehension of early deictic gestures). Within this same time frame, typically developing young children begin to comprehend simple print materials based on pictures that accompany text. Children initially do not directly associate printed words with the story being presented in a book and may only marginally attend to key, emphasized spoken function words within the story being read (Koppenhaver & Yoder, 1992).

Comprehension becomes decontextualized during the second year of life as a child is able to recognize the meaning of words outside familiar or routine contexts. The literature has identified a developmental progression of comprehension from person and object names to actions, from present to absent person and object names, and from single words to multiword combinations (Benedict, 1979; Huttenlocher, 1974). Miller, Chapman, Branston, and Reichle (1980) conducted a cross-sectional study of language comprehension in 48 children from 10 to 21 months of age. The children were instructed verbally, using no gestural cues, to identify people or objects and to carry out actions with objects. The authors found the following developmental patterns. By 1 year of age, children understood the names of familiar individuals who were present at the time of the comprehension opportunity. At this same time, 42% of children between 10 and 12 months of age comprehended names of common objects with which they played. By approximately 16 months, 100% of children understood common objects and 33% were beginning to comprehend the names of simple actions. At this same time, approximately 80% of children demonstrated the ability to comprehend some two-word constructions involving possessor + possession relationships. Other two-word constructions continued to present a formidable challenge. At 21 months of age, only 58% of children sampled understood agent + action combinations with even fewer understanding three-word constructions such as agent + action + object. These findings provide support for a developmental progression of the comprehension of semantic relations and indicate that even by 21 months of age, children are not able to rely on word order to comprehend multiword utterances.

Fenson and colleagues (1994) presented extensive data on the composition of early vocabulary comprehension based on normative studies from the CDI, which are consistent with the findings of Miller and colleagues (1980). They found that the most common categories of the first 50 words in children's receptive vocabularies were people (e.g., Mommy, Daddy, child's own name), games and routines (e.g., Peekaboo, bye, hi), familiar objects (e.g., household items, toys, clothing), animals, body parts, and action words.

Relationship Between Comprehension and Production

The traditional assumption about typical development has been that language comprehension precedes production. There is substantial evidence to support this assumption, particularly during the one-word stage (Greenfield & Smith, 1976; Huttenlocher, 1974; Oviatt, 1980). Goldin-Meadow, Seligman, and Gelman (1976) reported that some children understand far more words than they produce during the acquisition of the first 50 words. Benedict (1979) reported that children comprehend 50 words by the time they produce 10 words. Snyder et al. (1981) studied early lexical development in 32 children at 13 months of age using an extensive maternal interview, which was a preliminary version of the CDI, to determine language comprehension and production vocabulary. For these 13-month-olds, Snyder et al. (1981) found a mean comprehension vocabulary of 45 words (range of 11–97) compared with a mean production vocabulary of 11 words (range of 0–45). Bates, Bretherton, and Snyder (1988) reported a study that compared the interview data with a laboratory measure of comprehension obtained with the same children studied by Snyder et al. (1981) at 13 months of age. Eight different familiar objects were presented two times in sets of three. Bates et al. (1988) found that the laboratory measure of comprehension was significantly correlated (+.52; $p < 01$) with the interview measure of total comprehension, providing validation of the interview measure.

The normative data from the CDI provide more precise patterns in the relationship between early receptive and productive vocabularies. Fenson and colleagues (1994) reported that there was a substantial overlap between words comprehended and words produced. About half of the first 50 words comprehended also appeared on the production list and vice versa. Furthermore, comprehension showed a developmental advantage for most children. Comprehension of the first 50 words was reported for half of the children before production of the first 4 words. The authors also noted two major differences in the composition of the first 50 words to appear in vocabulary comprehension and production. First, verbs were totally absent from the production list but accounted for about 14% of the comprehension vocabulary. Second, the category of sound effects and animal sounds accounted for about 20% of the production list and for only 6% of the comprehension list.

Although it would be easier for practitioners if language comprehension and production vocabularies were isomorphic, there is further evidence suggesting that, for many children, such is not the case. Studies of typically developing children's vocabulary comprehension and production (Goldin-Meadow et al., 1976; Huttenlocher, 1974; Snyder et al., 1981) and grammatical constructions (Chapman & Miller, 1975) indicate that comprehension does not always precede or surpass production. Children may produce words that they do not accurately comprehend (Fenson et al., 1994; Leonard, Newhoff, & Fey, 1980). The relationship between comprehension and production may change with age. Snyder et al. (1981) found that comprehension and production vocabulary had a low correlation (+.29; $p < 0.11$) at 13 months of age. They identified three different patterns of comprehension/production abilities in the thirty-two 13-month-old children: 1) high comprehension/high production, 2) high comprehension/low production, and 3) low comprehension/low production. Snyder et al. (1981) suggested that these patterns may reflect individual variation in language styles. Children using an *analytic style* were more advanced in lexical development and showed a relatively high comprehension vocabulary. Snyder et al.'s findings indicate that comprehension and production proceed through similar developmental sequences but that the developmental discrepancy between them varies across children and at different points in development (Bloom & Lahey, 1978; McLean & Snyder-McLean, 1978; Owens, 1992; Snyder et al., 1981).

At a practical level, it makes sense that children's early comprehension and production vocabulary would differ. Often, children's interest in what they want to express may differ greatly in topic from the language that they hear from familiar others in their environment. For example, children may have a large number of opportunities to learn to understand the words "bath time" but have few opportunities when there is any motivation for talking about baths. Even though there is support for viewing comprehension and production as separate but intertwined processes, it is plausible that developing production skills may facilitate comprehension skills. Whenever a child produces a communicative act to mark an event, an opportunity is created for the child's communicative partner to produce a spoken word that corresponds directly to the referent. For example, a child points to a desired toy, and the adult, in turn, produces the name of the toy (either as a communication check or overt teaching opportunity). That the child may be highly motivated at this moment increases the probability that the child will attend to the association between the spoken word and the referent. Among children who use an electronic communication aid that produces digitized speech output, the advantage just described may be extremely likely. Each time a child selects a graphic symbol(s), a spoken message will be produced immediately. As a consequence, the proportion of communicative production opportunities in which spoken words are modeled that correspond to a reference may be greater than the opportunities that occur for typically developing children. However, if the utterance produced by the electronic communication aid user does not correctly match the referent being discussed, the learner would create an opportunity in which he or she might begin to associate incorrect spoken vocabulary with a referent event.

Studies of children's extensions have demonstrated both similarities and differences between production and comprehension. Most words overextended in production are not found to be overextended in comprehension (Kuczaj, 1986). Snyder et al.'s (1981) examination of the contextual flexibility and composition of the lexicon in the thirty-two 13-month-old children found that 60% of the vocabulary items comprehended were context restricted, as determined by maternal reports that these items were only comprehended with contextual cues. They also found that the percentage of nominal vocabulary comprehended averaged 34%, with a range of 14%–66%. The proportion of nominals that were contextually flexible ranged from 0% to 100%, with an average of 32%. They found a strong positive correlation (+.51; $p < 0.003$) between comprehension of context-flexible actions and total production vocabulary. These findings suggest that the flexible comprehension of names of people and objects as well as actions is a more robust indicator of the comprehension of word meanings and may be associated with the transition to symbolic communication expressively. In a longitudinal study of six children 6–24 months of age, Harris, Yeeles, Chasin, and Oakley (1995) found that words that were contextually flexible in production were also contextually flexible in comprehension. It can be concluded that lexical acquisition entails both comprehension and production, that mastery in one modality does not ensure mastery in the other, and that mastery in comprehension may aid contextually flexible production.

Much of the same trends described in the relationship between comprehension and production appear to hold true for young children developing gestural mode communication systems with notable caveats. Deictic gestures, such as pointing, appear to emerge earlier in productive communicative repertoires than comprehension of pointing (see Chapter 4). In the graphic mode, comprehension and production may involve the same stimuli and response topography for the learner. For example, with line-drawn symbols, an elicited comprehension assessment task might involve showing the learner a line drawing and providing an opportunity to find the object that matches from an array of referents. Production would involve showing the learner a referent and providing the opportunity to locate the line drawing that best corresponds. Researchers are only beginning to describe the relationship between comprehension and production for a child relying primarily on a graphic mode communication system to both receive and produce communicative utterances.

THE ACQUISITION PROCESS OF SYMBOLIC COMMUNICATION

It is interesting to reflect on the acquisition process and consider how and why children learn to talk. What is the impetus for moving through the transition to symbolic and ultimately linguistic communication? Bloom (1993) posited that the "child's intentionality drives the acquisition of language" (p. 5). Children acquire language to share their ideas, thoughts, and feelings. When children begin to talk, they use words to communicate the same meanings for the same purposes as they did through preverbal communicative means (Bates, 1976; Lahey, 1988). As their ideas and needs become more complex, a more explicit system of communicating is required. The emergence of the ritualized, context-bound first words sets into motion the development of a symbolic, referential language system.

Tomasello and colleagues (Tomasello, 1992; Tomasello, Kruger, & Ratner, 1993) presented a theory of human cultural learning to account for the precision with which humans can transmit information and learn from one another that is not evident in nonhuman animals. Rooted in the theory of Vygotsky (1934/ 1986) that the acquisition of communicative symbols is a social enterprise, Tomasello (1992) suggested that two components are essential for a child to develop language: 1) development within a cultural context that structures events for the child and 2) the child's special capacity to learn from this cultural structuring. The structuring for language acquisition entails routine cultural activities that employ coordinated attention and delineated roles. The child's capacity requires the social-cognitive skills of being able to attribute intentions to others and to see the event from the others' perspectives.

Bloom (1993) suggested that children are guided in their efforts to learn to talk by three principles of word learning: relevance, discrepancy, and elaboration. These three principles provide a developmental framework for targeting first words. First, the principle of relevance states that a child learns words when they are relevant to what the child has in mind. This suggests that the selection of words for an initial lexicon should reflect what captivates the child's attention and the important meanings that a child wants to share. The critical role of joint attention episodes in language learning supports this principle (see Chapter 2). Second, the principle of discrepancy states that what a child has in mind goes beyond that information known to others or anticipated from the context. Young children have an impressive ability to consider what information is needed by the listener and to provide it. When children first use words, they are likely to talk about things that are evident from the context. As children approach the vocabulary burst, they talk more about events that they anticipate but that are not evident to someone else. Thus, it is critical to design language-learning contexts in which there is a real communicative need to share information. Third, the principle of elaboration states that as a child's mental representations expand, the child is required to learn more words to express these ideas. Efforts to expand a child's vocabulary would be well placed on building a child's knowledge about objects, actions, agents, and recipients of actions. During the transition from symbolic communication to linguistic communication, a child's conceptual and emotional development promote the capacity and need for language learning.

Golinkoff, Mervis, and Hirsh-Pasek (1994) posited that the lexical principles proposed by Bloom (1993) describe children's behavior but fail to explain how children map the meanings of words onto mental representations of concepts. They formulated a two-tier set of specific lexical principles to characterize children's increasing linguistic sophistication. The first-tier principles of reference, extendability, and object scope are sufficient to initiate the infant's use of words but word learning is a "deliberate and laborious task" (Bloom, 1993, p. 125). The second-tier principles of categorical scope, novel name–nameless category, and conventionality enable the rapid acquisition of lexicon. These more advanced principles combine and alter the character of the lexical acquisition process.

Adding to these principles is the principle of response efficiency that has been derived from matching theory (Mace & Roberts, 1993). A principle of response efficiency suggests that the learner must select a communicative symbol and means of expressing that symbol that are most efficient for both the child and the listener. For example, immediacy of reinforcement represents an aspect of efficiency. Once a child has experience with the spoken word "apple," reinforcement will be obtained more quickly by saying "apple" rather than by saying "that" in the presence of a cluster of desired objects that includes an apple. The child's increasing competence in using more complex utterances will further disambiguate messages directed to his or her listener, thereby making them more efficient (see Chapter 17 for an in-depth description of several variables that influence response efficiency among users of graphic and gestural symbols).

In a treatise based on the work of Tinbergen (1951) in the field of ethology, Locke (1996) explored why infants begin to talk. There are four components to answer completely the question of why an animal or infant behaves as it does:

> One can ask an evolutionary question about HOW the capability evolved in the species. One can ask a developmental question about HOW immature members of the species develop the capability. One can ask a mechanistic question about WHAT happens in the nervous system when the behavior takes place. And finally one can ask a functional question about WHY a particular animal behaves as it does when in a particular circumstance. (Locke, 1996, p. 252)

Locke stated that language researchers have addressed the first three of Tinbergen's questions but have not yet adequately considered the question of why infants begin to talk. To explore what causes the infant to talk, researchers need to understand the consequences of behaviors that are precursors to language, including joint attention, vocal development, and lexical imitation. Locke posited that there are primary consequences for these behaviors, including the infant receiving comfort, reducing anxiety, and sharing emotional experience, as well as secondary consequences, including learning the prosodic cues of linguistic units and lexical development and discovering utterance structure.

CLINICAL AND EDUCATIONAL IMPLICATIONS

The developmental patterns described in this chapter provide a road map to assist practitioners in selecting initial areas to target for prelinguistic children and in planning language stimulation and intervention strategies. The transition to symbolic communication entails learning shared meanings derived from sociocultural activities. This transition has been characterized as having two major shifts: 1) first word acquisition, which is based on linking or associating words to events and is supported by ritualized sociocultural activities involving coordinated attention; and 2) a vocabulary burst that is triggered by the capacity to decontextualize word meanings and is supported by ostensive as well as nonostensive learning contexts. For the majority of children, appropriate exposure to and modeling of language and communicative behavior in daily interactions are the context of successful language acquisition.

In contrast to the emphasis on the sociocultural context of language acquisition in the developmental literature, many clinical assessment tools simply determine the presence or absence of comprehension and production skills that are relatively context free (Crais, 1995; Wetherby & Prizant, 1992). However, assessing criterion performance represents only a starting point. With young children who are at risk for delays in acquiring language, practitioners need to consider assessing first words and communicative functions in a highly familiar context by using parent reports to determine lexicon and by expanding the roles of caregivers in assessment (see Chapters 10 and 12). By carefully considering the contexts that support early comprehension and production, the interventionist will be in a better position to facilitate increasingly decontextualized language comprehension and production.

For children who are just beginning to learn first words, caregivers are in an optimal role to facilitate early communicative competence by providing large numbers of opportunities for repetitive routines to establish event representations. During these interactions, the literature suggests that it is critically important to follow the child's lead and both label objects that the child visually regards and describe actions to anticipate what will happen next within the activity. Once routines are well established, introducing variations and creating opportunities to delineate roles within activities and extend the activity themes will foster the decontextualization of language and serve the child well.

Rosch's (1978) notion of how children develop vocabulary concepts, described previously in this chapter, is very compatible with a behavioral interventionist's concept of general case instruction (Horner, McDonnell, & Bellamy, 1986; O'Neill & Reichle, 1993). In general case instruction, the interventionist's goal is to identify a set of practical teaching examples that adequately samples the range of positive attributes of the concept. Furthermore, other teaching examples are identified that sample the range of exceptions to the concept that are most likely to result in under- or overextensions if not addressed. A general case instructional strategy attempts to anticipate typical under- and overextensions and create discriminable teaching opportunities to help the development of word meanings.

The literature suggests that acquisition in gestural and graphic modes occurs somewhat concurrently with acquisitions in the vocal/aural mode. This has significant implications for children who may be temporary or long-term users of augmentative communication systems. Interventionists and parents often seek to demonstrate failure in the vocal mode before considering additional emphasis on graphic or gestural mode communication. However, virtually all children concurrently acquire communication in each of these modes. (See Chapters 4 and 7 for a discussion of the role of gestures and gestural repairs in early language development.) The extent to which acquisition in one influences the development of others varies. However, available literature suggests that taking advantage of vocal, gestural, and graphic modes concurrently represents the recommended practice in social-communicative interactions. Comparisons of acquisition rate of different symbol types across modalities should be used to understand the individual learner's strengths and needs and to determine the efficacy of intervention efforts.

All early communication, by nature, is contextually bound. Until communication becomes less contextually dependent, children engage in a variety of extensions in word meanings. Although typically developing children appear to progress to flexible use easily and quickly, some children with developmental disabilities appear to have far greater difficulty making adjustments in their use and understanding of communication as it becomes less contextualized. The developmental framework suggests that the size of lexicon and pace of word acquisition should guide the intervention context. First words should initially be taught within routinized meaningful contexts, and words should be mapped onto the child's communicative intentions. As word learning begins to accelerate, these contexts should be expanded to develop knowledge of role relations. (See Chapter 16 for information on facilitating the transition from prelinguistic to linguistic communication.)

The traditional view of comprehension has been somewhere between a precursor and prerequisite for communicative production. Theory and supporting evidence suggest that comprehension develops somewhat independently from production but in a very intertwined manner. Vocabulary frequently directed to young children may differ significantly from objects and actions that serve as the motivation for productive utterances. Correspondingly, interventionists should consider separately how well natural environments support opportunities for comprehension and production in selecting initial vocabulary and the mode to be emphasized initially in teaching that vocabulary.

The relationship between comprehension and production has important implications for the practitioner working with prelinguistic children. Bloom and Lahey (1978) suggested that waiting to teach production of a particular word, concept, or rule until comprehension has developed is not a prudent clinical practice. Children who are typically developing as well as children with language impairments have been found to produce words that they do not comprehend (see Leonard et al., 1982). The few intervention studies that have been done have found that teaching comprehension does not transfer to production skills (Guess & Baer, 1973; Leonard et al., 1982; Miller, Cuvo, & Borakove, 1977) but that teaching production does transfer to comprehension (Miller et al., 1977). Most available literature addressing issues of spontaneity and generalized use of newly established vocabulary suggests that the most logical intervention strategy involves teaching vocabulary that the learner is most apt to want or need to produce or comprehend. This logic suggests that early comprehension vocabulary and production vocabulary may be quite different. As discussed previously, "bath" may be a salient vocabulary to comprehend but is unlikely to be the focus of early production unless it is a preferred activity. Although further research is needed to explore the relationship between comprehension and production, the evidence suggests that comprehension and production should be taught concurrently.

Hart and Risley (1995) addressed the critical role that stimulating home environments can have when they occur early in life and over an extended period of time. However, many families cannot adequately support even the most obvious features of environments that promote language acquisition. It is critically important to develop intervention strategies that foster the role of the caregiver and concentrate on intervention directed at the language-learning environment rather than focusing too narrowly on only the learner (see Chapter 11). Furthermore, with the recognition of importance of understanding multicultural differences in family values, professionals will need to contend with how cultures differ in the amount that talk is valued in the home and the role of talk in teaching skills to children (van Kleeck, 1994).

DIRECTIONS FOR FUTURE RESEARCH

Although rapid progress has been made in describing the emergence of communication in children, each new answer opens a plethora of unanswered questions. It is known that children tend to use gestures just before intentional vocal behavior. Furthermore, at about 1 year of age, gestures and vocal behavior begin to be better coordinated. Although graphic symbols are used by children both to comprehend and produce communication, relatively little is known about the degree to which young children recognize graphic symbols or the contexts in which they tend to rely on graphic symbols to engage in communication.

Children's initial use of communicative symbols is highly contextualized. Although between 12 and 24 months of age children's propensity to use decontextualized symbols dramatically increases, relatively little work has examined exactly how the natural environment facilitates this mastery. Using symbols to refer to past or impending future events among the youngest communicators has received relatively little attention, even though most parents readily identify situations in which their 12- to 18-month-old communicated about the immediate future or past in the absence of any observable referents.

Much of the intervention literature has focused on communicative production. We believe that viewing comprehension and production as independent but intertwined competencies offers a number of opportunities for fruitful research. We know that young children rely a great deal on contextual cues offered by others; however, we do not know whether parents, caregivers, and teachers naturally fade this context or whether children simply become increasingly able to respond without it. Although pragmatic taxonomies drive the description of early communicative production, researchers have not placed enough effort on developing a corresponding taxonomy to examine early comprehension. Most comprehension assessment instruments examine semantic rather than pragmatic classes of communication and do not address aspects of the sociocultural context.

One aspect of pragmatic production that has received significant attention is conversational exchange. However, assessment strategies must more clearly examine the influence that production and comprehension vocabulary have on an individual's propensity to participate in communicative exchanges. Furthermore, if an individual does not have sufficient production or comprehension vocabulary, what pragmatic skills apart from vocabulary will allow him or her to maintain or shift the topic of a communicative exchange?

A number of semantic classes that emerge during the transition to symbolic communication pave the way for decontextualized language. Although we are beginning to get a better idea of how children combine vocabulary, we do not have a particularly good picture of the effect that communicative mode has on these acquisitions. With respect to actions, there is limited evidence to suggest that actions may be easier to represent gesturally than graphically. At the level of combining vocabulary into two- and three-word utterances, graphic display may be advantageous in that graphic representations may be held in a buffer as the utterance is formed. This allows the learner to monitor what symbols are part of the utterance being constructed. Having ongoing graphic representation and not operating under real-time constraints may represent a significant advantage in learning to combine relations. However, little research has explored the role that communicative mode has on the acquisition of traditional language forms and content.

CONCLUSION

A child's ability to use conventional signals intentionally to communicate forms the foundation for symbolic communication. The course of symbolic communication development has been characterized by two major shifts: first words and a vocabulary burst. This twofold process of learning shared meanings is rooted in sociocultural activities. The provision of early intervention to increasingly younger children and to individuals with more severe disabilities has created the impetus to view communication in terms of gestural and graphic and vocal/verbal mode acquisitions. There have been remarkable advances in the knowledge of how children produce and comprehend a beginning communicative repertoire. The developmental literature provides a rich body of information to guide intervention efforts in understanding a child's strengths and needs and in planning contexts for language learning. The challenge ahead lies in the ability to find strategies to determine among the most rudimentary communicators which mode(s) provides sufficient efficiency and readability to their communicative partners to enable natural environments to become the nurturing context that supports the growth of an initial social communicative repertoire and expansion of a symbolic communication system.

REFERENCES

Acredolo, L., & Goodwyn, S. (1990). Sign language among hearing infants: The spontaneous development of symbolic gestures. In V. Volterra & C. Erting (Eds.), *From gesture to language in hearing and deaf children* (pp. 68–78). New York: Springer-Verlag.

Barrett, M.D. (1986). Early semantic representations and early word-usage. In S. Kuckaj & M.D. Barrett (Eds.), *The development of word meaning: Progress in cognitive development research* (pp. 39–67). New York: Springer-Verlag.

Barrett, M.D., Harris, M., & Chasin, J. (1991). Early lexical development and maternal speech: A comparison of children's initial and subsequent use of words. *Journal of Child Language, 18,* 21–40.

Bates, E. (1976). *Language and context: The acquisition of pragmatics.* New York: Academic Press.

Bates, E. (1979). *The emergence of symbols: Cognition and communication in infancy.* New York: Academic Press.

Bates, E., Bretherton, I., & Snyder, L. (1988). *From first words to grammar: Individual differences and dissociable mechanisms.* Cambridge, England: Cambridge University Press.

Bates, E., O'Connell, B., & Shore, C. (1987). Language and communication in infancy. In J. Osofsky (Ed.), *Handbook of infant development* (pp. 149–203). New York: John Wiley & Sons.

Benedict, H. (1979). Early lexical development: Comprehension and production. *Journal of Child Language, 6,* 183–200.

Bloom, L. (1983). *One word at a time.* The Hague, The Netherlands: Mouton.

Bloom, L. (1993). *The transition from infancy to language.* New York: Cambridge University Press.

Bloom, L., & Lahey, M. (1978). *Language development and language disorders.* New York: John Wiley & Sons.

Bonvillian, J., Orlansky, M., & Folven, R. (1990). Early sign language acquisition: Implications for theories of language acquisition. In V. Volterra & C. Erting (Eds.), *From gesture to language in hearing and deaf children* (pp. 219–232). New York: Springer-Verlag.

Boudreau, D. (1994, June). *The use of environmental print in reading instruction with students with developmental disabilities.* Paper presented at Fourth Annual Literacy and Disabilities Symposium, Chapel Hill, NC.

Braem, P.B. (1990). Acquisition of the hand shape in American Sign Language: A preliminary analysis. In V. Volterra & C. Erting (Eds.), *From gesture to language in hearing and deaf children* (pp. 107–127). New York: Springer-Verlag.

Bruner, J. (1964). The course of cognitive growth. *American Psychologist, 19,* 9–15.

Bruner, J. (1981). The social context of language acquisition. *Language and Communication, 1,* 155–178.

Carpenter, R., Mastergeorge, A., & Coggins, T. (1983). The acquisition of communicative intentions in infants eight to fifteen months of age. *Language and Speech, 26,* 101–116.

Caseli, M., & Volterra, V. (1990). From communication to language in hearing and deaf children. In V. Volterra & C. Erting (Eds.), *From gesture to language in hearing and deaf children* (pp. 263–277). New York: Springer-Verlag.

Chan, S. (1994). Logos: The emblem of marketing wars. *Quintessence, 25,* 509–515.

Chapman, R. (1978). Comprehension strategies in children. In J. Kavanagh & W. Strange (Eds.), *Speech and language in the laboratory, school and clinic* (pp. 309–327). Cambridge, MA: MIT Press.

Chapman, R., & Miller, J. (1975). Word order in early two and three word utterances. Does production precede comprehension? *Journal of Speech and Hearing Research, 18,* 355–371.

Clark, E. (1973). What's in a word? On the child's acquisition of semantics in his first language. In T.E. Moore (Ed.), *Cognitive development and the acquisition of language* (pp. 65–110). New York: Academic Press.

Crais, E.R. (1995). Expanding the repertoire of tools and techniques for assessing the communication skills of infants and toddlers. *American Journal of Speech-Language Pathology, 4*(3), 47–59.

Daehler, M., Perlmutter, M., & Myers, M.A. (1976). Equivalence of pictures and objects for very young children. *Child Development, 47,* 96–102.

Dennis, R., Reichle, J., Williams, W., & Vogelsberg, T. (1982). Motoric factors influencing the selection of vocabulary for sign production programs. *Journal of The Association for Persons with Severe Handicaps, 7,* 20–33.

Dore, J. (1986). The development of conversation competence. In R. Scheifelbusch (Ed.), *Language competence: Assessment and intervention* (pp. 3–60). San Diego: College-Hill Press.

Fenson, L., Dale, P.S., Reznick, J.S., Bates, E., Thal, D., & Pethick, S.J. (1994). Variability in early communicative development. *Monographs of the Society for Research in Child Development, 59,* (Serial No. 242).

Fenson, L., Dale, P.S., Reznick, J.S., Thal, D., Bates, E., Hartung, J., Pethick, S., & Reilly, J. (1993). *MacArthur Communicative Development Inventories (CDI).* San Diego, CA: Singular Publishing Group.

Fenson, L., & Ramsay, D. (1980). Decentration and integration of the child's play in the second year. *Child Development, 51,* 171–178.

Fischer, P., Schwartz, M., Richards, J., Goldstein, A., & Rojas, T. (1991). Brand logo recognition by children 3 to 6 years: Mickey Mouse and Old Joe Camel. *Journal of the American Medical Association, 266*(22), 3145–3148.

Gentner, D. (1982). Why nouns are learned before verbs: Linguistic relativity versus natural partitioning. In S.A. Kuczaj (Ed.), *Language development: Vol. 2. Language, thought and culture* (pp. 301–334). Hillsdale, NJ: Lawrence Erlbaum Associates.

Gibson, E., & Schmuckler, M. (1989). The effects of imposed optical flow on guided locomotion in young walkers. *Behavioral Journal of Developmental Psychology, 2,* 193–206.

Goldin-Meadow, S., & Morford, M. (1990). Gestures in early child language. In V. Volterra & C. Erting (Eds.), *From gesture to language in hearing and deaf children* (pp. 249–262). New York: Springer-Verlag.

Goldin-Meadow, S., Seligman, M., & Gelman, R. (1976). Language in the two-year old: Receptive and productive stages. *Cognition, 4,* 189–202.

Golinkoff, R.M., Mervis, C., & Hirsh-Pasek, K. (1994). Early object labels: The case for a developmental lexical principles framework. *Journal of Child Language, 21,* 125–155.

Greenfield, P., & Smith, J. (1976). *The structure of communication in early development.* New York: Academic Press.

Guess, D., & Baer, D. (1973). An analysis of individual differences in generalization between receptive and productive language in retarded children. *Journal of Applied Behavior Analysis, 6,* 311–329.

Harding, C., & Golinkoff, R. (1979). The origins of intentional vocalizations in prelinguistic infants. *Child Development, 50,* 33–40.

Harris, M., Yeeles, C., Chasin, J., & Oakley, Y. (1995). Symmetries and asymmetries in early lexical comprehension and production. *Journal of Child Language, 22,* 1–18.

Hart, B., & Risley, T.R. (1995). *Meaningful differences in the everyday experiences of young American children.* Baltimore: Paul H. Brookes Publishing Co.

Horner, R.H., McDonnell, J.J., & Bellamy, G.T. (1986). Teaching generalized skills: General case instruction in simulation and community settings. In R.H. Horner, L.H. Meyer, & H.D. Fredericks (Eds.), *Education of learners with severe handicaps: Exemplary service strategies* (pp. 289–314). Baltimore: Paul H. Brookes Publishing Co.

Huttenlocher, J. (1974). The origins of language comprehension. In R.L. Solso (Ed.), *Theories in cognitive psychology* (pp. 331–368). Hillsdale, NJ: Lawrence Erlbaum Associates.

Johnston, S. (1992). *The influence of symbol size and array type on normal children's nonidentity matching skills.* Unpublished master's thesis, University of Minnesota, Minneapolis.

Kent, R.D. (1993). Speech intelligibility and communicative competence in children. In A.P. Kaiser & D.B. Gray (Eds.), *Communication and language intervention series: Vol. 2. Enhancing children's communication: Research foundations for intervention* (pp. 223–242). Baltimore: Paul H. Brookes Publishing Co.

Keogh, W.J., & Reichle, J. (1985). Communication intervention for the "difficult-to-teach" severely handicapped. In S. Warren & A. Warren-Rogers (Eds.), *Teaching functional language* (pp. 157–196). Baltimore: University Park Press.

Koppenhaver, D., & Yoder, D. (1992). Literacy issues in persons with severe physical and speech impairments. In R. Gaylord-Ross (Ed.), *Issues and research in special education* (pp. 156–201). New York: Teachers College Press.

Kuczaj, S. (1986). Thoughts on the intentional basis of early object word extension: Evidence from comprehension and production. In S. Kuczaj & M. Barrett (Eds.), *The development of word meaning: Progress in cognitive development research* (pp. 99–120). New York: Springer-Verlag.

Lahey, M. (1988). *Language disorders and language development.* New York: Macmillan.

Leonard, L., Newhoff, M., & Fey, M. (1980). Some instances of word usage in the absence of comprehension. *Journal of Child Language, 7,* 189–196.

Leonard, L., Schwartz, R.G., Chapman, K., Rowan, L., Prelock, P., Terrell, B., Weiss, A.L., & Messick, C. (1982). Early lexical acquisition in children with specific language impairment. *Journal of Speech and Hearing Research, 25,* 554–564.

Locke, A., Young, A., Service, V., & Chandler, P. (1990). Some observations on the origins of the pointing gesture. In V. Volterra & C. Erting (Eds.), *From gesture to language in hearing and deaf children* (pp. 42–55). New York: Springer-Verlag.

Locke, J. (1996). Why do infants begin to talk? Language as an unintended consequence. *Journal of Child Language, 23,* 251–268.

Mace, F.C., & Roberts, M.L. (1993). Factors affecting selection of behavioral interventions. In J. Reichle & D.P. Wacker (Eds.), *Communication and language intervention series: Vol. 3. Communicative alternatives to challenging behavior: Integrating functional assessment and intervention strategies* (pp. 113–134). Baltimore: Paul H. Brookes Publishing Co.

McLean, J., & Snyder-McLean, L. (1978). *A transactional approach to early language training.* Columbus, OH: Charles E. Merrill.

Mervis, C.B., & Bertram, J. (1993). Acquisition of early object labels: The roles of operating principles and input. In A.P. Kaiser & D.B. Gray (Eds.), *Communication and language intervention series: Vol. 2. Enhancing children's communication: Research foundations for intervention* (pp. 287–316). Baltimore: Paul H. Brookes Publishing Co.

Miller, J.F., Chapman, R.S., Branston, M., & Reichle, J. (1980). Language comprehension in sensorimotor stages V and VI. *Journal of Speech and Hearing Research, 23,* 284–311.

Miller, J.F., & Paul, R. (1995). *The clinical assessment of language comprehension.* Baltimore: Paul H. Brookes Publishing Co.

Miller, M., Cuvo, A., & Borakove, L. (1977). Teaching naming of coin values–comprehension before production versus production alone. *Journal of Applied Behavior Analysis, 10,* 735–736.

Mirenda, P., & Locke, P. (1989). A comparison of symbol transparency in nonspeaking persons with intellectual disabilities. *Journal of Speech and Hearing Disorders, 54,* 131–140.

Mizuko, M. (1987). Transparency and ease of learning symbols represented by Blissymbols, PCS, and Pic syms. *Augmentative and Alternative Communication, 3,* 129–136.

Musselwhite, C., & Ruscello, D. (1984). Transparency of three communication symbol systems. *Journal of Speech and Hearing Research, 27,* 436–443.

Mustonen, T. (1995). *The influence of sample type, sample size, choice array type and choice symbol size on the matching to sample performance of preschoolers with cognitive delay.* Unpublished doctoral dissertation, University of Minnesota, Minneapolis.

Nelson, K. (1973). Structure and strategy in learning to talk. *Monographs of the Society for Research in Child Development, 38* (Serial No. 149).

Nelson, K. (1991). Concepts and meaning in language development. In N. Krasnegor, D. Rumbaugh, R. Schiefelbusch, & M. Studdert-Kennedy (Eds.), *Biological and behavioral determinants of language development* (pp. 89–116). Hillsdale, NJ: Lawrence Erlbaum Associates.

O'Neill, R., & Reichle, J. (1993). Addressing socially motivated challenging behaviors by establishing communicative alternatives: Basics of a general-case approach. In J. Reichle & D.P. Wacker (Eds.), *Communication and language intervention series: Vol. 3. Communicative alternatives to challenging behavior: Integrating functional assessment and intervention strategies* (pp. 205–235). Baltimore: Paul H. Brookes Publishing Co.

Oviatt, S. (1980). The emerging ability to comprehend language: An experimental approach. *Child Development, 51,* 97–106.

Owens, R. (1992). *Language development: An introduction* (3rd ed.). Columbus, OH: Charles E. Merrill.

Piaget, J. (1970). *Genetic epistemology.* New York: Norton.

Platt, J., & Coggins, T. (1990). Comprehension of social-action games in prelinguistic children: Levels of participation and effect of adult structure. *Journal of Speech and Hearing Disorders, 55,* 315–326.

Poulin-Dubois, D., Graham, S., & Sippola, L. (1995). Early lexical development: The contribution of parental labeling and infants' categorization abilities. *Journal of Child Language, 22,* 325–343.

Prizant, B., & Wetherby, A. (1987). Communicative intent: A framework for understanding social-communicative behavior in autism. *Journal of the American Academy of Child Psychiatry, 26,* 472–479.

Reich, P. (1986). *Language development.* Englewood Cliffs, NJ: Prentice Hall.

Reichle, J. (1993). *Some observations on the acquisition of initial graphic and gestural mode communication systems.* Unpublished manuscript, University of Minnesota, Minneapolis.

Rosch, E. (1978). Principles of categorization. In E. Rosch & B.B. Lloyd (Eds.), *Cognition and categorization* (pp. 27–48). Hillsdale, NJ: Lawrence Erlbaum Associates.

Rosinski, R. (1977). *The development of visual perception.* Santa Monica, CA: Goodyear.

Schuler, A. (1980). Aspects of cognition. In W. Fay & A. Schuler (Eds.), *Emerging language in autistic children* (pp. 113–136). Baltimore: University Park Press.

Sigafoos, J., Doss, S., & Reichle, J. (1989). Developing mand and tact repertoires in persons with severe developmental disabilities using graphic symbols. *Research in Developmental Disabilities, 10,* 183–200.

Snyder, L. (1978). Communicative and cognitive abilities and disabilities in the sensorimotor period. *Merrill-Palmer Quarterly, 24,* 161–180.

Snyder, L., Bates, E., & Bretherton, I. (1981). Content and context in early lexical development. *Journal of Speech and Hearing Disorders, 24,* 262–268.

Steckol, K., & Leonard, L. (1981). Sensorimotor development and the use of prelinguistic performatives. *Journal of Speech and Hearing Disorders, 24,* 262–268.

Tardif, T. (1996). Nouns are not always learned before verbs: Evidence from Mandarin speakers' early vocabularies. *Developmental Psychology, 32,* 492–504.

Tinbergen, N. (1951). *The study of instinct.* Oxford, England: Clarendon Press.

Tomasello, M. (1992). *First verbs: A case study of early grammatical development.* New York: Cambridge University Press.

Tomasello, M., & Farrar, J. (1986). Joint attention and early language. *Child Development, 57,* 1454–1463.

Tomasello, M., & Kruger, A. (1992). Acquiring verbs in ostensive and non-ostensive contexts. *Journal of Child Language, 19,* 311–333.

Tomasello, M., Kruger, A.C., & Ratner, H.H. (1993). Cultural learning. *Behavioral and Brain Sciences, 16,* 495–552.

Tomasello, M., Strosberg, R., & Akhtar, N. (1996). Eighteen-month-old children learn words in non-ostensive contexts. *Journal of Child Language, 23,* 157–176.

van Kleeck, A. (1994). Potential cultural bias in training parents as conversational partners with their children who have delays in language development. *American Journal of Speech-Language Pathology, 31,* 67–78.

Vihman, M., & McCune, L. (1994). When is a word a word? *Journal of Child Language, 21,* 517–542.

Vygotsky, L. (1986). *Thought and language* (A. Kozulin, Ed., and Trans.). Cambridge, MA: MIT Press. (Original work published 1934)

Werner, H., & Kaplan, B. (1963). *Symbol formation.* New York: John Wiley & Sons.

Wetherby, A., Cain, D., Yonclas, D., & Walker, V. (1988). Analysis of intentional communication of normal children from the prelinguistic to the multi-word stage. *Journal of Speech and Hearing Research, 31,* 240–252.

Wetherby, A., & Prizant, B. (1989). The expression of communicative intent: Assessment guidelines. *Seminars in Speech and Language, 10,* 77–91.

Wetherby, A.M., & Prizant, B.M. (1992). Profiling young children's communicative competence. In S.F. Warren & J. Reichle (Eds.), *Communication and language intervention series: Vol. 1. Causes and effects in communication and language intervention* (pp. 217–251). Baltimore: Paul H. Brookes Publishing Co.

PART II

Assessment and Intervention Issues

10

Clinical Assessment
of Emerging Language
How To Gather Evidence
and Make Informed Decisions

Truman E. Coggins

ASSESSMENT IS A PROCESS OF gathering evidence and making informed judgments. Historically, the goal of clinical assessment, particularly the clinical assessment of emerging language, has been to identify children who exhibit delayed or deviant communication. Assessment findings are then compared against a norm, reference, or standard to decide whether the delay or deviance is meaningful or significant. The knowledge of typical development and interaction with typically developing children led to certain expectations that define the standard of "normal" against which a particular child is compared (Lund & Duchan, 1993).

In the 1990s, however, the utility of clinical assessment has come under fire. Experienced clinicians have become increasingly dissatisfied, disappointed, or discouraged with the theoretical and methodological context of conventional assessment approaches. The primary objection from professionals is that traditional assessment tools seem to provide little information of value (Korchin & Schuldberg, 1981) because the results fail to inform how, and in what specific ways, delay or impairment interferes with the child's activities of daily living. This growing sense of frustration also has been observed in the families of children with special needs.

This chapter examines how evidence is gathered, how informed decisions are reached, and how clinicians typically have approached the task of identifying infants and very young children with impaired language. Several nontrivial problems with respect to this traditional approach are highlighted that question the relevance of data typically gathered during an assessment. The chapter concludes by offering a new model and new measures to assist clinicians in gathering what is believed to be more clinically useful information.

DEVELOPMENT OF COMMUNICATION AND LANGUAGE

Traditional Stage Model of Development

Traditionally, development has been described in terms of stages. Stages capture the orderly progression of development that exists when the "grand sweep of development" is viewed (Thelen & Smith, 1994, p. xvi). The concept of stage has been strongly tied to theories of development and traditional assessment measures that examine language and communication in infants and young children. The basic premise of infant–toddler assessment is that children develop according to a relatively predictable pattern (Owens, 1995). In general, children go from being small and simple to being bigger and more complex.

Linguistically, children first produce sounds, then words, and then word combinations. Because this journey proceeds with remarkable orderliness in typically developing children, basic and applied researchers assigned children to organizational stages with confidence. Two children in the same stage of linguistic development, for example, are likely to have language production at the same level of constructional complexity (Brown, 1973).

In a typical stage model, the sequence of development is based on one behavior serving as the antecedent for the next behavior. The antecedent must occur for the ensuing behaviors to develop. The model assumes a predictable and lawful (i.e., invariant) sequence of development across individuals. As a result, most typically developing children are expected to reach important developmental milestones at or about the same age (Owens, 1995). Developmental predictability has allowed researchers and professionals to use deviation from average group performance as a standard against which to compare individual performance.

Limitations of Traditional Models of Communication and Language Development

There are several drawbacks in the way that stage models for assessing infants and young children are applied. First, most stages are not "true" stages in the Piagetian sense; that is, they do not represent qualitatively different changes of organization. Instead, they serve as a convenient means of organizing or classifying changing behaviors into prominent developmental milestones at particular points in time. Typically, stage-based models provide a general framework for organizing behavior. However, unless the clinician is constantly abreast of changes in descriptions of stages, he or she can be lulled into a simplistic view of emerging communication skills. For example, prespeech development was viewed in the 1970s as a monolithic stage children passed through on the way to first words. It is now widely believed that children pass through five or six distinct stages of early vocal development (see Stoel-Gammon, 1991; see also Chapter 5).

Second, stage models are based on the idea that an orderly developmental progression exists and that the sequence of stages is invariant. However, emerging behaviors often do not show systematic change that can be described in terms of traditional developmental stages. During the first 2 years of life, developmental trajectories often reveal "substantial variability, including sharp spurts, plateaus and drops" (Kitchner, Lynch, Fischer, & Wood, 1993, p. 894). Children's progression is not captured as a simple geometric progression. Clearly, there are spurts of development. Some of these are likely biologically influenced, whereas others may be environmentally driven. At a single point in time, the context of a situation in which behavior is sampled and/or the learner's state can influence the production and understanding of communicative behavior. Many traditional assessment measures that seem practical and convenient fail to account for the influence that child and/or contextual variables may have on the child's use of communication. Qualitatively sound assessment should attempt to account for everyday conversation in all its diversity (Chapman, 1992). A multitude of contextual factors can combine in myriad ways to influence the child's level of functioning (McCabe, 1989).

Third, instrumentation simplicity may have a negative impact on the validity of an assessment instrument. In a stage model of assessment, for example, tests are not generally concerned with the many contextual variables that may influence outcome. By their very nature and purpose, formal tests present specialized test items, in controlled situations, that have little resemblance to how children experience language in everyday contexts. Although it would be possible for clinicians to incorporate meaningful contexts into existing assessment protocols, to do so would create a nontrivial challenge to the standardization of the instruments. The goal of the assessment process from an interactive perspective is to examine how multidimensional aspects of language are influenced by a variety of features that comprise the context of a communicative environment. If there is to be an adequate fit between current theoretical models of communication and clinical practice, assessment strategies must address the interactive and dynamic nature of language (see Chapman, 1992; Mitchell, 1995; see also Chapter 12). Considering the effect that a milieu of context has on communicative events will enhance the social validity of assessment and intervention practices.

Social validity examines the acceptability or viability of evidence in relation to real-world settings (Schwartz, 1991). A socially valid assessment is one in which "an accurate and representative sample of the consumers' opinions is collected; then that information is used to sustain satisfactory practices or effect changes" (Schwartz & Baer, 1991, p. 190). Measures of social validity are valuable supplements to the data gathered by clinicians during their relatively brief interactions with the child. Including a child's caregivers in the assessment increases the likelihood of sampling real-life experiences and meaningful social contexts.

Clinical researchers have begun to propose models of communication and language that carefully address social validity (see Bricker, 1993; Fratalli, Thompson, Holland, Wohl, & Ferketic, 1995; Olswang & Bain, 1996; Rice, Sell, & Hadley, 1990; Yorkston, Beukelman, & Bell, 1988; Yorkston, Strand, & Kennedy, 1996). Bailey (1989), for example, called for an ecologically based assessment that would include all caregivers, avoid cultural bias (by taking into account cultural background, economic status, and the family's value system), and focus on skills that are necessary for the child to function in everyday situations. Bailey and Bricker (1986) contended that assessing children in routine settings while they participate in daily routines dramatically increases the likelihood of observing naturally occurring and functional behaviors.

OVERVIEW OF COMMUNICATION AND LANGUAGE ASSESSMENT METHODS

Purposes for Assessing Emerging Language

The purpose of assessment answers the question, "Why is this assessment being done?" There is near unanimous agreement among informed clinicians that the purpose of an assessment exerts a substantial influence on the process of assessment. Wachs and Sheehan (1988) aptly noted that "different decisions require different types of instruments and different types of assessment strategies....[I]t is the purpose and not the population that defines the instrument chosen" (p. 401). According to Bloom and Lahey (1978), "The answer to all perplexing problems in assessment is not always to search for another instrument, but to determine why more information is needed" (p. 307). Knowing why more information is needed, in turn, determines the methods to be used to obtain the necessary evidence. Four different purposes are typically cited for why assessment information is needed. The four purposes, described in detail in this section, include screening, identification or classification, intervention planning, and monitoring and evaluating intervention. These four assessment objectives form an inherent sequence in which each purpose serves as a prerequisite for the one that follows. Thus, assessment strategies become more focused and comprehensive as the purpose of the assessment moves from screening toward intervention.

Screening The purpose of a screening assessment is presumptive identification (Barnett, Macmann, & Carey, 1992). That is, the aim or intention of screening is to gather enough reasonable evidence quickly to decide whether a child is or is not likely to have a language impairment. Developmental screenings may be based on caregiver report, direct observations, or a blend of these two data-gathering strategies. Regardless of approach, however, a screening instrument does not specify the nature of a problem or identify children for special services but rather recognizes those for whom a more in-depth assessment is warranted (Cohen & Spenciner, 1994). Screening instruments are designed to provide broad pictures and general developmental information at specific points in time. Some children who do have disabilities may pass through the screening without being identified for more focused assessments. Infants and young children, particularly those at risk, should not be given a single screening test but instead should be reassessed on a regular basis.

Identification or Classification   The need to examine language and communication in greater detail sets the stage for an identification or classification assessment. Whereas the purpose of a screening assessment is to gather preliminary data to form a hypothesis, the purpose of an identification or classification assessment is to determine the degree of impairment a child displays on critical developmental functions. According to Crystal (1982), the reason for conducting this type of assessment is to identify a child's level of performance in relation to the level he or she should be achieving. The resulting data are used to estimate the existence and degree of developmental delay by comparing the child with a normative group of peers without disabilities. Thus, the findings from this type of clinical assessment are essential in establishing a child's initial and continuing eligibility for special services.

Intervention Planning   One particularly important purpose of assessment is to facilitate favorable intervention outcome. The degree to which assessment contributes to beneficial intervention is known as the intervention utility of assessment (Hayes, Nelson, & Jarrett, 1987). According to Paul (1995), clinicians should use assessment data to identify which intervention might best serve the needs of a particular client. Thus, it is reasonable to think of assessment directed at intervention planning as providing functional information that helps to move children from where they are to where they ought to be (Crystal, 1982).

Assessment data have two complementary roles to play in planning intervention. First, a decision must be reached regarding an intervention framework. That is, the interventionist must determine whether service delivery will be direct (i.e., the clinician is the primary agent for change) or indirect (i.e., clinician designates others to serve as the primary agent for change). Second, a set of teaching strategies must be adopted that closely match the child's needs. According to Olswang and Bain (1996),

> The decision regarding how to treat a language-impaired child grows out of the clinician's knowledge regarding assessment of children's current levels of performance and corresponding readiness for the acquisition of new behaviors, and the clinician's beliefs about the best way to bring about change. (p. 414)

Monitoring and Evaluating Intervention   Effective and accountable intervention involves ongoing assessment. It is imperative to document the process of change throughout the entire program of intervention because intervention requires ongoing problem solving as opposed to fixed answers to given questions (Schon, 1983). Empirical support provides the justification for moving from one intervention phase to the next, demonstrating that behaviors generalize beyond the intervention setting, and documenting the durability of change. Monitoring intervention also permits the provision of timely troubleshooting that

may be required for intervention strategies that are less successful than anticipated. Unless ongoing assessment occurs, clinicians have no way of knowing
whether intervention is effective. As Bricker (1993) stated, "To not evaluate
change over time will likely result in wasted efforts and the poor use of limited
resources" (p. 9).

In sum, the underlying reason or purpose for which a child is assessed dic-
tates different clinical outcomes. These outcomes may include finding children
at risk, confirming suspected impairment, agreeing on appropriate intervention,
and establishing effectiveness of intervention. Moreover, the purpose of a clinical assessment will ultimately define the methodologies needed to reach a specific decision about a particular child.

Procedures for Assessing Emerging Language

Although multiple methodologies are available for assessing the prelinguistic
and early linguistic abilities of young children (for a detailed review, see Paul,
1995), experienced clinicians continue to rely on two basic approaches for identifying language disorders: standardized and nonstandardized assessment.

Standardized assessment is the most widely used method for examining
either the status of children or their unique needs. This approach establishes the
presence of an impairment by referencing a child's deviation from average group
performance. To complement the information obtained from standardized tests,
many experienced clinicians routinely use nonstandardized measures to determine more precisely what children can and cannot do with their language. This
section briefly reviews both approaches.

Standardized Assessment Standardized assessment allows clinicians to
compare the skills, abilities, and achievements of an individual child with those
of a comparable (i.e., normative) referent group. Over the years, standardized
(i.e., norm-based) measures have been widely used for determining if a language
disorder exists and for determining its degree of severity. The long-standing pop-
ularity of norm-based standardized measures attests to their success in allowing
clinicians to make meaningful comparisons of performance among children.

There appear to be several reasons why standardized assessments have so
many proponents. On a practical note, standardized tests typically have clear
administration and scoring criteria that result in easily obtained tangible evidence (Prutting, 1982). In addition, standardized tests provide numeric data that
often are purported to be valid and reliable. Thus, clinicians can readily compare
the scores of one particular child to those of a large sample of children taking the
same test. This comparative ability is important in that standard scores are typically required to qualify a child for support services (e.g., speech and language)
in an educational system. Furthermore, it is possible to use standard scores to
examine general changes in performance over time (Bricker, 1993).

Nonstandardized Assessment Nonstandardized assessment procedures
do not have standardized stimuli or yield standard scores. These procedures are

carefully designed to meet the needs and unique characteristics of an individual child. Nonstandardized assessment methods allow clinicians the freedom to examine a specific communicative behavior in detail by systematically varying content and context. There is consensus among most speech-language pathology experts that a nonstandardized approach can provide valid indices of linguistic performance (James, 1993; Miller, 1981; Olswang & Bain, 1996; Paul, 1995).

The adapting and probing that are possible using nonstandardized procedures have allowed for fine-grain descriptions of language performance. These detailed descriptions typically are used to form baseline levels of functioning (Miller, 1981), to describe patterns of regularities in performance (Lund & Duchan, 1993), or to establish entry-level measurements across a range of pertinent domains (Bricker, Bailey, & Slentz, 1990). Nonstandardized approaches rely on the examiner to structure and organize the situational context based on the behavior of interest and the individual needs of the child. In addition, they allow the clinician to assess a particular behavior, multiple times, in a variety of relevant contexts to examine more precisely the nature of the presenting problem. Because nonstandardized procedures are flexible and child centered, they also "can be adapted to fit the needs and characteristics of the child being evaluated" (James, 1993, p. 204). This is a distinct advantage when faced with the limited attention span of a young child, the motoric limitations of a toddler with reduced muscle tone, or the restricted social interaction of a child with autism.

Naturalistic observation and structured elicitation tasks constitute two nonstandardized procedures that are often implemented to assess early linguistic and communicative abilities. Since the 1960s, naturalistic observation has been the predominant methodology for assessing language and communication production in typical and atypical children (e.g., Aram & Nation, 1982; Bloom & Lahey, 1978; Crystal, Fletcher, & Garman, 1976; Ingram, 1989; Miller, 1981). Much of what is known about language use in young children has been gained by observing children in natural or seminatural situations.

Elicitation tasks allow the interventionist to separate contextual and linguistic variables that may influence a child's ability to understand language (Miller, Chapman, Branston, & Reichle, 1980). Elicitation procedures have been used successfully with infants and toddlers to elicit social-action games (Platt & Coggins, 1990), relational meanings (e.g., MacDonald & Nikols, 1974; Olswang & Carpenter, 1982), and communicative intentions (Carpenter, Mastergeorge, & Coggins, 1983; Coggins, Olswang, & Guthrie, 1987; Snyder, 1978; Wetherby & Prizant, 1993; Wetherby & Rodriguez, 1992).

Limitations of Traditional Assessment Methods

Traditional assessment measures have often not considered important knowledge regarding prelinguistic and early linguistic development. Since the 1980s, child language specialists have produced a prodigious body of evidence regarding prelinguistic and early linguistic behaviors in typically developing children. We have learned that language and communication development are an integral part of infancy and are inexorably linked to changes in a variety of other domains, such as social, motor, cognitive, and perception (Bates, O'Connell, & Shore, 1987). However, this knowledge has not proliferated mainstream models of language assessment.

How Well Do Clinical Measures Reflect Clinical Research? The following constraints and limitations are inherent in many of the assessment measures used to identify at-risk children delineated by Olswang, Stoel-Gammon, Coggins, and Carpenter (1987) and Wetherby and Prizant (1992):

- Few test items reflect the literature on the relationship among linguistic, cognitive, and social-affective development.
- Most measures focus on form rather than function or intentions expressed.
- There is a decided lack of depth in assessing both prelinguistic communication and early linguistic forms of behavior presumed to be critical for typical language acquisition.
- Most tests are clinician directed, which limits the child's initiations and spontaneous utterances.
- It is difficult to interpret test results into clinically useful information.
- Rigid test administration guidelines make it difficult to use most measures with atypical children.
- Parents and/or caregivers typically are excluded from actively participating in the process.

Many of the preceding limitations compromise the ability to gather useful information. McCathren, Warren, and Yoder (1996) reviewed eight formal assessment instruments used by researchers and professionals to identify infants with suspected language impairment. They evaluated the instruments along two important dimensions. They explored the degree to which the instruments assessed important prelinguistic variables that child language researchers have shown to be closely related to language development. McCathren and colleagues wanted to know the degree to which these assessment measures reflected basic psychometric characteristics (i.e., reliability, validity, test administration, scoring) and could be used with clinical populations. The results revealed sparse correspondence between clinical research and clinical practice. The investigators found that five of the measures reviewed were of little use in early identification because they failed to assess important prelinguistic knowledge or lacked basic measurement integrity. According to McCathren and colleagues, the three measures that adequately assessed prelinguistic communicative development were Assessing Prelinguistic and Early Linguistic Behaviors in Developmentally Young Children (ALB) (Olswang et al., 1987), Communication and Symbolic Behavior Scales (CSBS) (Wetherby & Prizant, 1993), and the MacArthur Communicative Development Inventories (CDI)

(Fenson et al., 1993). However, both the ALB and CSBS take approximately 1 hour to administer and have involved scoring systems that may create a wariness among practicing clinicians.

How Representative Are Assessment Conditions? Often, infants and young children are assessed in unfamiliar rooms by clinicians who control the materials, atmosphere, and duration of the assessments. Furthermore, the parents of these children often are relegated to an observation room or, if allowed to remain in the testing suite, are usually asked to hold their child to minimize extraneous motor activity. Most clinical researchers and practitioners have assumed that a controlled assessment environment exerts "not only uniform but predictable specifiable influences" on language performance (Gallagher, 1983, p. 1). Because assessment contexts have been assumed to be static backgrounds, a clinician could exercise experimental control and still expect to obtain a representative sample of behavior.

The most important mission of any assessment is to provide information that is representative. A representative sample of behavior is one that provides exemplary information about the kinds of ideas or knowledge a child possesses and how well he or she can use this knowledge. Although there is unanimous agreement about the importance of a representative sample, researchers have not applied a uniform definition to the term. Clinical researchers have used the term *representative* to reflect two different aspects of knowledge and use. Representative has been used by some language specialists to portray a child's typical, usual, or everyday activities. In this context, a representative sample reveals information about a child's current, habitual, or independent level of performance. However, clinical researchers also have argued that a sample of behavior should capture a child's optimal or best possible display of abilities (McLean & Snyder-McLean, 1978). To this end, a clinician is obligated to determine the environmental or contextual conditions under which different communicative behaviors can be used in their most sophisticated, conventional form (Coggins & Olswang, 1987). When high levels of contextual support are readily available, children have been found to perform at a relatively high developmental level (Olswang, Bain, & Johnson, 1992).

Both views of representativeness may be critical for assessment. Traditional assessment strategies (i.e., standardized tests, nonstandardized procedures) have provided clinicians with important information concerning a child's typical level of performance at a particular point in time, in a controlled context. The results provide a sample of linguistic knowledge a child possesses and how well he or she can access that knowledge with little direct assistance from an adult. The information from traditional strategies is used by clinicians to identify children who might have an impaired communicative system.

In contrast, dynamic assessment procedures focus on whether the systematic modification of contextual cues (both linguistic and nonlinguistic) will contribute to a child's improved, if not optimal, performance (Olswang & Bain,

1996; Olswang et al., 1992). Dynamic assessment yields three types of useful clinical information: 1) the child's potential for learning, 2) contextual variables that influence performance, and 3) strategies to facilitate level of performance. In dynamic assessment, the clinician "gives considerable weight to the response that indicates the child is capable of performing at a higher, more conventional, more abstract, adultlike level" (Olswang et al., 1992, p. 195). The amount of demonstrated change between a child's typical and optimal level of performance is an indication of how modifiable a child is at a specific point in time, thus providing critical information for intervention planning.

An important function of an assessment is to provide an accurate and representative sample of information. Clinicians have been assured that they could obtain a representative sample of behavior in a controlled assessment environment. However, in light of the potential powerful influence of context, the gathering of one sample, in one setting, under one set of conditions no longer appears to be a realistic goal of assessment. A truly representative sample is one that samples a child's current level of performance as well as a child's potential for change.

Because communication occurs in the context of an interaction, it may be equally important to examine existing communicative behaviors produced by the child's communicative partner. This activity could be particularly important in assessments, such as the CSBS and ALB, that are intended to be used to facilitate intervention planning. In part, the child's potential for change may rest with the teaching strategies that a caregiver already uses and the frequency with which they are used. Although assessment instruments are beginning to consider the child's behavior in the milieu of a social context, few, if any, carefully scrutinize the behavior of the child's communicative partner.

How Well Do Results Predict Future Performance? The ability to render accurate, long-term predictions regarding the communicative development of typically developing children has been less than impressive. Trying to prognosticate developmental outcomes for children with known or suspected disabilities by sampling their current level of performance also has proven to be disappointing. In the absence of good predictive validity, the usefulness of assessment data for making informed intervention decisions remains a matter of considerate professional conjecture.

Why has the predictive validity of most formal assessment measures been so poor? First, infants and toddlers are genuinely difficult to assess. Children younger than the age of 2 years move in and out of alert states with dispatch. Trying to capture, focus, and sustain the attention of a 15-month-old child long enough to identify actions, follow simple directions, or manipulate objects often requires the perfect blend of skill, knowledge, and good fortune. Second, most developmental assessment measures depend heavily on motor and sensory abilities. As a result, any child with a compromised or immature motoric system, or a child with limited visual or hearing acuity, is at a decided disadvantage on norm-based or nonstandardized measures that require action-oriented responses to demonstrate cognitive or linguistic ability.

Interaction between a child and the social environment also exerts an influence on development. There is evidence to suggest that young children who are capable of initiating and sustaining interpersonal relationships are more socially sensitive; that is, better able to explain the feelings and actions of other people (Dunn, Brown, & Beardsall, 1991; Dunn, Brown, Slomkowski, Tesla, & Youngblade, 1991; Howe, 1991). Yet the items on most assessment measures focus exclusively on the child's problem-solving skills or motoric functioning without considering how those behaviors have been enhanced, impeded, or valued by the environment. For the most part, assessment methodology does not evaluate characteristics of temperament, social interpretation (e.g., thoughts, emotions, beliefs, desires), and the "goodness of fit" between the infant and the family. As a consequence, it is not surprising to find that predictability of most formal assessment measures is weak (Sargent & Coggins, 1992).

The remarkably weak predictive validity of most assessment tools places the clinician in an awkward position. For example, when assessment performance falls more than two standard deviations below the mean, a speech-language pathologist might argue that these findings support a "let's intervene now" approach. However, a developmental pediatrician might not be convinced that these communicative delays are of long-term significance and may advocate a "let's wait and see" approach. Because of the limited predictive validity of the assessment instruments, not only is it difficult to make an informed decision between these two fundamentally different perspectives, but adopting either has potentially serious consequences. By following the "let's wait and see" approach, one is at considerable risk of "under referring children and delaying potentially beneficial services" (Gibbs & Teti, 1990, p. 312). The "let's intervene now" approach, however, has the opposite drawback, that is, overreferring and inappropriately labeling children whose differences are within the range of normal variation.

Although the predictive validity of early formal assessment is clearly suspect, observation of children in their natural environments has given clinicians cause to be more optimistic. There is ample evidence to argue that the quantitative and qualitative aspects of language ability can be predicted from observing the performance of children at earlier stages. For example, Bates et al. (1987) found that well before children use communicative pointing, they give and show interesting objects to familiar adults. There is a robust correlation between the emergence of communicative pointing and the emergence of giving, showing, and ritualized request gestures (i.e., opening and shutting movement of the child's hand). Furthermore, these three gestures are highly correlated with the subsequent appearance of naming. There is also evidence from Snyder (1978) that the absence of these behaviors is associated with substantial delays in language development.

Based on their comprehensive review of the literature, McCathren et al. (1996) identified four prelinguistic variables that appear predictive of later language development irrespective of the presence or absence of other factors (e.g., Down syndrome, fragile X syndrome). Three of the variables are communicative in nature: babbling (i.e., amount and use of vocalizations), pragmatic functions (i.e., behavioral regulation, social interaction, joint attention), and language comprehension (i.e., level of vocabulary understanding). The fourth variable reflects development of play skills (i.e., combinatorial and symbolic). McCathren and colleagues argued that by assessing these prelinguistic predictors, clinicians can recognize a potential language impairment before a child fails to talk. The obvious implication of this early identification is that intervention efforts can commence during the first year.

How Variable Is Performance? Early cognitive, social, and linguistic development is remarkably variable. Investigators have reported wide performance variability across these developmental domains in relatively homogeneous groups of infants and young children (Coggins, 1991; Lahey, 1988; Platt & Coggins, 1990; Prutting, 1982; Stoel-Gammon, 1991; Thal, 1991; Wetherby & Rodriguez, 1992; Wetherby, Yonclas, & Bryan, 1989). Given the myriad ways in which contextual variables may influence the performance of infants and young children, a clinician needs to be confident that the scores obtained during an assessment are precise and stable.

A study by Coggins and Rosenbalm (1994) raised questions regarding the stability of early developing behaviors. Coggins and Rosenbalm (1994) examined the degree of constancy in the early prelinguistic (i.e., babbled utterances) and linguistic abilities, pragmatic functions, and play skills of 35 typically developing infants during the second year of life. Each infant and his or her mother were videotaped in low-structured play activities at 12, 15, 18, 21, and 24 months of age. Overall, the findings revealed that emerging behaviors exhibit different degrees of stability (i.e., temporal reliability) from 12–24 months. The domain presenting the most stable profile during the course of the second year was prelinguistic and early linguistic productions. This finding suggests that clinicians can be reasonably confident that the sounds, words, and early utterances they obtain during low-structured interactions are likely to remain constant over short periods of time. Pragmatic functions (i.e., requesting, commenting, answering) revealed an uneven pattern, with requesting being the most stable function throughout the second year. Finally, play skills were the least stable behaviors. Scores varied greatly over short periods of time even though the environment contained familiar elements, including materials, activities, and a well-versed social partner (i.e., the child's mother). Even by the end of the second year, reliability coefficients were not very stable.

In sum, most norm-based and nonstandardized measures operate under the assumption that a child's performance is relatively stable, particularly if data are collected in a more naturalistic context, such as play (Craig, 1983; Linder, 1993;

Nelson, 1993; Paul, 1995; Widerstrom, Mowder, & Sandall, 1991). The findings given previously suggest, however, that individual subjects were differentially sensitive to particular contexts, which resulted in considerable performance variability during the second year. The notable lack of behavioral stability during play would appear to compromise the clinician's ability to accurately determine a child's current developmental level across a range of important domains of behavior. The variability in children's social, communicative, and play behavior suggests that more active scrutiny of variables influencing child emotions could improve clinicians' abilities to accurately assess emerging communication skills.

A DYNAMIC, INTERACTIVE MODEL FOR DESCRIBING COMMUNICATION AND LANGUAGE DEVELOPMENT

The acquisition of language is an interactive, dynamic, and multifaceted process. To capture the complexity of this emerging system over time, new models of communication and language development have necessarily become multidimensional and multidirectional. The shift toward more dynamic and interactive paradigms appears to be a sensible means of exploring how emerging language can be both predictable and variable. Speaking to this point, Evans (1996) wrote:

> A dynamic systems account would predict that phonological, morphological, syntactic, semantic, and pragmatic components of language are all linked together and because the moment to moment interplay between all of these systems is continuously changing, the "state" of the child's linguistic knowledge during processing of language is dynamic—changing moment to moment and nonlinearly over time. From a dynamic systems framework, the interaction between the child's "state" of linguistic knowledge and the external constraints on the child's system should result in evolving and adaptive verbal behavior which under certain conditions will be stable and yet under others will be highly variable. (p. 241)

Fogel and Thelen (1987) proposed a dynamic systems model to account for the complex, constantly changing, and in some ways unpredictable nature of early development. New behaviors may emerge as a result of the interaction between domains (e.g., motor, cognition, communication) without the reliance on some underlying blueprint or a neural pattern (Thelen, 1993); that is, development often self-organizes. The idea of self-organization suggests that domains of development are not independent of one another. Instead, they influence one another, and through that influence new levels of development can be achieved. Thus, the dynamic systems approach provides an attractive alternative for moving away from traditional assessment models that consider developmental domains as separate entities developing in stages. Furthermore, the context and the problem a child is trying to solve play key roles in this model.

Principles of dynamic and interactive systems have emerged in the speech and language literature. Mitchell (1995), for example, attempted to enlighten some traditional thinking by constructing a dynamic, interactive developmental model of speech and language production. Chapman (1992) also created a model of early language learning from a dynamic and interactive perspective. The major claim of her Child Talk model is that early linguistic knowledge, in all of its diversity, is not separated or isolated from everyday experience but is "developed in the context of and embedded in world knowledge" (Chapman, 1992, p. 13). In other words, linguistic advances in both understanding and speaking are actively constructed out of dynamic interactions between the child and the everyday environment. Like Fogel and Thelen (1987), Chapman (1993) also contended that differing domains (in this case, linguistic domains) interact with each other in the formulation of new knowledge.

Implications for Clinical Assessment

Traditional stage-based models tend to emphasize language universals, predictable developmental stages, and noninteractive domains. In an effort to be as simple and as straightforward as possible, the assessment methods that follow from such a traditional perspective give little notice to individual differences, are designed to minimize the effects of context, assign children to developmental stages, and consider developmental domains separately. A dynamic systems interactive model assumes that knowledge is acquired in a dynamic relationship between the child and the environment, and assessment strategies consider context to be a critical variable, focus on the whole child during integrated activities, and assess interaction within and between conventional developmental domains (Mitchell, 1995). This section summarizes several ways in which selected principles of the dynamic, interactive model apply to early assessment and reveals how clinicians can arrive at new ways of thinking, gathering evidence, and making informed decisions with modest revisions of their existing beliefs.

Addressing the Importance of Context   Context plays a leading role in dynamic and interactive models. From this perspective, what children say and do, why and when they say and do things, and how they interpret what others say and do to them are believed to be conditioned by or contingent on the context. McCabe (1989) cautioned clinicians to not lose sight of the interactive nature of language and the context in which it occurs:

> As an interactive system, both parent and child influence the content as well as the form of communication. In considering the context of language interaction, we must recognize that the child has a host of characteristics in addition to that of being a language learner, and that each of these characteristics is a potential influence on the form and content of communication. (p. 6)

Although speech-language pathologists have become more cognizant of individual differences, most still behave as if context is not all that important with respect to assessment. Generally speaking, assessment revolves around selecting and administering standardized tests, recording and transcribing naturalistic language samples, or trying to elicit a particular behavior of interest. Little if any time is set aside to consider the ways in which contextual variables many influence or determine patterns of performance during an assessment.

For many clinicians, considering context has meant observing a child in a free-play situation, with a standard set of toys, where the adult (typically the mother) has been instructed, "Play with your child as you would at home." The implicit assumption underlying this instruction is that context exerts a consistent influence across children. However, communicative behavior varies substantially depending on the context. Thus, trying to use a single clinical context to measure a child's ability or potential no longer appears to be a realistic goal of assessment. Furthermore, traditional assessment measures that report a single summary statistic summed across contexts may obscure important differences in the ways different children use their language (Craig & Evans, 1993; Rice, 1995). Dynamic and interactive assessment strategies can be applied to both comprehension and production.

Assessing Emerging Comprehension Unlike spoken language that can be recorded on audio- or videotape for later analysis, comprehension is far less tangible because it is an "event that takes place privately within the mind of the listener" (Miller & Paul, 1995, p. 7). The major task in assessing early comprehension is appreciating the strong influence of context. This is challenging because context is a multidimensional construct that includes the physical context (e.g., layout of the room), the social context (e.g., the history people have with one another), the event context (e.g., why people have gathered together), the affective context (e.g., emotional state and goals of the participants), and the prior linguistic context (Lund & Duchan, 1993). Although these contextual variables are operative in the immediate situation, they also reveal the listener's experiences that, according to Milosky (1992), create "world knowledge and how selective aspects of world knowledge are activated in a given situation" (p. 21).

Children demonstrate their earliest comprehension by understanding a few words in specific and predictable contexts. Some of the initial evidence that children understand parental speech is reported during social-action games. For example, when the mother of a 9-month-old claps her hands together and says, "Pat-a-cake, pat-a-cake, baker's man," her child begins to clap; or when the father of a 12-month-old holds his son up to the window and says, "Wave bye-bye," the child shakes his hand. In each case, the child's apparent understanding of the game and the verbal request is intimately tied to the context and the parents' sensitivity to their repertoire of actions (Chapman, 1981).

Parents of young children typically scaffold important contextual variables until their children begin to master the linguistic form and content of a particular game as evidenced by their use of conventional behaviors associated with the game. By supporting their verbal messages with enough redundancy and context to ensure the child's understanding, parents may actually facilitate early language comprehension (Coggins & Olswang, 1987). Platt and Coggins (1990) found a positive relationship between the amount of structure parents provided during social-action games and their child's level of performance. This finding stresses the importance of assessing a young child's performance with varying degrees of contextual support to obtain an indication of not only what a child can do but also what a child may be capable of doing.

Given the context-dependent nature of emerging language, the most relevant clinical question is how infants and toddlers use context and their prior knowledge to comprehend messages. Chapman's (1978) investigations showed that infants and toddlers comprehend little of what they hear. Instead, they use strategies that are based on experience to "understand" adult speech. A comprehension strategy is a shortcut for arriving at the meaning of an utterance without "full marshaling of the information in a sentence" (Chapman, 1978, p. 309). Table 1 summarizes a set of strategies that have been observed in children from 9–24 months of age (based on Chapman, 1978; Paul, 1995). Clinicians must be aware of these strategies to not overestimate a child's level of understanding.

Comprehension delays may also reflect limitations in a child's ability to use context in processing information. Milosky (1992) argued that children with specific language impairments, by definition, have cognitive abilities within the normal range of variability. Furthermore, it is plausible that these children have had world experiences quite similar to their typically developing peers. However, rather than attributing delays solely to deficits in language, it is possible that "the nature and accessibility of knowledge representations may account for some of the language deficits" (p. 39). Stated differently, language impairments may be the result of a child's difficulty or inability to create contexts for remembering. Therefore, clinicians should exercise as much control and concern over the vari-

Table 1.   Summary of comprehension strategies observed during the first 2 years of life

Age (months)	Comprehension ability	Comprehension strategy
9–12	Understands a few words in a predictable context	1. Look at objects adults look at 2. Act on objects noticed 3. Imitate ongoing actions
12–18	Understands a few words outside familiar events; still depends on immediate context	1. Attend to objects mentioned 2. Give evidence of notice 3. Act in usual manner
18–24	Understands single words outside predictable context; knows a few two-word combinations	1. Locate objects mentioned 2. Put objects in containers (or on surfaces) 3. Act on objects in way mentioned

Sources: Chapman, R. (1978). Comprehension strategies in children. In J.F. Kavanaugh & W. Strange (Eds.), *Speech and language in the laboratory, school and clinic* (pp. 308–327). Cambridge, MA: MIT Press; and Paul, R. (1995). *Language disorders from infancy through adolescence: Assessment and intervention.* St Louis: C.V. Mosby.

ous aspects of context (e.g., situation, social, affective) during assessment as they do over the presentation of linguistic variables.

Given these contextual parameters, certain children may be expected to comprehend more in some situations than in others. For example, asking a child, "What do you want to drink?" at a fast-food restaurant where a soda machine is fully visible may be very different from asking the same question in the child's living room with no available objects to remind the child of possible responses. In addition, some adults are quite skilled in using supportive gestures and materials to facilitate comprehension opportunities. They typically wait to provide an utterance to comprehend until the child has disengaged from a distracting activity, they may create an interactive moment just before they verbally request a child's participation, or they may prosodically mark utterances to make them more discernible. Assessments of early comprehension skills will provide a more accurate and complete picture if they carefully sample a range of conditions that the child typically encounters during his or her daily routine.

Assessing Communicative Production The reason young children select a particular communicative gesture, vocalization, or word to encode is a function of their experience and the multifaceted aspects of the context as they perceive it. Therefore, the diversity, frequency, or even mode of a child's communication may vary depending on how an eliciting context is configured and perceived. For example, consider two 18-month-old boys with typically developing cognitive skills. Although their language comprehension is commensurate with their nonverbal problem solving, both of the boys have fewer than 10 words in their productive vocabularies. As part of a clinical assessment, each boy is being observed in a low-structured interaction with his mother. One mother is responsive and establishes routines and familiar social interactions that use familiar toys. The other mother is directive. Communicative utterances directed to her child reflect low "scriptedness" and a less familiar social context, novel toys and games, and restricted communicative opportunities. Differences in the language produced by the two children could as easily be a function of context as communicative abilities.

Contextual variables must be skillfully manipulated to reconcile variability in young children's emerging communicative productions. Based on a review of selected experimental research, Coggins (1991) identified six contextual variables that have the potential to substantially influence the performance of infants and toddlers. Five of these variables center on important nonlinguistic aspects of the environment and the sixth involves the adult's verbalizations. These six influential variables are summarized in Table 2.

Olswang et al. (1992) contended that the goal of infant–toddler assessment is to determine what the child is capable of expressing. To reach this objective, the clinician must establish the conditions under which communicative productions can be used in their most sophisticated, conventional form (Coggins & Olswang, 1987). By creating situations that vary the nonlinguistic and linguistic

Table 2. Contextual variables and levels of support that may influence performance

Contextual variable	Level of support	
Nonlinguistic	**Minimal**	**Maximal**
Purpose of an activity or interaction	Naturalistic	Contrived
Experience with communicative partner	Unfamiliar	Familiar
Nature of stimulus materials	Novel	Familiar/thematic
Familiarity of activities	New/original	Event/routines
Responsivity of the listener	Immediate	Delayed
Linguistic		
Availability cues or prompts	General statement	Elicited imitation

Adapted from Coggins (1991).

contexts along a continuum from minimal to maximal amounts of support (see Table 2), it is possible to gain insight into an individual child's modifiability or potential for change.

Assessment Strategies that Consider Communicative Strengths and Limitations

Clinicians and applied researchers have long been frustrated with the information that traditional assessment methods provide about atypical children. For example, because the rate of development in many children with language impairments is slow and gradual, items on standardized measures do not capture their small, albeit meaningful, changes. Furthermore, because most assessment methodologies have been designed to measure discrete skills on structured tasks in controlled environments, they do not consider abilities believed to be essential for infants and toddlers to function independently and cope with everyday environmental demands (Bricker, 1993). A growing number of clinical researchers have developed assessment tools that seek to provide accurate, reliable information on a child's behavioral repertoire in contexts that are meaningful for the child and the family. This view of a child's performance is consistent with a dynamic, interactive model of development.

Preschool Functional Communication Inventory Olswang (1996) crafted a functional communication assessment, called the Preschool Functional Communication Inventory (PFCI), that samples a child's communicative skills in meaningful, typical experiences and environments. A functional assessment measures the ability to receive or to convey a message, regardless of the mode, to communicate effectively and independently in a given (natural) environment (Fratalli et al., 1995). Functional assessment is exceptionally well-suited "to tap the skills that are important in the child's life, the skills the child has the most experience with and that are likely to be shaped by unique cultural forces" (Olswang, 1996, p. 6). A growing number of speech-language pathologists have embraced the clinical utility of functional assessment (Fratalli et al., 1995; Haley, Coster, Ludlow, Halltiwanger, & Andrellos, 1992; Rice et al., 1990).

The goal of the PFCI is to establish how well toddlers and young children can communicate with people who matter and in situations that matter. The assessment inventory is predicated on a conceptual framework that includes six important components: 1) behaviors of interest must be relevant to the everyday lives of youngsters; 2) stimuli must be operationally defined; 3) stimuli must be measured in natural communicative contexts; 4) results must provide evidence for a range of ages (i.e., 18–48 months) and impairments; 5) the protocol must be sensitive across gender, socioeconomic status, and culture; and 6) the inventory must be easily administered, interpreted, and understood.

The PFCI assesses a child's level of performance on four salient domains: 1) Social Communication, 2) Communication of Basic Needs, 3) Cognition–Play-Basic Concepts, and 4) Daily Routines. Each domain has a unique set of relevant behaviors that can be quantified by a speech-language pathologist who scores the child's emissions along a seven-point scale of independence. The scale of independence is designed to reveal the amount of environmental support that is required for a child to use different communicative functions in their most conventional form (i.e., 7—does with no assistance, 4—does with moderate assistance, 1—does not perform). For example, the second domain, Communication of Basic Needs, is composed of seven distinct dimensions, including expressing likes and dislikes, calling adult's attention, requesting assistance, responding to adult's queries, communicating hunger and thirst, communicating bathroom needs, and requesting help when injured.

In an effort to make the PFCI a more sensitive clinical instrument, the clinician rates a youngster's performance qualitatively. The quality of a child's communicative effort is scored for its adequacy (i.e., ability to appreciate the gist of a message and get a point across), appropriateness (i.e., relevancy of message to situation), timeliness (i.e., message occurs in suitable time), and sharing quality (i.e., responsiveness during social interactions). Qualitative judgments are made within and across domains.

Communication and Symbolic Behavior Scales Wetherby and Prizant (1993) constructed an assessment protocol, the CSBS, that explores emerging communicative development. Because this measure explores early communication from a social-interactive perspective, it provides clinicians with evidence relevant to a child's everyday uses of language during the second year of life. Furthermore, the CSBS is based on observing interactions between the parent (or caregiver) and child; thus, it provides an opportunity to observe the caregiver's behavior in the context of social exchange with the child.

The CSBS was designed primarily to assess communicative, social, and play behaviors. The measure samples performance in five related domains: 1) the range and distribution of communicative functions; 2) gestural, vocal, and verbal mode of expression; 3) reciprocal discourse strategies; 4) social-affective signaling; and 5) symbolic capacity of language comprehension, symbolic play, and constructive play. The CSBS provides cluster scores for measures of communicative abilities and an overall measure of symbolic development relatively independent of emerging linguistic and communicative behavior. According to McCathren and colleagues (1996), the CSBS is one of the few prelinguistic tools that assesses behavioral domains shown to be predictive of later language development.

The CSBS is a structured, yet flexible protocol. It allows clinicians to gather verbal and nonverbal behaviors from infants and toddlers using three different methodological perspectives. First, caregivers are requested to complete a questionnaire that focuses on how their child communicates in day-to-day situations. In addition, caregivers also respond to a series of questions at the end of the assessment regarding the typicality of the child's reactions and responses. Second, the child is observed in relaxed, relatively low-structured play activities that simulate natural adult–child interactions. Third, the clinician creates structured elicitation probes, or "communicative temptations," to entice the child to produce a desired behavior. For example, to elicit an intentional request, the clinician might place a favored object in a plastic jar and twist the lid so tight that the child cannot open it without assistance. Wetherby and Prizant (1993) maintained that these data collection strategies resemble natural, ongoing child–adult interactions, which can yield important information about the young child's everyday use of language.

The resulting information in each domain is converted to percentile ranks to create a communicative profile. The profile displays the relative strengths for the child in each of the communicative and symbolic domains. Because the CSBS provides information that can be used to explore important interactions within and between developmental domains, and because the measure can help in determining goals and contexts of intervention, it is consonant with the underlying assumptions of the dynamic, interactive model.

The Assessment, Evaluation, and Programming System for Infants and Children Bricker (1993) has crafted an integrated system of intervention that links early assessment with individualized educational programming. The *Assessment, Evaluation, and Programming System (AEPS) for Infants and Children* assesses functional skills and determines the conditions under which infants and toddlers are capable of using these skills to meet changing environmental demands. This assessment approach has allowed Bricker to establish a comprehensive profile of a child's abilities in everyday functional situations. More important, the AEPS can be used to evaluate the child's behavioral changes over time to determine whether intervention is producing desired outcomes. Ongoing monitoring provides clinicians with precisely the type of evidence they need to know when a child has reached a specific criterion and is ready to proceed with the next phase of intervention.

The AEPS is a criterion-referenced measure for children functioning between 1 and 36 months of age. It was designed to be used primarily as an observational tool during low-structured or naturalistic interactions. However, like the CSBS, the AEPS also uses elicitation probes and caregiver reports to gather assessment and evaluation information. The measure covers six developmental domains: 1) social, 2) fine motor, 3) gross motor, 4) adaptative, 5) cognitive, and 6) social-communication. Assessment goals and objectives within each domain have been carefully selected to establish the most efficacious sequence for learning new behaviors. For example, with respect to the social-communication domain, Bricker (1993) identified four hierarchically arranged assessment goals that include prelinguistic communicative interactions; transition to words; comprehension of words and sentences; and production of signals, words, and sentences. Within each of the four goals, Bricker also presented a set of operationally defined objectives. Thus, the transition to words goal has eight operationally defined objectives:

1. Gains person's attention and refers to object, person, or event
2. Responds with vocalizations and gestures to simple questions
3. Points to object, person, or event
4. Gestures and/or vocalizes to greet others
5. Uses gestures and/or vocalizations to protest actions or reject objects/people
6. Uses consistent word approximations
7. Uses consistent consonant–vowel combinations
8. Uses nonspecific consonant–vowel combinations and/or jargon

Assessment goals and objectives that the child does not perform become the content of intervention. Bricker (1993) contended that linking assessment with intervention in this manner produces educationally relevant outcomes and improves the timing of therapeutic experiences.

DIRECTIONS FOR FUTURE RESEARCH

Assessment is a process of gathering worthwhile information to reach informed decisions. Accumulating evidence that is worthwhile allows the possibility of reaching decisions that extend beyond normal curves, differential diagnosis, and the clinical setting. Clinicians who gather information of value explore, examine, and evaluate the effects of delayed, impaired, or deviant communication on a child's ability to meet the demands of everyday living. Thus, the justification for assessing language performance in infants and toddlers is to show how emerging language is enhanced or impeded by interactional effects between the child and environmental variables.

Researchers have begun to propose multidimensional models to account for the dynamic, complex, and multidimensional nature of language. In contrast to previous models that have traditionally focused on general trends or stages in development, these models focus on individual patterns of development and multivariate descriptions of the child. It is the fundamental, interactive nature of language and the strong influence of context that compromises the clinical utility of the data from traditional assessment methodologies.

The ultimate achievement in the acquisition of language is a communication system that can be used flexibly and frequently across linguistic and nonlinguistic contexts. Clinical researchers must seriously consider methodologies that go beyond z-scores, percentile ranks, and standard deviations as they attempt to characterize impairments in such a complex and vibrant system. Dynamic, interactive models provide a reasonable framework for meeting this challenge because they are designed for dealing with multiple and mobile variables that interact, influence, and change with each other over time. Future research should attempt to specify the dynamic relationships that exist among these interactive domains as the infant develops the ability to talk and understand the talk of others.

There is a tremendous need to carefully examine the individual and combined effect that contextual variables have on the development of an initial communicative repertoire. A related need is to carefully examine the effect that contextual variables have on the validity of assessment strategies. As the field increasingly moves toward dynamic assessment strategies, researchers carefully need to examine the relationship between standardized and nonstandardized assessment strategies in developing comprehensive assessment strategies that bridge the screening, identification, intervention, and evaluation functions served by a sound assessment process.

Finally, as the field strives to develop increasingly valid assessment tools, care must be given to the efficiency of the assessment instrument from the standpoint of those charged with the responsibility of its implementation. Researchers must carefully examine the cost-to-benefit ratio of comprehensive assessment strategies. Assessment instruments must be intuitively attractive to those charged with the responsibility of cultivating the emerging communicative repertoires of young children.

CONCLUSION

Instruments used to assess children's communicative behavior are becoming increasingly sensitive to the role that context plays in the ability to accurately represent a child's emerging competence. Examining the impact of contextual variables, in the short term, is likely to increase the complexity (and possibly length) of the assessment process unless better predictive control is gained. Because of the complexity of interactions among variables that influence a child's behavior, informal assessment will continue to represent a critical component of an interventionist's cadre of tools. Professionals must be thoroughly familiar with the range of contextual variables that are most critical to examine with any given learner. They must be familiar with standardized strategies that can be applied to all children that address a reasonable sampling of those variables. However, professionals must then be prepared to embellish the assessment protocol with systematic informal assessment strategies (see Chapter 13 for examples of such strategies). Sensitivity to contextual variables in assessment is of limited value, unless professionals design intervention protocols that address and are implemented in the milieu of important contextual features that influence communicative competence.

The professional field is becoming increasingly competent in improving the ability to identify children who may benefit from intervention. However, the price for progress is the identification of even more questions to answer. Clinicians are recognizing that their assessment responsibilities are not separate from but continue to be part of the intervention process. Consequently, assessment protocols must strive to examine not just the communicative forms that children understand and use but also the dynamic contexts in which communication occurs. As a result, assessment instruments are becoming increasingly sensitive to aspects of social validity in addition to reliability.

The explosion of information on the importance of early identification has resulted in a sensitivity to the important role that caregiver input can have in facilitating the assessment process. Furthermore, the need to serve increasingly younger children in the milieu of natural environments has resulted in clinicians more carefully considering the power of coordinating standardized with nonstandardized assessment protocols. This, in turn, has resulted in more contextually sensitive assessment instruments. However, clinicians recognize the limits of the predictive power of assessment but also foresee this as a critical area for further exploration. In summary, assessment capabilities have improved dramatically, and important answerable questions are on the horizon that should brighten service delivery for children and families.

REFERENCES

Aram, D., & Nation, J. (1982). *Child language disorders.* St. Louis: C.V. Mosby.

Bailey, D. (1989). Assessment and its importance in early intervention. In D. Bailey & M. Wolery (Eds.), *Assessing infants and preschoolers with handicaps* (pp. 1–21). Columbus, OH: Charles E. Merrill.

Bailey, D., & Bricker, D. (1986). A psychometric study of a criterion-referenced assessment instrument designed for infants and young children. *Journal of the Division for Early Childhood, 10,* 124–134.

Barnett, D., Macmann, G., & Carey, K. (1992). Early intervention and the assessment of developmental skills: Challenges and directions. *Topics in Early Childhood Special Education, 12,* 21–43.

Bates, E., O'Connell, S., & Shore, C. (1987). Language and communication in infancy. In J. Osofsky (Ed.), *Handbook of infant development* (2nd ed., pp. 149–203). New York: John Wiley & Sons.

Bloom, L., & Lahey, M. (1978). *Language development and language disorders.* New York: John Wiley & Sons.

Bricker, D. (1993). *Assessment, evaluation, and programming system (AEPS) for infants and children: Vol. 1. AEPS measurement for birth to three years.* Baltimore: Paul H. Brookes Publishing Co.

Bricker, D., Bailey, E., & Slentz, K. (1990). Reliability, validity and utility of the evaluation and programming system: For infants and young children (EPS-I). *Journal of Early Intervention, 14,* 147–158.

Brown, R. (1973). *A first language the early stages.* Cambridge, MA: Harvard University Press.

Carpenter, R., Mastergeorge, A., & Coggins, T. (1983). The acquisition of communicative intentions in infants eight to fifteen months of age. *Language and Speech, 26,* 101–116.

Chapman, R. (1978). Comprehension strategies in children. In J.F. Kavanaugh & W. Strange (Eds.), *Speech and language in the laboratory, school and clinic* (pp. 308–327). Cambridge, MA: MIT Press.

Chapman, R. (1981). Exploring intentional communication. In J. Miller (Ed.), *Assessing language production in children* (pp. 111–136). Baltimore: University Park Press.

Chapman, R. (1992). Child talk: Assumptions of a development process model for early language learning. In R. Chapman (Ed.), *Processes in language acquisition and disorders* (pp. 3–17). St. Louis: C.V. Mosby.

Coggins, T. (1991). Bringing context back into assessment. *Topics in Language Disorders, 11,* 43–54.

Coggins, T., & Olswang, L. (1987). The pragmatics of generalization. *Seminars in Speech and Language, 8,* 283–302.

Coggins, T., Olswang, L., & Guthrie, J. (1987). Assessing communicative intents in young children: Low structured observation or elicitation tasks? *Journal of Speech and Hearing Disorders, 52,* 44–49.

Coggins, T., & Rosenbalm, J. (1994, November). *Stability of emerging communicative behaviors.* Poster presented at the annual convention of the American Speech-Language-Hearing Association, New Orleans, LA.

Cohen, L., & Spenciner, L. (1994). *Assessment of young children.* White Plains, NY: Longman Publishing Group.

Craig, H. (1983). Applications of pragmatic language models for intervention. In T. Gallagher & C. Prutting (Eds.), *Pragmatic assessment and intervention issues in language* (pp. 101–127). San Diego, CA: College-Hill Press.

Craig, H., & Evans, J. (1993). Pragmatics and SLI: Within-group variation in discourse behaviors. *Journal of Speech and Hearing Research, 36,* 322–337.

Crystal, D. (1982). *Profiling linguistic disability.* London: Arnold.

Crystal, D., Fletcher, P., & Garman, M. (1976). *The grammatical analysis of language disability: A procedure for assessment and remediation.* London: Arnold.

Dunn, J., Brown, J., & Beardsall, L. (1991). Family talk about feeling states and children's later understanding of others' emotions. *Developmental Psychology, 27,* 448–455.

Dunn, J., Brown, J., Slomkowski, C., Tesla, C., & Youngblade, L. (1991). Young children's understanding of other people's feelings and beliefs: Individual differences and their antecedents. *Child Development, 62,* 1352–1366.

Evans, J. (1996). Plotting the complexities of language sample analysis: Linear and nonlinear dynamic models of assessment. In K.N. Cole, P.S. Dale, & D.J. Thal (Eds.), *Communication and language intervention series: Vol. 6. Assessment of communication and language* (pp. 207–256). Baltimore: Paul H. Brookes Publishing Co.

Fenson, L., Dale, P., Reznick, J.S., Thal, D., Bates, E., Hartung, J., Pethick, S., & Reilly, J. (1993). *MacArthur Communicative Development Inventories (CDI): User's guide and technical manual.* San Diego, CA: Singular Publishing Group.

Fratalli, C., Thompson, C., Holland, A., Wohl, C., & Ferketic, M. (1995). *The American Speech-Language-Hearing Association: Functional assessment for communication skills.* Rockville, MD: American Speech-Language-Hearing Association.

Fogel, A., & Thelen, E. (1987). Development of early expressive and communicative action: Reinterpreting the evidence from a dynamic systems perspective. *Developmental Psychology, 23,* 747–761.

Gallagher, T. (1983). Pre-assessment: A procedure for accommodating language variability. In T. Gallagher & C. Prutting (Eds.), *Pragmatic assessment and intervention issues in language* (pp. 1–28). San Diego, CA: College-Hill Press.

Gibbs, E.D., & Teti, D.M. (1990). Issues and future directions in infant and family assessment. In E.D. Gibbs & D.M. Teti (Eds.), *Interdisciplinary assessment of infants: A guide for early intervention professionals* (pp. 311–320). Baltimore: Paul H. Brookes Publishing Co.

Haley, S., Coster, W., Ludlow, L., Halltiwanger, J., & Andrellos, P. (1992). *Pediatric evaluation of disability inventory.* Boston: New England Medical Center Hospitals, Inc.

Hayes, S., Nelson, R., & Jarrett, R. (1987). The treatment utility of assessment: A functional approach to evaluating assessment quality. *American Psychologist, 42,* 963–974.

Howe, N. (1991). Sibling-directed internal state language, perspective taking, and affective behavior. *Child Development, 62,* 1503–1512.

Ingram, D. (1989). *First language acquisition: Method, description and explanation.* Cambridge, England: Cambridge University Press.

James, S. (1993). Assessing children with language disorders. In D. Bernstein & E. Tiegerman (Eds.), *Language and communication disorders in children* (3rd ed., 185–228). New York: Macmillan.

Kitchner, K.M., Lynch, C.L., Fischer, K.W., & Wood, P.K. (1993). Developmental range of reflective judgment: The effect of contextual support and practice on developmental stage. *Developmental Psychology, 29,* 893–906.

Korchin, S., & Schuldberg, D. (1981). The future of clinical assessment. *American Psychologist, 36,* 1147–1158.

Lahey, M. (1988). *Language disorders and language development.* New York: Macmillan.

Linder, T.W. (1993). *Transdisciplinary play-based assessment: A functional approach to working with young children* (Rev. ed.). Baltimore: Paul H. Brookes Publishing Co.

Lund, N., & Duchan, J. (1993). *Assessing children's language in naturalistic contexts* (3rd ed.). Englewood Cliffs, NJ: Prentice Hall.

MacDonald, J., & Nikols, M. (1974). *Environmental language inventory manual.* Columbus: Ohio University Press.

McCabe, A. (1989). Differential language learning styles in young children: The importance of context. *Developmental Review, 9,* 1–20.

McCathren, R.B., Warren, S.F., & Yoder, P.J. (1996). Prelinguistic predictors of later language development. In K.N. Cole, P.S. Dale, & D.J. Thal (Eds.), *Communication and language intervention series: Vol. 6. Assessment of communication and language* (pp. 57–75). Baltimore: Paul H. Brookes Publishing Co.

McLean, J., & Snyder-McLean, L. (1978). *A transactional approach to early language training.* Columbus, OH: Charles E. Merrill.

Miller, J. (1981). *Assessing language production in children: Experimental procedures.* Baltimore: University Park Press.

Miller, J., Chapman, R., Branston, M., & Reichle, J. (1980). Language comprehension in sensorimotor stages V and VI. *Journal of Speech and Hearing Research, 23,* 284–311.

Miller, J.F., & Paul, R. (1995). *The clinical assessment of language comprehension*. Baltimore: Paul H. Brookes Publishing Co.

Milosky, L. (1992). Children listening: The role of world knowledge in language comprehension. In R. Chapman (Ed.), *Processes in language acquisition and disorders* (pp. 20–44). St. Louis: C.V. Mosby.

Mitchell, P. (1995). A dynamic interactive developmental view of early speech and language production: Application to clinical practice in motor speech disorders. *Seminars in Speech and Language, 16*(7), 100–109.

Nelson, N. (1993). *Childhood language disorders in context: Infancy through adolescence*. New York: Macmillan.

Olswang, L. (1996). *The Preschool Functional Communication Inventory*. Seattle: University of Washington Speech and Hearing Clinic.

Olswang, L., & Bain, B. (1996). Assessment information for making treatment decisions: Predicting upcoming change in language production. *Journal of Speech and Hearing Research, 39*, 414–423.

Olswang, L., & Carpenter, R. (1982). The ontogenesis of agent: Linguistic expression. *Journal of Speech and Hearing Research, 25*, 306–314.

Olswang, L., Stoel-Gammon, C., Coggins, T., & Carpenter, R. (1987). *Assessing linguistic behaviors*. Seattle: University of Washington Press.

Olswang, L.B., Bain, B.A., & Johnson, G.A. (1992). Using dynamic assessment with children with language disorders. In S.F. Warren & J. Reichle (Eds.), *Communication and language intervention series: Vol. 1. Causes and effects in communication and language intervention* (pp. 187–215). Baltimore: Paul H. Brookes Publishing Co.

Owens, R. (1995). *Language development: An introduction* (3rd ed.). Columbus, OH: Charles E. Merrill.

Paul, R. (1995). *Language disorders from infancy through adolescence: Assessment and intervention*. St. Louis: C.V. Mosby.

Platt, J., & Coggins, T. (1990). Comprehension of social-action games in prelinguistic children. *Journal of Speech and Hearing Disorders, 55*, 315–326.

Prutting, C. (1982). Pragmatics as social competence. *Journal of Speech and Hearing Disorders, 47*, 123–134.

Rice, M., Sell, M., & Hadley, P. (1990). The social interactive coding system: An on-line clinically relevant tool. *Language, Speech & Hearing Sciences in Schools, 21*, 2–14.

Rice, M.L. (1995). Grammatical categories of children with specific language impairments. In R.V. Watkins & M.L. Rice (Eds.), *Communication and language intervention series: Vol. 4. Specific language impairments in children* (pp. 69–90). Baltimore: Paul H. Brookes Publishing Co.

Sargent, L., & Coggins, T. (1992). Obtaining and using new knowledge: Determining the relationship between theory and practice. *Topics in Early Childhood Special Education, 12*(1), 44–53.

Schon, D. (1983). *The reflective practitioner: How professionals think in action*. New York: Basic Books.

Schwartz, I. (1991). The study of consumer behavior and social validity: An essential partnership for applied behavior analysis. *Journal of Applied Behavior Analysis, 24*, 241–244.

Schwartz, I., & Baer, D. (1991). Social validity assessments: Is current practice state of the art? *Journal of Applied Behavior Analysis, 24*, 189–204.

Snyder, L. (1978). Communicative and cognitive abilities in the sensorimotor period. *Merrill-Palmer Quarterly, 24*, 161–180.

Stoel-Gammon, C. (1991). Normal and disordered phonology in two-year-olds. *Topics in Language Disorders, 11*, 21–32.

Thal, D. (1991). Language and cognition in normal and late-talking toddlers. *Topics in Language Disorders, 11,* 33–42.

Thelen, E. (1993). Early motor skill acquisition. In G. Tukewitz & D. Devenny (Eds.), *Developmental time and timing* (pp. 85–104). Hillsdale, NJ: Lawrence Erlbaum Associates.

Thelen, E., & Smith, L. (1994). *A dynamic systems approach to the development of cognition and action.* Cambridge, MA: MIT Press.

Wachs, T., & Sheehan, R. (Eds.). (1988). *Assessment of young developmentally disabled children.* New York: Plenum.

Wetherby, A., & Prizant, B. (1993). *Communication and Symbolic Behavior Scales manual: Normed edition.* Chicago, IL: Applied Symbolix.

Wetherby, A., & Rodriguez, G. (1992). Measurement of communicative intentions in normally developing children during structured and unstructured contexts. *Journal of Speech and Hearing Research, 35,* 130–138.

Wetherby, A., Yonclas, D., & Bryan, A. (1989). Communication profiles of preschool children with handicaps: Implications for early identification. *Journal of Speech and Hearing Disorders, 54,* 148–158.

Wetherby, A.M., & Prizant, B.M. (1992). Profiling young children's communicative competence. In S.F. Warren & J. Reichle (Eds.), *Communication and language intervention series: Vol. 1. Causes and effects in communication and language intervention* (pp. 217–253). Baltimore: Paul H. Brookes Publishing Co.

Widerstrom, A., Mowder, B., & Sandall, S. (1991). *At-risk and handicapped newborns and infants: Development, assessment, and intervention.* Englewood Cliffs, NJ: Prentice Hall.

Yorkston, K., Beukelman, D., & Bell, K. (1988). *Clinical management of dysarthric speakers.* Austin, TX: PRO-ED.

Yorkston, K., Strand, E., & Kennedy, M. (1996). Comprehensibility of dysarthric speech: Implications for assessment and treatment planning. *American Journal of Speech-Language Pathology, 5,* 55–66.

11

Role of Caregivers
in the Assessment Process

Elizabeth R. Crais and Stephen N. Calculator

THE IMPORTANCE OF CAREGIVERS IN the intervention efforts for children and older individuals with special needs is undeniable and has become a basic principle in most communication intervention activities. The interactionist perspective held by many professionals (Girolametto, 1988; MacDonald & Gillette, 1988; Mahoney & Powell, 1986; McLean & Snyder-McLean, 1978; Norris & Hoffman, 1990; Warren & Kaiser, 1988) focuses on the reciprocal nature of communication and the importance of caregivers in establishing basic communication skills (Wilcox, 1992). Although different primary agents may participate in intervention, most approaches use the child's familiar communication partners. Furthermore, for young children, the central role of the family in developing and implementing intervention plans is a major component of the Individuals with Disabilities Education Act (IDEA) of 1990 (PL 101-476), and the intent of the legislation reflects the theoretical perspectives inherent in the interactionist perspective. This chapter discusses principles and strategies useful for developing collaborative relationships with caregivers of both young children and older individuals who are making the transition from prelinguistic to linguistic and preintentional to intentional levels. For ease of reference and because of the overlap in information, this chapter primarily uses the term *children,* however, the chapter uses the term *older individuals* when information is exclusive to this latter group. In addition, the authors use the term *caregiver* to broadly represent parents and other individuals (e.g., relatives, child care workers) who spend considerable time with the child and who serve the functions of caregiving.

In planning intervention efforts there has been increased recognition of the need for children to develop skills within natural environments. In particular, attention has been drawn to issues related to the acquisition and generalization of skills that are useful to children in meeting their daily communication demands. With this recognition has come consensus concerning limitations of traditional pull-out or one-to-one professional–child models of intervention and a focus on magnifying the role of caregivers in the intervention process (Rosenberg &

Robinson, 1988). For children, the centerpiece of IDEA is its focus on caregiver participation; the mechanism for ensuring caregiver–professional collaboration is the individualized family service plan or individualized education program (IEP) process (Winton, 1990). Although the services provided to older individuals with special needs may not be mandated by federal legislation, the role of caregivers continues to be prominent.

A critical influence in developing most intervention plans is the role played by the assessment process and, more specifically, the role of caregivers in that process. Although there are a number of general references in the literature on the need to involve caregivers in the assessment process, there is typically a lack of specificity in delineating concrete ways that caregivers may participate more actively in assessment activities. Thus, this chapter addresses strategies to enhance the active participation of caregivers in the assessment process.

RATIONALE FOR ACTIVE CAREGIVER PARTICIPATION

Before moving into explicit strategies for enhancing caregiver participation in assessment, it is first useful to highlight several primary reasons for developing the strategies. The following is a brief overview of some of those reasons.

Historical Roles of Caregivers in Assessment

Caregiver's roles traditionally have been limited to observer or informant of developmental and health histories (Bailey, McWilliam, Winton, & Simeonsson, 1992). Professionals across a variety of disciplines have called for increased participation of caregivers *throughout* the assessment process (Andrews & Andrews, 1990; Bailey, 1989; Beukelman & Mirenda, 1992; Bloch & Seitz, 1989; Crais, 1992, 1993, 1995; Kjerland & Kovach, 1990; Neisworth & Bagnato, 1988; Sheehan, 1988; Sigafoos & York, 1991). For young children, increased parental involvement has included asking caregivers to identify their concerns and priorities, administer certain test items, and demonstrate typical interactions with their child. Once the assessment is complete, many professionals not only ask caregivers to help generate the goals for the child and family but also to help monitor the child's progress. For an older individual, caregivers may be asked to document the individual's preferences, identify target vocabulary, identify challenging or excessive behaviors, and complete some types of observation. Although these efforts may provide professionals with increased information and encourage caregivers to be more active in the process, they alone may not facilitate the development of truly collaborative relationships. When professionals ask caregivers to provide information regarding the child and then use that information to make decisions and recommendations *for* caregivers, little has changed other than that caregivers are now asked to provide more and varied types of information.

Ecological Perspective within Assessment

In considering the ecology of the child, many professionals refer to Bronfen-brenner's (1979) concept of the child nested within the family, which is itself embedded within a larger community system. A child with disabilities may be surrounded by a variety of caregivers and contexts. To promote shared knowledge and experiences, all the child's caregivers can be included as members of the assessment and intervention team. The child's differing ecologies (e.g., home, child care setting, center-based program, school), the child's interactions across these settings, and the facilitators and constraints inherent in those settings must be examined (see Chapter 18). In using the child's existing ecologies for assessment and intervention, many professionals have noted an increased ability of the child to transfer or generalize information, enhanced opportunities for people important to the child to learn about and be involved in intervention, and increased maintenance of skills (Bailey, 1989; Halle, 1988; Mirenda & Calculator, 1993).

Assessment and intervention activities must also match caregivers' perceptions of what is appropriate and important. As a consequence, caregivers' cultural backgrounds, economic statuses, and value systems must be taken into account. As suggested by Moore and Beatty (1995), the family's background and perspectives can be respected by doing the following: 1) recognizing diversity, including cultural differences and child-rearing practices, in assessment activities and interpretation; 2) interacting with the child and family in their native language; and 3) considering the use of socioculturally appropriate tests and techniques. For professionals who are not bilingual or who do not represent the family's cultural group, an interpreter or cultural mediator may be needed. Interpreters or cultural mediators can take many roles within assessment, such as liaison with parents, communication link between staff and parents, parental advocate, cultural gauge for what may or may not be relevant for the family, source of information for parents, interpreter during assessment and pre- or postassessment meetings, translator of all written materials (e.g., tests, reports), and referral source for the community (Moore & Beatty, 1995).

Assessment as Ownership Enhancement

Without active participation, caregivers may not assume "ownership" of the decisions made or the interventions planned (Beukelman & Mirenda, 1992). Furthermore, as suggested by Beukelman and Mirenda, if caregivers have been excluded from the assessment phase when team dynamics and interaction styles are established, they may not learn to participate as team members. To enhance ownership, Salisbury and Dunst (1997) suggested that caregivers should be given options regarding the frequency with which they provide input about the child, the medium through which this endeavor is carried out (e.g., through correspondence, telephone, personal contact), the location in which information will be exchanged, and their preferred type or level of involvement.

Assessment Aimed Toward Consensus Building

Beukelman and Mirenda (1992) suggested that a major goal of initial assessment should be the development of a process for long-term consensus building and management. Consensus is important in identifying the needs of the child and priorities for assessment, determining the child's levels of development, identifying the child's strengths and needs relative to intervention, determining whether and what type of intervention may be necessary, selecting child and caregiver outcomes and means to achieve those outcomes, and monitoring and evaluating the interventions and outcomes. As previous chapters highlight, for children with disabilities who are making the transition from preintentional to intentional communication or presymbolic to symbolic, communicative behaviors may not be as recognizable or consistently used as the behaviors of other children. Some children have behaviors that challenge or that interfere with communication efforts, thus making the achievement of consensus more difficult regarding overall developmental and communication levels. When both caregivers and professionals are active in the assessment of the child, a closer match between their individual views of the child may be obtained (Bloch & Seitz, 1989).

Critical Nature of Caregiver Input

The combined efforts of caregivers and professionals may achieve a larger sample of behaviors for analysis due to caregivers' unique knowledge about the child that is often unavailable to professionals (Bailey, 1989; Crais, 1993; McLean & McCormick, 1993). For some preintentional or presymbolic children who may have low activity levels, decreased responsivity, limited initiations, and infrequent eye contact, fewer communicative and affective cues may be available for both caregivers and professionals (Rosenberg & Robinson, 1988). Caregivers and professionals also may contribute different information to the assessment process. For example, Morrow, Mirenda, Beukelman, and Yorkston (1993) looked at caregivers', teachers', and speech-language pathologists' contributions to choosing vocabulary for children using augmentative systems. They noted that although there were many similarities in the words selected across the informants, these informants also contributed words that were unique to their interactions with the child. These findings indicate that no one informant group could have been left out of the vocabulary selection process and that professionals need to be aware of the expectations of caregivers.

Assessment Viewed as Intervention

In addition to what caregivers can contribute to assessment, they also can gain from their participation in the process. Taking care of any child with disabilities may be stressful and at times may place additional demands on caregivers (Turnbull & Turnbull, 1990). For caregivers of children or individuals who are preintentional or presymbolic, there may be increased caregiving issues and thus increased stress and frustration (Barber, Turnbull, Behr, & Kerns, 1988). As suggested by Barber et al., caregivers' awareness, knowledge, and understanding of a child's special needs are important factors in caregivers' overall adjustment to the child. As caregivers actively participate in assessment and receive support and information, they may gain an increased understanding of their child's special needs. In addition, as caregivers work together with professionals to build on their existing resources and generate strategies to address their concerns, caregivers may increase their ability to deal with stressful caregiving issues and to plan more effectively for their child (Dunst, Trivette, & Deal, 1988). Active participation in assessment also may increase caregiver awareness in specific areas. By completing a developmental assessment of their child, parents have been shown to increase their awareness of existing and future developmental milestones, are more likely to identify the child's strengths and needs, and take a greater role in intervention planning (Bloch & Seitz, 1989; Bricker & Squires, 1989; Brinckerhoff & Vincent, 1987).

Enhanced Assessment Efficiency with Caregiver Participation

The input of caregivers not only enhances the assessment process but can also shorten it. Across many disciplines and contexts, professionals are recognizing the reliability of caregivers to provide judgments of a child's behaviors and skills. Examples include high correlations between caregivers' concerns about their child's developmental status and the outcome of developmental screening measures (Bricker & Squires, 1989; Glascoe, McLean, & Stone, 1991); high correlations between maternal and professional estimates of the child's developmental status (Bloch & Seitz, 1989; Sexton, Thompson, Perez, & Rheams, 1990); and high correlations between caregivers' judgments of vocabulary and syntax levels and professional assessment using standardized testing and language sampling (Dale, 1991; Dale, Bates, Reznick, & Morisset, 1989). Thus, using caregivers as assessors is not only valuable for the information that it provides and promotes, but it also can also be viewed as an efficient strategy for gaining a greater amount and variety of information.

STRATEGIES AND TOOLS FOR GAINING ACTIVE CAREGIVER PARTICIPATION

In keeping with the view of assessment as a consensus-building process, the focus throughout this section is on highlighting strategies and tools for building consensus among professionals and caregivers. Beukelman and Mirenda (1992) suggested that there is scant attention in the literature to strategies that build consensus in the assessment process, despite various studies documenting the importance of these strategies. To further delineate possible consensus-building strategies, three critical steps are highlighted within the assessment process: 1) preassessment planning, 2) observation and assessment of the child by both caregivers and professionals, and 3) postassessment planning and decision making. Consensus building should take place throughout the assessment and intervention process and should be viewed as shaping all activities.

Preassessment Planning

Preassessment planning typically is identified as a process through which caregivers and professionals set the many parameters of an upcoming assessment (Crais, 1995; Kjerland & Kovach, 1990; McGonigel, Kaufman, & Johnson, 1991). Preassessment is both a time to gather information from caregivers and to provide caregivers with information to facilitate collaborative decision making. As described by Crais (1994), common goals for preassessment planning include identifying what caregivers want and need from assessment, identifying caregiver priorities and preferences for assessment activities, identifying areas and activities of strength for the child, and determining caregiver roles in assessment. Professionals can begin by gathering information about caregiver concerns or questions and identifying what caregivers want to gain from assessment. If an assessment is requested by someone other than the family, that individual is asked to meet with the team, including the family, and jointly formulate a list of three to five primary concerns or priorities for the assessment. The subsequent assessment then will be designed with the team's presenting concerns in the forefront, as will the subsequent report of results and suggested interventions. For children who have been assessed previously, it is helpful to ask caregivers about the kinds of activities that were performed, the types of activities that provided the most information, and what information from the previous assessment was most useful to them.

Other information gathered can include identifying the times and locations of the upcoming assessment, preferences for formal versus informal approaches, the child's favorite activities or toys, activities to avoid (e.g., ones that are too engaging or frustrating for their child), other people to include, and the order in which the activities will be conducted. For children who are moving from preintentional to intentional and presymbolic to symbolic behaviors, this type of parameter setting can be particularly useful, especially for planning the subsequent observations and data gathering that will take place in the child's natural environments.

Part of the preassessment planning activities also typically includes gathering information regarding the child's background (e.g., birth, medical, developmental histories) and existing behaviors (e.g., social, communicative, motor). Problems that may influence the validity of subsequent assessment procedures should be delineated, including, but not limited to, information about sensory status (including preferred learning modalities relative to input and output); present use of assistive technology; considerations related to optimal positioning of the child as well as manner of presenting materials; how the child prefers to be handled, approached, and prompted or cued; and average latency of response and ways of enhancing accuracy and efficiency of responding. In addition, the professional should explore the family's perceptions of the child's development, strengths, and needs. The perceptions and values held by the family regarding these areas are based on their own experiences and may be specific to their culture (Winton, 1996). As indicated by Winton, factors that shape family beliefs include, but are not limited to, ethnic background, socioeconomic status, religion, geographic location, and life experiences. Recognizing the emphasis families place on some behaviors or concerns, the events and activities in which they invest their time, and the reasons they give for making certain decisions can all provide important information about a family's beliefs and values (Winton, 1996). If assessment is to reflect the beliefs and values held by families about their children, then gathering this type of information is critical to the process.

Identifying Caregiver Roles   Using the preassessment planning time to identify caregivers' preferences for their roles and responsibilities in assessment is important. Following Owens and Rogerson's (1988) advice, caregivers should not only be present during the assessment but also should assist with activities and provide items that are familiar to the child (e.g., toys, books, personal belongings). In addition, caregivers may help identify the types of foods liked or disliked by the child that may be part of the assessment. As the parameters of the upcoming observation and assessment phase are set (e.g., informal versus formal approaches, identification of observation contexts and people who will be involved), professionals and caregivers can discuss the options available and decide which roles and responsibilities they each will take. Once the parameters have been set, the caregivers and professionals can identify the order of the activities (e.g., caregiver–child interaction then professional–child interaction, hearing screening then free play with toys and materials) and can build collaboratively the assessment plan. Throughout the assessment, it is important that caregivers be familiar with each task in advance of its being introduced to the child. This familiarity must extend beyond the content of the activity to its relevance in shedding light on those priority issues that originally prompted the assessment. This preassessment phase is an excellent time to discuss each assessment task and its relevance.

Throughout the assessment planning, it is important to take into consideration the sociocultural beliefs and values of the caregivers. Some caregivers may readily take an active role in assessment planning and implementation; others may be more hesitant and willing to allow the professionals to take the lead. As suggested by Winton and Bailey (1993), the kinds of questions and the way that they are asked can influence the degree to which caregivers take an active role in planning for their child. When professionals take the time to tap into and honor the knowledge that caregivers have about their child, the results can be far reaching. In situations in which an interpreter or cultural mediator is included, family preferences for the type of role played by this individual are important and the interpreter/mediator's membership on the assessment team is essential (Crais, 1996).

Identifying Child Preferences and Reinforcers   To begin the process of identifying preferences, Beukelman and Mirenda (1992) suggested asking questions, such as, "How do you know your child likes something, is happy, does not like something, or is unhappy or in pain?" However, as has been indicated with varied types of information, the manner in which information is gathered can be critical. One strategy that has been useful in other domains (e.g., documenting or selecting vocabulary, documenting syntactic or milestone development) is a recognition format that offers alternatives for caregivers and others to indicate the child's preferences. After caregivers identify initial preferences, others who interact with the child can be asked to react to and indicate their knowledge of the preferences and/or add ones not indicated on the list.

For older individuals, the types of preferred reinforcers also need to be identified and verified. In the identification of reinforcers, Reichle and Sigafoos (1991) suggested interviewing caregivers, teachers, peers, and significant others. However, as they noted, interviewing depends on the reliability of the information gathered, particularly the level of knowledge of these informants about the individual and how clearly the individual indicates preferences. Because of the problems associated with identifying preferences or reinforcers (e.g., reliability or familiarity of informant with individual, clarity of individual's signals, presence of motor disabilities, actual ability of item to strengthen behavior), Reichle and Sigafoos (1991) suggested using caregivers and others who spend significant time with the individual as a preliminary step to identify potential reinforcers, followed by rigorous and systematic assessment.

Identifying Behaviors or Situations of Concern   In regard to behaviors or situations of concern to caregivers, initial information could be gained about the characteristics of the behaviors, when and where they occur or do not occur, any contributing health problems, physiological influences, and child preferences (Doss & Reichle, 1991; Meyer & Evans, 1989). Following the suggestions of Winton and Bailey (1993), caregivers also can be asked to describe the kinds of things they have tried with these behaviors or situations and to talk about what worked or did not work. Asking caregivers to talk about the advice they have received from others regarding these situations also can be informative.

For children who exhibit challenging behaviors, it is critical before instituting intervention procedures to identify the relationship between a child's challenging behaviors and his or her communicative intents (Durand & Crimmins, 1988; Reichle, Mirenda, Lock, Piche, & Johnston, 1992). Teaching a communicative function that matches the social motivation of the challenging behavior may serve to replace the behavior (Reichle et al., 1992). Identifying this relationship may be difficult, however, for some children. Furthermore, as suggested by Reichle and colleagues, few empirically validated studies exist for deciding whether to shape an existing behavior into a communicative attempt, conditionally reinforce an existing behavior used commonly, or replace an existing behavior with a more conventional form. Thus, gathering information regarding the possible intent of challenging behaviors is crucial to intervention planning. The role of caregivers in making such decisions cannot be underestimated (see Chapter 16). To identify potential influences on excessive behaviors, caregiver-completed scales, such as the Motivation Assessment Scale (Durand & Crimmins, 1988), may be useful. This scale asks caregivers to indicate their agreement on four sets of items pertaining to requesting attention, requesting tangibles, escaping demands, and receiving sensory stimulation. As suggested by Doss and Reichle (1991), this type of scale can help focus the subsequent use of direct observation methods. As noted by Doss and Reichle (1991), any activities, peers, or caregivers that seem to lead to increased amounts of challenging behaviors can be discussed and, if necessary, pursued systematically through direct observations and further interviews.

Identifying Successful Interactions   During the early phases of information gathering, it is also helpful to ask caregivers what happens when activities go well (e.g., when the child is able to indicate needs, when challenging behaviors do not occur). In these instances, asking for a detailed description of the activity and what led to the successful interaction can be useful. In addition, asking who was present and what they did can give caregivers and professionals an idea of how the child responds to the efforts of others.

Identifying Family Preferences for Sharing Assessment Results   During the preassessment planning phase, time also should be spent discussing the "how, when, and where" of sharing assessment results. Caregivers can be asked their preferences about when and how the assessment results are shared and if there are others who may benefit from hearing and/or contributing to the results. The option of an additional follow-up meeting also may be useful for caregivers or others who cannot be present. Caregivers who will be performing observations or assessments themselves can be asked if they are comfortable sharing their findings during the postassessment meeting. Ideas for organizing these findings can be discussed or summary forms can be provided for caregivers to organize their results. Some caregivers may want to meet with one or more professionals before the actual sharing of results to discuss the findings and the way these might be presented to the team. Caregivers also need to be given the option of whether the assessment sharing and the development of an intervention plan are combined into one meeting or whether a follow-up meeting will be held to actually generate a plan.

Observation and Assessment by Caregivers

Caregivers have been asked to contribute to the assessment process by directly observing and assessing the child using various instruments. This section provides an overview of observational and assessment procedures as well as data that support the importance of caregiver participation.

Observations Caregivers participate in varied observational tasks, such as charting when particular behaviors occur, identifying the antecedents and consequences that surround certain behaviors, or indicating when and how the child is communicating intentionally. As suggested by Gradel, Thompson, and Sheehan (1981), pairing caregivers' natural observational abilities with the use of some type of discrete information gathering (e.g., checklists, behavioral observations) can provide detailed information on skill acquisition, skill maintenance, and generalization. The use of formats that provide some structure to the observations, such as those discussed by Beukelman and Mirenda (1992), Crais and Roberts (1991), and MacDonald (1989) (see also Chapter 16), may be useful. Judgment-based assessment approaches (Neisworth & Bagnato, 1988) are another means of using caregiver observational expertise along with interviews and observations by professionals. Some instruments typically administered by professionals encourage the presence of caregivers and can be used to solicit their perceptions during and after the assessment. Example instruments include the Communication and Symbolic Behavior Scales (Wetherby & Prizant, 1993) and the Infant-Toddler Language Scale (Rossetti, 1990).

Calculator (1984) used the term *prototypic partner* to refer to conversational partners who are most effective in engaging a child in reciprocal interactions in a particular setting. He suggested that assessment activities should be directed at delineating why some caregivers interacted more effectively than others with a child, under comparable circumstances; then this same information should be used as a basis for teaching other caregivers to adopt strategies that were already being employed naturally by the prototypic partner. An example tool that solicits input from multiple caregivers relative to a child's communicative abilities across three different settings is the Communication Repertoire Summary (Calculator, 1988). The settings are selected on the basis of the caregivers' consensus that the settings constitute situations in which opportunities and demands for communication are particularly significant. The responses of different caregivers, each of whom has opportunities to interact with the child in a specific setting, are compared with respect to types and relative effectiveness of modes of communication used by the child and themselves in that setting. Caregivers are asked to maintain a log entitled "Child's Communication with You," citing the form, content, and use of each message conveyed by the child over several days. These data can assist the team in identifying similarities and discrepancies in the communication skills of the child with different caregivers.

In addition to gaining caregivers' observations and perceptions of communication abilities, several instruments also can be useful in soliciting input from primary caregivers, other caregivers, and friends about instructional priorities and desired outcomes for a child. For example, the McGill Action Planning System, or MAPS (Vandercook, York, & Forest, 1989), and Personal Futures Planning (Mount, 1987) provide means by which a group can identify a child's strengths and needs relative to inclusion in his or her home community and then engage in systematic planning designed to promote networks of support for the child in existing and future settings that are deemed necessary to achieve certain goals or dreams for the child. Another tool, Choosing Options and Accommodations for Children, or COACH (Giangreco, Cloninger, & Iverson, 1993), includes a prescriptive procedure by which caregivers are assisted in identifying and then prioritizing their child's instructional needs. These goals are discussed by the team relative to how they can be addressed in an integrated manner in conjunction with the broader curriculum in which the child is participating.

These observational and instructional needs identification activities help to shape intervention planning in that they alert team members to the broader issues and concerns of families, friends, and other stakeholders. As such, these identification activities yield information that transcends discipline-specific boundaries, providing a forum through which team members can discuss their dreams and aspirations for a child and can conceive plans for actualizing such events. All of these procedures can complement more specific assessments by assisting team members to select tests, structure further observations and interviews, and interpret subsequent data relative to concerns revealed in the preassessment phase. These procedures also may be administered concurrent with or following more specific assessments of communicative status, as a supplementary source of data on which to base program development. They ensure that families will have significant input in the design of their children's programs, consistent with the concept of a collaboratively developed assessment and intervention plan.

Assessments   Another means through which caregivers may contribute actively to the assessment process is by directly assessing the child. For direct assessment of young children by caregivers and others (e.g., teachers, attendants, other professionals), instruments such as the following can be used: Ages & Stages Questionnaires (Bricker, Squires, & Mounts, 1995); Assessment, Evaluation, and Programming System (Bricker, 1993); Child Development Inventories (Ireland, 1992); MacArthur Communicative Development Inventories (Fenson et al., 1993); Parent/Professional Preschool Performance Profile (Bloch, 1987); and System to Plan Early Childhood Services (Bagnato & Neisworth, 1990). For more information on these instruments and their use by caregivers, see Crais (1993, 1995). For older individuals, an example of a parent-completed instrument is OLIVER: Parent-administered communication inventory (MacDonald, 1978), which provides caregivers with the opportunity to actually perform test exercises and report their results.

In asking or offering for caregivers to directly assess the child, a cautionary note needs to be addressed. Although many caregivers may be interested and willing to take varied roles in assessment (e.g., demonstrating feeding techniques, charting behaviors), not all will be comfortable assessing their child. As suggested by Sheehan (1988), there may be a minimum level of interest and skill exhibited by caregivers that may influence their participation in direct assessment. However, as argued by Diamond and Squires (1993), this hypothesized minimum level may vary with the content of the questions and the way that information is gathered (e.g., interview versus self-completion of a form, recall versus recognition format). As indicated by the work of Squires and Bricker (1991), even mothers who themselves were "at risk" (e.g., teenage mothers, those who had physically abused their child, those who had a history of substance use) were able to reliably complete developmental checklists when the questions were provided in a recognition format (e.g., "Does your child point to objects that she/he wants?").

A further example of the importance of the format used for gathering information is the work of Morrow et al. (1993), cited previously. In this study, three vocabulary selection methods were used to identify vocabulary for children with severe communication disorders and physical disabilities. The three tools were a blank page (e.g., informants were asked to write down all the words they thought were essential and useful), a categorical inventory (e.g., informants were given categories to complete, such as people, actions, places), and a vocabulary checklist (e.g., informants checked the words they thought were important and added any words not already included). The results indicated differences across the tools and informants in both satisfaction and words identified. For example, although the checklist received a slightly higher mean satisfaction rating, all the tools were selected by some informants as the most satisfactory. For most of the children, the checklist generated the greatest number of total words and different words (i.e., those not present on the other tools); however, the blank page generated the most for one child. Thus, when selecting assessment formats, the individual characteristics of the child and informant may be a better predictor of which type of tool to use. The use of multiple tools also can provide information not gained through the use of only one. Morrow et al. suggested for efficiency that a checklist format be used first, followed by a more open-ended tool (e.g., blank page, categorical inventory) to obtain unique words not found on the checklist.

Observations and Assessments by Professionals

Throughout the literature on the assessment of children who are making the transition from prelinguistic to linguistic or presymbolic to symbolic communication, there has been much focus on the professional scrutinizing the child's environment (Reichle et al., 1992). However, as Reichle and colleagues suggested, this kind of scrutiny may be less, rather than more, frequently used. In surveying interventionists on how to select vocabulary for users of augmentative and alternative communication (AAC) systems, Reichle (1983) revealed that only 12% of these professionals reported actually examining the child's existing and future environments and few used both professional and caregiver report.

The authors of this chapter were unable to locate findings to contradict Reichle's results, suggesting a persistence of this practice or applied researchers' failure to provide updated findings. Similar contrasts between the ideal and actual practices in observing children in natural environments can be found in the early intervention literature, although many professionals argue that to be ecologically valid, natural observations are necessary (Bailey, 1989; Bricker, 1993; Crais, 1995; Norris & Hoffman, 1990). It has become commonplace that intervention should take place in the natural environment; therefore, it is time that assessment be contextually appropriate as well.

Ecological Inventories One way to gather information in the child's natural settings is the use of ecological inventories. These inventories help identify the situations that call for communicative and nonsymbolic behaviors in those settings (e.g., fussing when toy is taken away) (Reichle et al., 1992). Sigafoos and York (1991) provided guidelines for conducting ecological inventories, which include first gathering an inventory of the demands and opportunities in the environment for the purpose of determining priority targets for instruction. Then, additional information can be gathered to delineate the natural cues and consequences derived from the environment. For each communication target, the professional analyzes the specific communicative intents to be taught, the mode of communication to be used, specific vocabulary, the natural cues and consequences to be highlighted, the time(s) of day when instruction should take place, and the way in which teaching opportunities can be used and sequenced (Calculator & Jorgensen, 1991; Mirenda & Calculator, 1993; Sigafoos & York, 1991).

The use of ecological inventories and discrepancy analyses, in which a child's repertoire of communication skills is compared with that which appears necessary to interact effectively with a range of partners in a particular setting, predicates that it is as important to examine environments in which interactions occur as it is to delve into any one child's proficiency of communication. Environments, and conversational partners, may be examined relative to a variety of factors, any one of which may later be targeted for intervention. Considerations include the following: 1) frequency of opportunities for interaction and proportion of interactions with adults versus peers, spontaneous versus engineered, and (for older individuals) paid versus unpaid adults; 2) opportunities to make choices and to indicate preferences; 3) responsiveness of others to the child's communicative attempts, which may be summarized in the form of a percentage of messages that are successful; and 4) physical structure (e.g., availability of motivating objects and events and degree to which they are accessible to the child).

Tools or protocols that combine interviews with observations include the ECO Environmental Scan (Gillette, in press) and those adapted for adults from child assessment tools, such as Owens' (1982) Caregiver Interview and Environmental Observation or Horstmeier and MacDonald's (1978) Environmental

Prelanguage Battery. As suggested by Owens and Rogerson (1988), use of these tools enhances the validity of further testing and encourages caregivers to become involved in the intervention process.

Analogue Assessments Analogue procedures offer a more direct means of involving caregivers in the assessment process (Calculator, 1994; Halle, 1993). The examiner sets up situations to increase the opportunity for a child to exhibit a behavior under investigation. For example, an examiner who is interested in how a child indicates choices may collaborate with a caregiver to modify an existing routine to afford opportunities for choice making and then note how the child responds to these opportunities. An opportunity to observe requests, for instance, may be facilitated by asking the child to perform a task when the materials necessary to comply are not available. For older children who have challenging or excessive behaviors, professionals need to examine many aspects of these behaviors. As suggested by Reichle et al. (1992), professionals need a continuum of assessment strategies aimed at matching social intentions to challenging behaviors, which need to be analyzed in the natural contexts through systematic manipulation of antecedents and consequences (see Chapters 13 and 14).

Professionals also need to observe and test information regarding a child's preferences; thus, Reichle and Sigafoos (1991) suggested the use of systematic preference testing, including watching a child approach an item and/or select an item, measuring the degree of effort exerted to gain access to an item, determining the rate at which an edible item is consumed, and testing the validity of the preference identified. Reichle and Sigafoos argued that these preferences must be tested empirically and, in most cases, this type of systematic testing would have to be organized by professionals; however, caregivers and others could help with the determination of both the items to test and the reactions of the child to the test items. Although there may be some evidence that preference testing in some areas (e.g., approach/nonapproach to items) may be more reliable than staff opinions regarding a child's likes and dislikes (Green et al., 1988), including staff and other caregivers in the testing may have a positive effect on their recognition and use of the favored reinforcers.

Dynamic Assessments Calculator (1994) also provided several examples of how dynamic assessment procedures can be used to gather assessment findings, especially with respect to a child's prognosis for benefiting from intervention. Through these procedures, different variables that are believed to be contributing to the occurrence or nonoccurrence of a desired behavior are systematically manipulated. These variables may occur as antecedents or consequences to the targeted behavior. The instructor monitors the corresponding impact of each intervention to determine its relative effectiveness in promoting positive changes in the child. In this way, team members are able to determine a child's responsiveness to intervention and thus gain insight concerning short- and long-term prognosis. The communication style of caregivers may also be modified and its effect on the child's success in responding monitored over time. In addition, a communication device may be modified in terms of content, means of access, output mode, and changes in frequency of initiation by the child then examined. (For additional information on dynamic assessment approaches, see Chapter 12).

Judgment-Based Approaches   The use of judgment-based assessment (JBA) procedures that involve collecting, structuring, and quantifying the impressions of professionals and caregivers about the child and critical environmental characteristics (Neisworth & Bagnato, 1988) also can help to develop collaborative partnerships in assessment. JBA, as proposed by Neisworth and Bagnato, is a process that combines the use of objective and subjective methods and relies heavily on interviews and self-report measures to corroborate the results of objective measures. JBA measures also can be used by professionals and caregivers to assess behavioral traits not typically evaluated on many tests, such as attention, motivation, goal directedness, temperament, and play style. Two example instruments for young children include the Carolina Record of Individual Behavior (Simeonsson, 1985), used to identify a child's behavioral state, and the Early Coping Inventory (Zeitlin, Williamson, & Szczepanski, 1988), used to identify a child's coping behaviors. Helpful resources on JBA include Bagnato and Neisworth (1990), Neisworth and Bagnato (1988), and an entire issue of *Topics in Early Childhood Special Education,* edited by Neisworth and Fewell (1990).

Postassessment Planning and Decision Making

The final phase of the assessment process is the sharing of findings and further decision making regarding the child. As a means of continuing to build consensus between caregivers and professionals, this step cannot be underestimated. Caregivers who have been dissatisfied with their assessment experiences often report that it is not the gravity of the information shared but the way the information was shared (Martin, George, O'Neal, & Daly, 1987; Tarran, 1981).

As with other phases, it is recommended that all those who can contribute to and gain from the sharing of the assessment information be present. In recognizing the wisdom of Beukelman and Mirenda (1992) in their suggestion to develop strategies to encourage participation by all team members during the assessment, the same suggestion may hold during the postassessment meeting. In contrast with traditional approaches where professionals do most of the reporting, alternatives include beginning the discussion by asking caregivers to give their impressions of the assessment activities, addressing the caregivers' concerns first, and asking caregivers what they view as the child's strengths or needs. Caregivers and others who have played a more active role in assessment (e.g., performing observations, completing checklists, conducting assessment activities) may be asked to provide an overview of their assessment results. Caregivers who have played a greater role in planning and assessing are more likely to be active in the sharing of results. Brinckerhoff and Vincent (1987) demonstrated this principle by asking caregivers to complete a family profile, a developmental checklist, and daily routine inventory before their child's IEP meeting. These caregivers also met with a school liaison before the IEP meeting to help organize their assessment findings. As indicated by Brinckerhoff and Vincent's findings, the caregivers who were more actively involved in assessment were more likely to contribute to intervention planning and decision making.

As suggested by McLean and Crais (1996), regardless of whether caregivers participate directly in assessment, they may be offered additional options that could help them prepare for the sharing session. For example, caregivers may be encouraged to think about or write down characteristics of the child, what they would like the child to do in the next month or year, and what ways they see possible to help their child achieve in these areas. When there is time between the assessment activities and the sharing session, caregivers may be given a list of questions that they may want to consider before the discussion (e.g., "What were your overall impressions of the assessment?" "What were the activities that went well?" "What were the activities that did not go as well?" "What areas would you like to discuss first?"). Consensus building also can be greatly facilitated by engaging caregivers in a process of validating assessment findings and corresponding interpretations of results. Caregivers are encouraged to support as well as to challenge examiners' impressions, comparing examiners' data to their own impressions. The sharing session is also a time in which results of assessment tasks can be tied to caregiver anecdotes, thus supporting the generalizability of results and, more important, others' abilities to relate what might otherwise be perceived as abstract impressions of day-to-day interactions and outcomes with a particular child.

Another strategy that may build consensus and contribute to a collaborative relationship is to share assessment information in an ongoing manner throughout the assessment process. In this way, as each task, tool, or series of tasks is completed, caregivers and professionals can discuss their findings and begin generating a list of ideas for either further assessment or later intervention planning. The ongoing sharing of assessment results may also reduce the amount of information that needs to be shared at the end (or at any one time) and thus may result in more accurate perceptions and understanding of what is shared.

Whether information is shared throughout or after the assessment, it is important that sharing be performed in a way that is useful to caregivers in decision making, that promotes feelings of competence and hope, and that facilitates consensus building. It may be useful at the end of an assessment to ask caregivers if their concerns and priorities were addressed and what, if anything, they still need from professionals. Returning to caregivers' original concerns expressed at the beginning of the process may be a way to revisit these issues and to direct further efforts to areas not addressed satisfactorily or still in question.

CLINICAL IMPLICATIONS

Caregivers can provide important information about how their child communicates, clarifying what might be missed or misinterpreted by a naive examiner. This would be particularly important for children whose existing means or forms of communication are idiosyncratic and highly ambiguous. Caregivers also can relate important information about the content of their child's communication, identifying meanings produced and understood by the child, and topics of high and low interest. Finally, the underlying intent, or purpose, of a child's messages can be interpreted by caregivers in preparation for enhancing or expanding these same uses of language.

This chapter has described strategies and tools for building consensus among professionals and caregivers throughout the assessment process. To gain active caregiver participation, it was recommended that, beginning during preassessment planning, professionals gather information about caregiver concerns and preferences, identify caregiver roles, and identify areas and activities of strength for the child. Procedures were described in which caregivers may contribute actively during direct child assessments and observations, and the importance of sharing findings and further decision making during postassessment planning as a means of continuing to build consensus was underscored.

To be most effective, the assessment process should be viewed as a series of consensus-building activities (Beukelman & Mirenda, 1992; Crais, 1991, 1992; Dunst et al., 1988). Without active participation, not only will valuable information be missed but caregivers may not assume ownership of decisions made. If assessment and intervention activities are to be owned by caregivers, the activities must match caregivers' perceptions of what is appropriate and important. The active participation of caregivers can enhance both the validity and reliability of the assessment through collaborative planning and implementation.

DIRECTIONS FOR FUTURE RESEARCH

Professionals working with both young children and older individuals who are making the transition from prelinguistic to linguistic and preintentional to intentional levels have recognized the critical role of the family in intervention efforts. Increased attention to the role of the family in the assessment process has been advocated by many (Bailey, 1989; Beukelman & Mirenda, 1992; Crais, 1993, 1995; Neisworth & Bagnato, 1988; Sigafoos & York, 1991). As a means to gather more ecologically valid information and to build a collaborative relationship with family members, active participation in assessment seems a natural choice. As indicated previously, however, few guidelines for recommended practices within assessment are available; furthermore, very few practices have been validated by empirical research. For example, little information is available as to the ways in which family members take part in assessment and their preferences for the type and amount of their participation, specifically, what types of choices within assessment are preferred by families, what the best ways are for professionals to gather information on the family's assessment preferences, what effects sociocultural factors have on the family's participation in assessment, and how professionals can better prepare families for more active roles in assessment. On the issue of ecological validity, how accurately do professionals' observations and interpretations of children's communicative behaviors match those of parents? To what extent do those behaviors judged significant by professionals correspond with parents' priorities?

The implications and ramifications for the child and family of the use of more active roles by family members within the assessment process have not been well delineated. For instance, what are the effects of differing levels of family participation on the assessment results, the ecological validity of the process, the satisfaction of family members and professionals, the family–professional relationship established, the outcomes identified for both child and family, and families' subsequent likelihood of participating actively as well as voluntarily in their child's intervention program? Although some efforts to examine family participation in assessment have yielded fruitful results (Bloch & Seitz, 1989; Brinckerhoff & Vincent, 1987; Crais & Wilson, 1996), more information is needed across assessment contexts, disciplines, and types of children and families.

CONCLUSION

The benefits of planning, performing, and sharing the findings of assessment in a collaborative manner cannot be underestimated. Benefits may come from the relationship and the roles and expectations developed among the caregivers, professionals, and others who interact routinely with the child. When caregivers and professionals work collaboratively in assessment, they set the tone for future interactions and begin the process of continuous consensus building. In addition, when caregivers are actively engaged in planning and conducting the assessment, the activities and results should better represent the child's typical functioning and be more consistent with the caregivers' views of the child. As suggested by Crais (1995), collaboratively planned assessments should also provide caregivers with more of what they want and need from assessment and, therefore, may be more useful to caregivers than traditional assessments. The roles of caregivers in the development and implementation of intervention efforts for any child are critical, but those roles and responsibilities become even greater for children who are making the transition from preintentional to intentional or presymbolic to symbolic communication. Thus, active participation of caregivers within the context of assessment becomes a beginning point for collaborative efforts throughout the intervention process. Although there is evidence that some professionals are offering more active roles to caregivers in assessment (Crais & Wilson, 1996), there are still many tasks and activities that could be performed by caregivers, if provided with the opportunity, the appropriate format, and the necessary support.

REFERENCES

Andrews, J., & Andrews, A. (1990). *Family-based treatment in communicative disorders*. Sandwich, IL: Janelle Publications.

Bagnato, S., & Neisworth, J. (1990). *System to Plan Early Childhood Services (SPECS)*. Circle Pines, MN: American Guidance Service.

Bailey, D. (1989). Assessment and its importance in early intervention. In D. Bailey & M. Wolery (Eds.), *Assessing infants and preschoolers with handicaps* (pp. 1–21). Columbus, OH: Charles E. Merrill.

Bailey, D., McWilliam, P., Winton, P., & Simeonsson, R. (1992). *Implementing family-centered services in early intervention: A team-based model for change*. Cambridge, MA: Brookline Books.

Barber, P.P., Turnbull, A.P., Behr, S.K., & Kerns, G.M. (1988). A family systems perspective on early childhood special education. In S.L. Odom & M.B. Karnes (Eds.), *Early intervention for infants and children with handicaps: An empirical base* (pp. 179–198). Baltimore: Paul H. Brookes Publishing Co.

Beukelman, D.P., & Mirenda, P. (1992). *Augmentative and alternative communication: Management of severe communication disorders in children and adults*. Baltimore: Paul H. Brookes Publishing Co.

Bloch, J. (1987). *Parent/Professional Preschool Performance Profile*. Syosset, NY: Variety Preschooler's Workshop.

Bloch, J., & Seitz, M. (1989, July). Parents as assessors of children: A collaborative approach to helping. *Social Work in Education, 226–244.*

Bricker, D. (1993). *Assessment, Evaluation, and Programming System (AEPS) for infants and children: Vol. 1. AEPS measurement for birth to three years*. Baltimore: Paul H. Brookes Publishing Co.

Bricker, D., & Squires, J. (1989). The effectiveness of parental screening of at-risk infants: The infant monitoring questionnaires. *Topics in Early Childhood Special Education, 9*(3), 67–85.

Bricker, D., Squires, J., & Mounts, L. (1995). *Ages & Stages Questionnaires (ASQ): A parent-completed, child-monitoring system*. Baltimore: Paul H. Brookes Publishing Co.

Brinckerhoff, J., & Vincent, L. (1987). Increasing parental decision-making at the individualized educational program meeting. *Journal of the Division for Early Childhood, 11,* 46–58.

Bronfenbrenner, U. (1979). *The ecology of human development: Experiments by nature and design*. Cambridge, MA: Harvard University Press.

Calculator, S. (1984). Prelinguistic development. In W. Perkins (Ed.), *Language handicaps in children* (pp. 66–71). New York: Thieme Stratton.

Calculator, S. (1988). Teaching functional communication skills to nonspeaking adults with mental retardation. In S. Calculator & J. Bedrosian (Eds.), *Communication assessment and intervention for adults with mental retardation* (pp. 309–339). Boston: Little, Brown.

Calculator, S. (1994). Designing and implementing communicative assessments in inclusive settings. In S. Calculator & C. Jorgensen (Eds.), *Including students with severe disabilities in schools: Fostering communication, interaction, and participation* (pp. 113–181). San Diego, CA: Singular Publishing Group.

Calculator, S., & Jorgensen, C. (1991). Integrating AAC instruction into regular education settings: Expounding on best practices. *Augmentative and Alternative Communication, 7,* 204–212.

Crais, E. (1991). Moving from "parent involvement" to family-centered services. *American Journal of Speech-Language Pathology, 1,* 5–8.

Crais, E. (1992). "Best practices" with preschoolers: Assessing within the context of a family-centered approach. *Best Practices in School Speech-Language Pathology, 2,* 33–42.

Crais, E. (1993). Families and professionals as collaborators in assessment. *Topics in Language Disorders, 14*(1), 29–40.

Crais, E. (1994). *Increasing family participation in assessing children birth to five* [In-service manual and audiotapes]. Chicago: Applied Symbolix.

Crais, E. (1995). Expanding the repertoire of tools and techniques for assessing communication skills of infants and toddlers. *American Journal of Speech-Language Pathology, 4*(3), 47–59.

Crais, E. (1996). Applying family-centered principles to child assessment. In P. McWilliam, P. Winton, & E. Crais (Eds.), *Practical strategies for family-centered early intervention* (pp. 69–96). San Diego, CA: Singular Publishing Group.

Crais, E., & Roberts, J. (1991). Decision making in assessment and early intervention planning. *Language, Speech, and Hearing Services in Schools, 22*(2), 19–30.

Crais, E., & Wilson, L. (1996). The role of parents in child assessment: Self-evaluation by practicing professionals. *Infant-Toddler Intervention, 6*(2), 125–143.

Dale, P. (1991). The validity of a parent report measure of vocabulary and syntax at 24 months. *Journal of Speech and Hearing Research, 34,* 565–571.

Dale, P., Bates, E., Reznick, S., & Morisset, C. (1989). The validity of a parent report instrument on child language at twenty months. *Journal of Child Language, 16,* 239–249.

Diamond, K., & Squires, J. (1993). The role of parental report in the screening and assessment of young children. *Journal of Early Intervention, 17*(2), 107–115.

Doss, L.S., & Reichle, J. (1991). Replacing excess behavior with an initial communicative repertoire. In J. Reichle, J. York, & J. Sigafoos (Eds.), *Implementing augmentative and alternative communication: Strategies for learners with severe disabilities* (pp. 215–237). Baltimore: Paul H. Brookes Publishing Co.

Dunst, C., Trivette, C., & Deal, A. (1988). *Enabling and empowering families.* Cambridge, MA: Brookline Books.

Durand, V., & Crimmins, D. (1988). Identifying the variables maintaining self-injurious behavior. *Journal of Autism and Developmental Disorders, 18*(1), 99–117.

Fenson, L., Dale, P., Reznick, J.S., Thal, D., Bates, E., Hartung, J., Pethick, S., & Reilly, J. (1993). *MacArthur Communicative Development Inventories (CDI).* San Diego, CA: Singular Publishing Group.

Giangreco, M.F., Cloninger, C.J., & Iverson, V.S. (1993). *Choosing options and accommodations for children (COACH): A guide to planning inclusive education.* Baltimore: Paul H. Brookes Publishing Co.

Gillette, Y. (in press). Collaboration with families in communication intervention. In T. Layton, L. Watson, & E. Crais (Eds.), *Handbook of early language impairments in children: Assessment and intervention.* Albany, NY: Delmar Publishers.

Girolametto, L. (1988). Improving the social-conversational skills of developmentally delayed children: An intervention study. *Journal of Speech and Hearing Disorders, 53*(2), 156–167.

Glascoe, F., McLean, W., & Stone, W. (1991). The importance of parents' concerns about their child's behavior. *Clinical Pediatrics, 30,* 8–11.

Gradel, K., Thompson, M., & Sheehan, R. (1981). Parental and professional agreement in early childhood assessment. *Topics in Early Childhood Special Education, 1,* 31–39.

Green, C., Reid, D., White, L., Halford, R., Brittain, D., & Gardner, S. (1988). Identifying reinforcers for persons with profound handicaps: Staff opinion versus systematic assessment of preferences. *Journal of Applied Behavior, 21,* 31–43.

Hale, J. (1988). Adopting the natural environment as the context of training. In S. Calculator & J. Bedrosian (Eds.), *Communication assessment and intervention for adults with mental retardation* (pp. 155–185). Boston: Little, Brown.

Halle, J. (1993). Innovative assessment measures and practices designed with the goal of achieving functional communication and integration. In L. Kupper (Ed.), *The Second National Symposium on Effective Communication for Children and Youth with Severe Disabilities: A vision for the future* (pp. 201–251). McLean, VA: Interstate Research Associates, Inc.

Horstmeier, D., & MacDonald, J. (1978). *Environmental Prelanguage Battery.* San Antonio, TX: The Psychological Corporation.

Individuals with Disabilities Education Act (IDEA) of 1990, PL 101-476, 20 U.S.C. §§ 1400 *et seq.*

Ireland, H. (1992). *Child Development Inventories.* Minneapolis, MN: Behavior Science Systems.

Kjerland, L., & Kovach, J. (1990). Family–staff collaboration for tailored infant assessment. In E.D. Gibbs & D.M. Teti (Eds.), *Interdisciplinary assessment of infants: A guide for early intervention professionals* (pp. 287–298). Baltimore: Paul H. Brookes Publishing Co.

MacDonald, J. (1978). *OLIVER: Parent-administered communication inventory.* San Antonio, TX: The Psychological Corporation.

MacDonald, J. (1989). *Becoming partners with children: From play to conversation.* Chicago: Riverside.

MacDonald, J., & Gillette, Y. (1988). Communication partners: A conversational model for building parent–child relationships with handicapped children. In K. Marfo (Ed.), *Parent–child interaction and developmental disabilities: Theory, research, and intervention* (pp. 220–241). New York: Praeger.

Mahoney, G., & Powell, A. (1986). *Transactional intervention program: A teacher's guide.* Farmington: University of Connecticut Health Center, Pediatric Research Training Center.

Martin, N., George, K., O'Neal, J., & Daly, J. (1987). Audiologists' and parents' attitudes regarding counseling of families of hearing-impaired children. *Asha, 29*(2), 27–33.

McGonigel, M., Kaufman, R., & Johnson, B. (1991). *Guidelines and recommended practices for the individualized family service plan* (2nd ed.). Bethesda, MD: Association for the Care of Children's Health.

McLean, J., & Snyder-McLean, L. (1978). *A transactional approach to early language training.* Columbus, OH: Charles E. Merrill.

McLean, M., & Crais, E. (1996). Procedural considerations in assessing infants and preschoolers with disabilities. In M. McLean, D. Bailey, & M. Wolery (Eds.), *Assessing infants and preschoolers with special needs* (pp. 46–68). Columbus, OH: Charles E. Merrill.

McLean, M., & McCormick, K. (1993). Assessment and evaluation in early intervention. In W. Brown, S.K. Thurman, & L.F. Pearl (Eds.), *Family-centered early intervention with infants and toddlers: Innovative cross-disciplinary approaches* (pp. 43–79). Baltimore: Paul H. Brookes Publishing Co.

Meyer, L.H., & Evans, I.M. (1989). *Nonaversive intervention for behavior problems: A manual for home and community.* Baltimore: Paul H. Brookes Publishing Co.

Mirenda, P., & Calculator, S. (1993). Enhancing curricula design. *Clinics in Communication Disorders, 3,* 43–58.

Moore, S., & Beatty, J. (1995). *Developing cultural competence in early childhood assessment.* Boulder: University of Colorado, Department of Communication Disorders and Speech Science.

Morrow, D., Mirenda, P., Beukelman, D., & Yorkston, K. (1993). Vocabulary selection for augmentative communication systems: A comparison of three techniques. *American Journal of Speech-Language Pathology, 2*(2), 19–30.

Mount, B. (1987). *Personal Futures Planning: Finding directions for change.* Ann Arbor: University of Michigan Dissertation Information Service.

Neisworth, J.T., & Bagnato, S.J. (1988). Assessment in early childhood special education: A typology of dependent measures. In S.L. Odom & M.B. Karnes (Eds.), *Early intervention for infants and children with handicaps: An empirical base* (pp. 23–49). Baltimore: Paul H. Brookes Publishing Co.

Neisworth, J.T., & Fewell, R. (1990). Judgment-based assessment. *Topics in Early Childhood Special Education, 10*(3).

Norris, J., & Hoffman, P. (1990). Language intervention within naturalistic environments. *Language, Speech, and Hearing Services in Schools, 21,* 72–84.

Owens, R. (1982). *Caregiver Interview and Environmental Observation. Program for the acquisition of language in severely impaired.* San Antonio, TX: The Psychological Corporation.

Owens, R., & Rogerson, B. (1988). Adults at the presymbolic level. In S. Calculator & J. Bedrosian (Eds.), *Communication assessment and intervention for adults with mental retardation* (pp. 189–238). Boston: Little, Brown.

Reichle, J. (1983). *A survey of professionals serving persons with severe handicaps.* Unpublished manuscript, University of Minnesota, Minneapolis.

Reichle, J., Mirenda, P., Lock, P., Piche, L., & Johnston, S. (1992). Beginning augmentative communication systems. In S.F. Warren & J. Reichle (Eds.), *Communication and language intervention series: Vol. 1. Causes and effects in communication and language intervention* (pp. 131–156). Baltimore: Paul H. Brookes Publishing Co.

Reichle, J., & Sigafoos, J. (1991). Establishing an initial repertoire of requesting. In J. Reichle, J. York, & J. Sigafoos (Eds.), *Implementing augmentative and alternative communication: Strategies for learners with severe disabilities* (pp. 89–114). Baltimore: Paul H. Brookes Publishing Co.

Rosenberg, S.A., & Robinson, C.C. (1988). Interactions of parents with their young handicapped children. In S.L. Odom & M.B. Karnes (Eds.), *Early intervention for infants and children with handicaps: An empirical base* (pp. 159–177). Baltimore: Paul H. Brookes Publishing Co.

Rossetti, L. (1990). *Infant-Toddler Language Scale.* East Moline, IL: LinguiSystems.

Salisbury, C.L., & Dunst, C.J. (1997). Home, school, and community partnerships: Building inclusive teams. In B. Rainforth & J. York-Barr (Eds.), *Collaborative teams for students with severe disabilities: Integrating therapy and educational services* (2nd ed., pp. 57–87). Baltimore: Paul H. Brookes Publishing Co.

Sexton, D., Thompson, B., Perez, J., & Rheams, T. (1990). Maternal versus professional estimates of developmental status for young children with handicaps: An ecological approach. *Topics in Early Childhood Special Education, 10*(3), 80–95.

Sheehan, R. (1988). Involvement of parents in early childhood assessment. In R. Sheehan & T. Wachs (Eds.), *Assessment of young developmentally disabled children* (pp. 75–90). New York: Plenum.

Sigafoos, J., & York, J. (1991). Using ecological inventories to promote functional communication. In J. Reichle, J. York, & J. Sigafoos (Eds.), *Implementing augmentative and alternative communication: Strategies for learners with severe disabilities* (pp. 61–70). Baltimore: Paul H. Brookes Publishing Co.

Simeonsson, R. (1985). *Carolina Record of Individual Behavior.* Chapel Hill: University of North Carolina, Frank Porter Graham Child Development Center.

Squires, J., & Bricker, D. (1991). Impact of completing infant developmental questionnaires on at-risk mothers. *Journal of Early Intervention, 15,* 162–172.

Tarran, E. (1981). Parents' views of medical and social-work services for families with cerebral palsied children. *Developmental Medicine and Child Neurology, 23,* 173–182.

Turnbull, A., & Turnbull, H. (1990). Family Information Preference Inventory. In A. Turnbull & H. Turnbull (Eds.), *Families, professionals, and exceptionality: A special partnership* (2nd ed., pp. 368–373). Columbus, OH: Charles E. Merrill.

Vandercook, T., York, J., & Forest, M. (1989). The McGill Action Planning System (MAPS): A strategy for building the vision. *Journal of The Association for Persons with Severe Handicaps, 14,* 205–215.

Warren, S.F., & Kaiser, A. (1988). Research in early language intervention. In S.L. Odom & M.B. Karnes (Eds.), *Early intervention for infants and children with handicaps: An empirical base* (pp. 87–108). Baltimore: Paul H. Brookes Publishing Co.

Wetherby, A., & Prizant, B. (1993). *Communication and Symbolic Behavior Scales* (1st ed.). Chicago: Applied Symbolix.

Wilcox, J. (1992). Enhancing initial communication skills in young children with developmental disabilities through partner programming. *Seminars in Speech and Language, 13*(3), 195–212.

Winton, P. (1990). A systematic approach to inservice training related to P.L. 99-457. *Infants and Young Children, 3,* 51–60.

Winton, P. (1996). Understanding family concerns, priorities, and resources. In P. McWilliam, P. Winton, & E. Crais (Eds.), *Practical strategies for family-centered early intervention* (pp. 31–53). San Diego, CA: Singular Publishing Group.

Winton, P., & Bailey, D. (1993). Communicating with families: Examining practices and facilitating change. In J. Paul & R. Simeonsson (Eds.), *Understanding and working with parents of children with special needs* (2nd ed., pp. 212–233). New York: Holt, Rinehart & Winston.

Zeitlin, S., Williamson, G., & Szczepanski, M. (1988). *Early Coping Inventory: A Measure of Adaptive Behavior.* Bensenville, IL: Scholastic Testing Service.

12

Prelinguistic Dynamic Assessment
A Transactional Perspective

Kary S. Kublin, Amy M. Wetherby,
Elizabeth R. Crais, and Barry M. Prizant

P ROFESSIONALS CONTINUE TO BE CHALLENGED by the chasm that exists between theories on child development and assessment practices commonly used with young children. Although there has been a proliferation of research in infant communication and socioemotional development, most formal tools used for direct assessment of a child's communication and language have major limitations in the capacity to evaluate a child's communicative competence during natural interactions (Prizant & Wetherby, 1990; Wetherby & Prizant, 1993b). The richness in developmental theories that has been woven in the literature regarding the role of caregivers in communication development is not adequately translated into assessment tools and strategies. This chapter blends two theoretical frameworks: the transactional theory of communication development and the learning theory underlying principles of dynamic assessment. It also describes how dynamic assessment can be viewed from a transactional perspective and can contribute to the theory and practice of assessment with prelinguistic children and their families.

TRANSACTIONAL THEORY
OF COMMUNICATION DEVELOPMENT

The process of communication development has been characterized from a transactional perspective since the 1970s (McLean, 1990; McLean & Snyder-McLean, 1978). Sameroff and colleagues (Sameroff, 1987; Sameroff & Chandler, 1975; Sameroff & Fiese, 1990) addressed the complex developmental interdependencies among children, caregivers, and social contexts in a transactional model. Sameroff and Chandler (1975) proposed a model for conceptualizing development that revolutionized the way developmental researchers consider relationships among child characteristics, caregiver characteristics, and environmental influences over time. In this transactional model, developmental outcomes at any point in time are seen as a result of a continuous dynamic interplay among child behavior, caregiver responses to the child's behavior, and environmental variables that may influence both the child and the caregiver.

The transactional perspective has been fueled by pragmatic and social-interactive theories, which have placed great emphasis on the context of social interaction in language development (Bates, 1976; Bloom, 1993; McLean & Snyder-McLean, 1978). Children are viewed as active participants who learn to affect the behavior and attitudes of others through active signaling and who gradually learn to use more sophisticated and conventional means to communicate through caregivers' contingent social responsiveness (Dunst, Lowe, & Bartholomew, 1990). The quality and nature of the contexts in which interaction occurs are considered to have a great influence on the successful acquisition of language and communicative behavior. Proponents of pragmatic theory believe that development can be understood only by analysis of the interactive context, not simply by focusing solely on the child or the caregivers, because successful communication involves reciprocity and mutual negotiation (Bates, 1976; Bruner, 1978).

Dunst et al. (1990) presented a model of the development of communicative competence that is transactional in nature, based on Goldberg's (1977) model of mutual efficacy in caregiver–child interaction. Dunst et al.'s model emphasizes the bidirectionality of contingent social responsiveness on the part of a caregiver and young child. Factors affecting a caregiver (e.g., psychological well-being, social support) as well as the child's biological capacity to engage in social exchanges will influence the caregiver's availability and responsivity to the young child (Dunst et al., 1990). Over time, when a young child's social behavior can be accurately interpreted or read by a caregiver, and the caregiver is able to respond in such a way as to meet the child's needs or to support social exchange, both caregiver and child develop a sense of efficacy. A cumulative effect of positive contingent responsiveness is that interactions become more predictable as expectancies and contingencies increase. Therefore, development is influenced by a child's ability to produce readable signals, a caregiver's ability to respond appropriately to the child's signals, and the routinization of such patterns.

The broad acceptance of a transactional model of development along with legislative mandates recognizing the central role of the family in the child's life have triggered a movement toward family-centered practice within the field of speech-language pathology (Crais, 1993; Dunst, Trivette, Starnes, Hamby, & Gordon, 1993). Family-centered principles—starting with family members' own perceptions of their situation and expectations for their child, respecting family members' priorities and preferences, planning for active participation of family members in assessment and intervention, building consensus, and sharing decision making—have helped to question traditional practices and provide a rationale for considering different ways to view the role of professionals.

Although professional discourse has delivered family-centered philosophy as an ideal worth striving toward and has produced rallying cries for changes to service delivery systems, a discrepancy still exists between common practice and recommended practice (Kagan & Neville, 1994). In assessment, though there are broad ways of understanding how to incorporate family-centered ideals, some of the practicalities remain fuzzy and ill defined. For this reason, an instrumental link was found between the principles of dynamic assessment and those of family-centered practice. Dynamic assessment offers a way of systematically approaching assessment within the individualized and context-specific assessment activities of family-centered practice, and family-centered principles add a transactional perspective.

LEARNING THEORY UNDERLYING DYNAMIC ASSESSMENT

Dynamic assessment is a term used for assessment protocols in which support is provided to test participants for completing tasks that would otherwise be too difficult for them to accomplish independently. Dynamic assessment theory is derived from the 1930s writings and lectures of Lev Vygotsky (1933/1978, 1934/1986) on the nature of learning. Vygotsky (1934/1986) described learning as being embedded within social events and occurring as a child interacts with people, objects, and events in the environment (van der Veer & Valsiner, 1991; Wertsch & Rogoff, 1984). He believed intelligence testing could account for the role of the social context if one could identify a child's *zone of proximal development* (ZPD), defined as the distance between a child's independent performance on a task and the child's performance when assisted by an adult or more capable peer (Vygotsky, 1933/1978, 1934/1986).

Vygotsky (1934/1986) believed that if a child's ZPD could be located, something of the child's potential for change over time could be known. Drawing on Vygotsky's theories, Feuerstein and others (Feuerstein, Miller, Rand, & Jensen, 1981; Feuerstein, Rand, & Hoffman, 1979; Lidz, 1991; Peña & Iglesias, 1993) presented dynamic assessment as tapping into a child's learning process and learning potential. Although traditional assessment approaches only judge a child's independent performance, dynamic assessment compares a child's assisted and unassisted performances, thereby locating learning within the social context of the help provided and offering hypotheses about the child's learning in situations beyond the assessment. It introduces scaffolding (Wood, Bruner, & Ross, 1976) into assessment activities, requiring practitioners to fine-tune their assistance to the type of help or support that will eventually enable the test participant to perform the task independently. Many draw on Vygotsky's theory to argue that performance on assessment tasks is modifiable because performance is influenced by the social context within which the test items are presented (Feuerstein et al., 1981; Lidz, 1991; Peña & Iglesias, 1993; van der Veer & Valsiner, 1991).

Our interest in dynamic assessment began with questions about how communication assessments reflect the ways in which children learn to communicate within a social context and how we can truly interpret a child's performance on such assessment activities. In this chapter, we interpret information gathered throughout assessment as determined by the social and interpersonal contexts of assessment activities. First, we contrast dynamic assessment with more static assessment approaches and provide an overview of variations within dynamic assessment. We look at how the concept of dynamic assessment has affected speech and language assessment with specific reference to the limitations of existing assessment tools. Second, we devote the remainder and majority of the chapter to our own reframing of dynamic assessment from a transactional perspective for prelinguistic children, including interpreting Vygotsky's ZPD for collaborative efforts of gathering and sharing information with families and ways to build a profile of a prelinguistic child's communicative competence through the application of dynamic assessment principles.

LIMITATIONS OF ASSESSMENT TRADITIONS

Many assessment tools used with developmentally young children do not incorporate the interactive nature of communication development into their assessment activities, thus leaving a disparate gap between them and the developmental theories previously presented in this chapter. Several limitations have been identified in the most frequently used formal communication assessment instruments for young children (Crais, 1995; Wetherby & Prizant, 1992). Most instruments do not allow for families to collaborate in decision making about the assessment process or to participate to the extent that may be desired by the family. With many instruments involving direct child assessment, activities are primarily clinician directed and designed to identify skills the child fails to perform. The activities often place the child in a respondent role, thereby limiting observations of spontaneous, child-initiated communication (Wetherby & Prizant, 1992). Most emphasize language milestones and forms of communication (e.g., number of different gestures, sounds, words, word combinations) rather than the social-communicative and symbolic foundations of language. Finally, few instruments focus on communication in day-to-day activities and therefore provide limited information that can be directly applied to intervention planning (Crais, 1995).

Many theories on how children acquire language embrace a transactional perspective (Bates, 1976; Bloom, 1993; McLean, 1990) and suggest that the following features are critical to assessment of language and communication in young children:

- Communication and language should be assessed within an interactive, meaningful context in which a child is encouraged to initiate communication.
- A child's caregiver should be integrally involved in the assessment as an active participant interacting with the child, as an informant providing infor-

mation about the child's competence and performance, and as a collaborator in decision making.

• Diagnostic assessment and assessment for program planning should not only identify relative developmental limitations, but they also should provide information about a child's relative strengths in communication and related areas of development.

• Assessment should be viewed as an ongoing, dynamic process in which a child's capacity for developing communicative competence is explored over time.

These features are pertinent not only to young children but also to older learners who are functioning at emerging intentional or symbolic communication levels. Dynamic assessment can address these features by exploring how a child's and family's capabilities are influenced by the many dimensions of the social context.

Dynamic versus Static Assessment

The "dynamic" part of dynamic assessment implies that the process is interactive and distinct from more static assessment activities. Static assessment procedures are usually formal in nature and place the child in a passive role with practitioners directing responses (Wetherby & Prizant, 1992). They generally require that practitioners avoid cueing or consequating the child (Campione, 1989) and classify any assistance provided to the child as a violation of the protocol on which the test was developed and standardized. One of the primary purposes of many of these tools is to provide a number score representing the child's overall behavior (Campione, 1989; Peña & Iglesias, 1993). They often require practitioners to make categorical decisions concerning the child's behaviors and competencies (e.g., pass versus fail, behavior present or behavior absent).

Static assessment procedures rely on products of learning gathered at one point in time (Peña, 1996) and often may reveal more about what a child *cannot* do rather than what that child *can* do or what the child has the *potential* to do. This snapshot approach to assessment can leave practitioners feeling constrained by the protocol and frustrated that the measure does not adequately represent what the child knows or is capable of doing. This is especially true for children with disabilities because a child's performance is compared with children who are typically developing. When only static assessment procedures are used, families and practitioners may voice concerns that the approach is focused on deficits rather than abilities and that valuable information about the child is lost or not acquired.

In contrast, the purpose of dynamic assessment is to explore the process of learning by gathering information about the type of support needed to change the child's behavior (Peña, 1996). Dynamic assessment is designed to identify a child's developmental strengths as well as limitations in relation to the learning context (Lidz, 1991; Missiuna & Samuels, 1989). Because practitioners work toward the child's successful performance on tasks that are attainable, the practitioner is always gauging what a child can do with what he or she is learning to do. By comparing a child's independent and assisted performances, practitioners may see that a child's strengths cluster around a developmental area (e.g., using positive and negative affect to clarify communicative messages) or that a child's strengths cluster around certain types of activities (e.g., building and stacking in constructive play) or ways of learning (e.g., imitation, gestural cues, arrangement of the environment to encourage initiating communication).

Dynamic assessment procedures promote active participation by both the practitioner and the child. The child's interests and attentional focus determine both the nature of the assessment activities and the help or support practitioners provide (Burns, Vye, Bransford, Delos, & Ogan, 1987; Wertsch & Rogoff, 1984). Practitioners are free to use their own intuitions and judgments about what will most help a child demonstrate his or her abilities (Lidz, 1991; Missiuna & Samuels, 1989). Descriptive information is usually generated, which can be further qualified by details of the social circumstances surrounding the assessment activities. Although informal assessment techniques are regularly used for dynamic assessment, formal tools also can be used dynamically by providing assistance to children for portions of the test that are within their ZPD (i.e., tasks they are able to complete with assistance) and by reporting these nonstandard results in a narrative or descriptive manner to supplement standardized test scores.

Links to the Instructional Literature

Dynamic assessment introduces aspects of what has traditionally been considered intervention into an assessment process by providing assistance to the child. Its principles reflect strategies found in both the behavioral and developmental literature. Some strategies, such as functional assessment, general case instruction, and milieu teaching, come from the behavioral literature describing systematic methods of assessment and instruction (see O'Neill & Reichle, 1993). Others, such as scaffolding and mediated learning, draw from Vygotsky's work. What they have in common is their assumption that a child's learning occurs within interactive situations.

The procedures used in *functional assessment* described in the behavioral literature are consistent with dynamic assessment. The purpose of a functional assessment is to identify functional relationships between particular behaviors displayed by a child and environmental variables that predict when a behavior will and will not occur (Dunlap & Kern, 1993; see also Chapter 13). The functional assessment process entails formulating hypotheses about functional relationships and testing the hypotheses by systematic manipulation of hypothesized variables. Functional assessment has been developed as a method to understand variables maintaining challenging behaviors in people with disabilities. Procedures used in functional assessment resemble dynamic assessment procedures in that specific efforts are made to understand how contextual variables support or assist that individual's behavior and learning.

General case instruction is a teaching approach also described in the behavioral literature in which systematic analysis of the features of stimulus classes is used to design effective teaching opportunities and to determine an instructional sequence (Horner, McDonnell, & Bellamy, 1986; O'Neill & Reichle, 1993). A general case approach emphasizes training sufficient exemplars and using natural consequences to promote stimulus and response generalization. This approach addresses the repertoire of opportunities necessary for successful learning. *Milieu teaching* is an instructional package embedded within ongoing interaction for the acquisition of early language and communication skills (see Chapter 15). It is characterized by allowing a child to initiate a tutorial interaction and responding to the child's communication using mand-model, time delay, and incidental teaching techniques (Hart & Risley, 1975; Kaiser, Yoder, & Keetz, 1992; Warren & Gazgag, 1990). These instructional strategies incorporate dynamic assessment procedures by delineating the range of teaching situations and prompts required for a child to acquire and generalize target skills.

Scaffolding is used in dynamic assessment and also is considered a teaching technique derived from parents' natural efforts to help their young children solve problems (Bruner, 1985). Wood et al. (1976) first used the term to connote the ways an adult may match his or her own notions of a child's abilities with components of the task being attempted. Adults scaffold for children by drawing them into particular tasks, presenting manageable elements of the task to them, helping them recognize the task goal and when it is achieved, and giving enough help so that they do not become frustrated (Stone, 1993). *Mediated learning* is a teaching strategy generally used with school-age children in which a teacher frames and focuses the learning situation to assist the student toward successful performance by using techniques such as guided questions and progressive hints (Burns et al., 1987; Feuerstein et al., 1979; Kaiser, 1993; Lidz, 1991; Peña, 1996). Both scaffolding and mediated learning entail systematic modification of the learning environment as the child acquires competence and independence. Dynamic assessment provides a way for doing this within the assessment context.

Dynamic assessment generally uses a test–teach–retest model in which the teaching phase of assessment consists of a series of graduated prompts (Peña, 1996). It incorporates interactive teaching strategies into assessment to delineate the range of teaching opportunities and to determine the child's responsiveness. Dynamic assessment yields information about the *modifiability* of the child by defining elicitation techniques and by understanding change through mediation (Ellis Weismer, Murray-Branch, & Miller, 1993; Olswang, Bain, & Johnson, 1992), similar to procedures used to determine *stimulability* for production of sounds (McReynolds & Elbert, 1978; Milisen, 1954). A child who is stimulable can usually imitate or produce the target sound, grammatical form, or word in a particular context. The assessment of modifiability identifies what level of graduated prompts is needed for the child to acquire and generalize a specified target sound, grammatical form, or word (Peña, 1996).

In the speech-language pathology literature there are several reports of the use of dynamic assessment, all with children who were already using words. Dynamic assessment has been used to address young children's potential for sound production, lexical acquisition, and acquisition of grammar (Bain & Olswang, 1992; Ellis Weismer et al., 1993; Guttierez-Clellan & Quinn, 1993; Olswang et al., 1992; Peña, Quinn, & Igelsias, 1992); it also has been used to identify effective instruction for teaching narrative skills and problem solving to older children (Burns et al., 1987; Butler, 1992; Campione & Brown, 1987; Campione, Brown, Ferrara, & Bryant, 1984; Diaz, Neal, & Vachio, 1991; Palincsar, Brown, & Campione, 1994; Pelligrini, McGillicuddy-Delisi, Sigel, & Brody, 1986). Dynamic assessment procedures have shifted the focus of assessment from the product to the process of learning and have contributed to removing the boundaries between assessment and intervention (see Peña, 1996, for a review and critique of dynamic assessment).

REFRAMING DYNAMIC ASSESSMENT

The studies cited previously provide an initial framework for the use of dynamic assessment procedures; however, none apply the framework to prelinguistic children or address the role of the family in the assessment process. These descriptions of dynamic assessment revolve around language tasks or target behaviors and do not address critical issues in family-centered assessments, such as creating meaningful contexts for assessment activities (Goodnow, 1993), providing help and support that is valued by the family and individualized to the child (Hatano, 1993), having a flexible agenda that is changeable according to the child's behavior during the assessment (Stone, 1993), and decision making with family members according to shared understandings created during the assessment process (Goodnow, 1993).

Another topic that is not adequately addressed in the literature on dynamic assessment for prelinguistic children concerns the nature and type of assistance available to support communication development. Test–teach–retest formats have traditionally been used in dynamic assessment, making them practitioner directed. Although the practitioner is responsive and supportive, the teaching phase often involves a predetermined set of behaviors that are hierarchically arranged. Because most of the dynamic assessment studies address children who are already speaking, they do not offer ideas for providing assistance during assessment to young children at preintentional or presymbolic levels. Considering the nature of the dynamic assessment context, it could be questioned whether a child's competence is constrained by his or her capacity to use the help and support provided by adults or whether it is constrained by adults' abilities to provide adequate assistance to the child (Goodnow, 1993; Litovitz, 1993).

In speech-language pathology, the conceptualizations of dynamic assessment have been drawn mostly from developmental psychology (e.g., Campione et al., 1984; Feuerstein et al., 1981; Hatano, 1993; Palincsar et al., 1994), where assessments regularly involve tasks that test participants are eventually expected to perform independently. However, communication is anything but an independent endeavor. The goal of developing communicative competence is to be able to participate in communication interactively and interdependently with others. Even speech intelligibility cannot be judged apart from the cooperative process involved in creating an understandable message (Kent, 1993). The burden of success for a communicative exchange is with both communicative partners, especially when one of those partners is developmentally young.

This section presents a framework for dynamic assessment of prelinguistic children. While preserving the principles of dynamic assessment, we have incorporated a transactional perspective. That is, in addition to the more conventional principles of dynamic assessment framed by Vygotsky with the ZPD (i.e., identifying a child's existing communication abilities and determining the help or support needed for that child to communicate at slightly higher levels), our version adds two components that extend its application. One component involves understanding the influence of the practitioner–family relationship on the family's sense of efficacy and, hence, on the child's development. The second involves assessing the influence of a host of contextual variables that may support the child's developing communicative competence.

To address the first component, we discuss ways in which we use dynamic assessment and family-centered principles to understand family members' perspectives on the goals and purpose of assessment. We describe ways of sharing assessment results dynamically throughout an assessment process and our reasons for doing this. Also, we explain how using dynamic assessment has helped us create contexts for shared decision making with families through collaborative problem setting and problem solving. To address the second component, we detail the parameters we use in identifying and exploring contextual variables that support a prelinguistic child's developing communicative competence and provide examples of this in a collaborative assessment process. Finally, we discuss definitions of communicative competence that can be created with family members and that are respectful of their cultural traditions and perspectives.

Prelinguistic Dynamic Assessment as a Collaborative Process with Family Members

We approach assessment as a process that occurs over time as we come to know a child within the context of his or her family and as we come to know family members' perceptions of their situation (Crais, 1993; Winton & Bailey, 1993).

Similarly, each family, over time, comes to understand the help and support that practitioners can provide. Thus, the practitioner–family relationship can be viewed as a variable influencing the family's sense of efficacy.

Understanding Family Members' Perspectives on the Goals and Purpose of Assessment We regularly begin our assessments by listening to family members' descriptions and definitions of their situation. Understanding a child's behavior begins with family members' stated reasons for participating in assessment. The value in seeking to understand family members' perspectives of their situation is allowing for the creation of a shared agenda for the time we spend together; in the end, the agenda is more efficient (Bailey & Henderson, 1993). This shared agenda is created by drawing on professional knowledge and expertise to suggest specific choices for assessment activities and by allowing family members' knowledge of their child to determine the actual activities that take place (Crais, 1992, 1993; Lidz, 1991). Practitioners and family members together can make decisions about what activities will be included, how the activities will proceed, and how the information gathered will be used.

Creating Contexts for Shared Decision Making with Families Through Collaborative Problem Setting and Problem Solving We have found that collaborative decision making with families cannot occur unless we share with families the process of problem setting as well as problem solving. Schön (1983) described problem setting as "the process by which we define the decisions to be made, the ends to be achieved, and the means which may be chosen" (p. 40). We effectively set situations when we acknowledge family members' immediate concerns, provide information to family members concerning the ways we are prepared to help, and use our specialized knowledge of communication development to translate family-stated goals (e.g., "I just want Rodney to be able to talk" or "We want Joyce to be able to communicate with people outside the family") into actual assessment activities and ways of interpreting assessment information. As described by Crais (1994), family members can provide information about their child (e.g., likes, dislikes, ways to see the best in the child), and practitioners can describe and offer options (e.g., formal versus informal assessment, professionals and/or parents assess the child, possible sequences of activities). Then families can choose options that meet their child's and their own needs and preferences. Table 1 provides possible ways practitioners can support and collaborate with families during assessments, which can enhance the family's efficacy of caregiving (Crais & Kublin, 1992).

If Vygotsky's concept of the ZPD is applied to interactions with families, the ZPD within the family–professional relationship is the distance between problem solving done alone by the family and that done collaboratively with others. Viewed another way, it could be the distance between what professionals could decide *for* families versus what could be decided *with* families. We propose an assessment framework that enables family members to have the choice of becoming both analyzers of their child's abilities and solution generators.

Table 1. Practitioner activities in assessment

Practitioners can

- Help caregivers understand their child's abilities (through describing, interpreting, and/or assessing their child)
- Provide information (e.g., about communication development, about what is typical, about what the small steps of communication development could be)
- Help caregivers believe that they are effective in understanding their child (e.g., by meeting their child's needs, sharing the world with their child)
- Help caregivers believe that they are promoting their child's further development (e.g., by identifying and reinforcing what caregivers already are doing to promote their child's communicative competence)
- Help caregivers understand and use opportunities for building communication (e.g., in daily caregiving routines, social games, play)
- Provide ideas to caregivers (e.g., about things to try that will facilitate communication development, about ways to understand their child's behavior as communicative)
- Help caregivers identify choices and priorities for decision making
- Help caregivers plan for the future by helping them imagine what to expect
- Help caregivers gain access to resources
- Support caregivers in the advocate role

Adapted from Crais and Kublin (1992).

Sharing Findings Dynamically Throughout an Assessment Process
We believe that sharing assessment findings can be accomplished dynamically throughout the assessment process rather than only at the end and provided exclusively by the practitioner. Family members and practitioners can build a collective view of the child's strengths and needs with ongoing dialogue about what each has observed during the assessment activities. For example, a practitioner might report to family members, "I noticed that Jessica turned her body toward you and looked at you when you added the gesture of reaching your hands out to her to ask her if she wanted to 'come up' into your arms for a hug." In this way, interpretations can be shared about the child's behavior (e.g., "Jessica seems to respond best if we add gestures to the things we say") and ideas can be generated for intervention throughout the assessment process (e.g., "Next time, let's try adding gestures to the words we use when giving her instructions or when playing social games with Jessica").

We have found it critical to recognize family members' own interpretations of the events that occur during an assessment process. These can come from family members' own definitions of communicative competence, what they perceive their child can do, and what they hope for their child. Families differ in how talking is valued, in how status is handled in interactions, and in beliefs about teaching language to children (van Kleeck, 1994). Differences between a family's and a professional's perceptions can come from values and beliefs that are linked to particular individual, family, or culture group identities.

Sharing assessment findings throughout an assessment process gives professionals the opportunity to reconcile what family members say is important with where their child is developmentally. For the family member who has said, "I just want Rodney to be able to talk," sharing assessment findings may mean discussing the ways Rodney intentionally communicated with gestures and sounds during the assessment activities, trying out various accommodations to expand or enhance Rodney's communicative attempts, and beginning to identify supportive contexts where these discussions can continue to take place. For the family who said, "We want Joycee to be able to communicate with people outside the family" and who taught us to read Joycee's facial expressions and head movements, sharing assessment findings could take the form of collaboratively identifying Joycee's most readable signals and the activities in which it would be easiest to introduce her to a new communication partner (e.g., teacher, aide, baby sitter, peer).

Illustration of How Dynamic Assessment Can Be Used Collaboratively

To describe how we used dynamic assessment collaboratively with one particular family, we have summarized three assessment events with Ronnie, a 3-year-old boy whose parents had been told by a psychologist that he has autism. When we met Ronnie's family, his parents had spent the last several months pursuing a diagnosis and were anxious to know what it meant for Ronnie. They also wanted to know what they could expect for the future.

Ronnie's mother: I eventually just came out and asked [the psychologist] would he go to school like a normal child....He said yeah, he will, BUT. . .

Ronnie's father: BUT...

Ronnie's mother: He may, of course. He's only 3, so you don't know how well...he's gonna do, so that's where the 'BUT' comes in. He may require special classes. Then again, since he's only 3, how do we know?

Ronnie's father: All I look at, at this point, is what can we do to help. Once we know what it is, what can we do to help? I neither expect miracles nor disaster.

As we talked with Ronnie's parents about what they wanted from the assessment, it seemed important to them to understand Ronnie's behavior in relation to the diagnosis of autism and in relation to what they could do "to help." They also wanted help in facilitating Ronnie's progress in his child care setting and in deciding whether speech-language therapy would be beneficial. When we asked them to talk about their concerns for Ronnie, some additional issues were raised.

Ronnie's mother: This is why Ronnie in some cases is spoiled...in a lot of ways. Because not knowing what he wants, you know. He's a normal child in a sense, but he can't talk to me. So, is he being really obnoxious and mean because he's just having a tantrum like every other kid? Or is he being…? Well, there's times you don't really know. It's a gray area. Okay, what do I do? The only thing I would like to see is that he becomes less frustrated. Because as he does get older, you can tell he does get more frustrated. Because, yeah…the kids at school can talk and he can't. And right now he's 3 and that's not that big a deal 'cause he's not all that tuned into that. But as he gets older it's going to become more of a problem. So it would be nice to have that a little bit eased up.

Ronnie's mother told us that she was unsure of how to interpret and handle Ronnie's challenging behaviors. She was seeking ways to decrease his frustrations and increase his communication skills. Our next step with Ronnie's parents was to identify assessment activities that would address their concerns and provide them with the information they needed to make further plans for Ronnie. In addition to the issues raised by Ronnie's family, we identified several areas we believed might be important to the process.

To focus our problem setting, we began with Ronnie's parents' self-identified need for information. We asked them to tell us a little of what they knew about autism. They had read a few articles in the newspaper and had seen the movie *Rain Man* (Guber-Peters & Levinson, 1988), but they were still unsure how all this fit with their son. They had been thinking about contacting an area program for children with autism and asked for our opinion. We described the materials the program offered and also gave them the telephone number for the local Parent-to-Parent Network, which supplies a variety of resources for parents. Then we began to plan assessment activities that would let us all see what Ronnie could do as well as give us opportunities to discuss his parents' concerns. Because Ronnie was not yet using words and relied on situation-specific gestures and actions to communicate his wants and needs, we suggested that we would like to see Ronnie in the settings and activities in which he was involved every day. His parents related that he spent a good deal of time at home and in a child care program 3 days per week. Together we decided that the home visit would be first, which would prepare us for what to look for in the child care environment.

During the home visit, it was agreed that both parents would play with Ronnie. They would also give him a snack and change his diaper so that we could see a range of his behaviors. In these activities we would try facilitating his communication through different kinds of support. We also asked Ronnie's parents if they would be interested in observing and providing more behavioral information about Ronnie than we could observe during one home visit. They agreed, so we introduced them to the parent interview for autism (Stone & Hogan, 1993) as one way to capture on paper ways to characterize Ronnie's behavior. His parents also made notes about what they saw during the home visit and during our interactions with Ronnie.

As we observed and interacted with Ronnie using familiar and unfamiliar toys and a few daily routines (e.g., snack, outside play, preparation for nap), and as we watched Ronnie play and go through his daily routines with his parents, we all discussed what we were seeing and thinking. As each activity occurred, we discussed Ronnie's strengths and his challenging behaviors, and we began to generate ideas for ways we might facilitate his communication and decrease the challenging behaviors. Together, we tried several of these options as we continued to interact with Ronnie throughout the home visit.

For the child care visit, we met first with Ronnie's parents and the child care staff. Together we identified several things that we could all look for in the child care setting (e.g., what kind of individual attention Ronnie was receiving, how the child care workers dealt with Ronnie's challenging behaviors, the strengths of the program for Ronnie, the kinds of communicating Ronnie did in this setting, what the staff did to facilitate Ronnie's communication). After the observation, we met again with Ronnie's parents and the staff to brainstorm about ways that his interactions and communication could be facilitated within that setting. Thus, his parents and child care workers were part of the identification of Ronnie's behaviors, strengths, and needs.

In summary, this collaborative approach made assessment with Ronnie's family a process and not a product; as such, it changed the way we gathered, interpreted, and shared information (Crais, 1993, 1995; Snow, 1994). We were aware of how observing what a child can do, particularly what that child can do with support, can change adult expectations for the child (Burns et al., 1987). For Ronnie's parents, taking such an active part in the assessment itself facilitated a larger role for them during the sharing of assessment information and intervention planning and contributed to their feeling of efficacy as caregivers. For further ideas about viewing assessment as a series of consensus-building activities, see Beukelman and Mirenda (1992); Crais (1996); and McLean and Crais (1996) (see also Chapter 11).

Dynamic Assessment of the Child's Communicative Competence

The second component of our reframed dynamic assessment process is more in line with other dynamic assessment approaches (e.g., Missiuna & Samuels, 1989; Olswang et al., 1992; Palincsar et al., 1994) and entails interactions within each assessment activity between the child and his or her communication partners. That is, the focus throughout assessment activities is to determine the child's communicative competence by identifying and exploring contextual variables that support the child's communication (see Snow, 1991). Instead of using a hierarchical cueing system, we draw on interactive behaviors that adults use with children, for example, waiting and looking expectantly, using repetitive words and gestures, and verbal expansions and extensions (Bornstein, 1989; Coggins, 1991; Norris, 1992; Platt & Coggins, 1990; van der Veer & Valsiner, 1991). We view prelinguistic dynamic assessment as including scaffolding, but we also see it as going beyond the use of models, questions, and imitations to include a range of contextual factors that influence interaction. This broader framework is particularly critical for children and older learners at the two transitions addressed in this volume—the transition to intentional communication and to symbolic communication.

Parameters Used in Identifying and Exploring Contextual Variables
To understand a child's developing competence, dynamic assessment needs to identify and explore contextual variables that support or impede the child's acquisition of communicative competence. For children who are at emerging intentional communication or symbolic communication levels, it is particularly critical to understand how the interactional context influences the child's communication. Before children acquire a large repertoire of referential words, their communication is bound to the interactional context. The meaning of their communicative signals can only be interpreted within the interactional context. Therefore, it is important to understand this relationship to enhance children's development of intentional communication and transition to symbolic communication.

From a transactional perspective, prelinguistic dynamic assessment of the child's communicative competence necessitates a dual focus on both the child and the communicative partner by considering the readability of the child's signals and how this is influenced by contextual variables (Dunst et al., 1990). The readability of a child's communication is a critical factor contributing to how the child's communicative partners will respond to communicative attempts and support communication growth. Important dimensions of the child's communication profile that contribute to readability are summarized in Table 2. These

Table 2. Dimensions of the child's communicative profile that contribute to readability

---

- *Social-affective communication:* Consider how the child uses directed eye gaze and facial expression to regulate interaction and indicate emotional state.
- *Range of communicative functions:* Consider whether the child's reasons for communication include indicating wants and needs (i.e., behavior regulation), drawing attention to self (i.e., social interaction), and directing attention to an object or event (i.e., joint attention).
- *Sophistication of communicative means:* Consider the repertoire and quality of gestures and vocalizations.
- *Rate of communicating:* Consider how frequently the child initiates and responds to communication.
- *Repair strategies:* Consider the child's ability to repeat or modify a communicative signal to clarify intentions when not understood.
- *Capacity to symbolize:* Consider the child's capacity to symbolize (i.e., ability to make one thing stand for and represent something else) across domains, including language comprehension, language production, symbolic play, and constructive play.

Adapted from Wetherby and Prizant (1993b).

dimensions are derived from the developmental literature presented in the chapters of Part I in this volume.

Prelinguistic dynamic assessment also needs to systematically explore how contextual support influences the child's communicative competence. Four major parameters are considered, which are listed in Table 3 and described in this chapter. It is presumed that these parameters interact such that their combined effect may exceed individual effects. For each parameter, we often observe a child in natural interactions, forming hypotheses about how these variables influence the child's readability and then testing the hypotheses by systematically engineering the environment to provide different kinds of contextual support (Goodnow, 1993). These steps are similar to those used in functional analysis and assessment of challenging behaviors (see Chapters 11 and 13).

The most basic parameter of the context is the nature of the opportunities for communication. Environments vary widely in regard to the quality and quantity of opportunities for initiating and responding to communication for a range of communicative functions (i.e., to request objects, to protest, to greet, to call, to comment, to request information [Wetherby & Prizant, 1993a]). The arrangement of the environment, the accessibility of materials, and the developmental appropriateness of activities will influence the opportunities for children to communicate. It is important to consider the balance of opportunities for a child to initiate communication and respond to social bids. Dynamic assessment should contrast how the child initiates communication in naturally occurring opportuni-

Table 3.   Parameters to systematically explore the influence of the interactional context on the child's communicative competence

---

Opportunities for communicating—Are there
- Opportunities for the child to communicate for a variety of reasons?
- Adequate arrangements and accessibility of materials?
- A balance of opportunities for the child to initiate communication and respond to social bids?
- Developmentally appropriate activities?

Structuring of the activity—Are there
- Exchangeable, cooperative roles?
- Clearly marked turns that the child can anticipate?
- Sequences of steps that are predictable to the child?

Interaction style of the communication partner—Is the partner
- Allowing the child to initiate?
- Responsive to the child's attempts to communicate?

Use of scaffolding to support or guide the child's behavior—Does the practitioner
- Use facial expressions, intonation, and gestures?
- Imitate the child's behavior?
- Interpret the child's emotional state or intention?
- Expand on the child's behavior or model a better behavior?
- Give verbal directions, ask a question, or offer help?

ties with ones that are engineered by the practitioner to understand what opportunities assist the child's initiation and to determine how to stimulate the child's use of the most readable communication for the broadest range of functions.

The next parameter is the *activity structure* and how it influences a child's communication in the framework of joint action routines. A *joint action routine* is a repetitive turn-taking activity in which there is mutual attention and mutual participation by both the child and the caregiver, exchangeable roles, and predictable sequences (Bruner, 1978; Snyder-McLean, Solomon, McLean, & Sack, 1984). Bruner (1978, 1981) suggested that joint action routines provide optimal opportunities for communication development and provide foundations for learning how to exchange roles in conversation. A prototypical example of a joint action routine for infants and toddlers is the game of Peekaboo (Bruner & Sherwood, 1976), which caregivers may play hundreds or thousands of times during the first 2 years of a child's life. Dimensions of activity structure to consider in prelinguistic dynamic assessment include the availability of exchangeable, cooperative roles; clearly marked turn taking; and a logical, predictable sequence of steps from beginning to ending. These dimensions allow the child to anticipate the nature and sequence of the activity and participate maximally; thus, they enhance communication (Platt & Coggins, 1990; Prizant & Bailey, 1992; Seigel-Causey & Wetherby, 1993; Snyder-McLean et al., 1984). Therefore, the assessment process should determine how these dimensions support or assist the child's ability to participate in communicative exchanges.

The next parameter considered is the *interaction style of communication partners.* The major questions explored concern how the child's communication partners allow the child to initiate and how the partners respond to the child's attempts to communicate. The developmental literature provides guidelines for assessing children at early stages of communication. The communicative partner's interaction style can be evaluated to determine if the following features are present: Does the partner wait for the child to initiate communication by pausing and looking expectantly, recognize the child's behavior as communication by interpreting the communicative function that it serves, and respond contingently to the child's communicative behavior in a manner that is consistent with the communicative intention of the child and that matches the communicative level of the child (MacDonald & Carroll, 1992)? It is important to consider the balance between the child and the partner; that is, whether the partner and the child each take an equal role in participating and responding meaningfully to the other person (MacDonald & Carroll, 1992). Caregivers who follow their child's lead, respond contingently, and systematically create a predictable communication environment provide help and support for their child to communicate more (Dunst et al., 1990).

The last contextual parameter is the *use of scaffolding to support or guide the child's behavior.* Scaffolding for prelinguistic children entails the following kinds of support: using facial expressions, intonation, and gestures; imitating the child's behavior; interpreting the child's emotional state or intention; modeling a more sophisticated behavior; expanding on the child's behavior; giving simple verbal directions; and asking a question or offering help. Practitioners and caregivers can draw on a large repertoire of support strategies and then individualize their support according to the behaviors of the child. Dynamic assessment should systematically explore how these different scaffolding techniques affect the child's communicative abilities when used spontaneously by the communicative partner or when simulated systematically during structured interactions.

One example of how we used scaffolding was with Bryan, a preverbal 2-year-old child identified as having pervasive developmental disorder. During a bubbles activity structured to entice communicative acts, we manipulated the use of scaffolding to explore what contextual support was needed from Bryan to initiate communication.

Bryan

After blowing bubbles, the clinician handed Bryan the closed bubble jar. Bryan looked up at the clinician, banged the jar, shook the jar, and looked at the clinician's hands. The clinician asked Bryan, "Need some help?" and waited (the standard procedure of offering support). Then the clinician said, "Watch, I'll help" and blew some bubbles to demonstrate. After closing the jar and handing it back to Bryan, the clinician put his hands in close proximity to Bryan and waited. After a short delay with Bryan looking around, back at the bubbles, and fleetingly at the clinician, the clinician again demonstrated by saying, "I'll help" and blowing more bubbles. This time when he handed the closed bubble jar back to Bryan, he put one hand just over the jar but not touching the lid, and Bryan pushed the clinician's hand down on the jar to request that more bubbles be blown.

This example illustrates how Bryan, who rarely initiated gestural communication, required the proximity of the clinician's hand with the jar to direct a signal to the clinician to get the jar open. The systematic increase in the support given to Bryan was highly informative for determining how to enhance Bryan's movement to intentional communication. It was not based on a predetermined hierarchy of cues but instead on an individualized repertoire of support being created for Bryan during the assessment process.

Illustration of Dynamic Assessment Procedures for Assessing Communicative Competence

The following example illustrates how we used dynamic assessment with a standardized assessment instrument, the Communication and Symbolic Behavior Scales (CSBS) (Wetherby & Prizant, 1993a). The CSBS was designed to provide a profile of young children's communicative, linguistic, social-affective, and language-related cognitive abilities. It involves systematic sampling procedures ranging from structured communicative opportunities that encourage the child to initiate communication (referred to as *communicative temptations*), to semistructured book sharing, to unstructured play activities. The sampling procedures were designed to resemble natural ongoing adult–child interactions and to provide opportunities for use of a variety of communicative behaviors (for more information on the CSBS, see Chapter 7).

When we met Alan, he was 3.5 years old and was described by his pediatrician as having a general developmental delay. The assessment information gathered from Alan illustrates how dynamic assessment allowed us to explore his abilities across domains of concern identified with his caregivers. With Alan, this process disclosed critical information about contextual support and structuring activities that guided the decision making for intervention planning.

Alan was referred to us by his parents and preschool teachers because of concerns about his language development and peer interactions. Alan had been attending a full-time preschool since about 6 months of age. We observed Alan at his preschool, which operates a model full-inclusion program using a developmentally appropriate play-based curriculum. During the observation, Alan was generally passive and nonverbal. He wandered and was primarily an onlooker; he did not initiate interactions with peers and did not engage in focused solitary or group play. Alan's preschool teacher indicated that his behavior during the observation was typical, and she asked for recommendations for developing his language and social interaction skills.

Next we saw Alan in a clinical evaluation with his mother. Alan's mother indicated that he began talking at 28 months of age and was also delayed in motor development. We used the CSBS (Wetherby & Prizant, 1993a) to better understand Alan's communication abilities, with his mother and the clinician as communicative partners. Alan's communicative behavior during the CSBS contrasted dramatically from that during the observation at preschool. During the structured contexts of the communication sample, Alan readily initiated communication for a full range of communicative functions, including requesting objects and actions, protesting, requesting a social routine, showing off, and commenting on objects and actions. He used a variety of gestures (i.e., giving, showing, pointing, reaching), including many distal gestures. He was able to coordinate gestures and vocalizations but also produced many vocal communicative acts without gestures. His vocalizations consisted of monosyllabic and multisyllabic utterances with a large variety of consonants. Alan's lexicon was greater than 15 words during the sample (e.g., "more bubbles," "pop," "open," "again"), and he produced a few two-word utterances (e.g., "more bubbles"), suggesting that he was emerging into the early multiword stage. He displayed frequent vocal imitation, some of which was used communicatively, which is typical of this language stage. He demonstrated comprehension of two-word combinations. His rate of communicating was high and was more consistent with a child in the multiword stage of language development. He was able to repair by repeating or changing a previous act to clarify his message. He demonstrated appropriate facial expression, eye gaze, and affect during the sample.

In contrast to his strengths in communication and language, Alan displayed very limited play skills during the CSBS. When given the feeding toy set and a stuffed Kermit the Frog, he initially did not pretend with the materials; instead, he organized them and stacked them. When given verbal directions by the clinician, "Alan, do you want to feed the froggy?" he touched the frog's mouth. He said "feed" and "eat." When given verbal directions by his mother, "The frog is hungry; can you give him something to eat?" again Alan just looked at Kermit. Finally, when the clinician gave Alan a spoon, putting it directly into his hand, he began to feed Kermit. Next, when the clinician gave him a cup, Alan also pretended to give the frog a drink without another verbal direction. Alan's motor delays may have contributed to his relative weakness in play but could not fully account for it because he displayed adequate manual dexterity to stack eight blocks, to carry out pretend actions with verbal directions, and to use gestures.

The dynamic nature of the assessment helped us to elucidate the discrepancy in communicative and language strengths Alan demonstrated during the CSBS evaluation compared with our observation of him at his preschool. All four parameters of dynamic assessment were manipulated: the nature of the opportunities, the structuring of activities, the interaction style, and the use of scaffolding. Alan's communication was most enhanced during the CSBS when there were ample opportunities to communicate that were highly structured. The communicative temptations used in the CSBS were designed to be optimal, brief joint action routines. In contrast, the interactional context at school involved loosely structured play activities, and Alan was not able to initiate communication in that context.

The interaction style of his communication partner also influenced Alan's language use. His communication was most enhanced by the facilitative interaction style used by the clinician during the communicative temptations, which involved waiting and following his lead. However, when the clinician used this interactional style during the loosely structured CSBS play sample, Alan rarely initiated communication. In more loosely structured activities, the clinician needed to be more directive. During the sharing books context, Alan's mother used a more directive interactional style and the following turns were exchanged:

Mother:	What's that? (while pointing to a picture)	Alan:	Frog.
Mother:	What's that?	Alan:	Bird.
Mother:	What's that?	Alan:	Horse.
Mother:	Those are owls. Can you say moon?	Alan:	Moo.
Mother:	These are bees. Can you say bees?	Alan:	Bees.

This style resulted in less sophisticated language than during exchanges with the clinician but more sophisticated than at school. Thus, it appeared that Alan's language use was minimized at preschool because most of his opportunities to interact with peers were during loosely structured play activities. The dynamic assessment findings provided critical information for designing the environment at Alan's preschool to enhance language and social interaction with peers and teachers as well as highlighting the importance of developing his play skills.

EDUCATIONAL AND CLINICAL IMPLICATIONS

We have suggested ways that the use of dynamic assessment can be broadened to include a number of communicative contexts, individualized repertoires of help and support, and shared decision making with families as to the purpose and content of the assessment activities. Family-centered dynamic assessment values the social constructs within which we communicate, building on a view of communication as the co-construction of messages. It is an assessment process that views a child's communication abilities as situated within specific contexts and events (Duchan, Hewitt, & Sonnenmeier, 1994) and one that fits the spirit and intent of the individualized family service plan process (Noonan & McCormick, 1993).

As described previously, assessment of a young child's communicative competence must begin with caregivers' perspectives: their own definitions of competence, what they expect from the communicative exchange, and their sense of efficacy as communication partners (van Kleeck, 1994; Westby, 1990). We have argued that formal and informal assessment activities can be used as tools for achieving consensus with family members about their child's communicative status and for exploring how communicative competence is influenced by context. Just as a child's communicative competence develops within social communicative exchanges, descriptions of competence develop within practitioners' and caregivers' communicative exchanges. Emphasis should be placed on the design of empowering activities that facilitate caregivers', practitioners', and young children's abilities or capacities to act in accomplishing shared goals (Ashcroft, 1987; Damico, 1994; Dunst et al., 1993).

In the day-to-day implementation of a dynamic assessment process, we have found it helpful to explain to family members the ways that we are prepared to provide help and support. Some families notice a marked contrast between our assessment approach and the ways they have dealt with other practitioners. Some families jump easily into a collaborative role, whereas other families may need more direction or guidance in the beginning (McBride, Brotherson, Joanning, Whiddon, & Demmitt, 1993). Empowerment and family decision making should be viewed as a choice. However, occasionally the situation arises when a family member says, "You're the professional. You tell me what to do." This situation may represent family members' experiences with other practitioners, previous situations outside of our assessment that usurped the family's decision-making power, or simply the need for more information. In these situations, we bring the conversation back to a discussion of choices, both within the assessment and for what will happen next. The pros and cons of each option should be provided, giving enough information, direction, and time for family members to feel they can make a reasonable decision.

A family-centered dynamic assessment process can help family members feel successful as caregivers and as advocates because their preferences for assessment activities, intervention, and support services can be directly identified and evaluated within the assessment and intervention planning process (Biro, Daulton, Szanton, & Garner, 1991; Kagan & Neville, 1994; Stone, 1993; Stonestreet, Johnston, & Acton, 1991). Some practitioners, however, may believe that this type of assessment process requires more time or a greater degree of flexibility than they can build into their protocols. In this case, we would encourage several things. First, the purposes in assessment should be clarified. If assessment is for intervention planning, then more than one session could be allowed to do this. Second, taking on these ideas is not unrealistic if approached in small manageable units. Ways to move the whole assessment team toward more family-centered practice should be considered, and resources should be collected for doing so (Crais, 1994; McWilliam, Winton, & Crais, 1996).

We believe the model presented is equally relevant across the life span of the individuals we assess because it draws on a definition of communicative competence that is created and mutually agreed on by those involved in the assessment activities. We believe it has particular usefulness for assessing individuals at prelinguistic levels because the interactive context for communication is systematically explored.

DIRECTIONS FOR FUTURE RESEARCH

There is a need for ongoing exploration of how dynamic assessment can be incorporated into different service delivery models. Practical constraints should be considered, such as the limited time allotted to building practitioner–family relationships and the organizational protocols required in many settings. Also, the effects of more dynamic and family-centered approaches within service delivery frameworks need to continue to be addressed with respect to those specifically reported by family members and experienced by the children themselves. We encourage research on preservice and in-service training that prepares practitioners to be collaborative problem setters and problem solvers in an effort to help move the field away from traditional, static, and tool-based assessment activities.

Using a dynamic assessment process may help to redefine what is meant by categorizing certain young children as being developmentally at risk. Instead of listing risk factors or eligibility criteria, research from a dynamic assessment perspective could involve understanding the child's many environments and identifying the help and support within those environments that would promote communicative competence. In addition, this research could provide insight into the roles of professionals in supporting families in the growth and development of their children.

CONCLUSION

In describing our approach to communication assessment with prelinguistic children and their families, we have presented a way to integrate transactional theory, family-centered principles, and dynamic assessment. Transactional theory offers a look at a young child's developmental process across caregiving relationships and interactional contexts. It emphasizes the mutual influence children and adults have on one another. Family-centered principles locate these ideas within the specific activities practitioners and caregivers do together, concentrating on the importance of meaningful contexts for assessment activities and the value of shared decision making. Dynamic assessment further describes how this can be done as an interactive process by systematically exploring the influence of help and support offered within the assessment context. We have suggested how dynamic assessment can incorporate a family-centered perspective, which is essential for prelinguistic children. Practitioners can recognize the ZPD created for problem setting and problem solving with family members when the support family members value most is attended to. Together practitioners and family members can explore the types of support, degree of structure, and contexts that will most benefit the child.

REFERENCES

Ashcroft, L. (1987). Defusing "empowering": The what and the why. *Language Arts, 64,* 142–155.

Bailey, D.B., & Henderson, L.W. (1993). Traditions in family assessment: Toward an inquiry-oriented reflective model. In D.M. Bryant & M.A. Graham (Eds.), *Implementing early intervention* (pp. 124–147). New York: Guilford Press.

Bain, B., & Olswang, L. (1992, November). *Examining readiness for learning two-word utterance: Dynamic assessment validation.* Poster session presented at the American Speech-Language-Hearing Association annual convention, San Antonio, TX.

Bates, E. (1976). *Language and context: The acquisition of pragmatics.* New York: Academic Press.

Beukelman, D.R., & Mirenda, P. (1992). *Augmentative and alternative communication: Management of severe communication disorders in children and adults.* Baltimore: Paul H. Brookes Publishing Co.

Biro, P., Daulton, D., Szanton, E., & Garner, C. (1991). Informed clinical opinion. *NEC*TAS Notes, December (4),* 1–4.

Bloom, L. (1993). *The transition from infancy to language.* New York: Cambridge University Press.

Bornstein, M.H. (1989). Between caretakers and their young: Two modes of interaction and their consequences for cognitive growth. In M.H. Bornstein & J.S. Bruner (Eds.), *Interaction in human development* (pp. 197–214). Hillsdale, NJ: Lawrence Erlbaum Associates.

Bruner, J. (1978). From communication to language: A psychological perspective. In I. Markova (Ed.), *The social context of language* (pp. 17–48). New York: John Wiley & Sons.

Bruner, J. (1981). The social context of language acquisition. *Language and Communication, 1*, 155–178.

Bruner, J. (1985). Vygotsky: A historical and conceptual perspective. In J.V. Wertsch (Ed.), *Culture, communication and cognition* (pp. 21–35). Cambridge, England: Cambridge University Press.

Bruner, J., & Sherwood, V. (1976). Early rule structure: The case of peekaboo. In J. Bruner, A. Jolly, & K. Sylva (Eds.), *Play: Its role in evolution and development* (pp. 277–285) London: Penguin Press.

Burns, M.S., Vye, N.J., Bransford, J.D., Delos, V.R., & Ogan, T. (1987). Static and dynamic measures of learning in young handicapped children. *Diagnostique, 12,* 59–73.

Butler, K. (1992, November). *Keeping the baby: Throwing out the bathwater: Dynamic assessment.* Miniseminar presented at the annual convention of the American Speech-Language-Hearing Association, San Antonio, TX.

Campione, J. (1989). Assisted assessment: A taxonomy of approaches and an outline of strengths and weaknesses. *Journal of Learning Disabilities, 22,* 151–165.

Campione, J.C., & Brown, A.L. (1987). Linking dynamic assessment with school achievement. In C.S. Lidz (Ed.), *Dynamic assessment: An interactional approach to evaluating learning potential* (pp. 82–115). New York: Guilford Press.

Campione, J.C., Brown, A.L., Ferrara, R.A., & Bryant, N.R. (1984). The zone of proximal development: Implications for individual differences in learning. In B. Rogoff & J.V. Wertsch (Ed.), *Children's learning in the "zone of proximal development"* (pp. 77–92). San Francisco: Jossey-Bass.

Coggins, T. (1991). Bringing context back into assessment. *Topics in Language Disorders, 11*(4), 43–54.

Crais, E. (1992). "Best practices" with preschoolers: Assessing within the context of a family-centered approach. In W. Second & J.S. Damico (Eds.), *Best practices in school speech-language pathology* (pp. 33–42). San Antonio, TX: The Psychological Corporation.

Crais, E.R. (1993). Families and professionals as collaborators in assessment. *Topics in Language Disorders, 14*(1), 29–40.

Crais, E.R. (1994). *Increasing family participation in assessing children birth to five.* Inservice manual and audiotapes. Chicago: Riverside.

Crais, E.R. (1995). Expanding the repertoire of tools and techniques for assessing the communication skills of infants and toddlers. *American Journal of Speech-Language Pathology, 4*(3), 47–59.

Crais, E.R. (1996). Applying family-centered principles to child assessment. In P.J. William, P.J. Winton, & E.R. Crais (Eds.), *Practical strategies for family-centered intervention* (pp. 69–96). San Diego, CA: Singular Publishing Group.

Crais, E.R., & Kublin, K.S. (1992, November). *Increasing family participation in assessment and intervention planning for infants/toddlers.* Short course presented at the annual convention of the American Speech-Language-Hearing Association, San Antonio, TX.

Damico, S.K. (1994). Empowering nonvocal populations: An emerging concept. *National Student American Speech-Language-Hearing Association Journal, 21,* 31–44.

Diaz, R.M., Neal, C.J., & Vachio, A. (1991). Maternal teaching in the zone of proximal development: A comparison of low- and high-risk dyads. *Merrill-Palmer Quarterly, 37*(1), 83–107.

Duchan, J.F., Hewitt, L.E., & Sonnenmeier, R.M. (1994). Three themes: Stage two pragmatics, combating marginalization, and the relation of theory to practice. In J. Duchan, L. Hewitt, & R. Sonnenmeier (Eds.), *Pragmatics: From theory to practice* (pp. 1–9). Englewood Cliffs, NJ: Prentice Hall.

Dunlap, G., & Kern, L. (1993). Assessment and intervention for children within the instructional curriculum. In J. Reichle & D.P. Wacker (Eds.), *Communication and language intervention series: Vol. 3. Communicative alternatives to challenging behavior: Integrating functional assessment and intervention strategies* (pp. 177–203). Baltimore: Paul H. Brookes Publishing Co.

Dunst, C.J., Lowe, L.W., & Bartholomew, P.C. (1990). Contingent social responsiveness, family ecology, and infant communicative competence. *National Student Speech-Language-Hearing Association Journal, 17,* 39–49.

Dunst, C.J., Trivette, C.M., Starnes, A.L., Hamby, D.W., & Gordon, N.J. (1993). *Building and evaluating family support initiatives: A national study of programs for persons with developmental disabilities.* Baltimore: Paul H. Brookes Publishing Co.

Ellis Weismer, S., Murray-Branch, J., & Miller, J. (1993). Comparison of two methods for promoting productive vocabulary in late talkers. *Journal of Speech and Hearing Research, 36,* 1037–1050.

Feuerstein, R., Miller, R., Rand, Y., & Jensen, M.R. (1981). Can evolving techniques better measure cognitive change? *Journal of Special Education, 15,* 201–219.

Feuerstein, R., Rand, Y., & Hoffman, M. (1979). *The dynamic assessment of retarded performers: The Learning Potential Assessment Device, theory, instruments and techniques.* Baltimore: University Park Press.

Goldberg, S. (1977). Social competence in infancy: A model of parent–infant interaction. *Merrill-Palmer Quarterly, 23,* 163–177.

Goodnow, J.J. (1993). Direction of post-Vygotskian research. In E.A. Forman, N. Minick, & C.A. Stone (Eds.), *Contexts for learning: Sociocultural dynamics in children's development* (pp. 369–381). New York: Oxford University Press.

Guber-Peters, United Artists, MGM/UA (Producer), & Levinson, B. (Director). (1988). *Rain man* [Film]. (Available from MGM/UA Home Entertainment)

Guttierez-Clellan, V.F., & Quinn, R. (1993). Assessing narratives from children from diverse cultural-linguistic groups. *Language, Speech and Hearing Services in the Schools, 24*(January), 2–9.

Hart, B., & Risley, T. (1975). Incidental teaching of language in preschool. *Journal of Applied Behavior Analysis, 13,* 407–432.

Hatano, G. (1993). Time to merge Vygotskian and constructivist conceptions of knowledge acquisition. In E.A. Forman, N. Minick, & C.A. Stone (Eds.), *Contexts for learning: Sociocultural dynamics in children's development* (pp. 153–166). New York: Oxford University Press.

Horner, R.H., McDonnell, J.J., & Bellamy, G.T. (1986). Teaching generalized skills: General case instruction in simulation and community settings. In R.H. Horner, L.H. Meyer, & H.D.B. Fredericks (Eds.), *Education of learners with severe handicaps: Exemplary service strategies* (pp. 289–314). Baltimore: Paul H. Brookes Publishing Co.

Kagan, S.L., & Neville, P.R. (1994). Parent choice in early care and education: Myth or reality? *Zero to Three, 14*(4), 11–18.

Kaiser, A.P. (1993). Introduction: Enhancing children's social communication. In A.P. Kaiser & D.B. Gray (Eds.), *Communication and language intervention series: Vol. 2. Enhancing children's communication: Research foundations for intervention* (pp. 3–10). Baltimore: Paul H. Brookes Publishing Co.

Kaiser, A.P., Yoder, P.J., & Keetz, A. (1992). Evaluating milieu teaching. In S.F. Warren & J. Reichle (Eds.), *Communication and language intervention series: Vol. 1. Causes and effects in communication and language intervention* (pp. 9–48). Baltimore: Paul H. Brookes Publishing Co.

Kent, R.D. (1993). Speech intelligibility and communicative competence in children. In A.P. Kaiser & D.B. Gray (Eds.), *Communication and language intervention series: Vol. 2. Enhancing children's communication: Research foundations for intervention* (pp. 223–242). Baltimore: Paul H. Brookes Publishing Co.

Lidz, C.S. (1991). *Practitioner's guide to dynamic assessment.* New York: Guilford Press.

Litovitz, B.E. (1993). Deconstruction in the zone of proximal development. In E.A. Forman, N. Minick, & C.A. Stone (Eds.), *Contexts for learning: Sociocultural dynamics in children's development* (pp. 184–196). New York: Oxford University Press.

MacDonald, J., & Carroll, J. (1992). Communicating with young children: An ecological model for clinicians, parents, and collaborative professionals. *American Journal of Speech-Language Pathology, 1,* 39–48.

McBride, S.L., Brotherson, M.J., Joanning, H., Whiddon, D., & Demmitt, A. (1993). Implementation of family-centered services: Perceptions of families and professionals. *Journal of Early Intervention, 17*(4), 414–430.

McLean, J.E., & Snyder-McLean, L.K. (1978). *A transactional approach to early language training.* Columbus, OH: Charles E. Merrill.

McLean, L.K. (1990). Communication development in the first two years of life: A transactional process. *Zero to Three, 11,* 13–19.

McLean, M., & Crais, E. (1996). Procedural considerations in assessing infants and toddlers with special needs. In M. McLean, D. Bailey, & M. Wolery (Eds.), *Assessing infants and toddlers with special needs* (pp. 46–68). Columbus, OH: Charles E. Merrill.

McReynolds, L., & Elbert, M. (1978). An experimental analysis of misarticulating children's generalization. *Journal of Speech and Hearing Research, 21,* 136–150.

McWilliam, P.J., Winton, P.J., & Crais, E.R. (1996). *Practical strategies for family-centered intervention.* San Diego, CA: Singular Publishing Group.

Milisen, R. (1954). A rationale for articulation disorders. *Journal of Speech and Hearing Disorders,* Monograph Supplement, *4,* 6–17.

Missiuna, C., & Samuels, M.T. (1989). Dynamic assessment of preschool children with special needs: Comparison of mediation and instruction. *Remedial and Special Education, 10*(2), 53–62.

Noonan, M.J., & McCormick, L. (1993). *Early intervention in natural environments.* Pacific Grove, CA: Brooks/Cole Publishing Company.

Norris, J. (1992). Assessing infants and toddlers in naturalistic contexts. In W. Secord & J.S. Damico (Eds.), *Best practices in school speech-language pathology* (pp. 21–32). San Antonio, TX: The Psychological Corporation.

Olswang, L.B., Bain, B.A., & Johnson, G.A. (1992). Using dynamic assessment with children with language disorders. In S.F. Warren & J. Reichle (Eds.), *Communication and language intervention series: Vol. 1. Causes and effects in communication and language intervention* (pp. 187–215). Baltimore: Paul H. Brookes Publishing Co.

O'Neill, R., & Reichle, J. (1993). Addressing socially motivated challenging behaviors by establishing communicative alternatives: Basics of a general-case approach. In J. Reichle & D.P. Wacker (Eds.), *Communication and language intervention series: Vol. 3. Communicative alternatives to challenging behavior: Integrating functional assessment and intervention strategies* (pp. 205–235). Baltimore: Paul H. Brookes Publishing Co.

Palincsar, A.S., Brown, A.L., & Campione, J.C. (1994). Models and practices of dynamic assessment. In G. Wallach & K. Butler (Eds.), *Language learning disabili-*

ties in school-age children and adolescents: Some principles and applications (pp. 132–144). New York: Macmillan.

Pelligrini, A.D., McGillicuddy-Delisi, A.V., Sigel, I.E., & Brody, G.H. (1986). The effects of children's communicative status and task on parents' teaching strategies. *Contemporary Educational Psychology, 11*(3), 240–252.

Peña, E.D. (1996). Dynamic assessment: The model and its language applications. In K.N. Cole, P.S. Dale, & D.J. Thal (Eds.), *Communication and language intervention series: Vol. 6. Advances in assessment of communication and language* (pp. 281–307). Baltimore: Paul H. Brookes Publishing Co.

Peña, E.D., & Iglesias, A. (1993, November). *Dynamic assessment: The model and its application to language assessment.* Short course presented at the American Speech-Language-Hearing Association Annual Convention, Anaheim, CA.

Peña, E.D., Quinn, R., & Iglesias, A. (1992). The application of dynamic methods to language assessment: A nonbiased procedure. *Journal of Special Education, 26*(3), 269–280.

Platt, J., & Coggins, T.E. (1990). Comprehension of social-action games in prelinguistic children: Levels of participation and effect of adult structure. *Journal of Speech and Hearing Disorders, 55*, 315–326.

Prizant, B.M., & Bailey, D.B. (1992). Facilitating the acquisition and use of communication skills. In D.B. Bailey & M. Wolery (Eds.), *Teaching infants and toddlers with handicaps* (pp. 299–361). Columbus, OH: Charles E. Merrill.

Prizant, B.M., & Wetherby, A.M. (1990). Toward an integrated view of early language and communication development and socioemotional development. *Topics in Language Disorders, 10*, 1–16.

Sameroff, A. (1987). The social context of development. In N. Eisenburg (Ed.), *Contemporary topics in development* (pp. 273–291). New York: John Wiley & Sons.

Sameroff, A., & Chandler, M. (1975). Reproductive risk and the continuum of caretaking causality. In F. Horowitz (Ed.), *Review of child development research* (Vol. 4, pp. 187–244). Chicago: University of Chicago Press.

Sameroff, A., & Fiese, B. (1990). Transactional regulation and early intervention. In S. Meisels & J. Shonkoff (Eds.), *Early intervention: A handbook of theory, practice, and analysis* (pp. 119–149). New York: Cambridge University Press.

Schön, D. (1983). *The reflective practitioner: How professionals think in action.* New York: Basic Books.

Seigel-Causey, E., & Wetherby, A. (1993). Nonsymbolic communication. In M. Snell (Ed.), *Instruction of students with severe disabilities* (4th ed., pp. 290–318). New York: Macmillan.

Snow, C.E. (1991). Diverse conversational contexts for the acquisition of various language skills. In J.F. Miller (Ed.), *Research in child language disorders: A decade of progress* (pp. 105–124). Austin, TX: PRO-ED.

Snow, C.E. (1994). Beginning from baby-talk: Twenty years of research on input and interaction. In C. Gallaway & B.J. Richards (Eds.), *Input and interaction in language acquisition* (pp. 3–12). Cambridge, England: Cambridge University Press.

Snyder-McLean, L., Solomon, B., McLean, J., & Sack, S. (1984). Structuring joint action routines: A strategy for facilitating communication and language development in the classroom. *Seminars in Speech and Language, 5*(3), 213–228.

Stone, C.A. (1993). What is missing in the metaphor of scaffolding? In E.A. Forman, N. Minick, & C.A. Stone (Eds.), *Contexts for learning: Sociocultural dynamics in children's development* (pp. 169–183). New York: Oxford University Press.

Stone, W.L., & Hogan, K.L. (1993). A structured parent interview for identifying young children with autism. *Journal of Autism and Developmental Disorders, 23*, 639–652.

Stonestreet, R.H., Johnston, R.G., & Acton, S.J. (1991). Guidelines for real partnerships with parents. *Infant-Toddler Intervention—The Transdisciplinary Journal, 1*(1), 37–46.

van der Veer, R., & Valsiner, J. (1991). *Understanding Vygotsky: A quest for synthesis.* Oxford, England: Blackwell.

van Kleeck, A. (1994). Potential cultural bias in training parents as conversational partners with their children who have delays in language development. *American Journal of Speech-Language Pathology, 3*(1), 67–78.

Vygotsky, L. (1978). *Mind in society: The development of higher psychological processes.* Cambridge, MA: Harvard University Press. (originally published in Russian in 1933)

Vygotsky, L. (1986). *Thought and language.* (A. Kozulin, Ed. and Trans. in 1934). Cambridge, MA: Harvard University Press.

Warren, S., & Gazgag, G. (1990). Facilitating early language development with milieu intervention procedures. *Journal of Early Intervention, 14*(1), 62–86.

Wertsch, J.V., & Rogoff, B. (1984). Editors' notes. In B. Rogoff & J.V. Wertsch (Eds.), *Children's learning in the "zone of proximal development"* (pp. 1–6). San Francisco: Jossey-Bass.

Westby, C. (1990). Ethnographic interviewing: Asking the right questions to the right people in the right ways. *Journal of Childhood Communication Disorders, 10*, 101–111.

Wetherby, A.M., & Prizant, B.M. (1992). Profiling young children's communicative competence. In S.F. Warren & J. Reichle (Eds.), *Communication and language intervention series: Vol. 1. Causes and effects in communication and language intervention* (pp. 217–251). Baltimore: Paul H. Brookes Publishing Co.

Wetherby, A.M., & Prizant, B.M. (1993a). *Communication and Symbolic Behavior Scales—Normed edition.* Chicago: Applied Symbolix.

Wetherby, A.M., & Prizant, B.M. (1993b). Profiling communication and symbolic abilities in young children. *Journal of Childhood Communication Disorders, 15*, 23–32.

Winton, P.J., & Bailey, D.B. (1993). Communicating with families: Examining practices and facilitating change. In J. Paul & R. Simeonsson (Eds.), *Understanding and working with parents of children with special needs* (2nd ed., pp. 210–230). New York: Holt, Rinehart & Winston.

Wood, D., Bruner, J.S., & Ross, G. (1976). The role of tutoring in problem-solving. *Journal of Child Psychology, 17*, 89–100.

13

Comprehensive Behavioral Support
Assessment Issues and Strategies

Robert O'Neill, Bobbie J. Vaughn, and Glen Dunlap

CARLY IS A 3-YEAR-OLD CHILD diagnosed as having developmental disabilities. She does not talk, although she does sometimes use gestures and loud vocalizations to communicate. Her family and preschool teachers are concerned because Carly engages in various kinds of self-stimulatory behavior (e.g., gazing at her fingers). She actively pushes adults and children away when they attempt to interact with her.

James is a 28-year-old man who has autism and moderate mental retardation. He talks rarely, but when he does he usually repeats what others have said to him (i.e., immediate echolalia). Sometimes James points to objects and occasionally screams when he does not appear to feel well. James produces a variety of troubling behaviors, including running away, screaming, pica (i.e., eating inedible objects), aggression toward others (e.g., hitting, kicking, biting, scratching), head banging, and destroying clothing, furniture, and other objects.

There are a number of differences between Carly and James, including their age and the socially acceptable and unacceptable behaviors they use to interact with others. What they have in common is a need for a comprehensive assessment of their communicative and problem behavior repertoires and the variables that influence them, followed by a comprehensive plan for promoting communicative and adaptive behavior (and reducing problem behavior). This chapter briefly describes and discusses characteristics of serious problem behaviors, introduces a framework for assessment and intervention referred to as *comprehensive behavioral support*, provides a description of a variety of functional assessment strategies, and demonstrates how such strategies can be used with people such as Carly and James.

Preparation of this chapter was supported by three projects funded by the U.S. Department of Education: 1) Cooperative Agreement No. H133B2004 from the National Institute on Disability and Rehabilitation Research (NIDRR); 2) Field Initiated Research Project No. H133G60119 from NIDRR; and 3) Outreach Project No. HO24D40006-95 from the Office of Special Education and Rehabilitative Services (OSERS). The opinions expressed are those of the authors, and no official endorsement by the U.S. Department of Education should be inferred.

SERIOUS PROBLEM BEHAVIORS

Children and adults with disabilities can present a variety of challenges to those attempting to provide educational and support services. Among the more serious of these challenges occurs when children or adults exhibit serious problem behaviors. Serious problem behaviors may vary widely in topography, frequency, and intensity but typically include such things as self-injury (e.g., head banging, hand biting), aggression (e.g., hitting and kicking others), and environmental damage or destruction (e.g., breaking windows, tearing up books). Such behaviors often result in more restrictive educational and residential placements (i.e., in institutions), greatly increased financial costs for providing support, and substantial stress for families and other caregivers (National Institutes of Health [NIH], 1991).

Conceptual and empirical work on the etiology, development, and maintenance of problem behaviors focuses on the separate and combined influence of biological/physical variables and behavioral/environmental variables (Thompson, Egli, Symons, & Delaney, 1994). The occurrence of problem behaviors in some people may have a close primary link to specific neurobiological dysfunctions (Nyhan, 1994; Schroeder & Tessel, 1994). Investigation also has focused on the behavioral or social functions that problem behaviors may serve for people, particularly those with very limited repertoires of conventional communicative skills. Engaging in problem behaviors may produce a variety of particular outcomes or effects that reinforce and maintain the behaviors (Iwata et al., 1994). Some of these effects may be more internal or private in nature (e.g., sensory stimulation, attenuation of pain from an ear infection), whereas others may be socially mediated (e.g., getting attention or a desired item from a caregiver). Behaviors that have such socially mediated environmental effects can be thought of as serving communicative functions in certain circumstances (Carr et al., 1994). The influence of such environmental or social variables may be augmented by the effects of various physical conditions (e.g., fatigue, hunger, various illnesses) that also can contribute to the development and expression of problem behaviors (Carr & Smith, 1995).

A tremendous amount of work remains to be done to elucidate the interrelationships among biological and environmental variables in the development and exhibition of serious problem behaviors (Guess & Carr, 1991; NIH, 1991). From a practical perspective, the current level of understanding directs practitioners to be aware of and consider both biological and environmental influences in assessing and developing support strategies for people exhibiting problem behaviors. Developing communicative skills as alternatives to problem behaviors will be a critical and effective approach for many people and receives substantial attention in this chapter (see also Chapter 14). In other cases, however, addressing physical or biological variables that influence problem behaviors will be a more appropriate and effective strategy. In many cases, a combination of approaches will be needed. The critical point is to try and logically match intervention and support strategies as closely as possible with the relevant variables that appear to be influencing the problem behaviors.

COMPREHENSIVE BEHAVIORAL SUPPORT

Since the early 1980s, there has been a substantial evolution in how people think about and provide support to individuals who exhibit problem behaviors. Approaches to figuring out problem situations and trying to make them better have been called by a variety of names, including nonaversive behavioral support (Horner et al., 1990), positive behavioral support (Bambara, Mitchell-Kvacky, & Iacobelli, 1994; Koegel, Koegel, & Dunlap, 1996), effective behavioral support (Bambara & Knoster, 1995), and positive approaches (Meyer & Evans, 1993). The authors of this chapter have chosen to use the term *comprehensive behavioral support* (CBS) to indicate that we are talking about an approach that takes a broad perspective with regard to important variables to consider in assessment and the full range of strategies that should be considered in developing and implementing a specific plan of support for an individual. A number of authors have delineated important characteristics of this type of approach (Bambara & Knoster, 1995; Dunlap, Ferro, & dePerczel, 1994; Hedeen, Ayres, Meyer, & Waite, 1996; Horner et al., 1990; O'Neill et al., 1997).

Assumptions and Characteristics of CBS

This section highlights some of the important aspects of CBS and characteristics to consider in developing and implementing a plan of support.

Focusing on Specific Behavioral Outcomes and Broader Lifestyle Impact Reducing the frequency and/or intensity of particular problem behaviors will always be an important outcome. However, it is also critical to consider the quality of life that a person is experiencing. The opportunity to have access to preferred places, activities, people, and events, both at home and in the community, is just as critical as changes in specific patterns of adaptive and problem behaviors.

Developing Support Plans Based on Assessment and Understanding One of the most critical aspects of CBS is that choosing strategies to promote communicative and adaptive behavior and to reduce problem behavior is based on a thorough assessment and understanding of the variables that influence the person's behavioral repertoire. This process often is referred to as functional assessment or functional analysis, as the emphasis is frequently on determining the motivations of problem behaviors or the functions that they serve for an individual (Neef & Iwata, 1994). The principles and procedures involved in such assessments are the focus of this chapter.

Developing Comprehensive Multicomponent Support Plans A hallmark of the CBS approach is the incorporation of many types of strategies into plans for supporting individuals (Hedeen et al., 1996; Horner, Close, et al., 1996). These strategies include more traditional behavior support techniques, such as arranging natural, positively reinforcing consequences for adaptive behavior and attempting to reduce or eliminate reinforcement for problem behavior. However, there is also consideration of a range of other strategies, including changes in general lifestyle (e.g., activity patterns, social interactions), problematic setting events (e.g., sleep patterns, medical illnesses), more immediate and specific antecedent events and variables (e.g., requests to perform difficult tasks), teaching and promoting positive adaptive behaviors, and emergency or crisis management procedures for responding to very serious occurrences of problem behavior. More detail on how these types of strategies are selected and implemented is provided in Chapter 14.

Teaching and Promoting Adaptive Behavior Much attention is paid to identifying and developing positive alternative behaviors during the comprehensive assessment and support process. Communicative repertoires have arguably received the most substantial attention. Conceptual work and subsequent research has focused on the perspective that problem behaviors can serve communicative or pragmatic functions for people (Reichle, 1991b). That is, people perform such behaviors because they result in particular reinforcing outcomes, many of which are socially mediated. Problem behaviors can thus be thought of as an alternative way of communicating messages, such as "I don't want to do this," "I want you to talk/interact with me," "Help me," or "I want more _____" (Doss & Reichle, 1991; Durand, 1986). Looking at problem behaviors from this perspective is not without controversy (Durand, 1990; Iwata, Vollmer, Zarcone, & Rodgers, 1993); however, it has proven to be a very effective conceptualization for assessment and intervention. A number of studies have documented that teaching learners functionally equivalent augmentative and alternative communicative responses (e.g., signing I WANT A BREAK; using an electronic device to say, COME TALK TO ME) as communicative replacements can result in substantial reductions in problem behavior and can lead to concomitant increases in communicative behavior (Carr et al., 1994; Durand, 1990; Durand, Berotti, & Weiner, 1993; Reichle & Wacker, 1993). Because it is critical to understand the behavioral or communicative functions that problem behaviors may be serving to select and teach appropriate equivalent alternative responses, communication strategies have been intimately tied to the functional assessment process.

Establishing socially acceptable communicative alternatives to challenging behaviors can be thought of as moving children and adults from more primitive to more conventional and to referential or symbolic communicative acts (McLean & Snyder-McLean, 1988). For example, Kenneth may currently rock in his chair and bite his wrist when he needs assistance to get more milk while at the dinner table. A more conventional communicative response to replace wrist biting might include holding up or pointing to his glass. Kenneth also could be taught symbolic responses, such as signing MILK or pointing to a picture of milk being poured into a glass. Reichle (1991b) offered a thorough discussion of issues relating to understanding, selecting, and teaching different levels of communicative acts.

Developing Technically Sound and Contextually Appropriate Support Plans It is critically important that behavior support plans be technically sound. That is, plans should be logically based on a thorough assessment and be in accord with established principles of behavior. However, they also need to be a good match with the values, skills, and resources of the people responsible for implementing them (Albin, Lucyshyn, Horner, & Flannery, 1996; O'Neill et al., 1997). If people receiving support, family members, and/or staff members are unwilling or unable to carry out planned strategies, then less than desirable outcomes should be expected.

Providing Long-Term Support Although in certain situations particular procedures may result in quick reductions in problem behaviors, it is clear that for many people effective behavioral support will involve an ongoing iterative process of assessment, strategy selection and implementation, and evaluation of outcomes. Understanding a person's unique perspective and his or her behaviors and helping to bring about substantial and enduring positive changes in a person's life will often require significant time and energy on the part of those providing support. This makes successful collaboration among people receiving support, friends and family members, and professionals a critical component of the process (Bambara & Knoster, 1995; Turnbull & Turnbull, 1996).

Comprehensive behavioral support is an evolving framework. However, at its core lies a focus on assessment and understanding of problematic situations as a critical first step in designing effective support. The next section describes the desired outcomes of and strategies for conducting such assessments.

FUNCTIONAL ASSESSMENT

Functional assessment has been described and defined in a variety of ways (Durand, 1993; Lennox & Miltenberger, 1989). From a broad perspective, it is a process for gathering information that will maximize the effectiveness and efficiency of behavior support plans (O'Neill et al., 1997). A more specific goal is to bring clarity and understanding to situations that may be confusing and chaotic. Systematic assessment can help identify the variables that influence a person's adaptive and problem behavior repertoire; that is, what things set the occasion for the occurrence (or nonoccurrence) of desired or difficult behaviors and what outcomes or consequences appear to be maintaining them.

Functional assessment methods include indirect approaches, such as the use of interviews or questionnaires with relevant informants (e.g., parents, teachers, residential staff); systematic direct observation of behaviors in typical settings; and functional analysis manipulations. *Functional analysis* is a term for a particular approach or subset of functional assessment procedures. Functional analysis involves conducting manipulations of specific antecedent and consequent variables and collecting systematic data to determine their effects on behavior (Neef & Iwata, 1994; Reichle & Wacker, 1993). Manipulations are usually carried out in the context of a structured experimental design. The terms *functional assessment* and *functional analysis* should not be used interchangeably, as sometimes happens, as they have different meanings in the literature and in their use by professionals and other people.

Typically, the assessment process would begin with information gathering via interviews or questionnaires. This step must be followed up with direct observations to attempt to validate and elaborate on hypotheses generated from the initial information. In many cases, information from these two initial steps (i.e., interviews and observations) will be sufficient to guide development and implementation of support strategies. However, more specific functional analysis manipulations also can be carried out as needed to clarify and substantiate information gathered with other methods. More details on and examples of specific functional assessment methods are presented later in this chapter.

Desired Outcomes of a Functional Assessment

In working with children and adults who exhibit serious problem behaviors and nontypical communicative repertoires, there are several desirable assessment outcomes. Table 1 presents five such outcomes.

Describing Behaviors At the conclusion of an assessment, interventionists need to have basic descriptive information about the problem behaviors a person exhibits and other behaviors that may be serving as nontypical forms of communication (e.g., idiosyncratic vocalizations or gestures) (Beukelman & Mirenda, 1992; Reichle, 1991a). Such information should include the specific topography or form of the behaviors, frequency and duration, and intensity or

Table 1. Five primary outcomes of a functional assessment process

1. Clear description of the problem behaviors and other nontypical communicative behaviors exhibited by the person, including classes or sequences of behaviors that frequently occur together
2. Identification of the events, times, and situations that predict when the problem behaviors and other nontypical communicative behaviors will and will not occur across the full range of typical daily routines
3. Identification of the consequences that maintain the problem behaviors and other nontypical communicative behaviors (i.e., what function[s] the behaviors appear to serve for the person)
4. Development of one or more summary statements or hypotheses that describe specific behaviors, a specific type of situation in which they occur, and the outcomes or reinforcers maintaining them in that situation
5. Collection of direct observation data that support the summary statements that have been developed

Adapted by permission from O'Neill et al. (1997); © Wadsworth.

severity when applicable (i.e., how much damage do the behaviors cause?). In addition, it is important to understand that a behavior may be related to another behavior or clusters of behaviors. If two or more behaviors are occurring for similar reasons (i.e., serving similar functions), intervention strategies should respond to them in a similar manner, even if they are topographically different (Sprague & Horner, 1992). A person may wave his or her hands, yell loudly, pound on the table, and throw objects, all of which may be related to recruiting attention or interaction. Similarly, a person may vocalize, tap his or her cheek, or aggressively push others against particular cabinets, behaviors that may serve the function of requesting particular food items.

Identifying Predictors of Behaviors   Identifying the contextual variables that predict or set the occasion for problem or nontypical communicative behaviors to either occur or not occur represents a critical area of information gathering. These contextual variables can be classified into two major categories: setting events and predictor events. *Setting events* are events that change the momentary value of reinforcers and punishers, thereby influencing the probability of behaviors that typically result in those consequences (Horner, Vaughn, Day, & Ard, 1996). Setting events typically do not directly provoke or set off a behavior, but they help to "set the stage" for behaviors to occur. (Setting events also are referred to as *establishing operations* by various authors and researchers.) Such events may occur some time before the occurrence of a problem behavior or may be happening concurrently with a more specific problematic situation (Halle & Spradlin, 1993; Horner, Vaughn, et al., 1996). Examples of such events include physical or medical conditions, such as hunger, fatigue, medication effects, or chronic illness (e.g., allergies, constipation, middle-ear infections); social events, such as previous negative interactions with parents, siblings, or peers; and other environmental factors, such as excessive heat, light, crowding, or noise in a classroom (Durand, 1993). Setting events combine with the second category of variables, which are more immediate antecedent or predictor events, to set the occasion for particular behaviors. More immediate antecedent variables include such things as specific tasks or activities, the presence or absence of certain people, and particular physical settings.

There are many situations in which setting events and more immediate antecedents or predictors may interact. For example, on most days Marika responds positively to her therapist's requests and encouragement to engage in range-of-motion exercises during physical therapy. However, if Marika has gotten very little sleep the previous night, or is experiencing an allergy-related sinus headache, the value of being left alone to rest and relax will be very high while the value of social praise and interaction for engaging in therapy may be relatively low. As a result, attempts to engage Marika in the exercises may be met with crying, scratching, and kicking, as she attempts to escape from the activity demands. As another example, when Jonathan is thirsty and he and his residential support person are in proximity to a soda machine, he may sometimes repeatedly tap on the machine with his knuckles. If he is not thirsty, such a response would be much less likely to occur.

It is important to understand the factors and situations that predict both the occurrence and nonoccurrence of behaviors, particularly problem behaviors (see Table 1). Examining and thinking about where problem behaviors are not occurring can be productive in identifying situations that work in a positive manner for the person. For example, if Tonya is consistently aggressive and disruptive during large-group activities but rarely acts out during small-group or one-to-one activities, it would be important to try to determine what accounts for this difference. Is it the increased social attention and interaction in the small-group and one-to-one contexts that reduce her aggressive and disruptive behaviors? Are the behaviors related to the types of tasks or activities that occur during the different situations? Or perhaps the higher levels of noise and confusion in large groups are aversive to her, relative to the smaller, calmer groups and dyads. Pursuing answers to these kinds of questions will lead to useful information that can ultimately be used in the program development process.

Identifying Outcomes or Consequences   Behaviors that are occurring on a consistent basis are happening because they are the most efficient strategies that an individual has acquired to either obtain desired outcomes or escape or avoid undesired outcomes. A primary purpose of functional assessment and analysis strategies is to identify the outcomes or reinforcers that are maintaining these behaviors. A number of authors have described classification schemes for communicative or behavioral functions of problem behaviors (Doss & Reichle, 1991; Iwata et al., 1993). Figures 1 and 2 provide examples of a branching scheme. The initial function of a behavior would be categorized as either obtaining desired events or avoiding or escaping undesired events. Each of these categories can be further examined with regard to whether they involve interacting with other people in the process (i.e., are they socially or nonsocially mediated?). Figures 1 and 2 provide specific examples of the types of outcomes or reinforcers that might be relevant in the different categories.

There are two critical points (among others) to consider. One is that the same events may have different effects on different people. For example, Jackson's loud screaming may be motivated by obtaining attention and interaction, while Anneke's aggressive pinching and scratching may be motivated by escaping or avoiding the same thing. The second point is that any particular individual may have multiple functions or motivations for different behaviors exhibited. Anneke may exhibit aggressive behavior when she wants people to leave her alone but also may exhibit self-injurious head banging when she wants to obtain a tangible item (e.g., food, drink). Such potential multiple functions are important to remember when conducting assessments and planning intervention strategies. Clinical experience and empirical data have demonstrated that if all of the different functions of a person's problem behaviors are not identified during assessment and addressed during the programming process (e.g., by teaching

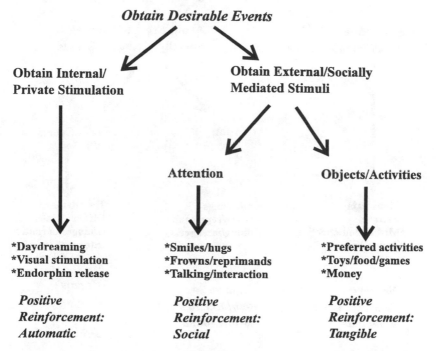

Figure 1. Examples of potential positively reinforcing outcomes that a person may want to obtain. (Adapted by permission from O'Neill et al. [1997]; © Wadsworth.)

multiple alternative communicative responses), then problem behaviors will continue to occur in at least some situations (Day, Horner, & O'Neill, 1994).

Developing Summary Statements or Hypotheses One useful strategy for pulling together assessment information is to develop concise summary statements or hypotheses that describe specific situations in which behaviors of concern are occurring, the specific behaviors that are happening in that situation, and the outcomes or reinforcers that appear to be maintaining those behaviors (Dunlap et al., 1993). Table 2 provides several examples of such summary statements. Some of the statements include references to both setting events and more immediate predictor events. The summary statements for Miguel illustrate a situation in which his self-injurious behavior appears to serve multiple functions. Summary statements should be developed for all the situations and functions that are relevant for an individual.

Validating Summary Statements with Direct Observation One strategy for collecting functional assessment information is to talk to relevant people, such as teachers and parents. Although this is a good approach, clinical experi-

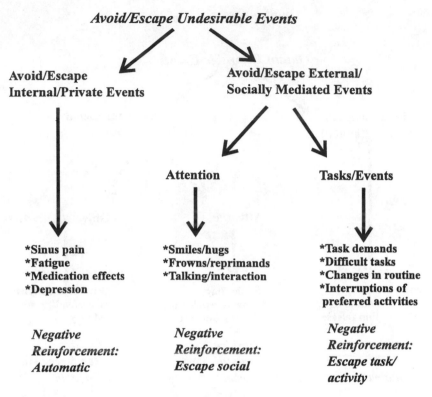

Figure 2. Examples of potential undesirable or aversive events that a person may want to avoid or escape (negative reinforcement). (Adapted by permission from O'Neill et al. [1997]; © Wadsworth.)

ence and empirical research have demonstrated that people closest to the learner and situations that provoke problem behavior are not always the most accurate observers and reporters of what is happening in particular situations (Iwata et al., 1993). Therefore, it is recommended that some level of systematic direct observation data collection be carried out in an effort to corroborate information obtained via interviews. The results of such observations allow those involved in the assessment process to confirm, revise, or eliminate summary statements or decide if new statements need to be added.

FUNCTIONAL ASSESSMENT STRATEGIES

There are three categories of strategies for collecting functional assessment information. These are collecting information from relevant people, collecting systematic direct observation data in typical settings, and carrying out specific functional analysis manipulations.

Table 2.   Examples of summary statements based on assessment information

- "When Perry is getting little attention in a large group in the classroom, he is likely shout profanities and throw things to get peer attention. This is more likely if he has not received much attention earlier in the day."
- "When Monique has slept less than 4 hours the night before and is asked to do independent assembly jobs at her work station, she is likely to tear up materials and hit her supervisor to escape from the task demands."
- "When Jacqueline is prompted to stop playing with the computer or record player in the play area, she is likely to fall on the floor and scream to try to continue to be allowed to play with the items."
- "In situations with low levels of activity or attention at home, Miguel will rock and begin to chew his wrist to produce self-stimulation."
- "When Miguel is asked to dress himself or do other nonpreferred self-care routines, he will begin to chew on his wrist to try to escape from the task demands."
- "If Andrea has received teacher reprimands earlier in the day and she begins to have difficulty with a reading or math assignment, she will put her head down, refuse to respond, and/or close her books to try to avoid having to complete the assignment."

Adapted by permission from O'Neill et al. (1997); © Wadsworth.

Informant Methods

Informant methods involve collecting information from people who know well the person of concern and his or her behavior patterns. Parents, teachers, vocational and residential service providers, and friends and acquaintances are examples of potential sources. Information may be gathered via informal or more structured interviews or instruments such as rating scales and questionnaires. For example, Durand and Crimmins (1992) developed the Motivation Assessment Scale (MAS), a 16-item questionnaire on which respondents are asked to rate how likely different types of situations are to affect a person's problem behavior. The focus is on trying to identify motivations or functions of the problem behavior (e.g., obtain attention, escape activity demands).

O'Neill et al. (1997) developed a comprehensive Functional Assessment Interview (FAI) format. This form provides a structure for an interview process and is focused on obtaining a wide variety of information relevant to the desired outcomes of the functional assessment process (see Table 1). Table 3 presents a summary of the key question areas from the FAI.

The FAI also includes a substantial emphasis on gaining information about the full range of a person's communicative repertoire. There are questions about both general expressive strategies and receptive communicative abilities. As an example, Figure 3 presents a matrix from the FAI for recording information about the different types of behaviors that a person might exhibit to serve a variety of communicative functions. To gather more supplemental detail on a person's communicative repertoire, practitioners could use one of a variety of more extensive interview instruments and protocols that have been developed for gathering information about communicative behavior (Beukelman & Mirenda, 1992; Calculator & Bedrosian, 1988; Halle, Chadsey-Rusch, Collet-Klingenberg, & Reinoehl, 1993).

Table 3. Summary of key question areas from the Functional Assessment Interview form and the Student-Assisted Functional Assessment Interview

Functional Assessment Interview Form[a]

1. Describe the behaviors with regard to topography, frequency, duration, and intensity.
2. Define ecological events (setting events) that predict or set up the problem behaviors.
3. Define specific immediate antecedent events that predict when the behaviors are likely and not likely to occur.
4. Identify the consequences or outcomes of the problem behaviors that may be maintaining them.
5. What is the relative efficiency of the problem behaviors in terms of physical effort and how often and how quickly people respond to them?
6. What are the primary ways that the person communicates with other people?
7. What are more general things to do and things to avoid in working with and supporting the person?
8. What are the things that the person likes and are reinforcing to him or her?
9. What is known about previous programs that have been attempted to decrease or eliminate the behaviors and the effects they had?

Student-Assisted Functional Assessment Interview[b]

1. In general, do you think your work is too hard/easy for you?
2. Do you think work periods for your subjects are too short/long?
3. Do you think you receive enough attention and rewards when you do a good job?
4. When do you have the fewest/most problems in school and why?
5. What changes could be made so that you would have fewer problems during certain times?
6. Rate how much you like the following subjects (Reading, Math, Social Studies, etc.).
7. What do you like/dislike about Reading, Math, Social Studies, etc.?

[a]Adapted by permission from O'Neill et al. (1997); © Wadsworth.

[b]From Kern, L., Dunlap, G., Clarke, S., & Childs, K.E. (1994). Student-assisted functional assessment interview. *Diagnostique, 19,* 29–39; adapted by permission.

Researchers and clinicians also have stressed the importance of considering the person exhibiting the behaviors of concern as a potential primary informant with regard to interviews. This will depend to some extent on the capabilities and willingness of particular individuals but should by no means be overlooked as an important part of the process. As examples of this, Kern, Dunlap, Clarke, and Childs (1994) and O'Neill et al. (1997) presented specific formats that can be used to structure interviews with school-age individuals about problem behaviors and related variables. Key question areas from the Student-Assisted Functional Assessment Interview (Kern et al., 1994) are presented in Table 3.

Whatever types of instruments or processes are used, it is important to keep in mind the critical outcomes of identifying behaviors, relevant setting events and antecedents, and maintaining outcomes or reinforcers. It is usually possible to generate one or more summary statements or hypotheses based on input from relevant people. However, it will be critical to collect direct observation data to attempt to validate or disconfirm these statements.

Communicative Functions	Complex speech (sentences)	Multiple word phrases	One word utterances	Echolalia	Other vocalizing	Complex signing	Single signs	Pointing	Leading	Shakes Head	Grab/reach	Gives objects	Increased movement	Moves close to you	Moves away or leaves	Fixed gaze	Facial expression	Aggression	Self-injury	Other
Request attention																				
Request help																				
Request preferred food/objects/activities																				
Request break																				
Show you something or someplace																				
Indicate physical pain (headache, illness)																				
Indicate confusion or unhappiness																				
Protest or reject a situation or activity																				

Figure 3.   Matrix for obtaining information about communicative repertoires. (From O'Neill, R.E., et al. [1997]. *Functional assessment and program development for problem behavior: A practical handbook* [2nd ed.]. Belmont, CA: Wadsworth; reprinted by permission.)

Direct Observation

Observations typically would be conducted in relevant settings during a person's usual routines, especially those that have been reported to involve problem behaviors or communicative attempts. The frequency and duration of observations may vary but would usually involve 1 or more hours per day for several days. Decisions about more time and effort would depend on the clarity and interpretability of the data being collected. It is often very useful to have the people who are specifically involved in situations collect data (e.g., parents, teachers). However, variables such as time constraints and complexity of data collection may make this difficult or impossible, in which case it may be necessary to have others (e.g., speech-language clinician, school psychologist) conduct the observations (Carr et al., 1994). There is a wide range of formats available for collecting direct observation data, which differ in their complexity and the level of detail they provide.

Scatterplot Grids   Touchette, MacDonald, and Langer (1985) presented a format for collecting basic information about where and when problem behaviors were occurring. An example of this format is present in Figure 4. Time interval information is provided by the rows of the grid, and different dates are represented by the columns. Various schemes can be used to fill in the squares to indicate the frequency of behaviors during a specific time period on a given date. The data for Alicia in Figure 4 were recorded using a slash to indicate one occurrence of behavior, an "X" to indicate two occurrences, and a filled-in block to

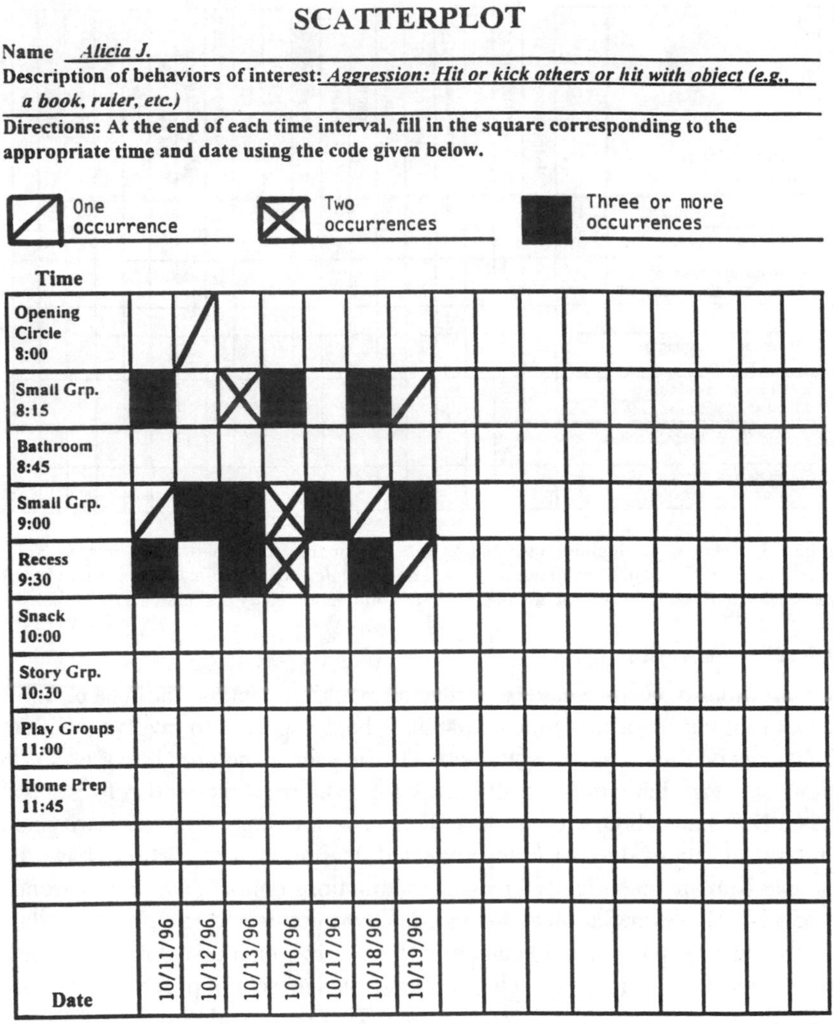

SCATTERPLOT

Name _Alicia J._

Description of behaviors of interest: _Aggression: Hit or kick others or hit with object (e.g., a book, ruler, etc.)_

Directions: At the end of each time interval, fill in the square corresponding to the appropriate time and date using the code given below.

◹ One occurrence   ⊠ Two occurrences   ■ Three or more occurrences

Time

	10/11/96	10/12/96	10/13/96	10/16/96	10/17/96	10/18/96	10/19/96
Opening Circle 8:00	◹						
Small Grp. 8:15	■	⊠	■		■	◹	
Bathroom 8:45				◹	■		
Small Grp. 9:00	◹		⊠	◹	■	■	
Recess 9:30	■		⊠	■	■	◹	
Snack 10:00							
Story Grp. 10:30							
Play Groups 11:00							
Home Prep 11:45							

Date

Figure 4. Example of a scatterplot data collection format. (Adapted by permission from Touchette, MacDonald, & Langer, [1985].)

indicate more than two occurrences. As can be seen in the figure, her behaviors were more frequent during time periods involving small-group work activities and during recess. Although scatterplots are not as demanding in terms of time and effort, they do not provide the detail that may be necessary to completely understand particular situations. For example, the data for Alicia in Figure 4 did not provide information about the specific antecedents and consequences that may be related to the behaviors in the problematic situations.

A-B-C (Antecedent-Behavior-Consequence) Formats When a behavioral incident occurs, the person collecting data writes down the behavior(s) of interest that occurred, the antecedent events or situations that were in effect immediately before the behavior(s), and the immediate events or consequences that occurred following the behavior(s). Such approaches provide more substantial detail relevant to the desired outcomes of a functional assessment process (Doss & Reichle, 1991; Reichle & Johnston, 1993). However, they are also more demanding in terms of the time and effort required to collect the data and summarize and interpret them.

Functional Assessment Observation Form The Functional Assessment Observation (FAO) Form assessment strategy, presented by O'Neill et al. (1997), combines elements of both scatterplot and A-B-C methods. However, instead of written descriptions of incidents, checkmarks or numbers are used to note the occurrence of specific behaviors and relevant antecedents and consequences. Based on initial interviews, this format allows a person to tailor the data collection process to be maximally relevant for a given individual. This form may be preferred by some practitioners over typical A-B-C formats, because it can provide similar detail but requires less writing during the data collection process. There also is no need to go through an extra step of reviewing and summarizing the data collected, as data are displayed on the form similar to a scatterplot and are readily available for inspection and interpretation.

Figure 5 presents an example of an FAO form that was used to collect data for Alicia during the same time periods and situations presented in Figure 4. The time periods are represented by the horizontal rows and are labeled with the different activities. The sections across the top of the form and related columns present spaces to record the occurrence of particular behaviors, different types of antecedent or predictor events, the perceived function that the behaviors were serving for the person, and the actual consequences that were provided. The far right column presents space for making notes or comments and for indicating (by use of initials) who was watching and recording data during different time periods.

Each episode of Alicia's aggressive behavior is represented by a number. The same number is used across the chart for a particular episode to indicate which behaviors occurred, the relevant antecedents and perceived functions, and the actual consequences. For example, during Episode 1, which occurred during small-group activity time, Alicia hit another student with her hand or fist and also hit a student with some type of object (e.g., book, ruler). The identified antecedent or predictor was a demand or request that was presented to Alicia. The perceived function of the aggression was to escape from the demand or request. As a consequence, Alicia was sent to sit in the corner. Each subsequent incident was recorded in a similar fashion by using successive numbers (2–14). As each episode was recorded, that number was crossed off in the Events row at

Functional Assessment Observation Form

Name: Alicia J.

Starting Date: 10/11/96   Ending Date: 10/12/96

Behaviors			Predictors						Perceived Functions								Actual Conseq.	

Behaviors: Hit/Kick others | Hit w/object | Demand/Request

Predictors: Difficult Task | Transitions | Interruption | Alone (no attention)

Perceived Functions — Get/Obtain: Attention | Desired Item/Activity | Self-Stimulation | Demand/Request; Escape/Avoid: Activity (/) | Person | Other/Don't Know

Actual Consequences: Redirect | Sit in corner

Comments: (if nothing happened in period) Write initials

Time	Hit/Kick others	Hit w/object	Demand/Request	Difficult Task	Transitions	Interruption	Alone (no attention)	Attention	Desired Item/Activity	Self-Stimulation	Demand/Request	Activity	Person	Other/Don't Know	Redirect	Sit in corner	Comments
Circle 8:00	1 8 / 2 9 / 3																P.O.
Small Grp. 8:15	1		1 8 / 2 9 / 3						1 8 / 2 9 / 3						8 1 / 2 9 / 3		P.O.
Bath-room 8:45																	J.A.
Small Grp. 9:00	4 10 / 11 12		4 10 / 11 12						4 10 / 11 12						10 4 / 12 11		J.A.
Recess 9:30	5 13 / 6 14 / 7					5 13 / 6 14 / 7		5 13 / 6 14 / 7							5 13 / 6 14 / 7		J.A.
Snack 10:00																	P.O.
Story 10:30																	P.O.
Play 11:00																	P.O.
Totals																	

Events: 1 2 3 4 5 6 7 8 9 10 11 12 13 14 15 16 17 18 19 20 21 22 23 24 25

Date: 10/11   10/12

Figure 5.   Example of a functional assessment observation form. (From O'Neill, R.E., et al. [1997]. *Functional assessment and program development for problem behavior: A practical handbook* [2nd ed.]. Belmont, CA: Wadsworth; reprinted by permission.)

the bottom of the form. The Events row and the Date row below it indicate that Episodes 1–7 occurred on October 11. Beginning on October 12, the first episode was recorded using the number 8, which was the next number in the sequence. As indicated, Episodes 8–14 occurred on October 12.

The data recorded over the 2 days provide important information about Alicia's behavior patterns. Her aggressive behavior during small-group activity times (Episodes 1–4 and 8–12) appears to be predicted by teachers asking her to engage in particular tasks or activities, and the apparent function of the behavior is to try to escape the task demands. Sometimes Alicia appears to be successful at producing this outcome, as she is made to sit in the corner away from the group. However, during the recess period the aggressive behavior occurs when she is by herself and not receiving any attention (Episodes 5–7 and 13–14). In this context, the perception is that the behaviors are functioning to recruit attention from others. Again, Alicia appears to be at least somewhat successful at achieving this outcome, as the data indicate that teachers or staff would typically interact with her while redirecting her to a more appropriate activity.

The data from the FAO example illustrate the increased level of detail that can be achieved using this type of format compared with a scatterplot approach. The FAO also does not require as much writing and time for interpretation as other methods (e.g., A-B-C charts). Alicia's data provide a good example of issues that were discussed previously in the chapter, with regard to potential multiple functions of behaviors. It should be ensured that intervention and support strategies were implemented to address both the escape and attention-getting motivations that were evident. For example, teachers could consider making changes in the curricular content or in the way in which task or activity demands were presented to Alicia in the small groups. In addition, she could be taught more appropriate means for requesting a break or an alternate activity, such as using an appropriate sign or gesture. Teaching more appropriate skills for initiating social interactions on the playground also would be necessary to attempt to affect that situation as well. These related types of programming issues and strategies are discussed more thoroughly in Chapter 14.

Many observation formats, including those described previously, are flexible enough to accommodate data collection on a wide range of behavioral and environmental events. Data can be collected on both adaptive communicative behaviors (both conventional and nontypical) and more problematic responses (which also may have communicative functions). Occurrences and characteristics of the physical and social setting that appear to serve as antecedent or consequent events can be recorded in relation to various behaviors. Although such flexibility may preclude the need for separate observational strategies focused solely on communicative behaviors, such formats are available if desired (Beukelman & Mirenda, 1992; Halle et al., 1993; Sigafoos & York, 1991).

The particular type of observation format that is used is not critical as long as it can accurately and validly generate the needed outcome information. Direct observation of communicative and problem behaviors should be used to determine if initial summary statements derived from interview assessment(s) make sense, if they need to be revised or deleted entirely, or if new statements need to be developed to accommodate information collected during the observation process (Carr et al., 1994).

Functional Analysis Manipulations

Functional analysis manipulations involve setting up specific situations to assess the impact of various antecedent situations and consequences on problem behaviors. Sessions are typically conducted in the context of an appropriate experimental design (e.g., a single-subject reversal or multielement design [Poling & Fuqua, 1986]), and systematic observational data are collected. An example of an antecedent manipulation was carried out with Juan, whose primary motivation for yelling and table pounding was suspected to be escaping from more difficult tasks. In Juan's case, specific sessions were arranged, some of which involved presenting more difficult tasks and some of which involved easier or more familiar tasks. If Juan yelled or pounded the table during the session, he was redirected to continue to attempt the tasks. Higher levels of problem behaviors consistently occurred during sessions involving difficult tasks, thereby supporting the summary statement or hypothesis.

Other approaches to functional analyses focus on consequence manipulations. For example, parents and teachers had hypothesized that Sarah's head slapping was maintained by attention from adults and others. During some assessment sessions, Sarah was asked to sit and play by herself while an adult sat nearby and pretended to be engaged in paperwork. If Sarah engaged in head slapping, the adult came over and stopped her, provided brief attention (i.e., "Sarah, please don't do that, you'll hurt yourself"), and then sat back down. During other comparison sessions, the adult engaged Sarah in ongoing play and social interaction. Rates of head slapping were high during sessions in which Sarah received contingent attention and quite low during play sessions, again confirming the initial hypothesis.

There are still other approaches that might include manipulations of both antecedents and consequences. For example, in Juan's case, in addition to the presentation of easy and more difficult tasks, the people working with him could have provided a brief break contingent on his disruptive behavior to help assess the potential escape-motivated properties of his behavior. Additional follow-up analyses also can be helpful in identifying effective intervention strategies, such as teaching communicative replacement behaviors. For example, in Juan's case, following the analysis focusing on task difficulty and escape motivation, additional manipulations could be carried out in which Juan is either provided with unsolicited assistance when he is presented with the difficult tasks or given no additional assistance with the tasks, as before. If the unsolicited assistance produces substantially lower rates of problem behaviors, then teaching Juan an appropriate communicative strategy (e.g., raising a hand, touching an arm, signing) for requesting such assistance is likely to be effective.

The technology for conducting functional analyses is well developed. Such analyses have been shown to be effective in identifying behavioral functions and guiding the implementation of effective interventions (Neef & Iwata, 1994). However, there are a variety of concerns with such approaches. For example, functional analyses have sometimes been conducted in situations that are not very similar to the typical daily situations in which people are involved, which raises concerns about the validity of the results. Conducting effective functional analyses requires substantial expertise and time on the part of those involved (as do many other assessment methods). Safety issues are also a primary concern, as the purpose of the assessment sessions is to attempt to provoke and observe the occurrence of the problem behavior. Ensuring that sessions are conducted so that the target person and support staff are kept safe is a critical consideration. It is important to consider the ethical issues created by the potential risks versus the information that may be obtained (Doss & Reichle, 1991; O'Neill et al., 1997).

There is a substantial need for further research on the comparative validity and reliability of different strategies for obtaining functional assessment information. Often, effective assessments in applied settings (e.g., classrooms, residential settings) can be carried out using informant methods and systematic direct observations. However, in some cases, functional analysis manipulations are necessary to ensure a thorough assessment. In such cases, appropriate guidelines and procedures should be followed (O'Neill et al., 1997). As with direct observations, the results of functional analyses should be used to evaluate the accuracy of initial summary statements and to prompt changes as needed. Conducting a functional assessment is not an end in itself. The entire purpose of the assessment is to serve as a basis for selecting and implementing effective intervention strategies that will make up a behavior support plan. As might be expected, often the assessment process will follow the order that has been described in this section. It will begin with collecting information from relevant people via interviews or other methods. Initial summary statements or hypotheses about various behaviors can then be generated. The validity of these statements is then assessed through systematic direct observation and functional analysis manipulations as needed.

APPLICATIONS TO INDIVIDUALS
EXHIBITING PROBLEM BEHAVIORS AND
NONTYPICAL COMMUNICATIVE REPERTOIRES

Comprehensive behavioral support emphasizes teaching and supporting appropriate communicative behaviors as alternatives to problem behaviors. It is very important that the assessment process provide a clear picture of the apparent communicative functions of targeted problem behaviors, the person's capabilities for exhibiting other conventional or nontypical (but less disruptive) communicative behaviors to serve various functions, the apparent antecedents and maintaining reinforcers for problem and communicative responses, and the person's ability to understand communicative acts produced by others (i.e., how well they respond to communicative initiations; whether they are spoken, signed, written, or involve the use of pictures or other graphics). To more fully illustrate the assessment process, we now return to Carly and James, who were introduced at the beginning of this chapter.

Carly

Carly, a 3-year-old with developmental disabilities, lives at home with her 6-year-old brother and both biological parents. Previous psychological tests have indicated that she has moderate intellectual disabilities. She also experiences low muscle tone in her trunk and upper extremities. Her parents reported that she has difficulty remaining seated or stationary for any length of time. Consequently, she spends a good deal of time wandering during activities and routines at home and in her preschool setting. Carly engages in self-stimulation, such as hand and finger gazing. She frequently tries to push other people (e.g., parents, siblings, teachers) away when they approach her, especially when she is engaged in the self-stimulatory behavior. Carly's nontypical and more conventional communicative behaviors at home and school include loud vocalizations, idiosyncratic gestures, iconic signs, and the use of objects, such as handing a cup to another person when she wants more juice. Her parents indicated it was sometimes difficult to take her on community outings because they felt uncomfortable with her loud vocalizations and self-stimulatory behavior.

Carly attends a private preschool where she is in a class with 11 other students. Although she is the only student with disabilities in her class, other students with disabilities are enrolled in other preschool classrooms at her school. Carly's school routine consists of an open center time, circle time, recess, lunch, and story time. The teacher reported that it is difficult for Carly to join in with the group and that she spent her time wandering, hand and finger gazing, vocalizing, and pushing other students away when they approach her to play. Both Carly's parents and her teacher are concerned with Carly's slow growth in the areas of socialization and communication. They are concerned that she spends too much time engaging in behaviors that prevent her from taking full advantage of the preschool curriculum, spending leisure time opportunities with family members at home, and socializing with students her own age.

Functional assessment interviews (based on O'Neill et al., 1997) were conducted with Carly's parents and her teacher. A summary statement subsequently was developed concerning her behaviors: "When Carly is in a situation that she finds difficult, confusing, or boring, she will wander, gaze at her hands or fingers, or push people away to escape from the situation." When Carly engaged in these behaviors it became difficult for the approaching adult or child to regain Carly's attention and participation. Peers usually became frustrated, which, in turn, shortened or terminated activities. In essence, Carly was able to escape or avoid the activity by engaging in problem behaviors (presumably reinforcing their occurrence). Carly did not appear to have any other viable communicative responses to exhibit in such situations. Instead, she resorted to what had always worked to get her out of these difficult or aversive situations. For Carly, problem behavior served to communicate "This is too hard" or "I don't know what I'm supposed to do." Interview assessments indicated that circle time and choice or center time were the most difficult situations at school, and family television watching and community outings were most problematic at home. The assessment interviews also provided information about other communicative behaviors in Carly's repertoire. Sometimes she used objects in a functional manner, such as handing a cup to an adult to request juice, and vocalized when she appeared to want something that was out of her reach.

Direct observation data were collected by Carly's teacher and other consultants on the occurrence of her behaviors and related environmental events using the functional assessment observation described previously. These observations confirmed that high rates of wandering and self-stimulatory behaviors occurred during circle time and choosing during open centers. Some open center activities required the use of fine motor movements, which Carly likely found difficult due to her lack of upper extremity strength. Carly did not appear to understand the choosing process during open center time and instead wandered from center to center. During circle time the children were required to wait their turn for participation. These turns were unpredictable in length and may have contributed to Carly's confusion and lack of interest. Staff would usually make repeated attempts to engage Carly in activities but would often give up and allow her to wander when she did not respond positively.

Home observations confirmed the reported difficulties when all family members were watching television and during community outings. Carly sat and watched animated videos but was not interested in prime-time television shows. During these, she wandered and gazed at her hands. Family members tried to get Carly to sit with them. These attempts typically involved chasing her several times, then eventually giving up and allowing her to wander. During community outings, problem behaviors occurred before getting in the car, during the ride, and getting out of the car. Carly's behavior interfered with family interactions and completing the outing. After Carly entered community settings (e.g., store, restaurant), her behaviors usually ceased as she apparently became entertained by the activity. Few demands were placed on Carly, except in regard to a few obligatory activities (e.g., eating in a restaurant).

The functional assessment interviews and observations led to a specific hypothesis about Carly's behaviors, which was confirmed both at home and at school. They also provided information about other aspects of Carly's communicative repertoire (e.g., use of objects in a communicative manner). This information provided her parents, teacher, and other interventionists with critical information for designing an effective plan of support to increase her adaptive communicative behaviors and reduce interfering problem behaviors (see Chapter 14 for more details on how this process was carried out).

James

James is a 28-year-old man diagnosed with autism and moderate to severe intellectual disabilities. James produces little or no spoken language, other than immediately repeating words in an apparently echolalic manner. Some apparently communicative behaviors include screaming or whining when he does not feel well or when he wants something he cannot have and pointing to obtain objects out of reach or to draw others' attention to the objects. James has a part-time job at a local university library. He lives on one side of a duplex by himself, with 24-hour one-to-one staff support. This intensive support is necessary because of the severity of James's problem behaviors, which include ritualistic behaviors such as straightening the silverware drawer or demanding that certain items remain in the same place all the time; running away; screaming and whining; assaultive behavior (e.g., hitting, scratching, biting, kicking); pica (i.e., eating inedible objects such as threads from clothing, shredded socks, or torn paper); self-injurious behavior (e.g., head banging on the wall); and property destruction (e.g., tearing his shirts or furniture upholstery, destroying any type of wall hanging). At the time of the initial assessment, James's destructive and assaultive behaviors at work and at home during mealtimes represented the primary concern of staff.

At work, James glues library card pockets in new books and repairs the bindings of old books. James works in 2-hour shifts because that is all his support staff believe he can tolerate. When he arrives at his work area there are usually tall stacks of books waiting. He repairs as many as he can within the 2-hour period. James usually takes one break during his shift. Staff reported that James rips and tears pages from the books. When they try to prevent this property destruction, he escalates to assaultive behaviors and has to be removed from the work setting. As a direct result of his challenging behaviors, James's position at the library is in jeopardy.

Staff reported that at home James had begun dumping food in the trash and ripping open food cartons or containers and scattering food. These episodes also escalate into dangerous assaultive behaviors. Assaultive behaviors usually require the use of brief physical restraint. James's behavior has led to several staff resignations as a result of the labor-intensive effort required in providing him with adequate support.

Functional assessment interviews were completed with James's support staff. Two primary hypotheses emerged from this process. The first hypothesis was "When James is asked to engage in a work activity and is unsure about how long it will last, he will engage in destructive and assaultive behaviors to escape from the activity demands." It appeared that when James walked into the library and saw a large stack of books waiting, it was probably not clear to him how much work he had to do or how long he had to do it. Tearing books or escalating to aggressive behavior effectively stopped the activity or resulted in his removal from the setting. This, in turn, resulted in a brief break or ended the activity completely. Hence, James's problem behaviors were sometimes maintained or reinforced by escaping from an aversive task situation.

A second hypothesis also emerged from the interviews. At home, staff members indicated that James was provided with verbal choices of available food items (e.g., "Do you want spaghetti or chicken for dinner?"). Often, he would repeat the last item named. After receiving this item, he frequently ripped, tore, or dumped it in the trash. Staff developed this hypothesis: "When James does not understand verbal choices offered to him and is presented with a non-preferred food item, he will exhibit destructive and/or assaultive behaviors to reject the initial item and attempt to get another item." James's problem behavior communicated a desire to obtain a different food item, which he apparently was unable to express with conventional spoken language.

Direct observations were conducted by James's support staff and other consultants using procedures described by O'Neill et al. (1997). These observations supported the two initial summary statements. James consistently exhibited destructive and assaultive behaviors at his work setting, which almost always resulted in work being stopped for a period or leaving the setting entirely. Similarly, a substantial proportion of mealtime routines included incidents of destructive and assaultive behaviors after James was given a particular food item to eat. When this occurred, staff often presented other choices of food items to attempt to determine what else, if anything, James wanted to eat.

James's situation is noteworthy in that the functional assessment interviews and observations indicated that his problem behaviors served more than one function. In one type of situation, his challenging behavior appeared to serve the purpose of escaping from aversive activities. In other situations, the same behaviors often resulted in the eventual acquisition of things that he wanted, such as preferred food items. In both instances, James was unable to communicate in more conventional ways, and his problem behaviors were reinforced by escaping from work and by obtaining desired food items. The functional assessment process provided the support staff with vital information for designing a comprehensive, effective support plan, including enhancing James's expressive and receptive communication skills (see Chapter 14 for more details on this process).

EDUCATIONAL/CLINICAL IMPLICATIONS

Conducting comprehensive functional assessments and analyses is a prerequisite step for developing and implementing intervention and support programs for children and adults exhibiting serious problem behaviors and has become an expected professional standard (O'Neill et al., 1997). A number of states (e.g., California, Florida, Minnesota, New York, Oregon, Washington, Utah) have instituted laws or regulations requiring a functional assessment before the implementation of significant behavioral interventions.

The challenge for parents, teachers, and other caregivers is how to use or adapt assessment tools and strategies to be effective in their particular settings and situations. People looking to carry out such assessments can often make use of the types of tools and procedures that have been referenced and described in this chapter. However, it is important not to lose sight that it is the *outcomes* that are critical, not the means for achieving them. People should not hesitate to alter, adapt, or modify forms and procedures to make them maximally useful in particular contexts, as long as they will still be effective in providing the needed information in a valid manner.

DIRECTIONS FOR FUTURE APPLICATION AND RESEARCH

Functional assessment procedures can be useful for a variety of situations and individuals who exhibit a wide range of communicative behaviors, some of which may be more disruptive or problematic than others. Although such assessment procedures have reached a stage of development at which they have much to offer, there are a number of areas that would benefit from further development and research.

One primary area of research need involves studies of the validity and utility of different assessment instruments and procedures, both singly and in combination. For example, different researchers have conducted studies in which the results from the MAS questionnaire (Durand & Crimmins, 1992) have been compared with results from more systematic direct observations and manipulations. Mixed results have been obtained, which indicate that responses on the MAS will not always be a reliable and valid indicator of behavioral functions of problem behaviors (Iwata et al., 1993). The inconsistent reliability and validity of the MAS indicates that researchers and clinicians should attend to the fact that similar instruments will sometimes provide accurate and valid results and to the need for continuing to assess the characteristics of different instruments and procedures to identify which strategies or combinations of strategies will be most helpful in different situations. From a logistical perspective, beginning with relevant informants will usually require less effort and be less time consuming than other approaches. However, following up on such information with more systematic procedures (e.g., direct observations) will usually be necessary to ensure its accuracy and comprehensiveness.

A second area for continued research is the application of functional assessment procedures to individuals with more sophisticated cognitive and communicative skills, such as students labeled as having emotional and behavioral disorders or adults with various diagnoses of mental illnesses (Durand, 1993).

Working with such individuals provides the opportunity to obtain information directly from them. Although this is a tremendous advantage and resource, multiple perspectives and strategies will continue to be important in developing the most valid picture of how a person is functioning and what affects him or her in different settings. Substantial strides have been made in these directions (e.g., Dunlap et al., 1993), but this will remain a vital area for continued research.

A third and final area concerns attention to and understanding of ethnic and cultural influences in the course of the assessment process. Such influences can clearly contribute to a person's perspectives and behavioral repertoires in a variety of ways (Warring, Hunter, & Zirpoli, 1993). Assessment procedures (e.g., interviews, observations) need to take into account and actively seek information about how a person's cultural background may have resulted in or may be maintaining patterns of behavior that are considered problematic by others (e.g., teachers). The incorporation of multicultural perspectives into the functional assessment process is clearly in its infancy and should be a substantial focus for researchers and clinicians.

CONCLUSION

The goal of functional assessment procedures is to obtain information that will enable the development and implementation of effective support plans for individuals. Achieving this goal requires the delineation of a comprehensive package of assessment strategies that involves interviews, direct observation, and environmental manipulations. In implementing assessment strategies, the goal is to formulate a testable hypothesis or hypotheses regarding the function or functions that challenging behavior serves for the individual being assessed.

Careful and thoughtful use of the continuum of assessment strategies described in this chapter dramatically increases the prospective interventionist's capability to design support strategies that can alter antecedents associated with challenging behavior or establish socially acceptable behavior that serves a social function equivalent to that served by challenging behavior. Both of these approaches represent important components of an overall behavioral support strategy (see Chapter 14 for a discussion of this strategy).

This chapter summarized an assessment logic that assumes that most challenging behavior is motivated to obtain more desirable contexts or escape or avoid less desirable contexts. These contexts may be socially driven (the desire to obtain attention) or non–socially driven (the desire to escape the pain of an earache). By carefully deriving function(s), the interventionist dramatically increases the probability that the intervention(s) will be more relevant to both the learner and those who spend time with him or her. Interventionists must continually scrutinize the contexts in which the learner participates in an effort to fine-tune a comprehensive plan of behavioral support. Although determining the function(s) served by problem behavior can be a particularly challenging task, the progress made in developing comprehensive assessment strategies can provide a theoretically sound yet practical initial step for improving the quality of life for people who engage in challenging behavior.

REFERENCES

Albin, R.W., Lucyshyn, J.M., Horner, R.H., & Flannery, K.B. (1996). Contextual fit for behavior support plans: A model for "goodness of fit." In L.K. Koegel, R.L. Koegel, & G. Dunlap (Eds.), *Positive behavioral support: Including people with difficult behavior in the community* (pp. 81–98). Baltimore: Paul H. Brookes Publishing Co.

Bambara, L.M., & Knoster, T.P. (1995). *Guidelines: Effective behavioral support.* Harrisburg: Pennsylvania Department of Education.

Bambara, L.M., Mitchell-Kvacky, N.A., & Iacobelli, S. (1994). Positive behavioral support for students with severe disabilities: An emerging multicomponent approach for addressing challenging behaviors. *School Psychology Review, 23,* 263–278.

Beukelman, D.R., & Mirenda, P. (1992). *Augmentative and alternative communication: Management of severe communication disorders in children and adults.* Baltimore: Paul H. Brookes Publishing Co.

Calculator, S.N., & Bedrosian, J.L. (1988). *Communication assessment and intervention for adults with mental retardation.* Boston: College-Hill Press.

Carr, E.G., Levin, L., McConnachie, G., Carlson, J.I., Kemp, D.C., & Smith, C.E. (1994). *Communication-based intervention for problem behavior: A user's guide for producing positive change.* Baltimore: Paul H. Brookes Publishing Co.

Carr, E.G., & Smith, C.E. (1995). Biological setting events for self-injury. *Mental Retardation and Developmental Disabilities Research Reviews, 1,* 94–98.

Day, H.M., Horner, R.H., & O'Neill, R.E. (1994). Multiple functions of problem behaviors: Assessment and intervention. *Journal of Applied Behavior Analysis, 27,* 279–289.

Doss, L.S., & Reichle, J. (1991). Replacing excess behavior with an initial communication repertoire. In J. Reichle, J. York, & J. Sigafoos (Eds.), *Implementing augmentative and alternative communication: Strategies for learners with severe disabilities* (pp. 215–237). Baltimore: Paul H. Brookes Publishing Co.

Dunlap, G., Ferro, J., & dePerczel, M. (1994). Nonaversive behavioral intervention in the community. In E. Cipani & F. Spooner (Eds.), *Curricular and instructional approaches for persons with severe handicaps* (pp. 117–146). Needham, MA: Allyn & Bacon.

Dunlap, G., Kern, L., dePerczel, M., Clarke, S., Wilson, D., Childs, K.E., White, R., & Falk, G. (1993). Functional analysis of classroom variables for students with emotional and behavioral challenges. *Behavioral Disorders, 18,* 275–291.

Durand, V.M. (1986). Self-injurious behavior as intentional communication. In K.D. Gadow (Ed.), *Advances in learning and behavioral disabilities* (pp. 141–155). Greenwich, CT: JAI Press.

Durand, V.M. (1990). *Severe behavior problems: A functional communication training approach.* New York: Guilford Press.

Durand, V.M. (1993). Functional assessment and functional analysis. In M.D. Smith (Ed.), *Behavior modification for exceptional children and youth* (pp. 38–60). Boston: Andover Medical Publishers.

Durand, V.M., Berotti, D., & Weiner, J.S. (1993). Functional communication training: Factors affecting effectiveness, generalization, and maintenance. In J. Reichle & D.P. Wacker (Eds.), *Communication and language intervention series: Vol. 3. Commu-*

nicative alternatives to challenging behavior: Integrating functional assessment and intervention strategies (pp. 317–340). Baltimore: Paul H. Brookes Publishing Co.

Durand, V.M., & Crimmins, D.B. (1992). *The Motivation Assessment Scale (MAS) administration guide.* Topeka, KS: Monaco & Associates.

Guess, D., & Carr, E.G. (1991). Emergence and maintenance of stereotypy and self-injury. *American Journal on Mental Retardation, 96,* 299–319.

Halle, J.W., Chadsey-Rusch, J., Collett-Klingenberg, J., & Reinoehl, R.B. (1993). *Communication assessment manual.* Unpublished manuscript, University of Illinois at Champaign, Department of Special Education.

Halle, J.W., & Spradlin, J.E. (1993). Identifying stimulus control of challenging behavior: Extending the analysis. In J. Reichle & D.P. Wacker (Eds.), *Communication and language intervention series: Vol. 3. Communicative alternatives to challenging behavior: Integrating functional assessment and intervention strategies* (pp. 83–109). Baltimore: Paul H. Brookes Publishing Co.

Hedeen, D.L., Ayres, B.J., Meyer, L.H., & Waite, J. (1996). Quality inclusive schooling for students with severe behavioral challenges. In D.H. Lehr & F. Brown (Eds.), *People with disabilities who challenge the system* (pp. 127–171). Baltimore: Paul H. Brookes Publishing Co.

Horner, R.H., Close, D.W., Fredericks, H.D.B., O'Neill, R.E., Albin, R.W., Sprague, J.R., Kennedy, C.H., Flannery, K.B., & Heathfield, L.T. (1996). Supported living for people with profound disabilities and severe problem behaviors. In D.H. Lehr & F. Brown (Eds.), *People with disabilities who challenge the system* (pp. 209–240). Baltimore: Paul H. Brookes Publishing Co.

Horner, R.H., Dunlap, G., Koegel, R.L., Carr, E.G., Sailor, W., Anderson, J., Albin, R.W., & O'Neill, R.E. (1990). Toward a technology of "nonaversive" behavioral support. *Journal of The Association for Persons with Severe Handicaps, 15,* 125–132.

Horner, R.H., Vaughn, B.J., Day, H.M., & Ard, W.R., Jr. (1996). The relationship between setting events and problem behavior: Expanding our understanding of behavioral support. In L.K. Koegel, R.L. Koegel, & G. Dunlap (Eds.), *Positive behavioral support: Including people with difficult behavior in the community* (pp. 381–402). Baltimore: Paul H. Brookes Publishing Co.

Iwata, B.A., Pace, G.M., Dorsey, M.F., Zarcone, J.R., Vollmer, T.R., Smith, R.G., Rodgers, T.A., Lerman, D.C., Shore, B.A., Mazaleski, J.L., Han-Leong, G., Cowdery, G.E., Kalsher, M.J., McCosh, K.C., & Willis, K.D. (1994). The functions of self-injurious behavior: An experimental-epidemiological analysis. *Journal of Applied Behavior Analysis, 27,* 215–240.

Iwata, B.A., Vollmer, T.R., Zarcone, J.R., & Rodgers, T.A. (1993). Treatment classification and selection based on behavioral function. In R. Van Houten & S. Axelrod (Eds.), *Behavior analysis and treatment* (pp. 101–125). New York: Plenum.

Kern, L., Dunlap, G., Clarke, S., & Childs, K.E. (1994). Student-assisted functional assessment interview. *Diagnostique, 19,* 29–39.

Koegel, L.K., Koegel, R.L., & Dunlap, G. (Eds.). (1996). *Positive behavioral support: Including people with difficult behavior in the community.* Baltimore: Paul H. Brookes Publishing Co.

Lennox, D.B., & Miltenberger, R. (1989). Conducting a functional assessment of problem behavior in applied settings. *Journal of The Association for Persons with Severe Handicaps, 14,* 304–311.

McLean, J., & Snyder-McLean, L. (1988). Application of pragmatics to severely retarded children and youth. In R.L. Schiefelbusch & L.L. Lloyd (Eds.), *Language perspectives: Acquisition, retardation, and intervention* (pp. 255–288). Austin, TX: PRO-ED.

Meyer, L.H., & Evans, I.M. (1993). Meaningful outcomes in behavioral intervention: Evaluating positive approaches to the remediation of challenging behaviors. In J. Reichle & D.P. Wacker (Eds.), *Communication and language intervention series: Vol. 3. Communication alternatives to challenging behavior: Integrating functional assessment and intervention strategies* (pp. 407–428). Baltimore: Paul H. Brookes Publishing Co.

National Institutes of Health (NIH). (1991). *Treatment of destructive behaviors in persons with developmental disabilities* (NIH Publication No. 91-2410). Bethesda, MD: U.S. Department of Health and Human Services.

Neef, N.A., & Iwata, B.A. (Eds.). (1994). Special issue on functional analysis approaches to assessment and treatment. *Journal of Applied Behavior Analysis, 27,* 196–420.

Nyhan, W.L. (1994). The Lesch-Nyhan disease. In T. Thompson & D.B. Gray (Eds.), *Destructive behavior in developmental disabilities* (pp. 181–197). Beverly Hills: Sage Publications.

O'Neill, R.E., Horner, R.H., Albin, R.W., Sprague, J.R., Storey, K., & Newton, J.S. (1997). *Functional assessment and program development for problem behavior: A practical handbook* (2nd ed.). Belmont, CA: Wadsworth.

Poling, A., & Fuqua, R.W. (Eds.). (1986). *Research methods in applied behavior analysis.* New York: Plenum.

Reichle, J. (1991a). Defining the decisions involved in designing and implementing augmentative and alternative communication systems. In J. Reichle, J. York, & J. Sigafoos (Eds.), *Implementing augmentative and alternative communication: Strategies for learners with severe disabilities* (pp. 39–60). Baltimore: Paul H. Brookes Publishing Co.

Reichle, J. (1991b). Describing initial communicative intents. In J. Reichle, J. York, & J. Sigafoos (Eds.), *Implementing augmentative and alternative communication: Strategies for learners with severe disabilities* (pp. 71–88). Baltimore: Paul H. Brookes Publishing Co.

Reichle, J., & Johnston, S. (1993). Replacing challenging behavior: The role of communication intervention. *Topics in Language Disorders, 13,* 61–76.

Reichle, J., & Wacker, D.P. (Eds.). (1993). *Communication and language intervention series: Vol. 3. Communicative alternatives to challenging behavior: Integrating functional assessment and intervention strategies.* Baltimore: Paul H. Brookes Publishing Co.

Schroeder, S.R., & Tessel, R. (1994). Dopaminergic and serotonergic mechanisms in self-injury and aggression. In T. Thompson & D.B. Gray (Eds.), *Destructive behavior in developmental disabilities* (pp. 198–210). Beverly Hills: Sage Publications.

Sigafoos, J., & York, J. (1991). Using ecological inventories to promote functional communication. In J. Reichle, J. York, & J. Sigafoos (Eds.), *Implementing augmentative and alternative communication: Strategies for learners with severe disabilities* (pp. 61–70). Baltimore: Paul H. Brookes Publishing Co.

Sprague, J.R., & Horner, R.H. (1992). Covariations within functional response classes: Implications for treatment of severe problem behavior. *Journal of Applied Behavior Analysis, 25,* 735–745.

Thompson, T., Egli, M., Symons, F., & Delaney, D. (1994). Neurobehavioral mechanisms of drug action in developmental disabilities. In T. Thompson & D.B. Gray (Eds.), *Destructive behavior in developmental disabilities* (pp. 133–180). Beverly Hills: Sage Publications.

Touchette, P.E., MacDonald, R.F., & Langer, S.N. (1985). A scatterplot for identifying stimulus control of problem behavior. *Journal of Applied Behavior Analysis, 18,* 343–351.

Turnbull, A.P., & Turnbull, H.R., III. (1996). Group action planning as a strategy for pro-viding comprehensive family support. In L.K. Koegel, R.L. Koegel, & G. Dunlap (Eds.), *Positive behavioral support: Including people with difficult behavior in the community* (pp. 99–114). Baltimore: Paul H. Brookes Publishing Co.

Warring, D.F., Hunter, S.M., & Zirpoli, T.J. (1993). Cultural influences on behavior. In T.J. Zirpoli & K.J. Melloy (Eds.), *Behavior management: Applications for parents and teachers* (pp. 471–514). Columbus, OH: Charles E. Merrill.

14

Comprehensive Behavioral Support

Application and Intervention

Glen Dunlap, Bobbie J. Vaughn, and Robert O'Neill

COMPREHENSIVE BEHAVIORAL SUPPORT IS A broad-based, multifaceted endeavor that is spawned by a commitment to the well-being and personal development of individuals with difficult behaviors, initiated through a process of functional assessment, and manifested by the implementation of a thorough plan of individualized intervention and support strategies. Whereas the previous chapter describes the essential features of the assessment process, this chapter focuses on the principal characteristics and procedures that compose components of a comprehensive intervention plan. The chapter begins with a discussion of the linkage between assessment and behavioral support strategies and with a review of the fundamental considerations in developing comprehensive support plans. The chapter also describes behavioral support components, including contextual and antecedent manipulations, and the development of functional alternatives to challenging behavior that include repertoires of functional communication. Subsequent sections include discussions of other support components as well as some concluding points regarding perspectives in assessment and intervention for difficult behaviors.

BASIC CONSIDERATIONS IN COMPREHENSIVE BEHAVIORAL SUPPORT

Developing support plans that are effective and optimally responsive to an individual's needs and characteristics requires careful attention to functional assessment data (Horner, O'Neill, & Flannery, 1993). To a large extent, the effectiveness of behavioral support is dependent on the scope and validity of

Preparation of this chapter was supported by three projects funded by the U.S. Department of Education: 1) Cooperative Agreement No. H133B2004 from the National Institute on Disability and Rehabilitation Research (NIDRR); 2) Field-Initiated Research Project No. H133G60119, also from NIDRR; and 3) Outreach Project No. H024D40006-95 from the Office of Special Education and Rehabilitative Services (OSERS). The opinions expressed are those of the authors, and no official endorsement by the U.S. Department of Education should be inferred.

the assessment data. Also important is the degree to which intervention plans are linked to the assessment data. This linkage implies that a capacity to obtain individualized assessment data and then tailor support plans to that assessment-based understanding is a central consideration of effective behavioral support (Horner, O'Neill, et al., 1993).

As Chapter 13 discusses, a functional assessment of problem behavior provides a breadth of information, which includes ideas about the operant functions of the behavior and messages about the individual's environment. With regard to the latter, problem behaviors can be interpreted as signals that an irritation is present in the context of the environment. The assessment process should be fairly specific in identifying the source of the irritation, whether it be a particular state of deprivation (e.g., a lack of sleep) or the presence of a discomforting stimulus (O'Neill, Horner, Albin, Storey, & Sprague, 1990). When the source is identified, a logical linkage from assessment to intervention is suggested; that is, the context can be modified through antecedent manipulations so that deprivation does not occur or so that the provoking event (e.g., teacher demand) is removed or ameliorated. This chapter later reviews the role of environmental context and various antecedent strategies that compose an important element of behavioral support.

The other clear message provided by a functional assessment involves the operant or communicative purpose of the problem behavior (Carr & Durand, 1985a, 1985b). Because the majority of problem behaviors can be viewed constructively as communicative acts that are maintained because they effect influence on the social environment, a crucial objective of the assessment process is to determine the intended function. When the function is distinguished, identifying an alternative communicative form (behavior) that can be established in lieu of the problem behavior (Carr et al., 1994; Doss & Reichle, 1991; Durand, 1990) becomes important. This instructional component of behavioral support is entirely dependent on the thoroughness of the assessment process. The process of functional assessment should result in the delineation of the specific communicative function of the problem behavior as well as features that can help in selecting the most reasonable form to develop as the functional alternative.

In addition to its linkage to the functional assessment process, comprehensive behavioral support is proactive, that is, its emphasis is placed during those times when problem behaviors are not occurring. The goal of comprehensive behavioral support is to *prevent* difficult behaviors from occurring by developing functional competencies (e.g., effective communications) and by creating an internal and external environment and lifestyle that are conducive to socially acceptable repertoires of behavior. Comprehensive behavioral support is an educative approach (Evans & Meyer, 1985) that achieves much of its power through personal empowerment and the establishment of functional skills. Comprehensive behavioral support also is distinguished by its explicit insistence that interventions and assistance be as typical as possible. Furthermore, all efforts to produce change should be conducted with full respect for the rights and dignity of all participants (especially the person who is the focus of the support program).

Behavioral Support Plans

Comprehensive behavioral support consists of strategies aimed at reducing problem behaviors while enhancing a person's quality of life. Enhancing quality of life includes opportunities to make choices, participate in a range of desirable and constructive activities, and engage in meaningful social interactions. A behavioral support plan specifies the results of the functional assessment, articulates objectives, presents the intervention and support components, identifies the roles and responsibilities of members of the support team, and lays out the procedures for monitoring, evaluating, and adjusting the plan. The behavioral support plan can be fairly complex with a large number of support strategies, or it can be relatively simple. In general, the intervention components found in behavioral support plans tend to cluster within categories that include the following:

- Setting factors, in which steps are taken to remediate health and medical problems and/or distal events that have been linked to problem behaviors
- Antecedent and contextual manipulations, in which changes are made to stimuli and stimulus combinations that have been implicated as being associated with high rates of problem behavior
- Functional communication training and other skill development, in which skills are taught that enhance a person's capacity to control his or her environment with a focus on developing communicative responses that serve the same function as the targeted problem behavior
- Reinforcement contingencies that ensure adequate levels and appropriate schedules of reinforcement are provided
- Self-management, in which instruction is designed to assist the person in controlling his or her own behavior
- Emergency (reactive) procedures, in which specific strategies are enacted to ensure that destructive episodes are concluded safely and as rapidly as possible
- Strategies to enhance lifestyles, in which efforts are made to support expanded and more meaningful relationships, work experiences, domestic routines, and other aspects of a person's life

In addition to these broad categories, there are systems issues, family support considerations, staff training, and assignment of appropriate personnel that can be incorporated in a support plan.

Despite attention to comprehensive behavioral support plans (Horner, O'Neill, et al., 1993; Horner, Sprague, & Flannery, 1993), there is not yet a specific, validated protocol for identifying intervention components and describing operational steps for implementation. Nevertheless, a number of considerations have emerged as important elements in support plan construction. Four of these considerations are discussed.

Develop Support Plans in the Context of Existing Goals and Activities
Behavioral support plans should not be isolated documents that do not relate to other aspects of a person's life. Rather, support plans should be fully integrated and consistent with individualized education programs, habilitation plans, and other descriptions of objectives and approaches. In this respect, comprehensive behavioral support is notably different from other forms of behavior management, in which the control of problem behavior was viewed as an endeavor distinct from educational and lifestyle considerations.

Personal futures planning (Kincaid, 1996; Mount, 1987; O'Brien, Mount, & O'Brien, 1991) provides a context that is especially valuable and congruent with the development of behavioral support plans. In Personal Futures Planning, a person's preferences, ambitions, strengths, and challenges are discussed by the person and his or her friends, family, and supporters in an effort to create a vision, direction, and actions that will result in a desirable and enhanced lifestyle. In many cases, the successful development and execution of a personal futures plan can accomplish many of the objectives of behavioral support. The interrelationships are substantial: An essential objective of behavioral support is to improve a person's lifestyle, and an improved lifestyle can reduce problem behaviors (Turnbull & Turnbull, 1990).

Design Support Plans in Partnership with the Person's Support Providers
When behavioral support programs fail, often it is because they are not implemented with adequate fidelity. A lack of fidelity is apt to occur when the programmatic requirements are incompatible with the investment, attitudes, values, resources, and routines that characterize the support providers and environments in which the program needs to be implemented (Albin, Lucyshyn, Horner, & Flannery, 1996). Albin and his colleagues described these issues as matters of "contextual fit" and argued that it is crucial for support plans to be designed with pervasive sensitivity to the individual and contextual constraints that occur in home, school, and community settings.

One strategy to help ensure contextual fit is to include all pertinent support providers (e.g., family, teachers) in the process of developing the support plan (Albin et al., 1996). By including these individuals as partners and collaborators, there is an increased likelihood that the plan will be feasible and consistent with existing contingencies and routines. It is important that the key personnel demonstrate a commitment to, and investment in, the success of the effort (Eno-Hieneman & Dunlap, in press). Although the process of full collaboration can be time consuming, the success of the program, especially in complex and intransigent circumstances, can depend on relevant input from those individuals who will be responsible for integrating the procedures into the context of their daily routines.

Derive Support Plans from the Process of Functional Assessment The process of functional assessment yields information regarding the probable purpose of the problem behavior and the specific circumstances under which the problem behavior is most and least likely to occur (O'Neill et al., 1990; Repp & Karsh, 1994). As Chapter 13 describes, this information enables the development of hypotheses or statements that summarize the best understanding of the function of the behavior. A number of authors have indicated that the elements of support plans should be hypothesis driven (e.g., Dunlap & Kern, 1993; Horner, O'Neill, & Flannery, 1993; Repp, Felce, & Barton, 1988; Repp & Karsh, 1994), and there is extensive evidence to support the value of assessment-based intervention plans (Koegel, Koegel, & Dunlap, 1996; Repp & Horner, in press).

Include Strategies for Rearranging Activity Patterns Associated with Problem Behavior One element that should be included in support plans in most circumstances involves the rearrangement of antecedent and reinforcing stimuli that occur within activities associated with problem behaviors (O'Neill et al., 1990). The support plan should describe specific ways in which the activity patterns can be rearranged by changing antecedent stimuli, developing new behaviors, and modifying the consequences.

Horner and colleagues (Horner & Billingsley, 1988; Horner, O'Neill, & Flannery, 1993) suggested a competing behaviors framework that offers a strategy for developing interventions from functional assessment data. The basic idea behind this framework is that alternative behaviors can compete successfully with existing problem behaviors if the relevant activity pattern is analyzed accurately and suitable adjustments are made to the antecedent stimuli and reinforcement schedules. The framework incorporates principles of functional equivalence, stimulus control, and setting events (i.e., events that alter the value of available reinforcers or punishers) (Gardner, Cole, Davidson, & Karan, 1984; Horner, Vaughn, Day, & Ard, 1996; Wahler & Graves, 1983) in a model designed to facilitate the construction of efficient and effective support plans.

The greatest challenge in building a comprehensive support plan is putting together an individualized, assessment-based program of support that is fashioned to meet the unique characteristics of the person with challenging behavior and the environments in which the individual operates. The following sections of this chapter discuss some of the numerous intervention components that can be considered as part of a support plan.

THE ROLE OF CONTEXT:
REARRANGING THE ANTECEDENT ENVIRONMENT

As Chapter 13 describes, antecedent stimulus and setting events are environmental phenomena that occur before or concurrent with a person's behavior and have an influence over the occurrence of the behavior. These events can be observable in the environment or they can be internal, physiological circumstances, such as fatigue or head pain. Some discrete events can be categorized as directly evoking a behavior (such events are identified as being discriminative for the behavior and are referred to as stimulus events), whereas other events are interpreted as contributing to the probability that a behavior will be produced (these are referred to as setting events). Often it is a combination of events that produces the behavior. For example, repeating an unpleasant demand might be responsible for an escape-related tantrum, but it might be best understood as a contribution to a complex and conditional instigation. If the demand is repeated only 4 or 5 times, the tantrum might not occur; however, if it is repeated more than 20 times, the probability of a tantrum is increased tremendously. The probability is heightened even further if the individual is tired, disturbed over a contentious social interaction, or suffering from a toothache (Horner et al., 1996). A challenge for behavioral support providers is to understand how these antecedent influences interact and combine to affect behavior.

An outcome of the functional assessment process is the identification of antecedent and contextual events that are associated with occurrences and nonoccurrences of problem behaviors (Doss & Reichle, 1991; O'Neill et al., 1990; Reichle, Halle, & Johnston, 1993). In particular, the assessment should implicate the antecedent stimulus and setting events that indicate a high probability of the problem behavior, and stimulus and setting events that are associated with an absence of the problem behavior (O'Neill et al., 1990). If the functional assessment is successful in specifying stimulus events, it may be possible to control or prevent the occurrence of the problem behavior. Such control can be achieved by removing or ameliorating those stimuli that are associated with the presence of the problem behavior and presenting those stimuli that are associated with the behavior's absence.

When an assessment identifies a stimulus or setting event, the event's offending features should be examined. For example, with an individual who has been observed to escape when requests are delivered, the actions requested may be excessively difficult, repetitive, painful, or noxious in some other manner. If the undesired features of requests can be detected, then adjustments in the stimulus presentations can be made (Horner et al., 1996). At other times, it might not be possible to identify the particular stimulus features responsible for occasioning the behavior. For example, when proximity of a particular peer or caregiver is associated with problem behavior, it may not be possible to identify the specific personal features that provoke the behavior. Whether the particular features can be detected, it is often possible and reasonable to remove the event from an individual's environment so that the problem behavior that had been evoked by the event no longer occurs (Horner et al., 1996).

An important aspect of behavioral support that has been exposed to systematic analysis involves the removal or amelioration of setting events (Horner et al., 1996) or establishing operations (Michael, 1982, 1993). In particular, internal factors (e.g., illness), discomfort arising from ecological variables (e.g., excessive noise, humidity), and events that occur before the target behavior (e.g., a fight with a sibling) are more frequently implicated as maintaining features influencing problem behavior (Dadson & Horner, 1993; Horner et al., 1996). An expectation of comprehensive behavioral support is that there is a sensitivity to such influences and that efforts are taken to eliminate or alleviate their impact. For example, if fatigue is an issue, steps can be taken to improve the person's sleep patterns, ensure that rest periods are available, and reschedule the most demanding or effortful activities so that they occur when fatigue is minimal. Similarly, efforts can be made to ensure that an individual is free from physiological pain and that anxiety-evoking circumstances are minimized.

When specific events or circumstances are identified as occasioning problem behavior, it is often possible to simply remove them from the person's environment. For example, problem behaviors in school often occur in the context of a particular activity. Upon examination, the activity may be inappropriate or unnecessary. In such situations, the problem behaviors can be eliminated by discarding the activity. If the activities are judged to be essential, the aversive qualities of the activity can often be ameliorated by infusing the activity with features that are preferred by the student (e.g., Clarke et al., 1995; Dunlap, Foster-Johnson, Clarke, Kern, & Childs, 1995; Dunlap & Kern, 1993; Foster-Johnson, Ferro, & Dunlap, 1994; Kern & Dunlap, in press). For example, an elementary school student with multiple disabilities was observed engaging in extraordinary amounts of disruptive behavior during fine motor exercises, but her disruptions were virtually eliminated when the activity was changed from the standard exercises conducted with the whole class to preparing drawings and cutouts for her personal photograph album. Dunlap and Kern (1993), Halle and Spradlin (1993), Horner et al. (1996), and Munk and Repp (1994) described various ways for removing or modifying stimuli to reduce problem behaviors.

It also is useful to consider ways to promote desirable behavior by presenting stimulus events that are associated with periods of appropriate responding. There usually are caregivers, teachers, or peers who occasion positive patterns of behavior. It may be possible to schedule the presence of these individuals so that they contribute to improved behavior during extended periods of time or during particularly challenging circumstances. Similarly, the process of functional assessment might identify other activities or stimuli, often idiosyncratic, that are discriminative for desirable behavior (Horner, Day, Sprague, O'Brien, & Heathfield, 1991). The presence or presentation of these stimuli can be a helpful adjunct to behavioral support efforts.

The use of antecedent and contextual manipulations can have powerful and rapid effects on the occurrence of problem behavior. A comprehensive, multifaceted, and assessment-based revision of antecedent circumstances has produced extensive and long-lasting benefits (Dunlap, Kern-Dunlap, Clarke, & Robbins, 1991; Kern, Childs, Dunlap, Clarke, & Falk, 1994). However, antecedent manipulations, by themselves, do not result in changes that can be expected to generalize across all settings or circumstances, and they do not provide new repertoires of competent performance that are necessary for lifelong lifestyle benefits. Therefore, comprehensive behavioral support should include strategies to teach a repertoire of skills that compete with the forms comprising a repertoire of problem behavior.

TEACHING: ESTABLISHING FUNCTIONAL COMMUNICATION

An outcome of the assessment process is an understanding of the maintaining consequences (i.e., reinforcers) of the problem behavior, and a vital implication of this understanding is that it leads to an instructional prescription. This implication comes from the concepts of response classes and functional equivalence (Carr, 1988). From an operant conceptualization, a problem behavior is strengthened and is maintained by a reinforcer. The function of the target behavior is to obtain the reinforcer. It is possible for that reinforcer to operate on various forms of behaviors. The group of these various topographies, governed by the same specific function (i.e., reinforcer), is known as a response class. All members of the response class function to secure the same reinforcer. Thus, the acts of throwing a dinner plate, engaging in a tantrum, and calmly requesting to be excused from the table are three members of the response class that produce the reinforcer of leaving (i.e., escaping from) the dinner table. These different behaviors are said to be functionally equivalent because, even though their forms are dissimilar, their functions (i.e., reinforcers) are identical.

A crucial aspect of functional equivalence is that, within a response class, some behaviors may be considered undesirable and antagonistic to optimal development, whereas other members of the same class may be socially and developmentally adaptive. Asking in a calm manner to be excused is a request form that is likely to be cherished by a child's parents; throwing dinner plates and engaging in tantrums are apt to be condemned. Another aspect of functional equivalence that is important in providing behavioral support is the inverse relationship among competing response class members. An increase in the occurrence of one member of the response class often will produce a decrease in other members. If requesting in a calm manner increases in frequency, throwing items and having tantrums will decrease. This covarying relationship between members of a response class has been demonstrated powerfully and frequently in the literature on functional communication training (Carr & Durand, 1985a; Durand & Carr, 1987; Sprague & Horner, 1992).

Functional communication training is a procedure based on the notion of functional equivalence and the perspective that interprets the functions of target behaviors as communicative (Carr et al., 1994; Donnellan, Mirenda, Mesaros, & Fassbender, 1984; Durand, 1990). That is, problem behaviors (e.g., engaging in a tantrum at the dinner table) are viewed as communicative acts that are functionally equivalent to alternative and more conventional members of the same response class, such as calm requesting (Durand & Crimmins, 1988). In a seminal study that established the validity of this framework, Carr and Durand (1985a) demonstrated the presence of individualized functions of children's problem behaviors. They showed that some of the children's behaviors were exhibited to solicit attention, whereas other behaviors were intended to terminate task demands. Subsequently, the authors taught the children to attain the same objectives (i.e., attention or escape) by employing more desirable forms of communication (e.g., speech). As the children used their alternative request forms, their problem behaviors subsided. Carr and Durand (1985a) referred to their procedure as functional communication training, and it has been shown in a large number of studies to be effective with a variety of target behaviors in diverse circumstances (e.g., Bird, Dores, Moniz, & Robinson, 1989; Carr & Kemp, 1989; Durand & Carr, 1991, 1992; Durand & Crimmins, 1988; Horner & Budd, 1985; Horner, Sprague, O'Brien, & Heathfield, 1990; Wacker et al., 1990).

Since the mid-1980s, there has been substantial research produced on functional communication training. This research has extended the range of behaviors and populations to which functional communication training has been applied, and it has addressed principles and parameters of assessment and implementation that relate to the effectiveness of the procedure. The impact of these investigations cannot be depicted adequately in this chapter; however, there are some considerations that merit attention. One issue pertains to the communicative form that is to be selected as a functionally equivalent alternative to the undesirable target behavior. Several authors (e.g., Doss & Reichle, 1991; Durand, 1990; Durand, Berotti, & Weiner, 1993) have provided helpful guidelines. One consideration is that the selected response should already be in the person's repertoire, or it should be extremely easy to develop (Reichle et al., 1993). First, if the response form is to replace the existing target behavior or strengthen existing communicative alternatives, it must be able to be produced readily, fluently, and spontaneously (Carr, Robinson, Taylor, & Carlson, 1990). Second, the response should require less effort to produce than the existing target behavior (Horner & Day, 1991). If a choice is to made about which communicative form to employ (e.g., a tantrum versus a spoken request), the selection could be based on the relative magnitude of physical or cognitive effort that is required to respond (Carr et al., 1990). Thus, other factors being equal, a one-word utterance would be more readily performed than a multiple-element sentence. Finally, it is important to select a form that will be comprehended by all members of the social environment to whom the communication might be directed (Carr et al., 1990). A gesture can be an appropriate form for a prelinguistic individual; however, it would be important for the gesture to be a salient expression and to have a generally understood meaning so that the message would be immediately detected and honored. Functional communication training cannot be successful unless the alternative, desirable form is effective in procuring the reinforcer at least as expediently as the existing behavior that is to be replaced (Carr et al., 1990).

OTHER COMPONENTS IN
COMPREHENSIVE BEHAVIORAL SUPPORT

Comprehensive behavioral support plans frequently include elements that are in addition to antecedent manipulations and the development of functional communicative alternatives to problem behaviors. This section delineates some of these principal categories of support components.

Positive Reinforcement

Although the promotion of educational and comprehensive approaches to behavioral support has tended to reduce the dominance of positive reinforcement as a distinct component of support programs, it remains a central principle and a crucial procedural ingredient. A major purpose of functional assessment is to identify a person's strongest reinforcers (O'Neill et al., 1990), and the concept of a behavioral function is directly translatable into traditional terms of reinforcement. The effective deployment of functional communication training can be described accurately as the skillful implementation of revised contingencies of reinforcement or the differential reinforcement of alternative responses. In a broader sense, the selective application of positive reinforcement is the essential vehicle through which all people learn the conditions under when and when not to use new communicative behaviors.

Positive reinforcement represents a distinct category of behavioral support because, in many cases, there is simply inadequate reinforcement in a person's environment to support desirable repertoires of behavior. Therefore, an important intervention strategy can be to infuse enrichment into these targeted environments by providing enhanced schedules of contingent or noncontingent reinforcement (Horner, 1980; Vollmer, Marcus, & Ringdahl, 1995). An additional consideration that has been discussed extensively yet continues to be a problem for many people in many settings is the assessment and identification of reinforcing stimuli. Two common concerns are pertinent. First, it is often the case that an impression of preference is regarded as equivalent to reinforcement. However, reinforcement is defined only on the basis of its effects on a behavior. Preference does not necessarily imply that a stimulus will function as a reinforcer. The second common mistake is to refer to reinforcement in procedural rather than functional terms. This error represents a core deficiency in many ineffective support efforts. As many authors have demonstrated (Dyer, 1987, 1989; Fisher et al., 1992), the identification and use of positive reinforcers can sometimes require a careful, systematic, and individualized process to be successful.

Reactive Procedures

When the behavior that is targeted for reduction is severe or intense enough that it poses a threat to the safety of the person or to others, support plans should include a clear description of procedures to contain and curtail the behavior while protecting all people from harm. These plans are sometime crisis management or emergency procedures. They are not inte intervention but are intended to deescalate and stabilize the situa tiously as possible. In cases in which the behavior constitutes a risk of harm, is important that reactive procedures be described in detail and that they include staff and other caregivers who are trained in appropriate emergency techniques.

In circumstances in which the undesirable behavior does not constitute a danger to people or property, instances of problem behavior can be ignored or regarded as an instructional opportunity. It is often fruitful to consider the occurrence of the problem behavior as an error and, thus, as an ideal time to provide correction in the form of a prompt (i.e., to produce the preferred mode of communication) and reinforcement following the desired communicative response. Although this is a viable strategy, the presentation of correction following the problem behavior must be used judiciously as it may reinforce the problem behavior. In other words, prompting may create a behavior chain in which problem behavior is followed by correction, a more desirable response form, and then reinforcement. The risk is that the reinforcer will increase the repetition of the entire chain rather than just the corrected performance. Furthermore, addressing problem behaviors as errors is an approach that assumes that a functional communication strategy has been developed and incorporated in the support plan.

Lifestyle Considerations

Although lifestyle considerations are presented in this chapter as a broad component of comprehensive behavioral support, this presentation runs the risk of doing a disservice to its true status. Lifestyle considerations are predominant variables that influence every aspect of a person's existence, including the presence or absence of significant problem behaviors. This group of issues is included in the discussion as a general element because it is important to explicitly consider these factors when developing and implementing plans for behavior support. Lifestyle considerations refer to a person's social life; the settings that a person inhabits; the activities that a person engages in at home, school, work, and in the community; and the extent to which the person has access to preferences, choices, and self-determination (Horner, Albin, & O'Neill, 1991). Important in this set of considerations are the person's interpersonal relationships and the extent to which a person experiences the multiple functions provided by interpersonal contact.

Deficiencies in a person's lifestyle can be a major factor in the occurrence of depression and in the likelihood of problem behaviors. There are times when substantial changes in a person's lifestyle should be the foremost ingredient of behavioral support. For some people, a change in residence, the active development of new friends, a change in jobs or classrooms, or an entry into a new hobby can be a decisive element in behavioral routines (Turnbull & Turnbull, 1990).

Other Skill Development

Although this chapter focuses on functional communication training and communication-based instruction as key components in behavioral support, other skill development also can be valuable to comprehensive programs of behavioral support. In general, the more competencies a person has available to have access to reinforcers and control his or her surroundings, the less problem behavior should be present (Dunlap, Johnson, & Robbins, 1990). Although there is an array of potential skills that can facilitate a person's social and community adaptation, some of the skills that may be most pertinent for behavioral support include self-management (Koegel, Frea, & Surratt, 1994) and leisure skills (Dattilo, 1991). Self-management, including self-monitoring, has been demonstrated to be useful in producing and maintaining reductions in a variety of difficult behaviors (Koegel & Koegel, 1990; Koegel et al., 1994; Koegel, Koegel, Hurley, & Frea, 1992), and leisure skills can be extremely important in developing social connections and in self-amusement for occupying oneself in an enjoyable and satisfying manner (Dattilo, 1991). Self-management techniques usually establish a performance criteria (e.g., behaviors, tasks, steps within a routine), often followed by a reinforcer for meeting performance criteria. This is usually recorded independently by the person with disabilities. Self-management builds self-efficacy because it is easy to see accomplishments and it offers a visual representation of the performance criteria (e.g., picture or orthographic representation) and of the reinforcer for accomplishing the criteria. Self-management also increases personal independence, decreases reliance on others, and promotes increased tolerance for delay of reinforcers.

The increase in leisure skills usually signifies more physical and social inclusion in school and community activities. It implies that activity preference and choice may occur as a result of the increase in leisure routines. This enhances overall quality of life and may effect decreases in problem behavior as a result of experiencing more control over activities, a more varied and exciting lifestyle, and the opportunities for successful social interactions around fun and exciting activities.

EDUCATIONAL IMPLICATIONS

This section returns to Carly and James, who were introduced and discussed in Chapter 13, and applies the previously discussed features of comprehensive behavioral support to their unique situations. In all situations involving comprehensive behavioral support, when possible, it is important to focus on the prevention of problem behavior. This usually involves the manipulation of antecedent or contextual variables. If these variables that set the occasion for the problem behavior are altered so that instead they set the occasion for conventional communicative behavior, then the person's need for the use of problem behavior has been eliminated.

Carly

Although Carly exhibited communicative behaviors, such as idiosyncratic signs, gestures, and the use of objects, she appeared unable to use these more conventional strategies to escape difficult situations. Carly needed additional supports to augment her existing communicative repertoire and contextual or environmental modifications to make activities more tolerable and more fun for her. Interventionists agreed that in school and at home Carly could use additional communication support pictures to augment her existing communicative repertoire. These pictures were used in two different ways. First, a schedule was established both at home and at school that would make activities and events more predictable. The second strategy involved combining both pictures and objects to offer choices in key activities.

For most children, a choice of activities is wonderful, but for Carly the number of choices was overwhelming. Carly's teacher provided her with a choice of two center activities at a time using picture and object representations. In this format, Carly was able to select her preferred activity by putting the pictures (i.e., one selected activity) of the chosen center on her schedule and proceeding to it. This helped Carly organize her environment (i.e., schedule of activities) into more meaningful chunks. Her parents used this same strategy at home and allowed Carly to select television programs and videos using both pictured and object representations. Selecting her preferred television shows increased Carly's attention to the activity. The subsequent placement of the selected picture on her schedule also provided her with clearer indications of the beginning and ending of activities. During circle time and community outings, a picture schedule also indicated what came before and after the difficult activity. Carly's teacher and parents also expanded her participation in home and school activities. At school during circle time, Carly was allowed to choose favorite songs and preferred portions of circle time (e.g., calendar, weather). Her teacher also allowed Carly to participate in setting up activities and assigned her a circle time "buddy" who helped her with difficult parts of the activity. For community outings, Carly had a portable picture schedule for store shopping. She used it to select and sequence items to buy for herself when going into stores. In addition, using her schedule, trips for ice cream were scheduled before returning home, so that Carly had something to look forward to when running errands with her mother.

Other comprehensive behavioral support procedures included teaching her to ask for a break during long or extended activities. Carly was given a red card with *break* printed on it that she could point to or pick up when she needed to escape briefly from activities. The card was chosen instead of the sign for BREAK because it was more efficient for her to pick up the card or point to it than to learn the sign. The sole use of signs was not an efficient response modality for Carly because of her difficulty with upper body strength. Often her signs were difficult to understand except by those who knew her well, and signs were difficult or cumbersome for her to use. In frustration, she often resorted to her problem behavior, which proved to be more efficient than signing. For Carly, the *break* card worked well and competed with the problem behavior in terms of efficiency. The card prompted an immediate response from the teacher or her peer buddy, and she was allowed to get a drink of water or go to the restroom. The picture schedule was used to return her to the activity.

In addition to antecedent and teaching manipulations, both Carly's teacher and parents made a more concerted effort to provide Carly with differential praise when she participated in activities. As a direct result of her negative responses to activities and people, both the teacher and her parents had inadvertently decreased the amount of praise they gave Carly. The combination of different teaching and support components virtually eliminated Carly's problem behavior and allowed her to have access to more activities and people. Her classmates spent more time socially engaged with her because she participated more in activities, and, as a result, they were more willing to support her in these activities. Both her teacher and parents introduced more new activities to Carly. As a result, her lifestyle expanded dramatically. Carly's life became much richer and she was a much happier child as a result of the process of providing comprehensive behavioral support.

James

Although James and Carly were different ages and had different repertoires of problem behaviors, they both shared a need for expanding their conventional communication, adaptive behaviors, and overall lifestyle. Many of the comprehensive behavioral support strategies that existed for Carly also worked well for James. As was discussed previously and in Chapter 13, James's destructive and assaultive behaviors served dual purposes. He escaped from lengthy or confusing activities, and he obtained preferred or desired food items (and rejected nonpreferred food items) for mealtimes.

Even though he was limited to single-word and echolalic productions, James used speech as a conventional means of communication. It was apparent that James's limited communicative repertoire meant that he needed augmentative or alternative methods of communication and additional methods of reorganizing his home and work environment. His staff first decided to break up his work into clearer chunks. At work, rather than gluing card pockets in seemingly endless stacks of books, he worked on stacks of five books at a time. The staff estimated his approximate rate of books per 2-hour work session and provided him with stacks of five that cumulatively equaled the amount he was typically able to finish in 2 hours. Any other books were removed from his work environment to avoid confusion on his part. They also saw this as a way to begin to increase his productivity and extend the length of his work time by indicating to James that he would be finished after five more books. Every 2 weeks, James's work demands increased by five more books. This chunking of the activity made the work look and seem less intimidating. In addition, the staff created a picture schedule for James with words beneath the pictures. This allowed them to schedule preferred activities following a successful work session. Because of James's echolalia and limited speech capacity, he used pictures as a means for choosing and scheduling preferred activities following his work. James's staff also offered pictures of either the water fountain or the restroom as a break choice from his work activities. Generally, breaks were offered after a stack of five books was completed. Breaks became more predictable for James and provided him with brief escapes from his work activities.

At home, the staff created a pictured menu of available food options for breakfast, lunch, and dinner. James not only responded verbally to the selection, but he also pointed to or selected the pictured food item. This helped clarify what James wanted for meals and also helped identify available food options. If the household was out of a food item, that pictured item did not appear on the menu. The use of a more concrete system of pictured food items augmented James's communication by helping him identify, through pictures, his preferred food items. The absence of food items also served as reminder to staff to visit the store for those items they needed for meals, rather than assuming an item was present with the result being James's display of problem behaviors. Because James could read some words, all pictured representations, both on his schedule and on the menu, were paired with the written representations.

In addition to pictures, James was taught to pair requests with oral language. At work he used the word *break* when he took a break from gluing, and at home James needed to say the name of, as well as point to, the pictured food representation. This technique was offered as a method of functional communication. Although pictures served as reminders for things he was unable to spontaneously request, such as a break or food, the hope was that he would eventually expand his oral language. The use of words with the pictures was introduced so that eventually James might move to a written schedule. However, the use of pictures proved to be more efficient than to rotely recall the names of food items and verbally request a break from work. These alternative methods of communication successfully competed with his destructive and assaultive behaviors in that the pictures served as stimuli for spoken language that was more difficult for James to use spontaneously and provided more instantaneous responses from staff.

Specific consequence strategies also constituted a component of the behavioral support plan for James. The first strategy took the form of increased use of general and specific praise for engaging in more conventional communicative behaviors and completion of work or other household chores. The second strategy involved the use of crisis management. At work, one consequence strategy consisted of reminders for James to take a break by pointing to his break pictures before he escalated to dangerous behaviors, reminding him of chosen reinforcers for finished work, taking longer breaks, and shortening work tasks. At home when the household had run out of an item or the item did not appear on the menu, the staff used the picture schedule with James to set up a time for a store visit, so that James would know the item would be there at a future time. Third, the staff taught him to express his disappointment of not having the desired food item.

The use of crisis management strategies usually consisted of emergency procedures. For example, if James's behavior escalated to dangerous levels, then he was escorted by staff to the car. Using a cellular phone, a staff member called to prepare other home staff for emergency procedures as well as for back-up staff to assist with the deescalation of dangerous behaviors. At home, if James's behaviors escalated (due to the absence of a preferred food item), he was escorted by staff to a safe area of the house, lowering demands and expectations until his destructive and assaultive behaviors subsided. When he was calm, James was returned to the menu for the continued selection of food and reminded of the upcoming trip to the store.

Overall, James's lifestyle changed dramatically with only rare episodes of destructive and assaultive behaviors. He was able to accompany staff on many more community outings and was able to make more frequent visits to others' houses because of the strategies developed within the framework of comprehensive behavioral support. James's lifestyle became much more enriched, and staff morale was greatly increased. Staff began to regard James as more of an equal and took him to concerts and other activities on their own personal time, thus expanding James's social circle tremendously.

Many similar comprehensive behavioral support strategies were used with Carly and James, although specific antecedent and teaching strategies varied. They were provided with ways to more efficiently communicate and thus had less need to communicate through the use of problem behavior. In both instances their lives changed dramatically, and people responded to them in very different and more positive ways. This was directly attributable to the use of a comprehensive method of behavioral support that included a thorough functional assessment and the subsequent development of key intervention strategies reflective of the features of comprehensive behavioral support.

DIRECTIONS FOR FUTURE RESEARCH

Comprehensive behavioral support is an enterprise that is young and dynamic; thus, there is an ongoing need for many directions of research. There is a need for basic research to inform program developers of fundamental mechanisms that determine the functional relations between environmental circumstances and patterns of behavior (Mace & Wacker, 1994), and there is a need for applied research that demonstrates, replicates, and evaluates the use of behavior support strategies in genuine community contexts (Horner & Carr, in press). There also is a need to refine and extend the procedures of functional assessment so that they will continue to claim enhanced validity and generality (see Chapter 13). Because comprehensive behavioral support is such a broad endeavor that affects so many aspects of a person's functioning, it is difficult to distinguish specific research emphases that are apt to be the most productive or beneficial. However, we have identified three research directions that we believe are especially important for concentrated research activity.

Setting Events

The field is beginning to form a conceptual basis and applied methodology for analyzing the impact of setting events on the occurrence of problematic forms of behavior (Carr, Reeve, & Magito-McLaughlin, 1996; Horner et al., 1996; Kennedy & Itkonen, 1993). Although the influence that various ecological, physiological, and distal events can exert on behavior is increasingly appreciated, there are as yet few illustrations in which specific effects have been isolated. There are even fewer reports that identify and then rectify problematic relations. This is clearly an area that warrants concerted attention.

Prevention

The focus of comprehensive behavioral support has been on assessing and remediating occurrences of significant problem behavior. The majority of research has addressed the problems after they have been established as serious and in immediate need of management. It can be argued that a preferable emphasis would be on directing intervention and research so that serious problem behaviors are prevented from occurring. One general approach that may have promise for longitudinal prevention is to provide focused, functional early intervention for children whose characteristics suggest a relatively high potential for the later development of serious problem behaviors (Dunlap & Fox, 1996; Dunlap et al., 1990). However, aside from a few demonstrations (Dunlap et al., 1990; Reeve, 1996), there has been essentially no research on this topic. Prevention research is challenging from a methodological perspective, and it can be expensive and logistically difficult to arrange for longitudinal analyses; however, the benefits of effective prevention efforts should justify the required costs and commitments.

Application Across Natural Contexts with Comprehensive Evaluation

Most research in the area of comprehensive behavioral support has addressed separable components of the endeavor and has employed narrow, specific measures with which to judge the effectiveness of the intervention. This is appropriate for building a technology, but it has yielded insufficient data regarding the feasibility, effectiveness, durability, and applicability of the approach in many circumstances. For example, there are relatively few reports of comprehensive behavioral support being applied in public community settings by families and other typical caregivers. There also are virtually no analyses that address the application of behavioral support strategies by individuals who represent diverse cultures, economic classes, or ethnic backgrounds. In general, there is a tremendous need for applied researchers to conduct systematic demonstrations in a variety of common circumstances in which problem behaviors affect the lifestyles of individuals with disabilities, their families, their caregivers, their friends, and the public at large. This research will be particularly useful if it demonstrates strategies that are effective from multiple perspectives, identifies barriers, and describes situational adjustments used to overcome the barriers. Demonstrations that explicitly extend the applicability of comprehensive support across environments and populations are apt to do more than any other type of research to promote the understanding and adoption of this orientation to problem behaviors.

CONCLUSION

Comprehensive behavioral support is a broad, multifaceted enterprise that is growing rapidly in the articulation and validation of its key features and in the operationalization of its processes. This chapter highlighted the major characteristics of comprehensive behavioral support. It is expected that future experience will bring refinement and new emphases that have not yet been incorporated in existing descriptions. For example, many questions remain regarding optimal strategies for promoting use of effective behavioral support strategies in complex community settings (e.g., Eno-Hieneman & Dunlap, in press). Systems issues and multicultural perspectives need to be explored in much greater depth and with more systematic analyses. It is certain that investigations into these areas will provide new and important insights in the efforts to provide effective, humane support for people with behavioral challenges.

REFERENCES

Albin, R.W., Lucyshyn, J.M., Horner, R.H., & Flannery, K.B. (1996). Contextual fit for behavioral support plans: A model for "goodness of fit." In L.K. Koegel, R.L. Koegel, & G. Dunlap (Eds.), *Positive behavioral support: Including people with difficult behavior in the community* (pp. 81–98). Baltimore: Paul H. Brookes Publishing Co.

Bird, F., Dores, P.A., Moniz, D., & Robinson, J. (1989). Reducing severe aggressive and self-injurious behaviors with functional communication training: Direct, collateral and generalized results. *American Journal on Mental Retardation, 94,* 37–48.

Carr, E.G. (1988). Functional equivalence as a mechanism of response generalization. In R.H. Horner, G. Dunlap, & R.L. Koegel (Eds.), *Generalization and maintenance: Life-style changes in applied settings* (pp. 221–241). Baltimore: Paul H. Brookes Publishing Co.

Carr, E.G., & Durand, V.M. (1985a). Reducing behavior problems through functional communication training. *Journal of Applied Behavior Analysis, 18,* 111–126.

Carr, E.G., & Durand, V.M. (1985b). The social-communicative basis of severe behavior problems in children. In J. Reiss & R.R. Bootzin (Eds.), *Theoretical issues in behavior therapy* (pp. 219–254). New York: Academic Press.

Carr, E.G., & Kemp, D.C. (1989). Functional equivalence of autistic leading and communicative pointing: Analysis and treatment. *Journal of Autism and Developmental Disorders, 19,* 561–578.

Carr, E.G., Levin, L., McConnachie, G., Carlson, J.I., Kemp, D.C., & Smith, C.E. (1994). *Communication-based intervention for problem behavior: A user's guide for producing positive change.* Baltimore: Paul H. Brookes Publishing Co.

Carr, E.G., Reeve, C.E., & Magito-McLaughlin, D. (1996). Contextual influences on problem behavior in people with developmental disabilities. In L.K. Koegel, R.L. Koegel, & G. Dunlap (Eds.), *Positive behavioral support: Including people with difficult behavior in the community* (pp. 403–423). Baltimore: Paul H. Brookes Publishing Co.

Carr, E.G., Robinson, S., Taylor, J.C., & Carlson, J.I. (1990). Positive approaches to the treatment of severe behavior problems in persons with developmental disabilities: A review and analysis of reinforcement and stimulus based procedures. *Monograph of The Association of Persons with Severe Handicaps, 4.*

Clarke, S., Dunlap, G., Foster-Johnson, L., Childs, K.E., Wilson, D., White, R., & Vera, A. (1995). Improving the conduct of students with behavioral disorders by incorporating student interests into curricular activities. *Behavioral Disorders, 20*(4), 221–237.

Dadson, S., & Horner, R.H. (1993). Manipulating setting events to decrease problem behaviors: A case study. *Teaching Exceptional Children, 25,* 53–55.

Dattilo, J. (1991). Recreation and leisure: A review of the literature and recommendations for future directions. In L.H. Meyer, C.A. Peck, & L. Brown (Eds.), *Critical issues in the lives of people with severe disabilities* (pp. 171–194). Baltimore: Paul H. Brookes Publishing Co.

Donnellan, A.M., Mirenda, P.L., Mesaros, R.A., & Fassbender, L.L. (1984). Analyzing the communicative functions of aberrant behavior. *Journal of The Association for Persons with Severe Handicaps, 9,* 201–212.

Doss, L.S., & Reichle, J. (1991). Replacing excess behavior with an initial communicative repertoire. In J. Reichle, J. York, & J. Sigafoos (Eds.), *Implementing augmentative and alternative communication: Strategies for learners with severe disabilities* (pp. 215–237). Baltimore: Paul H. Brookes Publishing Co.

Dunlap, G., Foster-Johnson, L., Clarke, S., Kern, L., & Childs, K.E. (1995). Modifying activities to produce functional outcomes: Effects on the problem behaviors of students with disabilities. *Journal of The Association for Persons with Severe Handicaps, 20*(4), 248–258.

Dunlap, G., & Fox, L. (1996). Early intervention and serious problem behaviors: A comprehensive approach. In L.K. Koegel, R.L. Koegel, & G. Dunlap (Eds.), *Positive behavioral support: Including people with difficult behavior in the community* (pp. 31–51). Baltimore: Paul H. Brookes Publishing Co.

Dunlap, G., Johnson, L.F., & Robbins, F.R. (1990). Preventing serious behavior problems through skill development and early intervention. In A.C. Repp & N.N. Singh (Eds.), *Perspectives on the use of nonaversive and aversive interventions for persons with developmental disabilities* (pp. 273–286). Sycamore, IL: Sycamore Press.

Dunlap, G., & Kern, L. (1993). Assessment and intervention for children within the instructional curriculum. In J. Reichle & D.P. Wacker (Eds.), *Communication and language intervention series: Vol. 3. Communicative alternatives to challenging behavior: Integrating functional assessment and intervention strategies* (pp. 177–203). Baltimore: Paul H. Brookes Publishing Co.

Dunlap, G., Kern-Dunlap, L., Clarke, S., & Robbins, F.R. (1991). Functional assessment, curricular revisions, and severe behavior problems. *Journal of Applied Behavior Analysis, 24,* 44–57.

Durand, V.M. (1990). *Severe behavior problems: A functional communication training approach.* New York: Guilford Press.

Durand, V.M., Berotti, D., & Weiner, J.S. (1993). Functional communication training: Factors affecting effectiveness, generalization, and maintenance. In J. Reichle & D.P. Wacker (Eds.), *Communication and language intervention series: Vol. 3. Communicative alternatives to challenging behavior: Integrating functional assessment and intervention strategies* (pp. 317–340). Baltimore: Paul H. Brookes Publishing Co.

Durand, V.M., & Carr, E.G. (1987). Social influences on self-stimulatory behavior: Analysis and treatment application. *Journal of Applied Behavior Analysis, 20*, 119–132.

Durand, V.M., & Carr, E.G. (1991). Functional communication training to reduce challenging behavior: Maintenance and application in new settings. *Journal of Applied Behavior Analysis, 24*, 251–264.

Durand, V.M., & Carr, E.G. (1992). An analysis of maintenance following functional communication training. *Journal of Applied Behavior Analysis, 25*, 777–794.

Durand, V.M., & Crimmins, D.B. (1988). Identifying the variables maintaining self-injurious behavior. *Journal of Autism and Developmental Disabilities, 18*, 99–117.

Dyer, K. (1987). The competition of autistic stereotyped behavior with usual and specially assessed reinforcers. *Research in Developmental Disabilities, 8*, 607–626.

Dyer, K. (1989). The effects of preference on spontaneous verbal requests in individuals with autism. *Journal of The Association for Persons with Severe Handicaps, 14*, 184–189.

Eno-Hieneman, M., & Dunlap, G. (in press). Issues and challenges in implementing community-based behavioral support: Two illustrative cases. In J.R. Scotti & L.H. Meyer (Eds.), *Behavioral intervention: Principles, models, and practices*. Baltimore: Paul H. Brookes Publishing Co.

Evans, I.M., & Meyer, L.H. (1985). *An educative approach to behavior problems: A practical decision model for interventions with severely handicapped learners*. Baltimore: Paul H. Brookes Publishing Co.

Fisher, W., Piazza, C.C., Bowman, L.G., Hagopian, L.P., Owens, J.C., & Slevin, I. (1992). A comparison of two approaches for identifying reinforcers for persons with severe and profound disabilities. *Journal of Applied Behavior Analysis, 25*, 491–498.

Foster-Johnson, L., Ferro, J., & Dunlap, G. (1994). Preferred curricular activities and reduced problem behaviors in students with intellectual disabilities. *Journal of Applied Behavior Analysis, 27*, 493–504.

Gardner, W.I., Cole, C.I., Davidson, D.P., & Karan, O.C. (1984). Assessment of setting events influencing functional capacities of mentally retarded adults with behavior difficulties. *Education and Training of the Mentally Retarded, 21*, 3–12.

Halle, J.W., & Spradlin, J.E. (1993). Identifying stimulus control of challenging behavior. In J. Reichle & D.P. Wacker (Eds.), *Communication and language intervention series: Vol. 3. Communicative alternatives to challenging behavior: Integrating functional assessment and intervention strategies* (pp. 83–109). Baltimore: Paul H. Brookes Publishing Co.

Horner, R.D. (1980). The effects of an environmental "enrichment" program on the behavior of institutionalized profoundly retarded children. *Journal of Applied Behavior Analysis, 13*, 473–491.

Horner, R.H., Albin, R.W., & O'Neill, R.E. (1991). Support students with severe intellectual disabilities and severe challenging behaviors. In G. Stoner, M.R. Shinn, & H.M. Walker (Eds.), *Interventions for achievement and behavioral problems* (pp. 269–287). Washington, DC: National Association of School Psychologists.

Horner, R.H., & Billingsley, F.F. (1988). The effect of competing behavior on the generalization and maintenance of adaptive behavior in applied settings. In R.H. Horner, G. Dunlap, & R.L. Koegel (Eds.), *Generalization and maintenance: Life-style changes in applied settings* (pp. 197–220). Baltimore: Paul H. Brookes Publishing Co.

Horner, R.H., & Budd, C.M. (1985). Acquisition of manual sign use: Collateral reduction of maladaptive behavior, and factors limiting generalization. *Education and Training of the Mentally Retarded, 20,* 39–47.

Horner, R.H., & Carr, E.G. (in press). Behavioral support for students with severe disabilities: Functional assessment and comprehensive interventions. *Journal of Special Education.*

Horner, R.H., & Day, H.M. (1991). The effects of response efficiency on functionally equivalent competing behaviors. *Journal of Applied Behavior Analysis, 24,* 719–732.

Horner, R.H., Day, H.M., Sprague, J.R., O'Brien, M., & Heathfield, L.T. (1991). Interspersed requests: A non-aversive procedure for reducing aggression and self-injury during instruction. *Journal of Applied Behavior Analysis, 24,* 265–278.

Horner, R.H., O'Neill, R.E., & Flannery, K.B. (1993). Building effective behavior support plans from functional assessment information. In M. Snell (Ed.), *Systematic instruction of persons with severe handicaps* (4th ed., pp. 184–214). Columbus, OH: Charles E. Merrill.

Horner, R.H., Sprague, J.R., & Flannery, K.B. (1993). Building functional curricula for students with severe intellectual disabilities and severe problem behaviors. In R.V. Houten & S. Axelrod (Eds.), *Behavior analysis and treatment* (pp. 47–71). New York: Plenum.

Horner, R.H., Sprague, J.R., O'Brien, M., & Heathfield, L.T. (1990). The role of response efficiency in the reduction of problem behaviors through functional equivalence training: A case study. *Journal of The Association for Persons with Severe Handicaps, 15,* 91–97.

Horner, R.H., Vaughn, B.J., Day, H.M., & Ard, W.R., Jr. (1996). The relationship between setting events and problem behavior: Expanding our understanding of behavioral support. In L.K. Koegel, R.L. Koegel, & G. Dunlap (Eds.), *Positive behavioral support: Including people with difficult behavior in the community* (pp. 381–402). Baltimore: Paul H. Brookes Publishing Co.

Kennedy, C., & Itkonen, T. (1993). Effects of setting events on the problem behavior of students with severe disabilities. *Journal of Applied Behavior Analysis, 26,* 321–327.

Kern, L., Childs, K.E., Dunlap, G., Clarke, S., & Falk, G.D. (1994). Using assessment-based curricular intervention to improve the classroom behavior of a student with emotional and behavioral challenges. *Journal of Applied Behavior Analysis, 27,* 7–19.

Kern, L., & Dunlap, G. (in press). Assessment-based interventions for children with emotional and behavioral disorders. In A.C. Repp & R.H. Horner (Eds.), *Functional analysis of problem behavior: From effective assessment to effective support.* Pacific Grove, CA: Brooks/Cole.

Kincaid, D. (1996). Person-centered planning. In L.K. Koegel, R.L. Koegel, & G. Dunlap (Eds.), *Positive behavioral support: Including people with difficult behavior in the community* (pp. 439–465). Baltimore: Paul H. Brookes Publishing Co.

Koegel, L.K., Koegel, R.L., & Dunlap, G. (Eds.). (1996). *Positive behavioral support: Including people with difficult behavior in the community.* Baltimore: Paul H. Brookes Publishing Co.

Koegel, L.K., Koegel, R.L., Hurley, C., & Frea, W.D. (1992). Improving social skills and disruptive behavior in children with autism through self-management. *Journal of Applied Behavior Analysis, 25*(2), 341–353.

Koegel, R.L., Frea, W.D., & Surratt, A.V. (1994). Self-management of problematic behavior. In E. Schopler & G. Mesibov (Eds.), *Behavior issues in autism* (81–97). New York: Plenum.

Koegel, R.L., & Koegel, L.K. (1990). Extended reductions in stereotypic behavior through a self-management in multiple community settings. *Journal of Applied Behavior Analysis, 1,* 119–127.

Mace, F.C., & Wacker, D.P. (1994). Toward greater integration of basic and applied behavioral research: An introduction. *Journal of Applied Behavior Analysis, 27,* 569–574.

Michael, J.L. (1982). Distinguishing between discriminative and motivational functions of stimuli. *Journal of Experimental Analysis of Behavior, 37,* 149–155.

Michael, J.L. (1993). Establishing operations. In *Concepts and principles of behavior analysis.* Kalamazoo, MI: Society for the Advancement of Behavior Analysis.

Mount, B. (1987). *Personal futures planning: Finding directions for change.* Unpublished doctoral dissertation, University of Georgia, Athens.

Munk, D.D., & Repp, A.C. (1994). Behavioral assessment of feeding problems of individuals with severe disabilities. *Journal of Applied Behavior Analysis, 27,* 215–240.

O'Brien, J., Mount, B., & O'Brien, C. (1991). *Framework for accomplishment: Personal profile.* Decatur, GA: Responsive Systems Associates.

O'Neill, R.E., Horner, R.H., Albin, R.W., Storey, K., & Sprague, J. (1990). *Functional analysis of problem behavior.* Sycamore, IL: Sycamore Publishing Company.

Reeve, C.E. (1996). *Prevention of severe problem behavior in individuals with developmental disabilities.* Unpublished doctoral dissertation, State University of New York at Stony Brook.

Reichle, J., Halle, J., & Johnston, S. (1993). Developing an initial communicative repertoire: Applications and issues for persons with severe disabilities. In A.P. Kaiser & D.B. Gray (Eds.), *Communication and language intervention series: Vol. 2. Enhancing children's communication: Research foundations for intervention* (pp. 105–136). Baltimore: Paul H. Brookes Publishing Co.

Repp, A.C., Felce, D., & Barton, L.E. (1988). Basing the treatment of stereotypic and self-injurious behaviors on hypotheses of their causes. *Journal of Applied Behavior Analysis, 21,* 281–289.

Repp, A.C., & Horner, R.H. (in press). *Functional analysis of problem behavior: From effective assessment to effective support.* Pacific Grove, CA: Brooks/Cole.

Repp, A.C., & Karsh, K.G. (1994). Hypothesis-based interventions for tantrum behaviors of persons with developmental disabilities in school settings. *Journal of Applied Behavior Analysis, 27,* 21–31.

Sprague, J.R., & Horner, R.H. (1992). Covariation within functional response classes: Implications for treatment of severe problem behavior. *Journal of Applied Behavior Analysis, 25,* 735–745.

Turnbull, A.P., & Turnbull, H.R. (1990). *Families, professionals, and exceptionality: A special partnership* (2nd ed.). Columbus, OH: Charles E. Merrill.

Vollmer, T.R., Marcus, B.A., & Ringdahl, J.E. (1995). Noncontingent escape as treatment for self-injurious behavior maintained by negative reinforcement. *Journal of Applied Behavior Analysis, 28,* 15–26.

Wacker, D., Steege, M., Northrup, J., Sasso, G., Berg, W., Reimers, T., Cooper, L., Cigrand, K., & Donn, L. (1990). A component analysis of functional communication training across three topographies of severe behavior problems. *Journal of Applied Behavior Analysis, 23,* 417–429.

Wahler, R.G., & Graves, M.B. (1983). Setting events in social networks: Ally or enemy in child behavior therapy. *Behavior Therapy, 14,* 19–36.

15

Facilitating the Transition from Preintentional to Intentional Communication

Steven F. Warren and Paul J. Yoder

THE ONSET OF INTENTIONAL COMMUNICATION late in the first year of life marks infants' active entry into their culture and ignites important changes in how others regard and respond to them. It would be hard to underestimate the importance of the accomplishment of intentional communication, given that a good deal of the child's future social and cognitive development is dependent on its occurrence. A significant delay in the onset of intentional communication is a strong indicator that the onset of productive language also will be delayed (McCathren, Warren, & Yoder, 1996). Such a delay may hold the infant in a kind of developmental limbo because the onset of intentional communication typically triggers a series of transactional processes from which productive language emerges within a few months.

A premise of this chapter is that infants with developmental delays can be actively assisted in their efforts to achieve intentional communication. Procedures have been developed to directly facilitate the transition from preintentional to intentional communication. The systematic application of these procedures may shorten the time it takes for infants with developmental delays to achieve intentional communication and to set off important transactional changes in how adults respond to them.

This chapter describes an approach its authors have developed for facilitating the transition from preintentional to intentional communication. The authors first provide a brief description of the transition from preintentional to intentional communication. (This process is thoroughly described in Part I of this volume.) This section focuses on some key parameters of this transition process that

Support for the preparation of this chapter and for the authors' research was provided by Grant No. RO1 HD27594 from the National Institute of Child Health and Human Development and Grant No. HO23C20152 from the Office of Special Education Programs of the U.S. Department of Education. However, the opinions expressed are solely those of the authors.

have direct relevance for our intervention model. Next we present the basic conceptual foundations of our approach and describe how to facilitate intentional communication. We describe the goals and procedures of our intervention and conclude the chapter with brief discussions of relevant cultural issues, clinical and educational implications, and future research directions.

TRANSITION FROM PREINTENTIONAL TO INTENTIONAL COMMUNICATION

During the final 3 months of their first year of life, most infants begin to intentionally communicate their desires and interests to others. The onset of coordinated attention occupies a "pivotal" juncture in this process (see also Chapter 2). Before the emergence of coordinated attention, an infant's intention is very difficult to discern (Bates, Benigni, Bretherton, Camaioni, & Volterra, 1979; Sugarman, 1984; Yoder & Munson, 1994).

Almost simultaneously with the emergence of coordinated attention, the child begins to move from preintentional to intentional communication. Requesting and commenting episodes provide the earliest contexts in which intentionality is demonstrated (Bates, O'Connell, & Shore, 1987). Both functions require the infant to shift his or her attention between his or her partner and an object. *Requesting* (also termed imperatives and proto-imperatives in the literature) is commonly defined as behavior that clearly indicates that the child wants something. Requesting is typically sustained until the goal is reached or becomes unreachable (Rogoff, Mistry, Radziszewska, & Germond, 1992). *Commenting* (also termed joint attention, indicating, declarative, and referencing in the literature) is the act of drawing another's attention to or showing a positive affect about an object or interest (Bates et al., 1987).

Although other communicative functions also emerge during this period (e.g., greeting, protesting), requesting and commenting are considered the fundamental pragmatic building blocks of both prelinguistic and linguistic communication (Bates et al., 1979; Bruner, Roy, & Ratner, 1980). They are also the two most frequent functions expressed during the prelinguistic period (Wetherby, Cain, Yonclas, & Walker, 1988). However, they are not mastered simultaneously. Requesting usually emerges around 9–10 months of age, whereas commenting typically emerges around 12 months of age (Bates, Camaioni, & Volterra, 1975; see also Chapter 2). Commenting indicates an interest in another person's attention, not to gain some object or service but to share affective states (see Chapter 6). This distinction between the functions of commenting and requesting is important to understanding why some children request but rarely comment (e.g., many children with autism). These two functions necessitate somewhat different intervention tactics, which this chapter discusses later.

Clarity and frequency are important attributes of intentional communication. Coordinated attention adds clarity to an infant's communication attempts.

Yoder and Munson (1994) found a positive relationship between the amount of coordinated attention children showed and the number of times their mothers said that the children communicated during a videotaped mother–child play session. The addition of gestures (e.g., pointing, holding an object up to an adult, reaching) and concurrent vocalizations can further clarify intent (Kim, 1996; Yoder & Warren, 1996). Kim (1996) and Yoder and Warren (1996) found that communication acts with coordinated attention and gestures, or vocalizations, were responded to more than acts with just coordinated attention or with gestures and vocalization but without coordinated attention. Frequency and clarity of communication are probably closely related because more frequent communication typically elicits more input and feedback by adults, leading to greater clarity of communication (Wilcox, 1992; Yoder, Warren, & Kim, 1997). The frequency with which children intentionally communicate predicts their later language development (McCathren et al., 1996), supporting the notion that frequent communication is both a source of further learning and an indicator of progress and should itself be an intervention target with low-rate communicators. Furthermore, research has indicated that rates of communication acts need to approach approximately one per minute on average for children to make the transition from prelinguistic to initial symbolic communication (Wetherby & Prizant, 1993; Wetherby, Yonclas, & Bryan, 1989; Wilcox, 1993).

Children at risk for mental retardation typically show delays in the onset of coordinated attention and in the onset of basic communication functions (see Berger, 1990; Landry, 1995; McCathren et al., 1996; see also Chapter 2). The length of these delays will vary from child to child, based on the nature of the disability and the responsiveness of the environment. In the experience of this chapter's authors, we often see children with general developmental delays who are approaching their second birthday, who still rarely engage in coordinated attention and who display very low rates of intentional communication.

CONCEPTUAL BASIS FOR PRELINGUISTIC COMMUNICATION INTERVENTION

What can be accomplished by teaching an infant or young child to intentionally communicate (assuming such an ambitious goal can be achieved)? Research on prelinguistic communication intervention is still in its infancy. Therefore, it can only be speculated what implications "turning on" intentional communication through intervention might have for the long-term development of a child. However, some findings combined with the increasing knowledge of the importance of early linguistic input and experience suggest the implications could be profound for many children. The discussions in this section of the transactional model of development and the cumulative deficit hypothesis are intended to establish a conceptual context for evaluating and interpreting the effects of prelinguistic communication intervention.

Transactional Model of Development

The transactional model of development undergirds much of the research presented in Part I of this volume (see especially Chapters 2 and 3). The general transactional theory of development (McLean & Snyder-McLean, 1978; Sameroff, 1983; Sameroff & Chandler, 1975) posits that the combination of both child variables and family variables will produce a more accurate model for predicting individual differences in later child development than either type of variable alone. The fundamental assumption of the transactional model is that development is facilitated by a bidirectional, reciprocal interaction between the child and his or her environment. A change in the child may trigger a change in the environment, which in turn affects the child and so on. In this way, both the child and the environment change over time and affect each other in a reciprocal fashion, and early achievements pave the way for subsequent development.

Transactional effects between infants and caregivers typically begin shortly after birth in the course of establishing initial handling, sleeping, and eating routines (Hanson, 1984). As development proceeds, a potentially powerful transactional effect often originates with the onset of clear, frequent intentional communication by an infant. This change in the infant's behavior elicits a substantial increase in linguistic mapping by many parents. Linguistic mapping of child communication refers to an adult verbally marking what the child is communicating nonverbally. For example, if a child reached for a cup and then looked at the adult, the adult's verbal response "You want the cup" is a linguistic mapping of what the child intended to communicate. An increase in linguistic mapping, triggered by the onset of clear, frequent communication by the child, may facilitate vocabulary development because the child is already attending to the referent of the words that the adult is modeling (Nelson, 1989). Research has indicated that both typically developing children (Tomasello & Farrar, 1986) and atypically developing children (Yoder, Kaiser, Alpert, & Fischer, 1993) acquire vocabulary, particularly object labels, more readily as a result of linguistic mapping.

The Transactional Effects of Prelinguistic Milieu Teaching Milieu teaching is a well-established early language intervention approach that has been extensively investigated (Kaiser, Yoder, & Keetz, 1992; McLean & Cripe, 1997; Warren & Kaiser, 1988). Prelinguistic milieu teaching (PMT) represents an extension and adaptation of the basic milieu model that suits the unique developmental characteristics of the prelinguistic period (Yoder & Warren, 1993). The distinguishing characteristics of the milieu model (i.e., focusing on following the child's attentional lead, embedding instruction within ongoing interaction, arranging the environment to elicit child responses, focusing on specific target behaviors, using discrete prompts when deemed necessary) are maintained in PMT.

In our initial explorations of the effects of PMT (Warren, Yoder, Gazdag, Kim, & Jones, 1993; Yoder, Warren, Kim, & Gazdag, 1994), we demonstrated that increases in the frequency and clarity of prelinguistic requesting covaried with substantial increases in linguistic mapping by teachers and parents. We have conducted an experimental analysis of the transactional effects of intentional communication on maternal linguistic responsivity (Yoder & Warren, 1997) in which 58 prelinguistic children with developmental delays and their parents participated in a randomized group experiment with excellent internal validity. To increase intentional communication, we provided 28 of the children with PMT for 20 minutes per day, 3 or 4 days per week, for 6 months. The other 30 children were assigned to an alternative intervention; a small, highly responsive play group. To control for possible inadvertent direct effects on maternal interaction style, mothers were kept naive to our methods, measures, records of child progress, and child goals.

The results of our analysis indicated that PMT facilitated greater use of intentional communication than the responsive small group did, but only for children whose mothers showed slightly above average maternal responsivity before the intervention. After controlling for pretreatment responsivity, PMT mothers responded linguistically to significantly more of their children's communication acts after the intervention than did mothers of children in the responsive play group. Finally, after controlling for the number of intentional communication acts at postintervention, the main effects of intervention on parent linguistic responsivity to the child became nonsignificant; that is, the intervention effect of PMT on maternal linguistic responsivity was in part the result of increases in intentional communication.

What are we to make of these results? It is clear that we can increase the clarity and frequency of young children's prelinguistic intentional communication; that is, we can activate intentional communication in young children with developmental delays. It is also clear that such increases can trigger an important transactional effect in adults—substantial increases in linguistic mapping. These are the kinds of effects that theory and research suggest should then lead to enhanced vocabulary development in children (see Chapter 3). However, such transactional effects appear to be dependent on a responsive caregiver who is sensitive to changes in the child's development and adjusts his or her own behavior to the child accordingly. Thus, a constraining influence on the occurrence of the types of transactional effects (Yoder & Warren, 1993) may be the general responsivity of caregivers. There is correlational evidence that many parents who are impoverished and poorly educated tend to be less responsive to their children and that this lowered responsiveness may have important long-term effects on their children's development (Hart & Risley, 1995). However, there is little evidence that parent responsivity is an unalterable trait and much evidence that parents can be taught to be responsive to changes in their children (e.g., Girolametto, 1988; Wilcox, 1992).

Low parental responsivity, in general, is only one of the factors that may reduce the probability that caregivers will increase their linguistic responsivity when their children's intentional communication increases. The clarity and frequency of the communication acts that are acquired and the general developmental level of the child may also influence whether a caregiver changes his or her interaction style in response to changes in the child's communication skills. These factors may combine to minimize or enhance transactional effects as children move from preintentional to intentional communication.

Acquiring the basic communication functions of requesting and commenting provides children with their first effective means of intentional communication, a powerful tool for controlling any environment they inhabit. Furthermore, these communication acts are acquired against a backdrop of the restricted repertoire of behavior that characterizes this early developmental period. This small repertoire may make it relatively easy for adults to recognize and respond differentially to specific occurrences of new behavior. These emerging communication acts require parents to do something that they presumably want to do, which is to be responsive to the child's interests and needs. Increases in clarity and frequency of requesting and commenting against the backdrop of the child's restricted behavioral repertoire help the parents notice the act, correctly interpret its intent, and respond appropriately.

The transition from preintentional to intentional communication may represent a period during which transactional effects can have a substantial impact on development. Adults have relatively dramatic changes to respond to, and the child's behavior and brain development may be most susceptible to alteration, both positive or negative, by environmental input and social responsiveness. During this period, the transactional model may be used by an interventionist to multiply the effects of a relatively circumscribed intervention (e.g., PMT) and perhaps alter the course of a child's development. However, the efforts of the interventionist, unless they are swift, effective, and continuing, may gradually be undercut and minimized by the child's own accumulating history. The next section discusses the role of the cumulative deficit hypothesis.

The Cumulative Deficit Hypothesis

Hart and Risley (1995) argued that language-learning experiences during the first 3 years of life have particularly strong effects on later vocabulary development and measures of intelligence in part because there is a huge cumulative input deficit that occurs in children who experience impoverished early input. To get a sense of how an input difference on a daily basis could accumulate into an overwhelming advantage or disadvantage for a child, consider the following: An input difference of 100 language-enhancing interactions per day (an average of slightly more than 7 such interactions per waking hour) would result in an input difference of 109,500 such interactions over a 3-year period. This type of cumulative difference across the first 3 years of life, coming at a time when evidence suggests that the brain may be most influenced by environmental input (Beckwith & Parmelee, 1986; Chugani, 1994; Locke, 1993), and during which most basic communication and language skills are acquired, can create an experiential lag that may be virtually impossible to overcome by later intervention efforts (Hart & Risley, 1995).

What evidence exists that such large cumulative deficits occur and that they play havoc with language development? Although the evidence is almost all correlational, it is also compelling. There is substantial evidence that typically developing young children experience large differences in terms of the quantity and quality of linguistic input they receive, and these differences generally correlate with important indicators of development later in childhood (e.g., vocabulary size, IQ, reading ability, school achievement) (Feagans & Farran, 1982; Gottfried, 1984; Hart & Risley, 1992; Prizant & Wetherby, 1990). Because they often display low rates of initiation and responsiveness (Rosenberg, 1982; Yoder, Davies, & Bishop, 1994), young children with developmental delays also may experience input that differs substantially in quantity and quality from the input that high-achieving, typically developing children receive, despite the best intentions of their caregivers.

Perhaps the effects of input differences would be muted if humans acquired language equally well at all ages; however, this is not the case. Instead, early childhood appears to be an optimal period for language acquisition in terms of concurrent brain development (Bates, Thal, & Janowsky, 1991; Locke, 1993) and in terms of the types of playful, carefully adapted, and fine-tuned language-enhancing experiences children naturally encounter on a daily basis when they have sensitive, responsive caregivers and teachers providing them with language-enhancing interaction (Bruner, 1981; Gallaway & Richards, 1994; Sokolov, 1993). As this optimal period draws to an end, children face what can be an exceedingly difficult barrier to cross if they have accumulated a large experiential deficit: the implicit and explicit language requirements of the first grade in primary classrooms throughout the literate, industrialized world. Mild mental retardation, learning disability, school failure—any of these designations and their consequences—may await the child with an insufficient language base at the beginning of primary school.

The best way to minimize the consequences of a large cumulative deficit in the quantity and quality of language input is to address it early, which in this case means much earlier than is typically meant by early intervention. Even during the 1980s and early 1990s, the preponderance of published research on early intervention has concerned children age 3 years or older. Yet a typical 3-year-old has already acquired most of the basic language system and is often a voluminous talker. It is noteworthy that the large cumulative experiential language deficits reported by Hart and Risley (1995) occurred by the time the children in their study were 3 years of age. Therefore, "early" needs to mean "as early as possible," before deficits grow too large and while interventionists can still harness the synergistic potential of transactional interaction effects on communication development. The next section considers how the development of frequent, clear, intentional communication can be facilitated.

FACILITATING INTENTIONAL COMMUNICATION

There are two general approaches to facilitating intentional communication: 1) Attempt to directly teach communication functions, and 2) teach adults who interact frequently with the child to be highly responsive to the child's communication attempts. If parents are already highly responsive to their infant's development, then the second tactic need not be specifically programmed. If parents are not highly responsive, then responsiveness should be taught because the potential of the transactional model depends on the provision of a suitably responsive environment (see Chapters 3 and 16). This section describes the specific procedures used in PMT to directly teach communication functions. The approach can be used to facilitate movement from preintentional to intentional communication and the development of symbolic communication skills. However, the focus of this chapter is solely on the transition from preintentional to intentional communication. The chapter also describes intervention goals, the provision of enabling contexts, specific teaching procedures, and basic strategies for teaching requesting and commenting.

Intentional Communication Goals

The onset and frequency of prelinguistic communication functions predicts later language development (McCathren et al., 1996). Therefore, our intervention efforts focus on increasing the frequency and clarity of children's requesting and commenting. This also results in an implicit focus on the development of coordinated attention. Because of the desire for children to talk as early as possible, it is tempting to target spoken words as goals as soon as a child begins to communicate. However, our position is that building a broad base of prelinguistic communication skills is a more important goal for children who are intentionally communicating less than once per minute in a structured communication protocol such as that provided by the Communication and Symbolic Behavior Scales (CSBS; Wetherby & Prizant, 1993). Prelinguistic children with low communication rates (less than once per minute) who have had linguistic communication as their primary goal have not appeared to benefit very much from intervention (Tannock & Girolametto, 1992; Wilcox, 1993). The PMT procedures described in this section offer an alternative to linguistic interventions for children with low rates of communication.

Enabling Contexts

Enabling contexts refers to a set of procedures intended to provide an optimal environment for the use of specific PMT techniques. These procedures are arranging the environment, following the child's attentional lead, and building social routines. They are to be used continuously to ensure a high degree of engagement by the child and to support frequent, developmentally progressive interactions between the child and adult. The basic formats for these procedures were developed for use in naturalistic early language intervention approaches such as milieu teaching (Warren, 1991) and responsive interaction teaching (MacDonald, 1989). They are also basic to the prelinguistic intervention approach described in Chapter 16.

Arranging the Environment The value of attending to and specifying the arrangement of the child's immediate environment rests on the fact that children are most likely to initiate about things they need or want or find interesting (Hart & Risley, 1968; Warren, 1991). This implies that the child inhabits a stimulating, interesting, developmentally appropriate environment. More specifically, arranging the environment involves placing desired materials (e.g., food, toys) either out of reach of the child or in a context in which adult assistance is necessary to gain access to them. For example, toys might be kept in clear plastic containers with lids that require adult assistance, crayons might be placed on the floor next to the adult where the child can see them but cannot easily reach them, or extra cupcakes might be placed in clear view but on a shelf beyond the child's reach.

The very predictability and order of a setting also can provide communication opportunities when this order is violated by silly, strange, or sabotaged events. These events can be either planned by an adult to set the stage for communication or unplanned events can simply be used for this purpose. The novelty of these events may create excellent opportunities for modeling and teaching commenting.

Positioning concerns how the adult places his or her body in relation to the child's body and a focal object. The adult should directly face the child and the focal object at the child's eye level (Musselwhite, 1986). With infants and toddlers, this may mean that the adult will need to sit or even lie on the floor. If a child is in a wheelchair, this will mean leaning down or sitting to achieve the child's eye level. This type of close, face-to-face contact facilitates coordinated joint attention between the adult and child (MacDonald, 1989). Sitting behind or above the child makes this type of interaction difficult.

Following the Child's Attentional Lead The quality of a child's attention is substantially greater to objects or events of the child's choosing, rather than to objects or events of the adult's choosing (Bruner et al., 1980). Furthermore, young children have difficulty deploying their attention on command for more than very short periods (Goldberg, 1977). Thus, following the child's attentional lead, a universal tenet of virtually all naturalistic early communication and language intervention approaches (Hepting & Goldstein, 1996) is employed to sustain the child's interest in activities and social interaction. In practice, this means that the adult plays with toys or engages in activities of interest to the child (typically selected by the child from an array of choices) in a manner similar to the child's play. Children who are passive and engage in low rates of action can make it challenging to maintain this procedure. Over time, adults can easily drop into directive styles in which they dominate most interaction episodes with the child. Experience suggests that if the goal is to build initiations, then it is far better for the adult to simply adapt his or her behavior to the child's initiation rate.

Contingent motor imitation is a helpful technique with a child who seldom initiates. *Contingent motor imitation* is an exact, reduced, or slightly expanded imitation of the child's motor production, which is performed by the adult immediately following the child's motor production. It represents a specific form of following the child's attentional lead. This simple technique is typically used at the start of intervention to establish a primitive form of turn taking between the child and adult that over time can be transformed into interaction and play routines. Contingent imitation may benefit the child because it allows him or her to regulate the amount of social stimulation received, increases the probability that adult input will be easily processed and understood (Dawson & Lewy, 1989), may encourage the child to imitate the adult's behavior (Snow, 1989), and may result in more differentiated play schemes (Dawson & Adams, 1984).

Contingent vocal imitation offers many of the same advantages and benefits as contingent motor imitation. It occurs when the adult follows a child's vocalization with a partial, exact, or modified vocal imitation. For example, the child might say "ba," which the adult might immediately imitate as "ba" or "ba ba." Contingent vocal imitation (like motor imitation) allows the child to regulate the amount of social stimulation received and may encourage the child to increase his or her rate of vocalization to imitate adult vocalizations.

Building Social Routines   Arranging the environment and following the child's lead support the development of social routines. Social routines, in turn, provide an excellent context for facilitating intentional communication. Social routines are repetitive, predictable turn-taking games and rituals, such as Peekaboo and Pat-a-Cake. They can be established in the course of daily activities such as feeding, bathing, and dressing as well as in games and toy play. Social routines can be unconventional and unique to a given child, may last from a few seconds to several minutes and may occur with a wide range of frequency. An individual may engage in a specific routine for a few days or a few years. The predictable structure of social routines may help children learn and remember new skills. Once a child learns a predictable role in a routine, he or she can devote greater attention to analyzing adult models of new ways to communicate (Conti-Ramsden & Friel-Patti, 1986; Nelson, 1989). In addition, the effectiveness of models may be enhanced because slight variations in the routine may create a "moderately novel" situation that is particularly salient to young children (Piaget & Inhelder, 1969).

Research with children who are developing typically and with children who have mental retardation has shown that social routines are particularly powerful elicitors of linguistic (Snow, Perlmann, & Nathan, 1987; Yoder & Davies, 1992) and prelinguistic (Bakeman & Adamson, 1984) communication. Once a social routine is well established with a child, adults can often elicit a high rate of requests and comments by interrupting or modifying the routine. Social routines also provide a natural context for modeling these communication functions and related skills, such as turn taking.

Specific Techniques

The establishment of one or more social interaction routines sets the stage for the use of specific techniques to prompt, model, and consequate clear, frequent intentional communication. These techniques also can be used in nonroutine interactions. The occasion for the use of any specific technique is determined by the quality of the child's engagement with an object of interest and/or his or her conversational partner. Prompts are used only when motivation to communicate is high (e.g., when the child is intently engaged in social interaction). Additional consequences can follow any intentional communication attempt. Specific teaching episodes should be brief, positive, and embedded in the ongoing stream of interaction.

Prompts   Prompts are used to elicit intentional communication attempts by the child or to elicit specific components of intentional communication. Two types of prompts, time delay and verbal prompts, are used to elicit communication attempts. A time delay for initiation is a nonverbal prompt that often functions as an interruption of an ongoing turn-taking routine. For example, if a child and adult were rolling a ball back and forth, the adult might interrupt this routine by withholding the ball and looking at the child expectantly until he or she initiates a request to continue the routine. Verbal prompts for communication can be open-ended questions (e.g., "What?") intended to elicit communication responses. Verbal prompts also can be used to elicit a specific component of communication. For example, when a child is requesting without eye contact, the directive statement "Look at me" can be used to elicit eye contact. Intersection of gaze is a technique that allows the adult to establish eye contact, an essential component of coordinated joint attention. To intersect the child's gaze, the adult moves his or her head into the gaze of the child. This technique is faded out as the child begins to regularly initiate and maintain eye contact.

Models   Models are used to support and enhance the vocal and gestural topography of the child's intentional communication attempts. Vocal models of sounds that the adult has heard the child use (e.g., "ba") are used to emphasize the vocal component of communication and attempt to increase the rate of child vocalization. Gestural models are used to encourage the child to use and imitate gestures. For example, when an airplane passes overhead, the adult might point to it as a model for the child to use pointing as an element of commenting.

Additional Consequences   Child communication attempts, such as requests and comments, should be consequated in accordance with their intent; that is, the child should receive whatever he or she has requested, and comments should elicit adult attention to the child's topic. Continued attention and interaction by the adult are assumed. These natural consequences may be supplemented with specific acknowledgment or linguistic mapping. Specific acknowledgment is provided by a smile and comment, which specifies the desired communication behavior that was used, after the child has used a targeted intentional communication component. For example, when a child makes eye contact with an adult in the course of initiating a request, the adult might smile and comment, "You looked at me!" while responding to the child's request. Frequent use of specific acknowledgment may disrupt the flow of interaction, and praise statements tend to lose their value for recipients if used too frequently. Therefore, these statements should be used primarily when a child is first acquiring a new behavior and then only in response to some occurrences.

Linguistic mapping occurs when the adult verbally states the core meaning of the immediately preceding communication act. For example, a child might hold up a doll for the adult to see (a comment), and the adult might respond, "It's a baby." As noted previously in this chapter, research with both typically and atypically developing children has indicated that linguistic mapping can be a powerful contributor to vocabulary development. Therefore, adults are encouraged to frequently use linguistic mapping as part of their response to intentional communication attempts.

Teaching Intentional Communication

The specific techniques described are meant to be embedded into ongoing interactions and to be used as dictated by the context and the child's communication goals. Some specific techniques may be used frequently (e.g., linguistic mapping) and others only until the child begins to intentionally communicate (e.g., intersection of gaze). However, the enabling procedures of arranging the environment, following the child's attentional lead, and building social routines are to be used at virtually all times during intervention.

We have worked with more than 70 young children who were in the process of moving from preintentional to intentional communication and then to symbolic communication. With the majority of these children, we specifically targeted increasing the clarity and frequency of their prelinguistic requests and comments as initial intervention goals. Our staff worked with these children three or four times per week, 20 minutes at a time, first developing some initial play routines; then concentrating on establishing clear, frequent requests; and finally establishing clear, frequent comments. The next section presents examples that demonstrate integrated use of intentional communication procedures.

Teaching Requesting It is helpful to first establish one or more social routines that involve turn taking between the adult and child. The number of sessions this requires depends on the child. Once the routine has been established and a particular instance of the routine has occurred for at least two turns, the adult may stop the routine by withholding his or her turn and looking expectantly at the child (i.e., time delay for initiation). A verbal prompt might also be given, such as "What?" (i.e., to start the activity) or "Do you want this?" (while holding an object the child needs to resume the activity). If there is not an appropriate response to the interruption of the routine, or if the child's response is incomplete (i.e., it is missing a component necessary to be considered intentional communication), then the adult may provide further assistance to the child. For example, if the child looked at the toy and displayed a discrete action or provided a vocalization but did not make eye contact with the adult, then the adult might prompt "Look at me" and/or intersect the child's gaze. The adult also might provide a gestural model if needed to complete the communication act. Prompts, models, and specific acknowledgments should be faded out as the child begins to intentionally request across different routines, but linguistic mapping should continue as part of the adult's response to the requests.

Teaching Commenting Commenting is taught in a different manner from requesting. The primary motivation for commenting is to recruit another's attention and to share affective states with the other person. It is usually necessary for young children to first develop a positive relationship with adults before they will comment to them with any frequency. Thus, we recommend waiting until such a relationship has been established before directly attempting to teach commenting. Of course, commenting may be modeled at any time.

Commenting is taught by modeling and by providing situations likely to elicit its use. One such situation is the introduction of novel events or objects. This can take many forms, including the addition of new toys or items within routines (which can be done on a daily basis) or the occasional occurrence (planned or unplanned) of silly or unusual events or even a sabotaged routine. The adult should model commenting concurrent with novel events. Another technique is for the adult to begin occasionally paying less attention to the child. For example, the adult could physically back off from the child or could turn his or her attention to another child or activity. This creates a situation in which the child may comment to gain the adult's attention, particularly if something novel occurs that the adult seems not to notice. Another approach is to let the child have the run of the room for a few minutes but with the adult clearly observing him or her from a short distance. As the child discovers novel items in this manner, he or she then may comment to the adult.

Direct efforts to teach clear forms of commenting and requesting should continue until a child is using these functions at an average of greater than one occurrence per minute in the course of a structured assessment protocol (e.g., the CSBS). Once a child has met or surpassed this criterion, training efforts may begin to focus on initial symbol acquisition (i.e., signs or spoken words) using procedures described in Chapter 16 or using milieu language teaching techniques (e.g., Warren, 1992).

CULTURAL CONSIDERATIONS

The communication functions that emerge near the end of the first year of life— requesting, commenting, protesting, greeting—are probably cultural universals that are unlikely to vary in any significant way across societies. Research indicates that the developmental progression of babbling to speech and the onset of coordinated attention are also universal across cultures and languages (see Chapters 2 and 5). Nevertheless, how adults from different cultures interact with young children may vary in some potentially important ways (van Kleeck, 1994).

There is very little research on the effects of cultural differences on intervention outcomes. For example, it is not known if individuals from the same cultural groups react the same or differently (from each other or from other cultural groups) to the same intervention. Heterogeneity of intervention effects across cultures may suggest that some cultural variables could override intervention effects, assuming there is greater variability across cultural groups than within these cultural groups. It is also plausible that cultural variables (e.g., language and dialect differences) have greater effects on the validity of assessments than the effectiveness of interventions per se. Attempts to get answers to these and other questions is complicated by the rapid changes going on within and across the cultures of the world (e.g., increased cultural blending, rapidly changing cultural standards, increasing literacy, overriding effects of industrialization and urbanization) (Phinney, 1996). Furthermore, research indicates that individual differences within cultures are often greater than differences between cultures (e.g., Jones, 1991; Zuckerman, 1990). Nevertheless, the potential value of research on cultural differences as they may affect early communication intervention efforts is substantial.

The intervention we have described reflects a set of biases emanating from our cultural view of young children and the appropriate roles of caregivers and interventionists. The acceptability of these procedures, and hence their ultimate effectiveness, may vary in some cases because of cultural differences. We presume that potential sources of bias can be limited through the careful collection and consideration of information on individual family values, beliefs, and desires (e.g., Coll & Meyer, 1993). This information then can be used to modify intervention strategies to enhance their acceptability and, thus, their effectiveness. This consideration of individual differences should be taken with all families, irrespective of their cultural or ethnic backgrounds. This perspective is completely congruent with the notion of individualizing efforts to meet the unique needs of the family and child, a widely accepted tenet of early intervention practices in many countries (Odom & McLean, 1996).

EDUCATIONAL AND CLINICAL IMPLICATIONS

The increasing knowledge of infant development and the bases of language acquisition are leading us into a new era. We now have the knowledge to predict which infants are most likely to experience delays in later language development (McCathren et al., 1996), and we have a first generation of comprehensive early communication assessments with predictive validity (e.g., CSBS). There are procedures that are potentially effective in enhancing a child's transition from preintentional to intentional communication and from intentional to symbolic communication (see also Chapter 16). These assessments and intervention protocols are being developed and evaluated at the same time that the knowledge of the effects of children's early social-communication environments and of brain development is reinforcing the critical nature of the first years of life. An important implication of these advances is that, when the need is indicated due to assessment or a preexisting condition (e.g., Down syndrome), communication intervention should begin as early in the second year of life as possible, much earlier than is often the case. Furthermore, intervention should be intensive and focused on developing clear, frequent prelinguistic communication. If necessary, a second focus of intervention should be increasing the responsiveness of the child's caregivers to his or her communication attempts. Transactional theory and research suggest that efforts to establish clear, frequent communication are facilitated by responsive caregivers who notice such changes in their children and reinforce and support their development.

Can parents and interventionists be too responsive with young children? If, in their eagerness to assist the child, they preempt his or her initiations, anticipate and respond to his or her presumed needs before he or she has had a chance to clearly indicate them, or so dominate interaction that the child has few real chances to take a communication turn, then the answer is yes. The ability of interventionists and parents to wait for the child to initiate and to match their social affect to the child's is often an underappreciated skill. Learning to truly *follow* the child's attentional lead and to use techniques such as time delay can help mitigate the tendency to be too responsive. Knowledge of the child's communicative abilities also is important. Research suggests that with a backdrop of responsivity to the children's clearest communication behaviors, mothers who negotiate the meaning of less clear communication attempts have children who use relatively more frequent, clear communication (Kim, 1996).

Finally, if the procedures being developed are going to affect more than a handful of children, speech-language pathologists and early interventionists will need to become competent in applying and modifying them, in training others to apply them, and in evaluating their effects. This will require the development and dissemination of suitable training materials.

FUTURE RESEARCH DIRECTIONS

In many respects, research on methods to facilitate prelinguistic communication development is still in its infancy. The number of published studies remains relatively small, considering the large amount of research that has been published on early language intervention. More important, the ultimate potential of prelinguistic communication intervention is not known. In our own work, we have not attempted to determine the actual efficacy of PMT in its most powerful form and context. For example, the Yoder and Warren (1997) study included a number of experimental controls likely to limit the actual efficacy of the intervention. Parents and teachers were kept naive as to the specific goals of the procedures used in the study so that we could investigate the transactional effects generated by increases in the children's intentional communication. Also, the amount of intervention children received was limited to a total of 60–80 minutes per week for a 6-month period. A true efficacy study would likely involve all individuals with a substantial stake in the child's future in the intervention and use the intervention procedures more frequently than we did. These limitations of our own work suggest that PMT may have substantial potential, perhaps far beyond what our research thus far has indicated. Full-scale efficacy studies are needed, especially on the potential effects of combining PMT with training to enhance the responsiveness of children's caregivers. Such research needs to be longitudinal in nature and should attempt to measure the effectiveness of comprehensive intervention on later language development.

Research and development targeted on translating PMT procedures into user-friendly protocols and materials suitable for practitioners in the field also is needed. One focus of such research should be on appropriate materials for parents. Another focus might be on devising culturally sensitive materials suitable for use in different cultural contexts. This type of work might consider the nature of the specific training techniques as well as culturally appropriate object–play schemas. Finally, research on PMT and other early communication interventions will continue to be informed by the type of developmental research reflected in many of the chapters in Part I of this volume, by research on the relationship of early brain and language development, and by research on the effects of the cumulative experiential deficits and ways to mitigate them.

CONCLUSION

The transition from preintentional to intentional communication is a developmental milestone second to none. It marks children's entry as full participants in the social milieu around them and triggers other transactional processes that in a short time lead to symbolic communication. Any substantial delay in this transition may cause other delays along the developmental path, the effects of which may further multiply to the overall detriment of the child. This is a risk that interventionists want to minimize or eliminate altogether. Therefore, the provision of effective prelinguistic communication intervention, implemented as soon as there are any reasonable concerns about the infant's developmental trajectory, needs to become both a research and a practice priority.

REFERENCES

Bakeman, R., & Adamson, L. (1984). Coordinating to people and objects in mother–infant and peer–infant interaction. *Child Development, 55,* 1278–1289.

Bates, E., Benigni, L., Bretherton, I., Camaioni, L., & Volterra, V. (1979). *The emergence of symbols: Cognition and communication in infancy.* New York: Academic Press.

Bates, E., Camaioni, L., & Volterra, V. (1975). The acquisition of performatives prior to speech. *Merrill-Palmer Quarterly, 21,* 205–226.

Bates, E., O'Connell, B., & Shore, C. (1987). Language and communication in infancy. In J. Osofsky (Ed.), *Handbook of infant development* (pp. 149–203). New York: John Wiley & Sons.

Bates, E., Thal, D., & Janowsky, J.S. (1991). Early language development and its neural correlates. In I. Rapin & S. Segalowitz (Eds.), *Handbook of neuropsychology: Vol. 7. Child neuropsychology* (pp. 107–179). New York: Elsevier/North Holland.

Beckwith, L., & Parmelee, A.H. (1986). EEG patterns of preterm infants, home environment, and later IQ. *Child Development, 57,* 777–789.

Berger, J. (1990). Interactions between parents and their infants with Down syndrome. In D. Cicchetti & M. Beeghly (Eds.), *Children with Down syndrome: A developmental perspective* (pp. 101–146). Cambridge, England: Cambridge University Press.

Bruner, J. (1981). The social context of language acquisition. *Language and Communication, 1,* 155–178.

Bruner, J., Roy, C., & Ratner, R. (1980). The beginnings of request. In K.E. Nelson (Ed.), *Children's language* (Vol. 3, pp. 91–138). New York: Gardner Press.

Chugani, H.T. (1994). Development of regional brain glucose metabolism in relation to behavior and plasticity. In G. Dawson & K.W. Fischer (Eds.), *Human behavior and the developing brain* (pp. 153–175). New York: Guilford Press.

Coll, C., & Meyer, E. (1993). The sociocultural context of infant development. In C. Zeanah (Ed.), *Handbook of infant mental health* (pp. 56–69). New York: Guilford Press.

Conti-Ramsden, G., & Friel-Patti, S. (1986). Mother–child dialogues: Considerations of cognitive complexity for young language learning children. *British Journal of Disorders of Communication, 21,* 245–255.

Dawson, G., & Adams, A. (1984). Imitation and social responsiveness in autistic children. *Journal of Abnormal Child Psychology, 12,* 209–226.

Dawson, G., & Lewy, A. (1989). Reciprocal subcortical-cortical influences in autism: The role of attentional mechanisms. In G. Dawson (Ed.), *Autism: Nature, diagnosis, and treatment* (pp. 144–173). New York: Guilford Press.

Feagans, L., & Farran, D.C. (1982). *The language of children reared in poverty: Implication for evaluation and intervention.* New York: Academic Press.

Gallaway, C., & Richards, B.J. (Eds.). (1994). *Input and interaction in language acquisition.* Cambridge, England: Cambridge University Press.

Girolametto, L. (1988). Improving the social-conversational skills of developmentally delayed children: An intervention study. *Journal of Speech and Hearing Disorders, 53,* 156–167.

Goldberg, S. (1977). Social competence in infancy: A model of parent–infant interaction. *Merrill-Palmer Quarterly, 23,* 163–177.

Gottfried, A.W. (Ed.). (1984). *Home environment and early cognitive development: Longitudinal research.* New York: Academic Press.

Hanson, M.J. (1984). Parent–infant interaction. In M.J. Hanson (Ed.), *Atypical infant development* (pp. 179–206). Baltimore: University Park Press.

Hart, B., & Risley, T.R. (1968). Establishing the use of descriptive adjectives in the spontaneous speech of disadvantaged preschool children. *Journal of Applied Behavior Analysis, 1,* 109–120.

Hart, B., & Risley, T.R. (1992). American parenting of language-learning children: Persisting differences in family–child interactions observed in natural home environments. *Developmental Psychology, 28*(6), 1096–1105.

Hart, B., & Risley, T.R. (1995). *Meaningful differences in the everyday experience of young American children.* Baltimore: Paul H. Brookes Publishing Co.

Hepting, N.H., & Goldstein, H. (1996). What's "natural" about naturalistic language intervention? *Journal of Early Intervention, 20,* 250–265.

Jones, J. (1991). Psychological models of race: What have they been and what should they be? In J. Goodchilds (Ed.), *Psychological perspectives on human diversity in America* (pp. 3–46). Washington, DC: American Psychological Association.

Kaiser, A.P., Yoder, P.J., & Keetz, A. (1992). Evaluating milieu teaching. In S.F. Warren & J. Reichle (Eds.), *Communication and language intervention series: Vol. 1. Causes and effects in communication and language intervention* (pp. 9–48). Baltimore: Paul H. Brookes Publishing Co.

Kim, K. (1996). *Maternal behavior related to prelinguistic intentional communication in young children with developmental delays.* Unpublished doctoral dissertation, Vanderbilt University, Nashville, TN.

Landry, S.H. (1995). The development of joint attention in premature low birth weight infants. In C. Moore & P. Dunham (Eds.), *Joint attention: Its origin and role in development* (pp. 223–250). Hillsdale, NJ: Lawrence Erlbaum Associates.

Locke, J.L. (1993). *The child's path to spoken language.* Cambridge, MA: Harvard University Press.

MacDonald, J. (1989). *Becoming partners with children: From play to conversation.* San Antonio, TX: Special Press.

McCathren, R.B., Warren, S.F., & Yoder, P.J. (1996). Prelinguistic predictors of later language development. In K.N. Cole, P.S. Dale, & D.J. Thal (Eds.), *Communication and language intervention series: Vol. 6. Advances in assessment of communication and language* (pp. 57–76). Baltimore: Paul H. Brookes Publishing Co.

McLean, J., & Snyder-McLean, L. (1978). *A transactional approach to early language training.* Columbus, OH: Charles E. Merrill.

McLean, L.K., & Cripe, J.W. (1997). The effectiveness of early intervention for children with communication disorders. In M.J. Guralnick (Ed.), *The effectiveness of early intervention* (pp. 349–427). Baltimore: Paul H. Brookes Publishing Co.

Musselwhite, C.R. (1986). *Adaptive play for special needs children.* San Diego, CA: College-Hill Press.

Nelson, K.E. (1989). Strategies for first language teaching. In M.L. Rice & R.L. Schiefelbusch (Eds.), *The teachability of language* (pp. 263–310). Baltimore: Paul H. Brookes Publishing Co.

Odom, S.L., & McLean, M.E. (1996). *Early intervention/early childhood special education recommended practices.* Austin, TX: PRO-ED.

Phinney, J.S. (1996). When we talk about American ethnic groups, what do we mean? *American Psychologist, 51*(9), 918–927.

Piaget, J., & Inhelder, B. (1969). *The psychology of the child.* New York: Basic Books.

Prizant, B., & Wetherby, A. (1990). Toward an integrated view of early language and communication development and socioemotional development. *Topics in Language Disorders, 10*(4), 1–16.

Rogoff, B., Mistry, J., Radziszewska, B., & Germond, J. (1992). Infants' instrumental social interaction with adults. In S. Feinman (Ed.), *Social referencing and the social construction of reality in infancy* (pp. 323–348). New York: Plenum.

Rosenberg, S. (1982). The language of the mentally retarded: Development, progress, and intervention. In S. Rosenberg (Ed.), *Handbook in applied psycholinguistics* (pp. 329–392). Hillsdale, NJ: Lawrence Erlbaum Associates.

Sameroff, A.J. (1983). Developmental systems: Contexts and evolution. In P.H. Mussen (Ed.), *Handbook of child psychology* (Vol. 1, pp. 237–294). New York: John Wiley & Sons.

Sameroff, A.J., & Chandler, M.J. (1975). Reproductive risk and the continuum of care-taking casualty. In F.D. Horowitz, M. Hetherington, S. Scarr-Salapatck, & G. Siegel (Eds.), *Review of child development research* (Vol. 4, pp. 187–244). Chicago: University of Chicago Press.

Snow, C.E. (1989). Imitativeness: A trait or a skill? In G.E. Speidel & K.E. Nelson (Eds.), *The many faces of imitation in language learning* (pp. 73–90). New York: Springer-Verlag.

Snow, C.E., Perlmann, R., & Nathan, D. (1987). Why routines are different: Toward a multiple factors model of the relation between input and language acquisition. In K.E. Nelson & A. van Kleeck (Eds.), *Child language* (Vol. 6, pp. 65–97). Hillsdale, NJ: Lawrence Erlbaum Associates.

Sokolov, J.L. (1993). A local contingency analysis of the fine-tuning hypothesis. *Developmental Psychology, 29*(6), 1008–1023.

Sugarman, S. (1984). The development of preverbal communication. In R.L. Schiefel-busch & J. Pickar (Eds.), *The acquisition of communicative competence* (pp. 23–67). Baltimore: University Park Press.

Tannock, R., & Girolametto, L. (1992). Reassessing parent-focused language intervention programs. In S.F. Warren & J. Reichle (Eds.), *Communication and language intervention series: Vol. 1. Causes and effects in communication and language intervention* (pp. 49–79). Baltimore: Paul H. Brookes Publishing Co.

Tomasello, M., & Farrar, M.F. (1986). Joint attention and early language. *Child Development, 57,* 1454–1463.

van Kleeck, A. (1994). Potential cultural bias in training parents as conversational partners with their children who have delays in language development. *American Journal of Speech-Language Pathology, 31,* 67–78.

Warren, S.F. (1991). Enhancing communication and language development with milieu teaching procedures. In E. Cipani (Ed.), *A guide for developing language competence in preschool children with severe and moderate handicaps* (pp. 68–93). Springfield, IL: Charles C Thomas.

Warren, S.F. (1992). Facilitating basic vocabulary acquisition with milieu teaching procedures. *Journal of Early Intervention, 16*(3), 235–251.

Warren, S.F., & Kaiser, A.P. (1988). Research in early language intervention. In S.L. Odom & M.B. Karnes (Eds.), *Early intervention for infants and children with handicaps: An empirical base* (pp. 89–108). Baltimore: Paul H. Brookes Publishing Co.

Warren, S.F., Yoder, P.J., Gazdag, G.E., Kim, K., & Jones, H.A. (1993). Facilitating prelinguistic communication skills in young children with developmental delay. *Journal of Speech and Hearing Research, 36,* 83–97.

Wetherby, A.M., Cain, D.H., Yonclas, D.G., & Walker, V.G. (1988). Analysis of intentional communication of normal children from prelinguistic to the multiword stage. *Journal of Speech and Hearing Research, 31,* 240–252.

Wetherby, A.M., & Prizant, B. (1993). *Communication and Symbolic Behavior Scales: Normed edition.* Chicago: Applied Symbolix.

Wetherby, A.M., Yonclas, D., & Bryan, A. (1989). Communicative profiles of handicapped preschool children: Implications for early identification. *Journal of Speech and Hearing Disorders, 54,* 148–158.

Wilcox, M.J. (1992). Enhancing initial communication skills in young children with developmental disabilities through partner programming. *Seminars in Speech and Language, 13*(3), 194–212.

Wilcox, M.J. (1993, November). *Issues regarding linguistic readiness in young children with developmental disabilities.* Paper presented at the annual convention of the American Speech-Language-Hearing Association, Anaheim, CA.

Yoder, P.J., & Davies, B. (1992). Do children with developmental delays use more frequent and diverse language in verbal routines? *American Journal on Mental Retardation, 97*(2), 197–208.

Yoder, P.J., Davies, B., & Bishop, K. (1994). Adult interaction style effects on the language sampling and transcription process with children who have developmental disabilities. *American Journal on Mental Retardation, 99*, 270–282.

Yoder, P.J., Kaiser, A.P., Alpert, C., & Fischer, R. (1993). The effect of following the child's lead on the efficiency of teaching nouns with preschoolers with mental retardation. *Journal of Speech and Hearing Research, 35*, 1–35.

Yoder, P.J., & Munson, L. (1994). The effect of adult continuing wh-questions on conversational participation in children with developmental disabilities. *Journal of Speech and Hearing Research, 37*(1), 193–204.

Yoder, P.J., & Warren, S.F. (1993). Can developmentally delayed children's language development be enhanced through prelinguistic intervention? In A.P. Kaiser & D.B. Gray (Eds.), *Communication and language intervention series: Vol. 2. Enhancing children's communication: Research foundations for intervention* (pp. 35–62). Baltimore: Paul H. Brookes Publishing Co.

Yoder, P.J., & Warren, S.F. (1996). *Effects of prespeech milieu teaching or intentional communication: A transactional analysis.* Unpublished manuscript, Vanderbilt University, Nashville, TN.

Yoder, P.J., & Warren, S.F. (1997, April). *Experimental analysis of the transactional effects of intentional communication and maternal linguistic responsivity.* Poster presented at the biannual conference of the Society for Research in Child Development, Washington, DC.

Yoder, P.J., Warren, S.F., & Kim, K. (1997). *Maternal responsivity to communicative acts of varying types.* Submitted for publication.

Yoder, P.J., Warren, S.F., Kim, K., & Gazdag, G.E. (1994). Facilitating prelinguistic communication skills in young children with developmental delay: II. Systematic replication and extension. *Journal of Speech and Hearing Research, 37*, 841–851.

Zuckerman, M. (1990). Some dubious premises in research and theory on racial differences. *American Psychologist, 45*, 1297–1303.

16

Facilitating the
Transition from Prelinguistic
to Linguistic Communication

M. Jeanne Wilcox and Michelle S. Shannon

DURING THE PRELINGUISTIC PERIOD, MOST children develop a rich and complex system of communication abilities characterized by increasing competence in conveying messages to their interactive partners. As is apparent from chapters in Part I, children's emerging skills (e.g., play, gestures, babbling, coordinated attention) and environmental factors (e.g., adult responsivity) interact to facilitate and support the emergence of a highly functional communication system. These early communication skills appear to form a necessary basis for initial language use. That is, for children with well-established communication systems, the acquisition of language has enormous utility; messages are generally exchanged more efficiently with language. Children who do not have well-established communication systems may have little motivation to acquire language because a gestural system may appropriately meet their limited communication needs.

While many children make the transition from prelinguistic to linguistic communication with relative ease, others require specific facilitation efforts, or intervention, to assist the emergence of language. It is these children who serve as the focus of this chapter, which discusses selected issues concerning early language acquisition in children developing atypically, as well as specific strategies that may serve to facilitate a successful transition from prelinguistic to linguistic communication. The approach to this topic is organized into four sections, each of which reflects the belief that the most effective interventions evolve from some degree of reflection on the language acquisition process. The chapter begins with a brief overview of the authors' perspectives of the language acquisition process and then turns to issues regarding the onset of linguistic behavior, focusing on the nature of first words and the tasks a child faces in making the transition from prelinguistic to linguistic communication. This is followed by a

Preparation of this chapter was supported in part by U.S. Department of Education Grants No. H023C00126 and No. H029D1001. Information contained in this chapter does not necessarily reflect views of the U.S. Department of Education and no official endorsement should be inferred.

discussion of possible relationships between prelinguistic and linguistic behavior and specific communication behaviors that may signify readiness for language intervention. The final section focuses on the design and implementation of initial language interventions, including selection of target behavior, intervention approaches, the relative effectiveness of specific intervention strategies, and important considerations when providing intervention to young children from varying sociocultural backgrounds.

A PERSPECTIVE ON THE LANGUAGE ACQUISITION PROCESS

Consensus has not been achieved regarding the process or processes underlying children's acquisition of language abilities, and a full discussion of relevant issues is beyond the scope of this chapter. Although there is no *single* account of the language acquisition process that is sufficient to guide approaches to early intervention (see Rice, 1995, for a discussion), it is essential for language interventionists to have an understanding of the complexity of the behaviors to be acquired as well as the ease with which most children undertake language acquisition during the preschool years. The ease with which most children master complex language behavior reflects the likelihood of specialized biological mechanisms designed for the purpose of language acquisition. At the same time, interventionists must consider ways to design and implement effective interventions based on characteristics of the social interactive context *known* to promote and facilitate language development. Few resources are available that integrate the relatively distinct perspectives of the biological and environmental contributions to language acquisition. The brief discussion in this chapter of the language acquisition process is motivated by the necessity of integrating these two perspectives to most efficiently and effectively provide early language intervention services.

First, although some language skills follow a parallel, and at times interdependent, path with regard to other developmental accomplishments (e.g., sitting, walking, formation of attachments, means–ends manipulations, symbolic play), language should be viewed as having a unique and independent acquisition process (e.g., Curtiss, 1989; Fowler, 1990; Levy, Amir, & Shalev, 1994; Rondal, 1994). Second, while language is typically studied through the various behaviors it manifests, language acquisition is largely the product of a biologically governed process. Following Lenneberg (1967), the human capacity for language is taken to be directly attributable to a uniquely human neural organization. Similarly, following Wakefield and Wilcox (1995), many aspects of language acquisition during the early years are primarily a function of brain maturation. Evidence regarding the genetic bases of language impairments (Gopnik & Crago, 1991; Lahey & Edwards, 1995; Tallal, Ross, & Curtiss, 1989; Tomblin, 1989) provides additional support in this regard. In adopting a biological view of the acquisition process, the intent is not to minimize the importance of an environmental contribution, as the environment plays a key role in providing a child with a language to acquire as well as a role in facilitating the acquisition process. Rather, the intent of including this discussion is to lay the theoretical foundations for specifying the biological conditions under which environmental contributions are operative in language acquisition.

The third point regarding the language acquisition process pertains to the nature and timing of intervention efforts. Specifically, to the extent possible, it is important to consider neurobiological readiness when making decisions regarding intervention targets and methods. Consider, for example, an intervention targeting the transition from prelinguistic to linguistic communication. On the theoretical framework adopted in this chapter, a child whose brain has not reached the state of maturation compatible with verbal representations will derive minimal benefit from an intervention strategy that targets language acquisition. With such children, the most effective intervention might be one that targets the enhancement of nonlinguistic communication skills, building the motivational foundations for later language acquisition (e.g., Wilcox, 1992; Wilcox, Hadley, & Ashland, 1996).

The comments of the authors of this chapter pertain to the nature and timing of interventions and not to the decision as to a given child's need for intervention. Hence, we are not suggesting that interventionists should wait for a particular state of neurobiological maturity or readiness before providing intervention. Any young child evidencing difficulty with the communication or language acquisition process should be provided with appropriate intervention. Our concern is with *appropriateness*; it is important for intervention techniques and goals to *match* a child's maturational capabilities, at least to the extent that a given child's abilities in this regard are known. We recognize that basing aspects of developmental intervention decisions on a particular state of neurobiological readiness is not without difficulty, particularly when evidence regarding the specific neurological bases of language is in an emergent phase. However, as discussed in a subsequent section on readiness and initial language interventions, there are various behavioral indicators that language interventionists may use to infer neurobiological readiness.

The final point regarding the process of language development is that language unfolds within a broader social and neural organization that is shaped by experiences encountered in the environment (for a review, see Greenough, Black, & Wallace, 1987). Accordingly, children's emerging linguistic abilities should be viewed as deriving from the interplay of their biological potentials and environments. Furthermore, biological potentials and environments vary, and although children with typical potential may acquire necessary skills in any social context, children with atypical potential often require special or extraordinary contextual support. Herein lies the role of the language interventionist, to facilitate language acquisition through the provision of essential environmental support that is matched, to the extent possible, with children's innate abilities and experiences.

THE NATURE OF EARLY LINGUISTIC COMMUNICATION

There is variation in interpretation as to what constitutes a child's transition to linguistic communication. For example, some equate the onset of linguistic behavior with a child's production of his or her first word, and others define the onset of linguistic behavior with reference to evidence of rule-governed productions (i.e., word combinations; lexical categories such as noun, verb). Still others focus on comprehension and define the onset of linguistic behavior with respect to a child's language comprehension abilities. It is important for interventionists to consider and specify what constitutes the onset of linguistic behavior to select appropriate target behaviors and design effective interventions. For the purposes of this chapter, we are defining *initial linguistic behavior* as a child's first word production with *word* defined as a spontaneously produced form that is phonetically consistent and used to convey a consistent meaning. We view these first words as symbolic, yet not fully linguistic (as a rule-governed system has not yet emerged). Accordingly, we regard the period corresponding to a child's development of a first lexicon of approximately 50 different word productions as the transition from prelinguistic to linguistic communication. Typically, after children have established this first lexicon, evidence for rule-governed behavior is observed and the transition to fully linguistic communication has been achieved. This chapter is concerned with the period before the transition to linguistic communication, or with the transitional period; thus, it is necessary to give some consideration to the nature of first words (see Chapter 9 for a more in-depth discussion of this transitional period).

First words are generally restricted to a single, highly specific interactive context (Barrett, Harris, & Chasin, 1991; Bloom, 1993) and, as such, are considered context bound. As noted by Wilcox, Hadley, et al. (1996), context-bound words are acquired as children encounter repeated and specific input in the course of daily activities, such as feeding, bathing, and social play routines. These activities create opportunities for children to form associations between words and specific objects, actions, or events. Although the acquisition of context-bound words reflects a critical initial step in language acquisition, to gain a productive expressive ability, the word must be separated from the context in which it was learned. This process has been referred to as decontextualization (Barrett, 1986) and requires a child to form associations between words and more generalized concepts. Decontextualization is facilitated by exposure to words in different contexts representing varying communication functions. As children gain this understanding of language, previously context-bound words either disappear or take on a new status and are used productively in a broad base of communication contexts. However, not all first words appear as contextualized productions. Some words, such as those learned receptively through exposure to numerous exemplars, may first appear as decontextualized productions. For many initial words, though, the task a child faces in effecting a transition from prelinguistic to linguistic communication includes shifting from contextualized to decontextualized word use. The very first words, as highly restrictive and often context-bound productions, may be best conceptualized as entry-level symbolic behaviors, representing a bridge between contextually rooted prelinguistic and relatively decontextualized linguistic communication.

READINESS AND INITIAL LANGUAGE INTERVENTIONS

A key factor in the success of initial language interventions, or for any developmental language intervention, is the extent to which a child demonstrates readiness for the selected linguistic target. As noted by Long and Olswang (1996) in their analysis of readiness and growth patterns of young children with specific expressive language impairments, improved understanding and knowledge regarding readiness patterns and indicators can serve to refine intervention practices substantially. Readiness for linguistic communication may be relatively easy to discern in some prelinguistic children. For example, those who have not yet acquired the ability to communicate intentionally are unlikely to be ready to use language as a means of communication. In recognition of the fact that a system of nonverbal communication is a precursor to verbal communication, intervention with such children typically targets intentional nonverbal expression of such meanings as request or comment (Wilcox, 1992; Wilcox, Shannon, & Bacon, 1996). Similarly, children who have begun using words to communicate have demonstrated probable readiness for additional word acquisition. The issue is more complicated for the large number of prelinguistic children who demonstrate intentional nonverbal communications in the absence of any word approximations. The authors view such children as members of a "fuzzy set" in terms of readiness for initial lexical training; some may be ready and some may not. With these types of children, readiness, or lack thereof, is often inferred by the success or failure of initial language intervention efforts, that is, a trial-and-error process. However, with this sort of approach readiness cannot really be differentiated from poorly implemented or ineffective interventions. Ideally, we should be able to ascertain readiness prior to a trial period of language intervention through procedures such as dynamic assessment (e.g., Bain & Olswang, 1995; Olswang, Bain, & Johnson, 1992) and/or clinical analyses of children's current abilities and known relationships to subsequent language growth.

Various characteristics of a child's prelinguistic behavior may indicate readiness for initial lexical acquisition. Furthermore, certain aspects of the child's environment may facilitate a transition to linguistic communication. In general, as interest in prelinguistic intervention procedures has grown, so has attention to potential relationships between prelinguistic and linguistic communication in young children with varying developmental problems. An understanding of these relationships is important because interventionists may learn strategies that enable them to more efficiently approach the task of facilitating the transition to linguistic communication.

From an intervention perspective, we believe that any attempt to understand prelinguistic–linguistic relationships requires consideration of three related issues: 1) the extent to which prelinguistic communication may serve to indicate readiness for linguistic communication, 2) the extent to which aspects of prelinguistic communication behavior may serve to predict linguistic outcomes, and 3) the extent to which certain aspects of prelinguistic behavior and interactions may serve to facilitate subsequent linguistic communication. Although these issues are similar, they have different implications for intervention. For example, an aspect of children's prelinguistic communication may be viewed as an indicator of linguistic readiness (e.g., tendency to initiate interpersonal interaction) but is not, in and of itself, likely to be causally related to subsequent linguistic development. This would imply that although interventionists may want to profile linguistic readiness through careful attention to aspects of a child's prelinguistic communication interactions and behavior, they would not necessarily expect these behaviors to serve as predictors for linguistic outcome, nor would they view them as prerequisites that, if absent, must be trained. However, if it turns out that certain prelinguistic communication behavior predicts aspects of linguistic outcome, then interventionists may profile prelinguistic communication for early identification of those children at risk for language disorders. However, predictors are not necessarily causal agents; thus, an absence of a particular predictor would not necessarily confirm a future language problem nor would it mean that a given predictive behavior serves as a prerequisite and must therefore be added to a child's repertoire. Finally, if it can be shown that aspects of prelinguistic communication facilitate linguistic outcomes, then intervention protocols could be designed with these facilitative behaviors in mind. Therefore, we are interested in identifying such things as *indicators* of linguistic readiness so that we can commence lexical training at the most optimal time, *predictors* for linguistic outcome so that we can construct reliable early identification protocols, and *facilitators* of linguistic behavior so that our intervention techniques can be designed in the most efficient manner.

Although the transition from prelinguistic to linguistic communication has received substantial attention for children developing typically, for children developing atypically the investigative history is less thorough. Hence, aspects of the empirical database are in an emergent phase, and the ensuing discussion is appropriately viewed as a status report. Primary candidates meriting consideration in prelinguistic behavior–initial linguistic relationships, as discussed in Part I, include phonology, intentional nonverbal communication and gestures, play, joint attention, and adult responsivity. This section briefly summarizes relevant research in each of these areas, with an eye toward the issues under consideration (i.e., readiness, prediction, and facilitation).

Phonology

All young children demonstrate limited phonetic inventories during vocal production of their first 50 words. They maximize their limited capabilities through preferential acquisition of words that contain consonants within their expressive phonetic inventories and selective avoidance of words that do not (e.g., Schwartz & Leonard, 1982; Stoel-Gammon, 1985; see also Chapter 5). This phonological selectivity also has been established during initial lexical acquisition for children who demonstrate specific receptive and expressive language impairment (SLI–RE) (Leonard et al., 1982). In addition, predominantly prelinguistic children with specific expressive language impairment (SLI–E), when compared with age-matched typical peers, have been found to demonstrate reduced consonantal inventories and reduced frequency of vocalizations that contain consonants (Paul & Jennings, 1992; Rescorla & Ratner, 1996). The Rescorla and Ratner investigation, which included more detailed phonetic analyses, revealed similar usage of phonemes appearing in initial positions for the children with SLI–E and for the typically developing children. However, the children with SLI–E demonstrated a marked reduction in use of final-position consonants as well as a preponderance of earlier developing syllabic shapes.

It would appear that phonological selectivity, in conjunction with a reduced consonantal repertoire and lower frequencies of consonantal vocalizations, serves to further constrain initial lexical acquisition in young children with language impairment. In their review of research pertaining to predictors for early language development, McCathren, Warren, and Yoder (1996) concluded that prelinguistic vocalization frequency and consonantal use consistently predicted vocabulary development and amount of speech. Accordingly, it is reasonable to hypothesize that those children who demonstrate prelinguistic vocal behaviors that include frequent vocalizations, consonantal productions, and a relatively diverse phonetic repertoire can be expected to achieve better expressive language outcomes, at least in the speech modality. This receives support from an investigation conducted by Whitehurst, Smith, Fischel, Arnold, and Lonigan (1991) in which they examined potential relationships between babbling and subsequent language outcome (5 months postinitial assessment) in a group of 37 children with SLI–E who were in the initial stages of lexical acquisition (their average productive vocabulary sizes were less than 18 words). Expressive language outcome was measured by the Expressive One-Word Picture Vocabulary Test (Gardner, 1981) and the verbal expression subtest of the Illinois Test of Psycholinguistic Abilities (Kirk, McCarthy, & Kirk, 1968). Results indicated that the single best predictor for expressive language outcome was the proportion of consonantal to vowel babble. Vowel babbling was found to impede language growth whereas consonantal babbling was viewed as facilitative.

Overall, it would appear that the phonological behavior of prelinguistic children provides important information regarding readiness indicators as well as predictors of linguistic outcome. In particular, children's phonetic repertoires (i.e., mastered consonants) and consonantal productions (e.g., vowel–consonant [VC], consonant–vowel [CV], CVC, CVCV) should be considered in determining readiness for acquisition of initial words in the speech mode. An extremely limited consonantal repertoire is likely to constrain initial speech-word acquisition and, if other readiness indicators are present, would suggest that initial word acquisition should emphasize a speech-mode alternative (e.g., sign). In contrast, assuming the presence of other readiness indicators, a relatively diverse phonetic repertoire, as indicated by a variety of consonantal vocalizations, would suggest the likelihood of success with initial speech-word acquisition.

Nonverbal Communication

During prelinguistic communication development, children develop a rich system of meanings and nonverbal modes for conveyance of those meanings. It is generally agreed that these early communication skills formulate a necessary (although certainly not sufficient) basis for initial language use. That is, children cannot be expected to use language as a tool for communication if they have not first learned to communicate. Therefore, children's nonverbal intentional communication abilities become a prime candidate when considering readiness issues. Early language interventionists have recognized the need to facilitate intentional communication function *before* targeting initial lexical acquisition. However, little is clear beyond this fact. For example, few guidelines exist regarding such concerns as the amount of intentional communication and the number of different communication functions regarded as sufficient, or the relative importance of communication function types (e.g., request, comment, answer). Comparisons of children developing language typically with those demonstrating language disorders (of varying etiologies) have revealed delays in the onset of intentional nonverbal communication as well as differences in communication behavior types and uses (e.g., Mundy, Sigman, Kasari, & Yirmiya, 1988; Thal & Tobias, 1992, 1994; Wetherby, Yonclas, & Bryan, 1989). Investigators also have found a relationship between certain aspects of nonverbal communication and subsequent language abilities in young children with Down syndrome (Mundy, Kasari, Sigman, & Ruskin, 1995; Smith & von Tetzchner, 1986). In the Smith and von Tetzchner investigation, analyses of nonverbal requests and comments revealed that the complexity of requests (e.g., reach versus reach plus a vocalization) produced by prelinguistic children with Down syndrome ($n = 13$) was related to subsequent expressive language abilities as measured by the Reynell Developmental Language Scales (Norwegian adaptation) (Reynell, 1985). No patterns were noted for other communication functions (i.e., nonverbal comments). Mundy et al. (1995), in their longitudinal study of predominantly prelinguistic children with Down syndrome ($n = 37$), found patterns consistent with those reported by Smith and von Tetzchner (1986). Nonverbal communication assessments included appraisal of social-interaction behavior (e.g., eliciting attention or physical contact with others), joint attention bids, responses to joint attention, and requests. Results indicated that nonverbal requests and social-interaction behaviors were predictors of subsequent expressive language abilities, and no patterns were evident with regard to receptive language abilities.

When comparing the Mundy et al. (1995) and the Smith and von Tetzchner (1986) investigations, the findings are consistent with respect to nonverbal requesting ability and the children with Down syndrome. Thus, nonverbal requesting ability may be a useful prognostic indicator for young children with Down syndrome in that higher degrees of complexity and production frequency are associated with more positive expressive language outcomes. Furthermore, the Mundy et al. (1995) investigation suggests that social interaction behavior, as measured by ability to elicit attention, may also prove to be a prognostic indicator for children with Down syndrome.

Research also indicates that rate of intentional nonverbal communication merits consideration with regard to prognosis for children who demonstrate communication and language delays. Wilcox (1993) conducted a preliminary examination of varying aspects of children's prelinguistic behavior that might contribute to later linguistic development. Subjects for the longitudinal inquiry were 30 prelinguistic children who demonstrated general developmental delays of undetermined etiology. The children were observed at 6-month intervals over a 2-year period and were assigned to one of four groups that were differentiated by the point at which onset of word use was noted: 1) 12 who were prelinguistic at Observation 1 and symbolic (i.e., in the phase of initial lexical acquisition) at Observation 2; 2) 6 who were prelinguistic at Observations 1 and 2 and symbolic at Observation 3; 3) 5 who were prelinguistic at Observations 1, 2, and 3 and symbolic at Observation 4; and 4) 7 who never demonstrated word use, that is, were prelinguistic at all observation points. Dependent measures were the children's rate of intentional communication, number of productive communication functions (e.g., request, comment, protest, answer, acknowledge), rate of word use (when appropriate), and rate of gestural indicating behavior (e.g., point, give, show, reach). All rate measures were computed as use per 10-minute observation unit. Analysis focused on the measurement point at which children demonstrated onset of words and the point immediately before word onset. For children who never produced words during the 2-year time period, analysis was conducted with data from all measurement points.

No trends were noted with respect to indicating behavior (e.g., reach, point, give, show) or to the number of productive communication functions. However, a consistent trend was revealed with rate of intentional communication and rate of word use. Specifically, for the three groups of children who eventually made the transition to linguistic communication ($n = 23$), a mean rate of at least 9.0

intentional communication acts per 10-minute unit was observed in the measurement point *immediately prior* to onset of words. This trend was consistently replicated across the three groups of children who demonstrated initial word acquisition. The group of children who did not acquire words during the observation period never demonstrated a rate of intentional communication acts per 10-minute unit that approached 9.0; that is, their rate of intentional communication behavior was below 4 acts per 10-minute unit for all measurement points.

The Wilcox (1993) study was preliminary, and the sample was small in three of the groups; however, the consistent replication of the rate trend across the groups lends support to the validity of the findings. Furthermore, the findings regarding rate of intentional communication are consistent with those reported by others (e.g., Wetherby & Prizant, 1993; Wetherby et al., 1989). Specifically, Wetherby and colleagues (1989) reported that rates of intentional communication acts approach 1.0 act per minute as children are making the transition from prelinguistic to initial symbolic communication. Although the rate noted by Wilcox (1993) converts to a slightly lower per-minute figure (i.e., 0.9) than that reported by Wetherby et al. (1989), the findings are congruent. Thal and Tobias (1992) also reported a relationship between rate of nonverbal communication and language outcome. In their longitudinal investigation of young children who evidenced delays in expressive language development, they found that "truly delayed" (i.e., SLI–E) versus "late bloomers" could be differentiated with regard to preverbal use of communicative gestures. Specifically, the late bloomers produced higher rates of intentional nonverbal communication than did children who proved to be SLI–E as well as a group of typically developing age-matched controls.

Given the research conducted, it would seem that rate of intentional communication serves as an indicator of readiness for the transition to linguistic communication. It may be that expressive language, as a far more efficient means of communication, is motivated by a threshold rate of nonverbal communication. That is, as children's nonverbal communication behaviors increase, children may come to realize the need for a more conventional means of communication to avoid misunderstandings typical of nonverbal communication systems and/or to communicate a broader range of messages. Higher rates of intentional nonverbal communication may also result in higher rates of facilitative input (i.e., verbal models of a nonverbal communication act) from people in the environment. This possibility receives support from an investigation conducted by Yoder, Warren, Kim, and Gazdag (1994) in which they found that mothers and teachers of prelinguistic children were more likely to provide verbal models of children's nonverbal intentional versus preintentional communication acts.

It also has been suggested that higher rates of intentional nonverbal communication may serve as a compensatory mechanism for children who experience a temporary barrier in oral-language acquisition (e.g., Acredolo & Goodwyn, 1988; Thal & Tobias, 1992). In particular, Thal and Tobias (1992) hypothesized that the late bloomers in their study used communicative gestures to compensate for their temporary expressive language limitations, thereby allowing continued communication development and ultimately typical oral-language acquisition patterns.

Overall, it appears that three conclusions can be drawn regarding the role of preverbal intentional communication and the readiness issues of concern. First, rate of preverbal intentional communication may serve as an indicator of linguistic readiness. Children who demonstrate rates that approach 1.0 per minute may be signifying readiness to begin the transition from prelinguistic to linguistic communication. Second, rate of intentional communication may be a useful prognostic indicator, at least for children with SLI–E. In this population, high rates of intentional preverbal communication are suggestive of a child who will eventually outgrow his or her communication delay. Third, for children with Down syndrome, limited nonverbal requesting abilities as well as selected social-interactive behaviors (i.e., attention elicitation strategies, turn taking with objects) may be important indicators of subsequent expressive language difficulties. Although it is well established that children with Down syndrome have expressive language difficulties, they are not a homogeneous group, and their expressive language outcomes demonstrate high degrees of inter-child variability. Therefore, an earlier indicator of those children who are likely to experience the most difficulty may allow earlier and more effective facilitation efforts.

Play

Young children's play, particularly symbolic play, has received investigative attention focusing on potential play–language relationships in children with a variety of developmental language problems (Beeghly, Weiss-Perry, & Cicchetti, 1990; Casby & Ruder, 1983; Leonard, 1987; Rescorla & Goosens, 1992; Thal & Bates, 1988; Thal, Tobias, & Morrison, 1991). Most research designs have included comparisons of children with age-matched and language-matched (or mental age–matched) controls who are developing typically. Associations between symbolic play and language acquisition (i.e., comprehension and expression) are apparent in the empirical database, although for prelinguistic children the strongest association appears to be with language comprehension.

Little evidence addresses the extent to which prelinguistic play may serve to predict and/or improve linguistic outcome, particularly with regard to initial lexical acquisition. Some indirect evidence is available in a study conducted by Yoder, Warren, and Hull (1995) in which they examined potential predictors of children's success in a prelinguistic intervention program that targeted nonverbal requesting. Subjects in the investigation included eight children with developmental delays of varying etiologies (e.g., Down syndrome, undetermined etiology, microcephaly, agenesis of the corpus callosum). Results indicated that higher levels of symbolic play were associated with better intervention outcomes, that is, greater increases in intentional nonverbal communication. In particular, the children's baseline levels of symbolic play with objects were positively correlated with increases in nonverbal requesting behavior.

The conclusion of the preceding section is that prelinguistic intentional communication rates were potential indicators of linguistic readiness. We further concluded, at least for children with SLI–E, that higher rates of intentional communication were good prognostic indicators. To the extent that symbolic play levels contribute to an increase in prelinguistic communication rates, it would seem that symbolic play can be viewed as an indirect indicator of readiness or as a parameter to consider in determining prognosis. In addition, there is a relatively substantial database that establishes associations among symbolic play, language comprehension, and initial use of communication symbols (i.e., words). Although an association should not be construed to mean prerequisite or precursory behavior, it is not unreasonable to conclude that, for some children, the associated behavior can be interpreted as evidence of a general readiness for representational behavior. Therefore, in combination with other indicators, symbolic play levels may serve to indicate a general readiness for acquisition of an initial lexicon.

Joint Attentional Processes and Adult Responsivity

There is a fair amount of variation in the conceptualization of joint attentional processes; variation is even more apparent in methods used to examine such processes in prelinguistic children. In our view, joint attentional processes include a child's ability to establish and maintain shared reference with an interactive partner as well as the ability to respond to a partner's attentional bids (see Chapters 2, 3, and 6 for further discussion of these topics). Our treatment of the issues, as presented in this chapter, are relatively brief and restricted to considerations of indicators, predictors, and facilitators.

The vast majority of research in early joint attentional processes has focused on children developing typically (see Moore & Dunham, 1995, for a review) and clearly establishes a link between time spent in and quality of adult–child joint attentional episodes and subsequent vocabulary development. In general, increased amounts of time spent in joint attention are associated with subsequent increases in vocabulary size. Furthermore, maternal behaviors (e.g., directives, comments) that follow a child's attentional focus have been shown to have a positive influence on children's language acquisition as measured by productive vocabulary size (e.g., Akhtar, Dunham, & Dunham, 1991). However, it should also be noted that although adults' provision of verbal labels corresponding to a child's focus of attention is important for initial word acquisition, children eventually demonstrate the ability to acquire new words under discrepant labeling conditions, that is, situations in which an adult verbal label does not correspond to a child's immediate attentional focus (Baldwin, 1993).

Studies of joint attentional processes in atypical populations have focused on children with varying etiologies and associated language difficulties, including those with autism (e.g., Sigman & Kasari, 1995), late talkers (Paul & Shiffer, 1991; Rescorla & Fechnay, 1996), infants at risk (Landry, 1995), those with Down syndrome (Newman, 1995), and those with general developmental delays (Shannon, Wilcox, & Bacon, 1993; Walentas, 1994). Children with autism have demonstrated marked deficiencies in all aspects of joint attentional interactions. Other children (i.e., children with Down syndrome, preterm low birth weight infants, children with developmental delays) have demonstrated difficulty in joint attention initiations but relative ease in appropriately responding to their interactive partners' attentional bids. Conflicting findings have been reported for young children identified as late talkers. Paul and Shiffer (1991) as well as Rescorla and Fechnay (1996) compared groups of late talkers (mean ages of about 25 months in each investigation) with their age-matched typically developing peers. Results of the Paul and Shiffer investigation indicated deficiencies in the late talkers' abilities to establish joint attention while Rescorla and Fechnay found that their late-talking children did not differ significantly from their typical peers. Although differences in coding systems might account for some variation in the findings, as noted by Rescorla and Fechnay, differences in the late talkers' receptive language abilities may serve as a more likely indicator. Approximately 25% of the children in the Paul and Shiffer investigation demonstrated receptive and expressive language problems; the remaining children presented with expressive delays in isolation. All children in the Rescorla and Fechnay investigation demonstrated age-appropriate receptive language skills; delays were only apparent in expressive language skills.

It would seem that among children with specific language impairment, a differentiation of receptive–expressive versus expressive-only subtypes may be required when considering joint attentional processes. Furthermore, it may be that early joint attentional processes are more closely linked with receptive language abilities, not just for children with specific language impairment but for other groups of children who demonstrate language and communication disorders (e.g., those with autism or general developmental delays). Support for such a relationship is provided in an investigation conducted by Newman (1995) in which she examined potential relationships between time spent in joint attention and subsequent language abilities for young children with Down syndrome. The investigation was a longitudinal inquiry in which 10 children with Down syndrome were measured at three points over a 12-month time period that generally corresponded to the acquisition of their first 50 words. Results indicated that when the children were prelinguistic, time spent in prelinguistic joint attention was correlated ($r = .59$) with subsequent receptive language abilities, as measured by the Sequenced Inventory of Communication Development (SICD) (Hedrick, Prather, & Tobin, 1975) administered 6 months following the joint attention measures. Once the children demonstrated some initial lexical acquisition, the time spent in joint attention was strongly correlated ($r = .83$) with expressive language abilities, also as measured by the SICD administered

6 months later. These results, at least for the expressive language finding, are consistent with results reported for typically developing children. Comparisons cannot be established in terms of prelinguistic joint attention and subsequent receptive language abilities because we are unaware of investigations of prelinguistic joint attentional processes and subsequent language ability in typically developing children.

The ability to establish joint attention as well as time spent in joint attention may prove to be useful prognostic indicators; however, at least equal consideration should be given to the quality of the joint attention episodes. One way to conceptualize such quality is with regard to adult responsivity. There are various ways in which responsive interaction has been found to facilitate early language acquisition (see Chapter 3), although it may be that for the most efficient results responsive interaction strategies should be combined with some strategy for elicitation of a targeted word. However, of concern here is initial lexical acquisition, or facilitating the transition from prelinguistic to linguistic communication. Studies by Wilcox, Shannon, and Bacon (1992, 1996) provided strong evidence for the role of adult responsivity by itself. In an attempt to evaluate linguistic benefits of a prelinguistic intervention protocol, Wilcox et al. (1992, 1996) examined longer-term language outcomes of children whose mothers completed a prelinguistic intervention program developed by Wilcox (1992). The program was designed to teach prelinguistic children's communication partners strategies for enhancing or establishing children's intentional communication productions. The intervention protocol incorporated such principles as following a child's attentional lead, identifying and responding to children's intentional communication behavior, identifying and responding to children's potential communication cues (i.e., those to be responded to as if they were intentional communication productions), using contextually appropriate responses, and applying strategies for natural elicitation of more complex communication behavior. Unlike most programs that train participants in responsive interaction strategies, the mothers were trained to identify and respond to specific child behavior. They were also trained in strategies for arranging the environment to create opportunities or a need for communication (e.g., providing toys that required adult assistance to create opportunities for requests, introducing novel items or events to create opportunities for comments) as well as strategies for natural elicitation of behavior (e.g., pretending to misunderstand in an attempt to elicit a desired behavior or a more complex behavior). However, direct elicitation strategies (e.g., "Can you do…?", "Show me…", "Tell me…") were discouraged.

Experimental methods in the investigation included comparisons of 10 children whose mothers participated in the training program with 10 standard practice control children. The children ranged in age from 19 to 38 months. All 20 children were enrolled in early intervention programs; however, only mothers of children in the experimental condition participated in the 6-month interaction training program. All children demonstrated prelinguistic communication abilities at recruitment for participation in the research. Intervals for comparison included pre- and postintervention and 6, 12, and 18 months following the conclusion of intervention. Dependent measures included rate of word production (single and multiword combinations) during mother–child sampling sessions and standard test scores. The standardized test information was available from comparisons of the scores obtained on the SICD that was administered before intervention and again at 18 months postintervention. Results revealed significantly greater use of words by children whose mothers took part in the experimental training program. Differences were also noted in the receptive and expressive SICD scores, with experimental children demonstrating significantly higher scores at the final measurement point. Control children did demonstrate word use but at lower production rates. These results support the idea that intervention in which mothers are trained in optimal interactive patterns, by itself, may facilitate later child language development, at least with respect to the transition from prelinguistic to linguistic communication. It also should be acknowledged that the sample size was relatively small and high individual variation was noted in both experimental and control children. Although rate data are useful, no information was provided on diversity of word use (e.g., productive vocabulary size), a measure that would seem to be important in examination of linguistic outcomes.

Overall, joint attention, in combination with adult responsivity, seems to have a role to play with respect to prediction and facilitation of linguistic outcomes. In general, it appears that as children's capacity for engaging in joint attention episodes increases, so does a more positive linguistic outcome in terms of vocabulary size. In addition, responsive interaction (e.g., following a child's lead, responding to communication behavior, natural elicitation of more complex behavior) appears to function as a facilitator for children's transition from prelinguistic to linguistic communication.

Word Production Capabilities

We previously suggested that children who demonstrate production of some words are typically assumed to be ready for initial linguistic training. Although this may be true in many cases, it is not universally so, and results of three investigations provide some guidance for further thinking in this regard. Kouri and Wilcox (1996) examined potential relationships between young children's lexical learning during intervention and their baseline abilities as determined through standardized testing and analyses of communication samples. Participants in the inquiry included a group of 27 children (mean age of 25 months) who demonstrated developmental delays and were estimated to have expressive vocabulary sizes of fewer than 25 true words (as determined by direct observation and detailed maternal interviews). All children were enrolled in an early intervention program that consisted of individual language intervention to facilitate acquisition of targeted lexical items. Analyses of the children's word learning after 3 months of intervention (i.e., 24 individual sessions) were conducted to determine the possible predictive value of baseline measures. Performance on standardized tests (i.e., SICD–Receptive, SICD–Expressive, Battelle Developmental Inventory [BDI]–Composite, BDI–Cognitive) did not predict the number of words acquired during intervention. However, the number of words a child had at baseline was found to be a predictor for acquisition of targeted lexical items, irrespective of the intervention method. Children who had more words at baseline acquired more words during intervention. Furthermore, children who had no words or few words (fewer than two) at baseline demonstrated minimal acquisition in either intervention condition. These findings are consistent with those reported previously for another population of young children, those with SLI–E (Whitehurst, Fischel, Arnold, & Lonigan, 1992; Whitehurst et al., 1991). Whitehurst and colleagues have indicated that 2-year-olds who present with a substantial expressive language delay are likely to make rapid, spontaneous progress if they demonstrate the ability to name a number of objects on request. Furthermore, Whitehurst et al. found that the rate of children's word production as well as estimated vocabulary size (as per maternal report) were positively correlated with subsequent expressive language outcome.

Children's vocabulary sizes at baseline (i.e., identification) may have uses as both predictors and indicators relative to expected linguistic outcome. In terms of a predictor, the work of Whitehurst et al. (1991, 1992) supports the idea that expressive vocabulary size may differentiate those children who are truly SLI–E from those who can be expected to outgrow a temporary expressive delay. In terms of an indicator, a child's expressive vocabulary size upon identification may serve as a primary factor to consider in determining readiness for initial linguistic behavior. The minimal learners ($n = 3$) in the Kouri and Wilcox (1996) investigation are of particular interest in this regard. These children presented with other assumed indicators of readiness for linguistic behavior, including productive communication functions and some consonant sounds in their phonetic repertoire. However, all three children demonstrated productive use of fewer than three of their target words, suggesting that these factors alone may not have been sufficient for a determination of readiness for linguistic intervention. The children's estimated baseline expressive vocabulary sizes were determined to range from zero to two word productions, which could have served as another factor to consider. Furthermore, rate of nonverbal intentional communication (which was not available for these children), when considered in conjunction with baseline words, may have contributed to a profile of children who were simply not ready to begin the transition to linguistic communication.

DESIGN AND IMPLEMENTATION OF INTERVENTIONS

Since the 1970s, a large amount of attention has been directed toward identification of effective language intervention strategies, and interventionists have a number of choices from among those judged as effective (see reviews in Fey, 1986; Kaiser & Gray, 1993). The basic efficacy has been established for several approaches, and it is clear that language intervention accomplishes the goal of improving acquisition over that which would be expected through maturation alone. Intervention research in the mid-1990s has shifted to address questions regarding the relative effectiveness of varying approaches. Although some research has conducted comparisons at a global level (i.e., effectiveness of one approach versus another for a given population), noted patterns of individual variation have prompted examination of issues associated with achieving a match between the selected approach and children with particular characteristics or at particular developmental levels. This is a critical issue confronting both early language interventionists and researchers. The following sections consider intervention approaches in this regard and discuss components common to all early language interventions, variations in intervention approaches, the relative effectiveness of approaches, and cultural considerations in the design and implementation of interventions.

Intervention Procedures: Similarities, Variations, and Effectiveness

There has been a strong emphasis on designing early language interventions that reflect that language emerges within a social context (e.g., Rice & Wilcox, 1995; Wilcox & Shannon, 1996). Three parameters are common to most early language intervention approaches designed from this perspective, including an emphasis on teaching to children's attentional focus, manipulation of the physical and/or linguistic environment to create opportunities for communication, and provision of natural consequences for communication or lack thereof. Although most early language intervention approaches are similar in terms of these basic principles, there are two key areas of variation. The first pertains to strategies for facilitating children's production of a response (e.g., no specific elicitation strategies, environmental arrangement to increase likelihood of a response, a specific direction to produce a particular response). The second area of variation focuses on the person who serves as the primary intervention agent (e.g., parent, professional). These differences have served as the basis for the bulk of research on the relative effectiveness of early language interventions.

Response Facilitation Strategies Intervention approaches can be classified into one of three groupings: 1) those that make specific provisions for elicitation of children's responses, 2) those that target specific child language behavior in an interactive context but do not attempt to elicit child responses, and 3) those that have a more global interactive focus and train children's partners in general language and communication facilitation strategies. The first group is referred to as *milieu teaching techniques,* the second as *responsive interaction techniques,* and the third as *global interaction techniques.*

The first group, milieu teaching techniques, comprises a set of strategies that can be embedded in typical activities, teaches to a child's attentional lead,

and includes provisions for elicitation of child responses through such mechanisms as requests for imitation (e.g., "You want the cup. Can you say cup?"),
questions (e.g., "What is this?"), or requests for verbal behavior (e.g., "Tell
me"). Specific strategies within milieu techniques include incidental teaching
(Hart & Risley, 1975), mand model (Warren, McQuarter, & Rogers-Warren,
1984), systematic commenting (Warren & Gazdag, 1990), and time delay
(Halle, Marshall, & Spradlin, 1979).

A large database documents the basic efficacy of milieu techniques for children of varying developmental levels, in both individual and classroom settings
(for a review, see Kaiser, Yoder, & Keetz, 1992). Overall, milieu teaching procedures consistently have been shown to increase frequency of communication
behavior, vocabulary, and use of specific language structures in young children
with communication and language delays. Milieu teaching techniques also have
been adapted for prelinguistic children and found to be effective in increasing
the frequency of children's nonverbal requests and comments (Warren, Yoder,
Gazdag, Kim, & Jones, 1993; Yoder et al., 1994). Although effects of prelinguistic milieu teaching on initial linguistic development have yet to be determined,
the approach shares important characteristics with the prelinguistic intervention
protocol developed and tested by Wilcox and colleagues (Wilcox, 1992; Wilcox
et al., 1992, 1996; see also Chapter 15). Given the similarity between the two
approaches and the longer-term language effects associated with the Wilcox et
al. (1992, 1996) protocol, it seems likely that prelinguistic milieu teaching will
prove to be similarly beneficial.

Responsive interaction techniques, the second group, have also been
referred to as focused stimulation (Leonard et al., 1982) and interactive modeling (Wilcox, Kouri, & Caswell, 1991). This group of procedures shares characteristics associated with milieu techniques, including provision of intervention
within the context of typical activities and following children's attentional leads.
However, responsive interaction techniques do not include provisions for elicitation of specific child responses. Rather, focused input is provided with reference
to children's attentional focus resulting in facilitation strategies that may include
provision of models, expansions, or recasts to increase saliency of targeted language behavior. Basic efficacy is well established for responsive interaction
techniques; they have been found to be effective facilitators for acquisition of
various grammatical forms (e.g., Bunce & Watkins, 1995; Camarata & Nelson,
1992; Fey, Cleave, Long, & Hughes, 1993) as well as initial lexicons (Leonard et
al., 1982; Wilcox, 1984; Wilcox et al., 1991). Furthermore, Wilcox and colleagues (Wilcox et al., 1992, 1996) demonstrated that prelinguistic children of
mothers who participated in a responsive interaction training program that targeted enhancement of children's intentional communication abilities had superior language outcomes compared with a group of standard practice controls
whose mothers did not receive such training.

The third group of approaches, global interaction techniques, includes those that train children's primary communication partners in strategies known to facilitate language acquisition but do not directly provide intervention to the children and do not have specific child language targets. Rather, the goal is general enhancement of communication ability (e.g., turn taking, conversational initiations), vocabulary, and word combinations, among others. These approaches have been referred to as the interactive model (Tannock & Girolametto, 1992), conversational model (MacDonald, 1985), and child-initiated interaction (Norris & Hoffman, 1990). Although these techniques have been linked with improvements in adult–child interactions, efficacy has not been established in terms of child language behavior (for a review, see Tannock & Girolametto, 1992). That is, change has been documented in adult-interactive strategies as well as in aspects of the children's participation in interaction (e.g., turn taking). However, as of the late 1990s, changes in child language behavior have not been attributable to global interaction techniques.

Intervention Agents   Another source of variation in early language interventions pertains to the intervention agents. Most of the intervention approaches described in the preceding section have been implemented with family members as well as a variety of early intervention personnel (e.g., speech-language pathologists, teachers, physical or occupational therapists). For example, parents have been taught to implement milieu teaching techniques (e.g., Hemmeter & Kaiser, 1994) as well as responsive interaction strategies (e.g., Wilcox, 1992), with positive changes in children's communication behavior noted in both applications. In addition, the global interaction techniques were designed for parent training, although, as noted previously, the efficacy of such programs is restricted to changes in parental behavior and general aspects of child communication interaction.

When considering a parent-training component as part of a particular child's intervention programming, specific communication behavior targets must be identified to facilitate parental models and responses. Furthermore, the length of the parent training must be sufficient to allow mastery of the interactive skills emphasized. For example, Wilcox (1992), in collaboration with parents, identified specific child communication targets and included a combination of group and individual training to allow parents time to master targeted interaction skills and reliably recognize response opportunities and targeted child behavior. Individual training sessions took place in the families' homes and included observation of mother–child interactions with subsequent review and "coaching." Similarly, Kaiser, Hemmeter, Ostrosky, Alpert, and Hancock (1995) found that although parents in their study varied in the time it took to master milieu teaching procedures, all parents required group instruction as well as intensive home training sessions to reach criterion levels of performance in the implementation of milieu techniques.

A concern of many interventionists regarding parent training is that such training by itself may be insufficient to effect desired change in children's behavior. An investigation by Kot and Law (1995) is pertinent to this concern. The study was designed to compare the effects of language interventions that were provided with and without a parent-training component. Participants included 14 children with SLI–RE who ranged in age from 3-0 to 3-6. The first group ($n = 7$) received direct child intervention in a group setting, and their parents also attended group sessions that emphasized increasing the use of labels and utterances related to the child's focus of attention. The second group ($n = 7$) received only the direct child intervention in a group setting. Results indicated that children in both groups demonstrated comparable language gains, but only parents who participated in the parent program demonstrated increased use of targeted interactive strategies. However, the postintervention measures were taken immediately after the 7-week intervention program, so information regarding a potential long-term benefit of the parent training is not available.

Relative Efficacy of Early Language Intervention Approaches

Comparisons of early language intervention protocols mostly have centered on issues associated with children's response requirements. Olswang, Bain, Rosendahl, Oblak, and Smith (1986) were among the first to address this issue and did so through an alternating interventions design in two preschool children with language impairments. At baseline, one child had an estimated productive vocabulary size of 10–12 words and the other, 2–3 words. Three intervention conditions were examined including modeling only, modeling plus an obstacle to facilitate a need to communicate, and modeling plus response elicitation. A different set of seven lexical items served as the intervention targets for each child in each of the three intervention conditions. Preintervention dynamic assessment procedures were conducted to determine which conditions might be most beneficial for each of the children. Results indicated that the model-plus-elicitation condition resulted in higher rates of correct productions for both children. However, experimental control could only be demonstrated for one child; thus, these results must be restricted to interpretation for a single child.

Ellis Weismer, Murray-Branch, and Miller (1993) also examined the relative effectiveness of modeling and modeling plus evoked production. Three young children with SLI–E, who had estimated productive vocabulary sizes of 13, 16, and 25 words, were included in the study. A single-case alternating intervention design was employed with different lexical items targeted in each condition. One child demonstrated essentially equal acquisition with both intervention conditions, although it was reported that he reluctantly participated in the model-plus-evoked-production condition and produced more spontaneous language during the model-only condition. Another child demonstrated no acquisition in either condition. The third child demonstrated learning in both conditions, but in the model-plus-evoked-production condition an advantage was noted with regard to lexical frequency and diversity.

Two studies have examined the relative effectiveness of milieu teaching and responsive interaction (Kouri & Wilcox, 1996; Yoder, Kaiser, et al., 1995). Yoder, Kaiser, et al. (1995) reported pre- and posttest measures in 38 children ages 2–7 years with mild to severe developmental delays. The children varied greatly in terms of language functioning; however, all were producing some single-word utterances and were able to verbally imitate 8 of 12 words. All children were enrolled in a classroom program in which the teachers facilitated language acquisition during typical classroom activities through either milieu teaching or responsive interaction. Because personnel in a given classroom implemented a particular procedure for all children in the class, the children were not randomly assigned to the different intervention conditions. All children had specific language targets. Analysis of pre- and posttest measures revealed that children with receptive language and vocabulary-age scores around 24 months of age made greater language gains in the milieu condition, and children with receptive language and vocabulary-age scores close to 36 months of age or older did better in the responsive-interaction condition.

Kouri and Wilcox (1996) also examined the relative effects of a milieu teaching strategy (i.e., mand model) and a responsive interaction protocol they termed interactive modeling. Participants included 27 young children with developmental language delays of undetermined etiologies who were randomly assigned to either the mand-model ($n = 12$) or interactive-modeling-intervention condition ($n = 15$). Intervention spanned a time period of approximately 3 months and included twice-weekly individual play sessions that were 45 minutes in duration. The play sessions took place in a room at an early intervention program that was designed to resemble a typical family room. All children demonstrated at least two productive communication functions and three consonant sounds within their phonetic repertoires and had fewer than 25 productive words at baseline (range of 0–25), as determined by a combination of maternal report and direct observation, clearly placing them in the period of development we have termed the transitional period with respect to acquisition of linguistic behavior. In addition to tracking acquisition of words in the intervention sessions, home generalization probes were conducted pre- and postintervention. Results indicated that children in both intervention conditions demonstrated acquisition of targeted words, but, overall, acquisition and generalization to home environments was superior for children in the mand-model condition, suggesting an advantage for a milieu teaching technique during initial lexical training.

The Kouri and Wilcox (1996) results are consistent with the findings reported by Yoder, Kaiser, et al. (1995) in which they found an advantage for milieu teaching with children at early stages of language development. They were also consistent with aspects of findings in the Ellis Weismer et al. (1993)

and the Olswang et al. (1986) investigations. Specifically, both investigations noted, for some children, a learning advantage for the modeling-plus-evoked-production condition, which was very similar to the mand-model milieu technique tested by Kouri and Wilcox (1996). Hence, it would seem reasonable to conclude that if a profile of readiness for initial lexical learning is apparent, a technique that provides some mechanism for response elicitation may be the most efficient procedure to use. This is not to say that modeling alone does not facilitate initial word learning; certainly evidence indicates that it does, and, for some children, it may prove to be a preferred method.

Early Language Interventions and Cultural Considerations

The interventions considered all make assumptions about typical activities and optimal parent–child or adult–child interactive strategies. These assumptions comprise potential sources of bias that must be considered when designing intervention programs for children of varying backgrounds and sociocultural experiences. It is critical for interventionists to think about the bases from which most early language facilitation techniques derive and adjust as necessary to avoid conflict with a given family's value system.

Early communication and language acquisition is inextricably bound to the interpersonal interactive context. The reality of this relationship is confirmed by the fact that the most efficacious communication and early language intervention protocols are those designed to integrate specific facilitation strategies within a meaningful social context (e.g., Fey, 1986; Rice & Wilcox, 1995; Wilcox & Shannon, 1996). As a result, almost all intervention protocols that target initial language acquisition (i.e., the transition from prelinguistic to initial linguistic communication) include a focus on children's communication interactions in typical settings (e.g., home, playgroup) and rely on adult-interactive techniques known to facilitate children's language acquisition. However, much of what is known about language development and adult–child interaction patterns has been derived from studies examining these variables in Anglo, middle-class cultures (Ochs & Schieffelin, 1984). Furthermore, cross-cultural research on communication and language acquisition provides extensive documentation that appropriate sociolinguistic behaviors (including facilitation techniques) and contexts comprise a significant source of variation across cultures (e.g., Crago, 1992; Harkness, 1975; Ochs & Schieffelin, 1984; Rogoff, Mistry, Goncu, & Mosier, 1991; Schieffelin & Ochs, 1986; Ward, 1971).

There are similarities in children's language acquisition across diverse groups. All children begin to acquire their native language at about the same age. Also, caregivers across all cultures use language in some way to interact with their children and support and guide their children's learning (Crago, 1992; Rogoff, 1990). Important differences among cultures include beliefs about how children learn language, the value placed on child talk, social contexts that are appropriate for caregiver–child interaction, and people who are available to guide children's learning and participation (Heath, 1989; Lynch & Hanson, 1992; Schieffelin & Ochs, 1986; van Kleeck, 1994). Almost all early language intervention approaches make assumptions that are potentially inappropriate about each of these areas of cross-cultural variation. In her review of early intervention procedures and cross-cultural data, van Kleeck (1994) concluded that most approaches for young children, particularly parent training programs, implicitly reflect mainstream Western cultural values. Accordingly, interventions have been based on what is assumed to be the universal course of language development and interactional patterns, but in reality they are restricted to a particular economic and ethnic group. For example, consider the primary goals of all early language intervention efforts: to increase a child's expressive language output. As simple and obvious as this goal may seem through the eyes of Western culture, it may be contrary to the value system of other cultures. Indeed, in her study of the Inuit, Crago (1990) found that "talkativeness" by a young child was viewed as a potential sign of a learning problem. Another common component of most programs is an adult–child dyadic focus, particularly in parent training protocols. In some cultures (e.g., Mexican American), adults infrequently engage in dyadic interactions with children; typical dyadic partners for a young child are older siblings (Langdon, 1992). Also, as noted by van Kleeck (1994), in some cultures (e.g., Mexican American, Kaluli) adult–child interactions that do occur are most likely to be triadic and include the mother, child, and another adult, with the mother prompting her child in what to say to the other adult.

Other essential components of intervention approaches considered in this chapter include following a child's attentional lead, responding to child initiations, and providing a verbal model (with or without a response requirement) that corresponds to a child's communication intent or attentional focus. Van Kleeck (1994) provided numerous citations and examples of cultures (e.g., rural Louisiana African American, Mexican American and other Hispanic populations, Native American, Pennsylvania Dutch, Western Samoans) in which some or all of these parameters have the potential for conflict with prevailing values, beliefs, or typical communication styles. Hence, any of these seemingly basic interaction components, whether taught as a parent-implemented strategy or provided by an interventionist, may be limited in effect because the underlying assumption regarding interaction may bear little resemblance to a given child's typical communication experiences. If early language intervention is to have the desired outcome, the actuality or potential for cultural conflict must be anticipated and avoided.

Fortunately, potential sources of bias can be minimized through careful gathering of information and development of goals and intervention strategies in collaboration with family members. An important initial step is for interventionists to develop an awareness as to which aspects of a particular intervention goal or strategy are based on assumptions that may not be held by all families. It is important to note that each child and family that comes to the intervention setting must be approached as unique and without preconceived assumptions regarding their values and beliefs. During the assessment and intervention processes, time must be spent establishing relationships with families to discover their values and beliefs, particularly with regard to their perceptions of the role of communication and language in their child's life and to their beliefs regarding communication and language development and teaching.

Once appropriate information is gathered, comparisons can be made between values promoted by specific intervention approaches and those held by families. When there appears to be a conflict between the two value systems, disagreement should be discussed openly and honestly with the families and solutions or alternative options should be explored. In this way interventionists and family members are in a position to determine if a particular aspect of an intervention strategy should be dropped but the basic strategy maintained, an alternative strategy should be identified, or the strategy should be implemented as designed, with the acknowledgment of the potential conflict and an appropriate plan designed for managing this conflict (e.g., Andrews & Andrews, 1990; van Kleeck, 1994).

EDUCATIONAL AND CLINICAL IMPLICATIONS

As noted throughout this chapter, myriad factors interact to affect and assist children's transition from prelinguistic to linguistic communication. In an ideal world the empirical database would provide sufficient information for early language interventionists to comprehensively profile prelinguistic children to determine the optimal timing of initial language intervention and the optimal intervention procedure. However, the world is far from ideal, and the present database is far too thin to offer such a direct and practical application. Hence, interventionists are restricted to a short list of clinical implications, or possibilities for application, all of which must be viewed as candidates for ongoing refinement from future researchers and interventionists.

From this cautionary perspective, we focus first on the notion of readiness. A child's individual capabilities are certainly a critical component to a successful transition to linguistic communication, and this chapter has considered several aspects of children's prelinguistic behavior that may serve as indicators of future language difficulties or predictors of language outcome. While the data are in an emergent state, there is sufficient information to suggest that children's phonological skills and rates of nonverbal communication production may serve as useful indicators of initial intervention success. In particular, children who are producing relatively high rates of nonverbal communication with higher proportions of consonantal babbling are those who may progress the most rapidly in our initial language intervention efforts. In contrast, children who communicate at lower rates (e.g., less than 1.0 act per minute) and have larger amounts of vowel babble may benefit from intervention efforts that have a focus on strengthening the communication basis for language.

A second consideration with regard to clinical implications pertains to facilitators, specifically those that would seem to ease or promote children's transition from prelinguistic to linguistic communication. Evidence indicates that caregiver responsivity plays a role in facilitating children's language gains. Optimal adult strategies include following a child's attentional lead, responding to intentional communication with contextually appropriate linguistic models, and creating opportunities for children to communicate. These strategies, which also correspond to components of many early language intervention procedures, can be easily integrated within most caregiving activities and may prove useful for parent training protocols.

Finally, the comparative efficacy data can be used to formulate preliminary guidelines for selection of a particular intervention protocol. First, it is apparent that the global interaction interventions, by themselves, are not likely to facilitate initial language acquisition. Hence, when we wish to train an initial lexicon, a milieu or responsive interaction approach is preferable. Furthermore, data suggest that a milieu approach may be more efficient than responsive interaction, although this effect is mediated by a child's baseline word production capabilities. As the number of baseline words increases, the differential effectiveness of milieu versus responsive interaction diminishes. Thus, when a child has few or no words, a milieu approach is likely to be most beneficial. As children move past the acquisition of the first 10–15 words, this benefit is less apparent. Finally, communication and language acquisition patterns vary substantially across children; there will always be those who do not fit the suggested trends, and interventionists are urged to observe carefully and modify their procedures accordingly.

DIRECTIONS FOR FUTURE RESEARCH

Potential areas for additional research were identified throughout the chapter; this section briefly highlights our perceptions of major needs. First, the extent to which a prelinguistic child demonstrates readiness for language acquisition merits future investigation in terms of biological readiness as well as behavioral indicators of such readiness. Although models of brain–early language relationships have been proposed (e.g., Wakefield & Wilcox, 1995), the empirical database providing support for such models is in an emergent state. Given that increasing evidence points to a strong biological basis for language acquisition, additional information regarding underlying neural substrates and biological readiness will facilitate the ability to provide the optimal intervention at the optimal time. Technological advances should greatly facilitate this line of inquiry and we look forward to the results of such efforts.

A second area for future research concerns behavioral indicators of linguistic readiness. Although increased knowledge of the biological bases for language acquisition may contribute to the intervention decision-making process, it is critical to continue exploration of prelinguistic–linguistic behavioral relationships. A better understanding of this relationship will prove useful to the assessment and intervention process. In the discussion of prelinguistic indicators, predictors, and facilitators, we identified some promising areas of inquiry (e.g., nonverbal communication rates, responsivity) but noted the specific and preliminary nature of most findings. The understanding of prelinguistic–linguistic behavioral relationships is advancing, but in many ways it is still quite rudimentary and largely has been restricted to delineation of single factors. As researchers and interventionists continue the quest to understand and identify prelinguistic indicators, predictors, or facilitators, it is unlikely that any single factor will prove constant either within or across populations. Thus, a productive direction for future inquiries might include a focus on understanding behavioral combinations for the purpose of establishing profiles of readiness for initial linguistic behavior.

A third area meriting additional investigative attention concerns the efficacy of initial linguistic interventions for multicultural families and their young children. As noted in the previous discussion of these issues, the interactional focus of most effective early language intervention approaches increases the likelihood of bias or conflict in applications with members of nondominant cultures. As awareness of this potential problem has increased, various investigators have described options for minimizing possible bias (e.g., Heath, 1989; Langdon, 1992; van Kleeck, 1994). These various suggestions have resulted in a heightened sensitivity among many service providers, particularly those in areas heavily populated with individuals from varying cultural backgrounds. Approaches to dealing with the problem must be individualized for a given family. However, research has yet to address the outcomes of such efforts, that is, the extent to which heightened sensitivity and appropriately individualized procedures result in improved outcomes for young children with developmental language disabilities. Given an ever-increasing diversity in the population of young children in need of early language intervention, this is a critical area for future research.

The final recommendation for future research focuses at a broader level, encompassing aspects of all preceding recommendations. Specifically, there is an acute need for continued investigation of early language intervention procedures and their relative effectiveness for varying groups of families and their young children. Overall, such research with prelinguistic or early linguistic children is sparse and has focused primarily on comparing one method with another for children with similar language needs. One exception is the Yoder, Kaiser, et al. (1995) investigation in which comparisons were made between methods across children at varying baseline language levels. Investigations of this sort represent a promising start, and continuation of research is needed that includes careful examination of intervention effects with respect to children's unique language needs and other characteristics. An important component of this line of investigation will be an emphasis on families and their young children from varying sociocultural backgrounds. However, it will be necessary to consider information such as this in conjunction with the multitude of effective intervention techniques and the numerous biological and behavioral parameters on which children can be expected to demonstrate individual variation. Ultimately, an empirical and clinical knowledge base is required that is capable of guiding an interventionist's selection of the most efficacious technique given a prelinguistic child's unique characteristics and circumstances. The authors anticipate that such work will and should progress slowly, as there are numerous factors to weave into a meaningful pattern of understanding.

REFERENCES

Acredolo, L., & Goodwyn, S. (1988). Symbolic gesturing in normal infants. *Child Development, 59,* 450–466.

Akhtar, N., Dunham, F., & Dunham, J. (1991). Directive interactions and early vocabulary development: The role of joint attentional focus. *Journal of Child Language, 18,* 41–50.

Andrews, J., & Andrews, M. (1990). *Family based treatment in communicative disorders.* Sandwich, IL: Janelle Publications.

Bain, B., & Olswang, L. (1995). Examining readiness for learning two-word utterances by children with specific expressive language impairment: Dynamic assessment validation. *American Journal of Speech-Language Pathology, 4,* 81–91.

Baldwin, D. (1993). Infants' ability to consult the speaker for clues to word reference. *Journal of Child Language, 20,* 395–418.

Barrett, M. (1986). Early semantic representations and early word usage. In S. Kuczaj & M. Barrett (Eds.), *The development of word meaning.* New York: Springer-Verlag.

Barrett, M., Harris, M., & Chasin, J. (1991). Early lexical development and maternal speech: A comparison of children's initial and subsequent uses of words. *Journal of Child Language, 18,* 21–40.

Beeghly, M., Weiss-Perry, B., & Cicchetti, D. (1990). Beyond sensorimotor functioning: Early communicative and play development of children with Down syndrome. In D. Cicchetti & M. Beeghly (Eds.), *Children with Down syndrome: A developmental perspective* (pp. 329–368). New York: Cambridge University Press.

Bloom, L. (1993). *The transition from infancy to language.* New York: Cambridge University Press.

Bunce, B.H., & Watkins, R.V. (1995). Language intervention in a preschool classroom: Implementing a language-focused curriculum. In M.L. Rice & K.A. Wilcox (Eds.), *Building a language-focused curriculum for the preschool classroom: Vol. 1. A foundation for lifelong communication* (pp. 39–72). Baltimore: Paul H. Brookes Publishing Co.

Camarata, S., & Nelson, K.E. (1992). Treatment efficiency as a function of target selection in the remediation of child language disorders. *Clinical Linguistics and Phonetics, 6,* 165–178.

Casby, M., & Ruder, K. (1983). Symbolic play and early language development in normal and MR children. *Journal of Speech and Hearing Research, 26,* 404–411.

Crago, M. (1990). Development of communicative competence in Inuit children: Implications for speech-language pathology. *Journal of Childhood Communication Disorders, 13,* 73–83.

Crago, M. (1992). Ethnography and language socialization: A cross-cultural perspective. *Topics in Language Disorders, 12,* 28–39.

Curtiss, S. (1989). The independence and task-specificity of language. In M. Bornstein & J. Bruner (Eds.), *Interaction in human development* (pp. 105–137). Hillsdale, NJ: Lawrence Erlbaum Associates.

Ellis Weismer, S., Murray-Branch, J., & Miller, J. (1993). Comparison of two methods for promoting productive vocabulary in late talkers. *Journal of Speech and Hearing Research, 36,* 1037–1050.

Fey, M. (1986). *Language intervention with young children.* Austin, TX: PRO-ED.

Fey, M., Cleave, P., Long, S., & Hughes, D. (1993). Two approaches to facilitation of grammar in children with language impairment: An experimental evaluation. *Journal of Speech and Hearing Research, 36,* 141–157.

Fowler, A. (1990). Language abilities in children with Down syndrome: Evidence for a specific syntactic delay. In D. Cicchetti & M. Beeghly (Eds.), *Down syndrome: The developmental perspective* (pp. 302–328). New York: Cambridge University Press.

Gardner, M.F. (1981). *Expressive One-Word Picture Vocabulary Test (EOWPVT).* Austin, TX: PRO-ED.

Gopnick, M., & Crago, M. (1991). Familial aggregation of a developmental language disorder. *Cognition, 39,* 1–50.

Greenough, W.T., Black, J.E., & Wallace, C.S. (1987). Experience and brain development. *Child Development, 58,* 539–559.

Halle, J., Marshall, A., & Spradlin, J. (1979). Time delay: A technique to increase language use and facilitate generalization in retarded children. *Journal of Applied Behavior Analysis, 12,* 431–439.

Harkness, S. (1975). Cultural variation in mother's language. *Word, 27,* 495–498.

Hart, B., & Risley, T. (1975). Incidental teaching of language in the preschool. *Journal of Applied Behavior Analysis, 8,* 411–420.

Heath, S.B. (1989). The learner as cultural member. In M. Rice & R. Schiefelbusch (Eds.), *The teachability of language* (pp. 333–350). Baltimore: Paul H. Brookes Publishing Co.

Hedrick, D.L., Prather, E.M., & Tobin, A.R. (1975). *Sequenced Inventory of Communication Development (SICD).* Seattle: University of Washington Press.

Hemmeter, M., & Kaiser, A. (1994). Enhanced milieu teaching: Effects of parent-implemented language intervention. *Journal of Early Intervention, 18,* 269–289.

Kaiser, A.P., & Gray, D.B. (Eds.). (1993). *Communication and language intervention series: Vol. 2. Enhancing children's communication: Research foundations for intervention.* Baltimore: Paul H. Brookes Publishing Co.

Kaiser, A.P., Hemmeter, M., Ostrosky, M., Alpert, C., & Hancock, T. (1995). The effects of group training and individual feedback on parent use of milieu teaching. *Journal of Childhood Communication Disorders, 16,* 39–48.

Kaiser, A.P., Yoder, P.J., & Keetz, A. (1992). Evaluating milieu teaching. In S.F. Warren & J. Reichle (Eds.), *Communication and language intervention series: Vol. 1. Causes and effects in communication and language intervention* (pp. 9–48). Baltimore: Paul H. Brookes Publishing Co.

Kirk, S., McCarthy, J., & Kirk, W. (1968). *Illinois Test of Psycholinguistic Abilities (ITPA).* Urbana: University of Illinois Press.

Kot, A., & Law, J. (1995). Intervention with preschool children with specific language impairments: A comparison of two different approaches to treatment. *Child Language Teaching and Therapy, 11,* 144–162.

Kouri, T., & Wilcox, M. (1996). *Initial lexical training in prelinguistic children with developmental delays: A comparison of two intervention approaches.* Unpublished manuscript, Arizona State University, Tempe.

Lahey, M., & Edwards, J. (1995). Specific language impairment: Preliminary investigation of factors associated with family history and with patterns of language performance. *Journal of Speech and Hearing Research, 38,* 643–657.

Landry, S. (1995). The development of joint attention in premature low birth weight infants: Effects of early medical complications and maternal attention-directing behaviors. In C. Moore & P. Dunham (Eds.), *Joint attention: Its origins and role in development* (pp. 223–250). Hillsdale, NJ: Lawrence Erlbaum Associates.

Langdon, H. (1992). Language communication and sociocultural patterns in Hispanic families. In H. Langdon & L. Cheng (Eds.), *Hispanic children and adults with communication disorders: Assessment and intervention* (pp. 99–131). Rockville, MD: Aspen Publishers, Inc.

Lenneberg, E.H. (1967). *Biological foundations of language.* New York: John Wiley & Sons.

Leonard, L. (1987). Is specific language impairment a useful construct? In S. Rosenberg (Ed.), *Advances in applied psycholinguistics: Disorders of first-language development* (Vol. 1., pp. 1–39). New York: Cambridge University Press.

Leonard, L., Schwartz, R., Chapman, K., Rowan, L., Prelock, P., Terrell, B., Weiss, A., & Messick, C. (1982). Early lexical acquisition in children with specific language impairment. *Journal of Speech and Hearing Research, 25,* 554–564.

Levy, Y., Amir, N., & Shalev, R. (1994). Morphology in a child with a congenital left-hemisphere brain lesion: Implications for normal acquisition. In H. Tager-Flusberg (Ed.), *Constraints on language acquisition: Studies of atypical children* (pp. 49–74). Hillsdale, NJ: Lawrence Erlbaum Associates.

Long, S., & Olswang, L. (1996). Readiness and patterns of growth in children with SELI. *American Journal of Speech-Language Pathology, 5,* 79–85.

Lynch, E.W., & Hanson, M.J. (Eds.). (1992). *Developing cross-cultural competence: A guide for working with young children and their families.* Baltimore: Paul H. Brookes Publishing Co.

MacDonald, J. (1985). Language through conversation: A model for intervention with language delayed persons. In S. Warren & A. Rogers-Warren (Eds.), *Teaching functional language* (pp. 89–122). Baltimore: University Park Press.

McCathren, R.B., Warren, S.F., & Yoder, P.J. (1996). Prelinguistic predictors of later language development. In K.N. Cole, P.S. Dale, & D.J. Thal (Eds.), *Communication and language intervention series: Vol. 6. Assessment of communication and language* (pp. 57–75). Baltimore: Paul H. Brookes Publishing Co.

Moore, C., & Dunham, P. (Eds.). (1995). *Joint attention: Its origins and role in development.* Hillsdale, NJ: Lawrence Erlbaum Associates.

Mundy, P., Kasari, C., Sigman, M., & Ruskin, E. (1995). Nonverbal communication and early language acquisition in children with Down syndrome and in normally developing children. *Journal of Speech and Hearing Research, 38,* 157–167.

Mundy, P., Sigman, M., Kasari, C., & Yirmiya, N. (1988). Nonverbal communication skills in Down syndrome children. *Child Development, 59*(1), 235–249.

Newborg, J., Stock, J.R., Wnek, L., Guidubaldi, J., & Svinicki, J. (1984*). Battelle Developmental Inventory (BDI).* Chicago: Riverside.

Newman, M. (1995*). Joint attentional processes and language development in children with Down syndrome.* Unpublished master's thesis, Arizona State University, Tempe.

Norris, J., & Hoffman, P. (1990). Comparison of adult-initiated vs. child-initiated interaction styles with handicapped prelanguage children. *Language, Speech, and Hearing Services in Schools, 21,* 28–36.

Ochs, E., & Schieffelin, B. (1984). Language acquisition and socialization: Three developmental stories and their implications. In R. Shweder & R. LeVine (Eds.), *Culture theory: Essays on mind, self, and emotion* (pp. 276–320). Cambridge, England: Cambridge University Press.

Olswang, L.B., Bain, B.A., & Johnson, G.A. (1992). Using dynamic assessment with children with language disorders. In S.F. Warren & J. Reichle (Eds.), *Communication and language intervention series: Vol. 1. Causes and effects in communication and language intervention* (pp. 187–216). Baltimore: Paul H. Brookes Publishing Co.

Olswang, L.B., Bain, B., Rosendahl, P., Oblak, S., & Smith, A. (1986). Language learning: Moving performance from a context-dependent to -independent state. *Child Language Teaching and Therapy, 2,* 180–210.

Paul, R., & Jennings, P. (1992). Phonological behavior in toddlers with slow expressive language development. *Journal of Speech and Hearing Research, 35,* 99–107.

Paul, R., & Shiffer, M. (1991). Communicative initiations in normal and late-talking toddlers. *Applied Psycholinguistics, 12,* 419–431.

Rescorla, L., & Fechnay, T. (1996). Mother–child synchrony and communicative reciprocity in late-talking toddlers. *Journal of Speech and Hearing Research, 39,* 200–208.

Rescorla, L., & Goosens, M. (1992). Symbolic play development in toddlers with expressive specific language impairment (SLI–E). *Journal of Speech and Hearing Research, 35,* 1290–1302.

Rescorla, L., & Ratner, N. (1996). Phonetic profiles of toddlers with specific expressive language impairment (SLI–E). *Journal of Speech and Hearing Research, 39,* 153–165.

Reynell, J. (1985). *Reynell Developmental Language Scales.* Los Angeles: Webster Psychological Services.

Rice, M.L. (1995). Language acquisition and language impairment. In M.L. Rice & K.A. Wilcox (Eds.), *Building a language-focused curriculum for the preschool classroom: Vol. 1. A foundation for lifelong communication* (pp. 15–26). Baltimore: Paul H. Brookes Publishing Co.

Rice, M.L., & Wilcox K.A. (Eds.). (1995). *Building a language-focused curriculum for the preschool classroom: Vol. 1. A foundation for lifelong communication.* Baltimore: Paul H. Brookes Publishing Co.

Rogoff, B. (1990). *Apprenticeship in thinking: Cognitive development in social context.* Oxford: Oxford University Press.

Rogoff, B., Mistry, J., Goncu, A., & Mosier, C. (1991). Cultural variation in the role relations of toddlers and their families. In M. Bornstein (Ed.), *Cultural approaches to parenting* (pp. 173–184). Hillsdale, NJ: Lawrence Erlbaum Associates.

Rondal, J. (1994). Exceptional cases of language development in mental retardation: The relative autonomy of language as a cognitive system. In H. Tager-Flusberg (Ed.), *Constraints on language acquisition: Studies of atypical children* (pp. 155–174). Hillsdale, NJ: Lawrence Erlbaum Associates.

Schieffelin, B., & Ochs, E. (Eds.). (1986). *Language socialization across cultures.* New York: Cambridge University Press.

Schwartz, R., & Leonard, L. (1982). Do children pick and choose? *Journal of Child Language, 9,* 319–336.

Shannon, M., Wilcox, M., & Bacon, C. (1993, November). *Joint attentional processes in young children with developmental disabilities.* Paper presented to the American Speech-Language-Hearing Association Convention, Anaheim, CA.

Sigman, M., & Kasari, C. (1995). Joint attention across contexts in normal and autistic children. In C. Moore & P. Dunham (Eds.), *Joint attention: Its origins and role in development* (pp. 189–204). Hillsdale, NJ: Lawrence Erlbaum Associates.

Smith, L., & von Tetzchner, S. (1986). Communicative, sensorimotor, and language skills of young children with Down syndrome. *American Journal of Mental Deficiency, 91,* 57–66.

Stoel-Gammon, C. (1985). Phonetic inventories, 15–24 months: A longitudinal study. *Journal of Speech and Hearing Research, 28,* 505–512.

Tallal, P., Ross, R., & Curtiss, S. (1989). Familial aggregation in specific language impairment. *Journal of Speech and Hearing Disorders, 54,* 167–173.

Tannock, R., & Girolametto, L. (1992). Reassessing parent-focused language intervention programs. In S.F. Warren & J. Reichle (Eds.), *Communication and language intervention series: Vol. 1. Causes and effects in communication and language intervention* (pp. 49–80). Baltimore: Paul H. Brookes Publishing Co.

Thal, D., & Bates, E. (1988). Language and gesture in late talkers. *Journal of Speech and Hearing Research, 31,* 115–123.

Thal, D., & Tobias, S. (1992). Communicative gestures in children with delayed onset of oral expressive vocabulary. *Journal of Speech and Hearing Research, 35,* 1281–1289.

Thal, D., & Tobias, S. (1994). Relationships between language and gesture in normally developing and late-talking toddlers. *Journal of Speech and Hearing Research, 37,* 157–170.

Thal, D., Tobias, S., & Morrison, D. (1991). Language and gesture in late talkers: A 1-year follow-up. *Journal of Speech and Hearing Research, 34,* 604–612.

Tomblin, J. (1989). Familial concentration of developmental language impairment. *Journal of Speech and Hearing Disorders, 54,* 287–295.

van Kleeck, A. (1994). Potential cultural bias in training parents as conversational partners with their children who have delays in language development. *American Journal of Speech-Language Pathology, 3,* 67–78.

Wakefield, J., & Wilcox, M. (1995). Brain maturation and language acquisition: A theoretical model and preliminary investigation. In D. MacLaughlin & S. McEwen (Eds.), *Proceedings of the 19th annual Boston University Conference on Language Development* (Vol. 2, pp. 643–654). Somerville, MA: Cascadilla Press.

Walentas, J. (1994). *Young children with developmental disabilities: Communication status and joint attention.* Unpublished master's thesis, Arizona State University, Tempe.

Ward, M. (1971). *Them children: A study in language learning.* Prospect Heights, IL: Waveland Press.

Warren, S., & Gazdag, G. (1990). Facilitating early language development with milieu intervention procedures. *Journal of Early Intervention, 14,* 62–86.

Warren, S., McQuarter, R., & Rogers-Warren, A. (1984). The effects of mands and models on the speech of unresponsive language-delayed preschool children. *Journal of Speech and Hearing Disorders, 49,* 43–52.

Warren, S.F., Yoder, P., Gazdag, G., Kim, K., & Jones, H. (1993). Facilitating prelinguistic communication skills in young children with developmental delay. *Journal of Speech and Hearing Research, 36,* 83–97.

Wetherby, A., & Prizant, B. (1993). *Communication and Symbolic Behavior Scales.* Chicago: Riverside.

Wetherby, A., Yonclas, D., & Bryan, A. (1989). Communicative profiles of handicapped preschool children: Implications for early identification. *Journal of Speech and Hearing Disorders, 54,* 148–158.

Whitehurst, G.J., Fischel, J.E., Arnold, D.S., & Lonigan, C.J. (1992). Evaluating outcomes with children with expressive language delays. In S.F. Warren & J. Reichle (Eds.), *Communication and language intervention series: Vol. 1. Causes and effects in communication and language intervention* (pp. 277–314). Baltimore: Paul H. Brookes Publishing Co.

Whitehurst, G.J., Smith, M., Fischel, J., Arnold, D., & Lonigan, C. (1991). The continuity of babble and speech in children with specific expressive language delay. *Journal of Speech and Hearing Research, 34,* 1121–1129.

Wilcox, M. (1984). Developmental language disorders: Preschoolers. In A. Holland (Ed.), *Language disorders in children* (pp. 101–128). San Diego, CA: College-Hill Press.

Wilcox, M. (1992). Enhancing initial communication skills in young children with developmental disabilities through partner programming. *Seminars in Speech and Hearing, 13,* 195–212.

Wilcox, M. (1993, November). *Issues regarding language readiness in young children with developmental disabilities.* Paper presented to the annual convention of the American Speech-Language-Hearing Association, Anaheim, CA.

Wilcox, M., Hadley, P., & Ashland, J. (1996). Communication and language development in infants and toddlers. In M. Hanson (Ed.), *Atypical infant development* (pp. 365–402). Austin, TX: PRO-ED.

Wilcox, M., Kouri, T., & Caswell, S. (1991). Early language intervention: A comparison of classroom and individual treatment. *American Journal of Speech-Language Pathology, 1,* 49–62.

Wilcox, M., Shannon, M., & Bacon, C. (1992, December). *From prelinguistic to linguistic behavior: Outcomes for young children with developmental disabilities.* Paper presented to the International Early Childhood Conference on Children with Special Needs, Washington, DC.

Wilcox, M., Shannon, M., & Bacon, C. (1996*). Longer-term outcomes of prelinguistic intervention.* Unpublished manuscript, Arizona State University, Tempe.

Wilcox, M.J., & Shannon, M.S. (1996). Integrated early intervention practices in speech-language pathology. In R.A. McWilliam (Ed.), *Rethinking pull-out services in early intervention: A professional resource* (pp. 217–242). Baltimore: Paul H. Brookes Publishing Co.

Yoder, P., Kaiser, A., Goldstein, H., Alpert, C., Mousetis, L., Kaczmarek, L., & Fischer, R. (1995). An exploratory comparison of milieu teaching and responsive interaction in classroom applications. *Journal of Early Intervention, 19,* 218–242.

Yoder, P., Warren, S., & Hull, L. (1995). Predicting children's response to prelinguistic communication intervention. *Journal of Early Intervention, 19,* 74–84.

Yoder, P., Warren, S., Kim, K., & Gazdag, G. (1994). Facilitating prelinguistic communication skills in young children with developmental delay: II. Systematic replication and extension. *Journal of Speech and Hearing Research, 37,* 841–851.

17

Implementing Augmentative Communication Systems

Joe Reichle, James W. Halle, and Erik Drasgow

B{ETWEEN} 9 {AND} 14 {MONTHS OF AGE}, most children use their first spoken word (Reich, 1986). However, individuals with developmental disabilities have far more difficulty than their typically developing peers in acquiring an initial repertoire of spoken words. This chapter focuses on the transition to intentional and subsequently to symbolic communication by children who have moderate to severe mental disabilities and who may require the use of an augmentative communication system.

Augmentative communication uses gestural and graphic modes. Gestural mode includes idiosyncratic gestures, natural gestures that are widely comprehended by individuals unfamiliar with sign, sign languages, sign systems, and fingerspelling. Graphic mode includes three-dimensional (e.g., empty soda can = drink, car keys = go for a ride) and two-dimensional (e.g., photos, line drawings, printed words) displayed representations. Two general techniques can be used to transmit graphic symbol selections to a listener. In a direct selection technique, an individual selects symbols by touching, giving, or pointing to them (including directing eye gaze). Individuals with severe physical disabilities who cannot self-select symbols may require a scanning selection technique. In a scanning selection technique, a partner or electronic cursor offers symbol choices from which the individual makes a selection. Augmentative communication applications can supplement both communicative production and comprehension. For example, a deaf individual may produce and comprehend American Sign Language. Among individuals with mental retardation, a communication board with photographic symbols may be used to enable the individual to produce utterances. If this individual is unable to comprehend spoken language, the same symbols may be selected by a communicative partner to enable the communication board user to understand messages. In a significant proportion of augmentative communication applications with individuals who have developmental disabilities, an augmentative communication system is used to replace or supplement speech production. Concurrently, spoken language produced by others represents the primary mode of comprehension. For many individuals with developmental disabilities, using sign or a communication board represents a primary means of communication with vocal utterances functioning as the augmentative communication system.

This chapter discusses shared perspectives of researchers who have influenced assessment and intervention practices for augmentative system users with moderate and severe disabilities and describes challenges in confirming early intentional communication. Subsequently, the process of how rudimentary intentional gestures can become more conventional gestural and graphic symbols is described. The chapter also addresses concerns in maximizing the efficiency of gestural and graphic communication modes in the consideration of how existing, more idiosyncratic communicative behavior may come to be replaced with more efficient forms. In addition, the relationship between comprehension and production for people who rely on augmentative communication systems is discussed.

PERSPECTIVES ACROSS THEORETICAL ORIENTATIONS FOR ILLOCUTIONARY COMMUNICATION

Illocutionary communication is purposeful and intends to influence a partner. Efforts to establish and expand illocutionary communication skills are often a primary focus of intervention with children and youth with severe disabilities (McLean & Snyder-McLean, 1991; Owens, 1995). The attainment of illocutionary communication is predictable, smooth, and rapid for youngsters following typical developmental paths. However, children and youth with severe disabilities do not proceed in development with the same ease (Bates, 1976; Bates, Camaioni, & Volterra, 1975; Coggins & Carpenter, 1981; Wetherby, Cain, Yonclas, & Walker, 1988) and often reflect a major developmental stumbling block (McLean & Snyder-McLean, 1991; Owens, 1995; Siegel-Causey & Guess, 1989).

Both cognitive and behavioral perspectives acknowledge a continuum of development in the acquisition of illocutionary communication (cf. Sachs, 1993). A continuum in the development of intentional communication is particularly well suited to children and youth with severe disabilities. Some children may demonstrate early features of intentionality, such as physical contact designed to influence a partner's behavior, but remain at this level for years. Furthermore, children and youth with developmental disabilities often exhibit restricted types and limited functions of communication (i.e., pulling away to protest an undesired activity or event). Finally, some aspects of intentional communication that are displayed by typically developing youngsters (e.g., alternating eye gaze) may never be consistently used by children with developmental disabilities. The progress of children with more severe disabilities along the identified continuum may be both slow and, in many instances, more idiosyncratic.

Delineating features that constitute an initial illocutionary repertoire require observing the learner in his or her natural environment. Over time and through the partner's history of response, nonpurposeful acts take on meaning and are gradually shaped into functional communication. Chapter 16 provides a detailed discussion of differences regarding the point in development at which the learner's partner plays the most critical role in communication acquisition.

There is general agreement that the goal of prelinguistic communication intervention is to establish, enhance, and expand communicative behaviors produced for the benefit of a listener. There is widespread agreement that successful communication intervention increases opportunities for intentional communication (both the number and diversity) and enhances the responsiveness of communicative partners. For interventionists, a critical feature of the assessment and intervention process involves a practical determination that those who produce perlocutionary acts learn to produce illocutionary communicative acts.

CHARACTERISTICS OF ILLOCUTIONARY COMMUNICATION FOR AN AUGMENTATIVE SYSTEM USER

A central point of confusion in the literature addressing the communicative status of individuals with developmental disabilities is how illocutionary communication can be differentiated from nonpurposeful or perlocutionary communication (Scoville, 1983; Sugarman, 1984; Wetherby & Prizant, 1989). Rather than relying on any single feature, most researchers use a collective set of criteria for determining whether a particular child's behavior is illocutionary. Although the specific criteria employed across investigations have differed (cf. Harding & Golinkoff, 1979; McLean, Snyder-McLean, Brady, & Etter, 1991; Wetherby & Prizant, 1989), there does appear to be some agreement (cf. Sachs, 1993).

Wetherby and Prizant (1989) defined intentionality as the deliberate pursuit of a goal. Bates (1979) described intentional communication as "signaling behavior in which the sender is aware a priori of the effect that a signal will have on his listener" (p. 36). Although seemingly straightforward, it is very difficult to directly measure intentional behavior. Instead, it must be inferred from the learner's behavior and his or her social partner's actions. One approach to inferring intentionality involves observing to see whether clusters of behaviors proposed as indicators of intentionality are produced. Wetherby and Prizant (1989) proposed indicators of intentionality that include the following: 1) alternating eye gaze between goal and listener; 2) persistent signaling until a goal is accomplished or failure is indicated; 3) waiting for a response from a listener; 4) changing the signal quality until the goal has been met; 5) ritualizing or conventionalizing communicative forms; 6) ceasing signal production when the goal is met; and 7) displaying satisfaction when the goal is met and dissatisfaction when it is not met.

Complicating the application of criteria that address intentionality is that, even after the child has begun producing intentional utterances, a number of acts interpreted as intentional will continue to have perlocutionary function. Applying criteria connoting intentionality is often challenging with both typically developing children and with individuals with developmental disabilities who require augmentative communication systems. For some individuals with developmental disabilities, the crux of communication difficulty is a motivational issue. To communicate about an object or event, an individual must have some active interest or disinterest. Although motivation is a potential stumbling block in assessing typically developing children, it may be more so, for two reasons, with people with severe developmental disabilities who require an augmentative communication system. First, typically developing children readily display curiosity and respond to stimulus novelty (Halle, 1987). Consequently, even though assessment tasks may not directly involve the use of identified reinforcers, brief bursts of participation may be attributable to the curiosity of a typically developing child. Second, typically developing children appear to be far more apt to be reinforced by the social actions and reactions of those around them. Thus, even if the actual activity is of limited interest, it is likely that adult enthusiasm will maintain brief intervals of engagement to "please" the partner with whom they are interacting. However, individuals with moderate or severe disabilities often distance themselves from others, choosing to spend their time alone, when permitted. When this occurs, communication is necessarily compromised. In addition to motivational challenges, a number of other challenges face the interventionist attempting to apply specific criteria to determine intentionality.

Alternating Gaze Between Goal and Listener

Visual regard requires that a learner shift his or her gaze between a referent and a listener. No doubt, the presence of this criterion assists in confirming the presence of intentionality. However, there is little evidence that it is a necessary prerequisite for illocutionary communicative acts. Gaze aversion constrains visual regard in a social interchange but should not be misconstrued as necessarily diminishing the intentional features of communication.

Among individuals who use a graphic mode augmentative communication system, the demands of the device's symbol display may make it more difficult for the individual to shift gaze, that is, coordinating speaking with eye gaze shifts between communicative partner and referent. A graphic mode communicator may be so occupied with selecting and displaying a message that gaze shifts are very asynchronous. In using graphic symbols, an individual must shift his or her gaze between the referent object or activity, his or her symbol display, and his or her communicative partner. Because speech has no visible display, the speaker need only coordinate his or her gaze between referent and listener. Reichle (1995) reported that, among successful beginning graphic mode system users, it is quite common to observe shifts in gaze between referent and symbol sequence without the individual directly shifting eye gaze to a listener. Significantly more often than their more successful counterparts, less successful beginning graphic system users shifted their gaze between referent and partner without directly examining their symbol displays. This in turn resulted in a greater propensity to engage in a position bias response in which a particular symbol was selected as a result of its physical position on a symbol display. It appears that among some graphic mode augmentative system users, coordinating eye gaze between listener and referent may be far more complex than it is for those who speak.

Persistent Signaling Until Goal Is Accomplished or Failure Is Indicated

Persistence may be very much related to communicative motivation. It consists of the speaker's continuing efforts to achieve a goal when the listener does not understand, misunderstands, or purposely fails to honor a communicative act. Because of the subtlety and idiosyncracy of strategies used by some augmentative system users who experience significant developmental disabilities, the persistence of communicative attempts may be easily missed. For example, because the physical effort expended to communicate may be so great, some people may fuss or increase body movement as a follow-up to the emission of an initial communicative utterance that is not consequated. Enhanced evidence of intentionality would result if a child were more persistent in emitting idiosyncratic behaviors when a listener was available compared with situations in which a listener typically is unavailable. Although this could be viewed as persistence, it may go unnoticed by the learner's listener. If this occurs repeatedly, the learner's persistence in making his or her message understood may be extinguished.

Also, extinction may account for what appear to be smaller and less diverse repertoires of communication, which would limit methods of repairing a communication breakdown. The authors of this chapter are working with a child who walks into the kitchen and waits for her mother to find the food item she wants. We believe that her walking into the kitchen is a communicative overture and her waiting may represent communicative persistence because of the consistency of her behavior in place and time and the consistency of the mother's response of providing food. If an interventionist does not identify waiting or coercive behavior as types of repair strategies, then the child's act will go unrecognized.

Sometimes parents and family members understand idiosyncratic signaling that is missed entirely by a general audience who has not had experience with the particular learner. Available evidence suggests that individuals with more severe disabilities are unlikely to encounter as many unfamiliar individuals as their typical counterparts (C. Lakin, personal communication, May 1995). Consequently, there may be fewer naturally available opportunities to demonstrate to an individual the need to acquire traditional communicative repair strategies.

Waiting for a Response from a Listener

Researchers generally agree that most parents are very responsive to their typically developing children's early vocal and gestural behavior. However, in some instances, mothers of children with developmental disabilities appear to be either overly responsive, thus suppressing opportunities for communicative emissions by their children, or less responsive to the communication signaling by their children. Several plausible explanations posited for differences in responsivity among parents and their children with developmental disabilities have focused on the low rate of utterances produced by some children; lack of child responsiveness; and parents' difficulties in interpreting their children's signals, which discourages reciprocal interaction and may promote episodic directiveness by mothers. Linfoot (1994) reported that some individuals appear to be relatively unresponsive to communicative overtures produced by children with developmental disabilities. When acting on an utterance produced by an individual with a severe developmental disability, individuals may be more likely to act on some communicative functions than others. Reichle (1995), observing the interactions between children with moderate intellectual disabilities and their teachers and parents, observed that adults were far more likely to consequate a proto-imperative than a proto-declarative. In addition, with both parents and teachers, preschool children with developmental disabilities were far more likely to repair proto-imperatives than proto-declaratives. Consequently, even though parents and teachers may not have been optimally responsive, they may have been taught to be more differentially attentive to proto-imperatives. However, the trend to be very responsive to proto-imperatives is not unique to populations with disabilities (S.F. Warren, personal communication, May 1994).

Despite the possible influence that communicative context may have on a partner's responsivity among users of communication boards, speaking communicative partners tend to interrupt before the augmentative system user has an opportunity to complete a communicative repair (see, e.g., Reichle, York, & Sigafoos, 1991). Because graphic mode communication use is so slow, a history may have developed in which familiar listeners may anticipate the function and meaning of a learner's message that should actually be repaired and may provide consequences that are hypothesized to match the speaker's intent. Partners may have learned through years of living with the individual what he or she likes to eat and drink, the clothes he or she likes to wear, and preferred daily activities. Although this phenomenon of preempting is not limited to children with severe disabilities, it is more pervasive in the lives of those with more severe disabilities. Entire days often are organized around particular routines that capitalize on this phenomenon. Due to the routinization of the schedule and the regularity of the environment, the need to communicate may be diminished, which, in turn, may promote learned helplessness (Guess, Benson, & Siegel-Causey, 1985; Seligman, 1975).

Changing the Signal Until the Goal Is Met

The observation that speaking partners of graphic mode augmentative communication system users frequently interrupt, at first, seems to contradict the previously mentioned observation that some caregivers and teachers may be less responsive to overtures emitted by people with severe developmental disabilities. With some children who use augmentative communication systems, a listener's attention may "wax and wane" as a function of the contexts in which communicative exchanges occur. When adults are attending to the child, they may overanticipate and allow few opportunities for repairs. However, when adult partners are preoccupied with other tasks, it may be very easy to miss communicative overtures. These inconsistent opportunities for repairs may make it more difficult for augmentative communication system users to learn the conditions that require conversational repair (see Chapter 7 for a more detailed description of the emergence of repair strategies used by typically developing children and preschoolers with disabilities). Future research should attend more closely to the longitudinal history of listener consequences provided for rudimentary communicative utterances.

Summary

Certain criteria used in determining intentionality may require careful consideration in their application to individuals with developmental disabilities who use augmentative communication systems. Although applicable, these criteria may not represent obligatory features of intentional utterances. Once children are producing some forms that they use consistently in the presence of some referents and are producing an increasing variety of communicative functions, the interventionist's attention increasingly begins to focus on the range of conventional communicative forms to teach.

FORMS USED TO EXPRESS
INITIAL COMMUNICATIVE FUNCTIONS

Most typical individuals rely primarily on speech production augmented with gestural and graphic mode symbols. However, for individuals who have extremely limited speech production, graphic and/or gestural modes may become primary avenues for communication. Once the child begins producing an increasingly greater proportion of intentional communicative utterances, interventionists can begin to focus on more decontextualized uses of new communicative forms. As this happens, more contextualized forms are used with decreasing frequency. This section discusses forms of early and simple graphic and gestural symbols and addresses assessment and intervention strategies that can be derived from this information.

Bates (1976) and Bates, Benigni, Bretherton, Camaioni, and Volterra (1979) differentiated diectic gestures, whose sole function is to establish reference, from representational gestures, whose function is to denote specific objects/events (see Chapter 4 for a description of the sequence of emergency communication gestures). The distinction between diectic and representational gestures has critical implications for early assessment and intervention. By definition, diectic gestures (e.g., pointing to an object) can be used to refer to a very wide range of referents and communication functions. Consequently, with beginning communicators diectic gestures may promote the identification of a wide range and number of teaching opportunities. Representational gestures (e.g., moving an imaginary cup to one's mouth) have the advantage of placing less of the communication responsibility on the learner's listener because they are more directly related to particular referents. This, in turn, tends to make interpersonal communication exchanges more efficient with fewer listener queries or learner repairs to complete a successful message transmission. Diectic gestures usually are considered developmentally simpler and are clearly presymbolic, whereas representational gestures emerge slightly later and, like first words, are more likely symbolic but highly contextualized.

Numerous sources (e.g., Werner & Kaplan, 1963) suggest that representational gestures emerge as a result of children's participation in well-scripted routines in which actions are increasingly used in the absence of related objects or in the presence of object substitutes. However, many natural contexts for learning representational vocabulary seem to be less available to individuals with severe developmental disabilities. Koppenhaver and Yoder (1992) suggested that children with severe disabilities receive far fewer opportunities to participate in play and early literacy activities than their typically developing peers. The limited opportunities for joint activity routines that accompany reading and play activities may significantly influence early representational symbol acquisition among people with developmental disabilities (see Chapter 9 for additional discussion).

With less exposure to well-scripted routines that promote the acquisition of representational gestures, it is possible that children with developmental disabilities may receive a proportionately greater exposure to diectic gestures. That is, parents may be actively pointing and using diectic gestures during brief episodic exchanges that call attention to referents. Many opportunities to learn diectic gestures may be initiated by the child in an effort to obtain positive reinforcers or avoid negative reinforcers. Because these episodes are rich with contextual cues for the child's listener, these opportunities may result in relatively brief exchanges that focus less around turn taking per se.

In addition to the experiential differences between typically developing individuals and those with developmental disabilities, there may be differences in the discriminations required to match diectic and representational gestures. Diectic gestures require a functional match between gesture and communication function, whereas representational gestures require a match between gesture and communicative function in addition to a match between the gesture and a specific referent class (e.g., the sign for ball must be matched to a round spherical object). Diectic gestures convey pragmatic functions but not semantic meanings.

Gestural representations comprise unique combinations of motor actions involving hand shape, movement of the hands and arms, and location where the sign is produced with respect to the rest of the learner's body (see Chapter 9). A number of investigators have found that during initial discrimination learning, it is helpful if the motor parameters of the signs being introduced are more maximally discriminable (Griffith & Robinson, 1980; McLean & Snyder-McLean, 1987; Stremel-Campbell, Cantrell, & Halle, 1977). For example, at mealtime it is quite common to see interventionists implementing procedures to teach signs representing both EAT and DRINK. These signs share similar hand shapes, locations, and movement patterns. This means that they may be less discriminable to a beginning communicator than two gestures that share fewer common features. It is also possible that the uniqueness of gestures represents a distinct advantage in establishing an initial communicative repertoire. If two gestures are produced very differently, they may be more discriminable to the learner than a graphic mode response that always involves touching a symbol.

In addition to experiences with gestures, young children are exposed to a wide array of graphic symbols that are available across home, community, and school environments. For example, corporate logos, such as those for McDonald's, Burger King, or Dairy Queen, are often recognized by young children around their second birthday. Other trademarks and corporate logos, such as those on wrappers of favorite candy, are also discriminated at early ages (See Chapter 9 for an extensive description of the various two- and three-dimensional symbols that can be implemented to augment communication in vocal and gestural modes.) Discussions of symbol selection strategies for individuals with developmental disabilities have been explicitly delineated in a number of summative works (Beukelman & Mirenda, 1992; Reichle, York, & Sigafoos, 1991). Deciding the relative emphasis to place on graphic and gestural modes has received relatively limited attention. Most practitioners and researchers seem to be in agreement that coordinating both graphic and gestural modes represents the most plausible strategy to create an efficient augmentative communication system (Reichle, York, & Sigafoos, 1991). Creating a well-coordinated system can begin by examining the relationship between early gestural and graphic representation.

Replacing Existing Idiosyncratic Communication Forms

One goal of the interventionist is to replace nonsymbolic and idiosyncratic communication forms (e.g., banging hand on a surface to get attention) with more conventional forms. It seems reasonable to use a learner's existing, less symbolic forms to identify function and intent. These forms then are replaced with new symbolic ones that preserve the function and intent of the previously used, more idiosyncratic forms. Thus, new communication forms established will be functionally equivalent to earlier and more idiosyncratic communication forms (Carr, 1988). Existing forms often can be altered by incorporating the old form into the new form or by expanding the old form (Reichle, Halle, & Johnston, 1993). For example, if an individual who does not speak requests by grabbing or reaching, these behaviors may be able to be readily prompted or shaped into the American Sign Language for WANT.

However, not all idiosyncratic communication is socially acceptable. Among populations with more severe disabilities, investigators have described consistently used forms associated with certain communication functions that are socially unacceptable (see, e.g., Carr, 1977; Carr & Durand, 1985a, 1985b). Carr (1977) described the communication hypothesis as the theoretical basis for associating certain forms of challenging behavior with specific communication functions. An extension of this hypothesis holds that it should be possible to establish acceptable communication behavior that replaces and serves the same function as socially unacceptable behavior. Communicative functions often associated with positive reinforcement include requesting desired objects, events, and attention. Functions associated with negative reinforcement include protesting/rejecting, requesting a break, commenting on task completion ("All done"), or requesting a work check.

If an individual uses a communicative form that is widely understood, effective, and is not challenging behavior, then why replace it? We offer several answers to this question. First, existing forms, such as leading or grabbing, may be acceptable to those familiar with the individual, but the use of these forms may be inappropriate with strangers, especially if they involve physical contact. Second, the lack of symbolic forms limits the individual to communicating only in the presence of actual referents. Two operational rules for interventionists are that the new communicative alternative must be functionally equivalent to the old socially unacceptable form, and the new communicative alternative should be more efficient than the behavior to be replaced.

Ensuring that New Communication Forms Are Functionally Equivalent and Maximally Efficient

Selecting an efficient symbol to teach is not a simple issue. Often the individual has existing nonsymbolic forms that are widely generalized (Drasgow & Halle, 1995). From the individual's perspective, these forms may be very efficient. Any new symbol form that is introduced must serve the same social function(s) of the communication form being replaced to be "functionally equivalent" (Carr, 1977). Furthermore, the new communication form must become efficient, from the user's perspective. Response efficiency is determined by criteria that include the amount of physical effort the response requires, the amount and/or quality of reinforcement as an outcome of the use of the response, the amount of time between the response and reinforcement, and/or the rate at which the learner must emit communication before it is consequated (Mace & Roberts, 1993; Horner, Day, Sprague, O'Brien, & Heathfield, 1991). For an individual with physical disabilities using a graphic communication system, the amount of physical effort required may be the most formidable challenge. For an individual using the gestural mode, which can only be consequated if emitted within view, the rate at which the communication utterances must be emitted before a response may be the formidable challenge. Each of these efficiency factors is discussed briefly.

Ensuring Immediacy of Consequences Delivered by Listeners As discussed previously, when individuals are acquiring a new communication behavior, it is important that their listeners are responsive. Among individuals who produce challenging behavior, listeners have a propensity to respond immediately. For example, if a child bangs her head on the floor, a parent tends to respond immediately with attention. Once a more socially acceptable attention-getting strategy has been taught, listeners may become progressively less immediately attentive to a communication overture. When this occurs, the new communication form is at risk of being less effective than the previous socially unacceptable communicative form. In the short term, the consequence of the ineffectiveness may result in the need for the learner to repeat the utterance before it is consequated. If this occurs over a short period of time, the learner may revert to the use of the old communication form (Horner & Day, 1991; Horner, Sprague, O'Brien, & Heathfield, 1990).

Ensuring Quality of Consequences Delivered by Listeners Several years ago we met a 2½-year-old who was receiving services in a center-based preschool setting. This little girl craved attention. She had discovered that if she screamed loudly, teachers would run to her side and often spend 10–15 minutes rocking her. In an effort to give her a socially acceptable alternative to screaming, we introduced a small microcassette recorder that was clipped to her waistband. She was taught to touch a button that immediately produced a spoken message, "Could you please come here," that was stored behind a single-response button. The child readily learned to use the symbol. During acquisition, the novelty of the tape loop appealed to educators as well as the child. It was common for people to spend 10–15 minutes with the child when she used the tape loop. Over the course of the next month, staff began to report that increasingly she was reverting to screaming. Observations revealed that when the tape loop was activated, the child typically received less than 15 seconds of attention. However, when she screamed, she received 10–15 minutes of attention. Subsequent intervention involved providing significantly less attention for screaming and significantly more attention for tape loop use. In this example, because only a single symbol was available, no discrimination between different symbols was required. Once the child learned that an intentional act of touching a symbol resulted in a desired action, additional symbol choices, each associated with a specific object or action, could be introduced. Consequently, what began as a simple intentional act could evolve into a repertoire of conditionally used symbols, each associated with a particular referent.

Demonstrating that augmentative communication can be maximally efficient creates a potential dilemma for the interventionist. New communicative utterances will be perceived as maximally efficient if the outcome matches the learner's desire on each occasion that an utterance is used. However, natural environments impose numerous restrictions on the conditions under which the social function of certain utterances can be fulfilled. If the interventionist is to teach new communicative skills in the milieu of a natural environment, care must be taken to ensure that the learner is accustomed to natural maintaining contingencies that may only conditionally reinforce communicative utterances.

CONDITIONAL COMMUNICATIVE UTTERANCES

Each time an individual chooses to communicate, there are two levels of conditional discriminations that must be made. First, he or she must discriminate whether conditions call for a communicative production. For example, in deciding whether to produce a request for a desired item, the individual first must decide whether the item is attainable. For example, a cola beverage can be made available at home after dinner but not in the middle of a church service. Second, if the desired item is available, an individual must consider whether it is attainable directly or whether mediation by another person is required. If no mediation is required, the individual may serve him- or herself. If mediation is required, the individual can produce a request.

Since the early 1980s, an instructional methodology addressing strategies to pursue in teaching the conditional use of behavior has emerged (see O'Neill & Reichle, 1993, for a discussion). General case instructional procedures provide a framework for interventionists to identify a range of conditions under which a newly taught behavior should be used (i.e., positive teaching examples) and a variety of key examples in which the learner should refrain from using the new behavior (i.e., negative teaching examples). If an individual decides to produce an utterance, he or she then must choose among the different forms that are available. For the most part, traditional intervention procedures have focused on teaching only *positive examples* or instances where a new behavior should be produced. *Negative examples* consist of those opportunities in which an individual should refrain from producing the behavior being taught. If both positive and negative teaching examples are not addressed, it is possible that a learner's ability to efficiently engage in the conditional use of newly established communicative behavior will be jeopardized.

Reichle, Sigafoos, and Remington (1991) reported on the implementation of a program to teach an individual with severe developmental disabilities a requesting skill. Only positive teaching examples were implemented. Each day when the learner approached snacktime at school, he received snack items contingent on producing a request. The interventionists documented that the learner's frequency of self-selecting snack items that were nearby steadily decreased. In a second example, Reichle (1995) reported teaching a woman with severe mental retardation to request assistance. Once again, only positive teaching examples were used. As the woman approached the activity in which she had difficulty, she was taught to request assistance. One of the tasks used in teaching her to request assistance was opening a jar of peanut butter to make a sandwich. During probes in which the lid of the jar had been removed, the individual continued to request assistance even though she was capable of continuing without any assistance. These preceding examples suggest that if interventionists fail to conditionally address the use of newly established communicative repertoires, the learner may begin to exhibit characteristics of learned helplessness, which characteristically have been associated with the lack of an efficient communication repertoire.

For a child developing typically, conditional use of newly acquired utterances occurs as a result of discriminative stimuli and consequences provided as the natural environment. It is unclear whether individuals with severe disabilities are exposed to insufficient examples or whether the discriminations required by natural teaching examples are too subtle. Carefully planned opportunities that ensure a critical range of positive and negative teaching examples are critical in teaching an individual to be a competent communicator.

RELATING COMPREHENSION TO PRODUCTION

Available evidence suggests that producing and understanding communicative behavior emerge as separate but often intertwined skills (see Chapters 4 and 9). Children learn to comprehend spoken words at the same time they learn to produce spoken words; however, lexical items produced and comprehended do not precisely correspond.

Among augmentative communication system users who rely exclusively on graphic mode symbols for both comprehension and production, the relationship between the two may be much more intertwined. What distinguishes comprehension from production is whether the focus of the partner's attention is the symbol or the referent. For example, in an elicited comprehension assessment task, the interventionist might offer a graphic symbol, and the learner would select the corresponding real object/event referent. In an elicited production task, the interventionist might offer an object referent, and the learner would locate a matching symbol. Assuming that the learner can match objects (i.e., referents) and symbols regardless of which is the sample and which is the choice, comprehension and production skills are likely to be comparable.

There is some evidence suggesting that among individuals with severe disabilities, the sample and choices may not yield the same performance when reversed (Brady & Saunders, 1991). However, Reichle (1995) demonstrated that if samples and choices in an object-to-graphic symbol-matching task are juxtaposed during intervention, learners with severe disabilities may begin to respond equally well to novel sets of stimuli when sample and choice roles are reversed. This finding suggests that if a vocabulary item to be taught will be functional for the learner's comprehension and production vocabulary, it may make sense to teach comprehension and production concurrently. A critical area for further empirical scrutiny is the degree to which comprehension and production are related in the exclusive application of the graphic mode.

Rarely do augmentative system users rely exclusively on graphic or gestural mode for both comprehension and production. Many individuals with severe developmental disabilities produce communication using gestural or graphic symbols and, at the same time, comprehend spoken language. The logic for such dual communication is compelling. If an individual can receive communication produced verbally, the potential range of opportunities for at least partial participation in social settings dramatically increases. Without this capability, the augmentative system user must rely on an interpreter to encode spoken messages into a mode that the learner can comprehend. Among young children with moderate and severe developmental disabilities, producing language using an electronic communication aid with digitized or synthesized speech output may facilitate the learner's acquisition of the comprehension of spoken language. Each time the learner produces vocabulary, he or she selects a graphic symbol. Touching a graphic symbol, in return, produces a spoken word or message. Assuming (and this is a rather large assumption) that the learner is attending to the spoken output, a relationship (i.e., correspondence) between graphic symbol and spoken word may be made. Assuming that this pairing results in the acquisition of comprehended spoken words, there may be several variables that lessen the probability that speech production output directly influences comprehension at the lexical (i.e., word) level. Communication devices usually are programmed so that a message unit (often consisting of an entire sentence) is produced when the learner selects a single symbol. When this occurs, it is unclear how and whether the learner segments the spoken message into meaningful units. When an older speech synthesis package (e.g., VOTRAX, Echo) with somewhat more limited intelligibility is used, the learner's ability to correspond artificial spoken utterances with slightly different-sounding real speech may be limited.

The preceding discussion might lead to the belief that augmentative system users rely primarily on single communicative modes within the domains of production and comprehension; this, however, is not the case. Some relationships between gestural and vocal modes in the acquisition of an early productive communication repertoire are outlined in Chapter 4. Relatively little is known about how the use of graphic symbols influences and interacts with gestural and vocal modes within either comprehension or production. There is a critical need to closely examine the relationship between comprehension and production among augmentative communication system users. Particularly important will be exploring how intervention in one communication mode influences acquisition in other modes.

IMPLICATIONS FOR CLINICAL PRACTICE AND EDUCATION

One implication of the advances in augmentative and alternative communication is the notion that communication interventions can be designed and implemented at very early ages. Evidence suggests that all children demonstrate contingent actions in response to social stimuli very early in their development. More important, others in the environment have the capability of responding contingently to the actions of augmentative system users. If these actions result in reinforcement for the augmentative system user, at some point the child is apt to more frequently and spontaneously produce these behaviors.

However, partners of augmentative system users may be too participative in interactions, reducing a conversation to yes/no response options for the augmentative user. Alternatively, the listener may be less responsive, perhaps as a result of low-rate initiations and conversational repairs offered by the augmentative system user. Some interventionists adhere to a very indirect, almost stimulation, model of teaching augmentative system use. Other interventionists advocate direct instructional procedures. Interventionists must place themselves in a position to determine systematically the specific intervention strategy from which any given learner will benefit.

Vygotsky's (1934/1986) zone of proximal development suggests that the young learner and his or her environment operate as a kind of unit. That is, the learner's propensity to use new behaviors may be influenced by the quantity and overt features of cues provided by the environment in which the learner operates. The communicator initially provides substantial support. Over time, the learner gradually assumes increasing responsibility as his or her competence grows. A special challenge in establishing spoken utterances is how to provide support (i.e., cues and prompts). Typically developing children tend to produce behavior that is acted on by others. Children and adults with developmental disabilities may produce far less behavior on which their communication partner can act. This means that other strategies must be considered to ensure that communication approximations occur.

Because communication is a social behavior, there is a propensity to hold the use of an augmentative communication system to the same social conventions of speech. This is not possible. Speech is far faster than graphic mode augmentative forms, which means that situations will arise in which the graphic mode augmentative system user will not be able to produce an utterance quickly enough (or have relevant messages stored to retrieve) to fully participate. The interventionist's role is to be as anticipatory as possible in planning messages with the learner and his or her family to maximize the range of conversations in which the learner can participate.

Visually referencing one's listener as well as the referent object or activity is an important feature of emerging conversational behavior; for a graphic mode system user, however, an additional layer of orientation is required to communicate. A graphic mode augmentative system user must transfer gaze among his or her listener, referent event, and his or her communicative device. During the early phases of intervention, it is important that the interventionist actively encourage and promote these shifts in reference to promote greater fluency.

Two inherent roles of natural interactions are violated frequently in the interactions between augmentative system users and their conversational partners. First, because many augmentative system users initiate less than their typically developing peers, it may be inherently more difficult to follow the child's attentional lead. Second, because of potentially fewer child-produced utterances, an interactional pattern that waxes and wanes between being overly directive and nonresponsive may occur. Interventionists must be diligent to contingently respond and shape communicative productions of augmentative system users and need to carefully consider situations in which conversational repair strategies other than yes/no questions are used to clarify messages generated by an augmentative system user.

Finally, it is important to consider the multimodal aspects of augmentative communication applications. There may be a temptation for interventionists to lock into a single augmentative communication mode. Graphic and gestural modes have inherently different (and in some cases almost reciprocal) advantages and disadvantages. Gestural mode is efficient with partners who understand gestures and in situations in which speed and portability are critical. Efficient communicators use gestural, graphic, and vocal modes.

Inherent in considering combining an augmentative communication mode with existing speech is the frequent parent concern that implementing an augmentative communication system will in some way discourage vocal mode development. However, experience has suggested that when intervention continues to encourage vocal behavior, the implementation of graphic and gestural mode communication does not impede vocal mode progress and, in some cases, may have assisted in vocal mode development. Interventionists must recognize parents' potential fears that recommending an augmentative communication mode may imply that the vocal mode has been abandoned and should be prepared to address this concern.

IMPLICATIONS FOR FUTURE RESEARCH

As an area of empirical inquiry, augmentative communication is very young. Few experimental investigations of graphic mode augmentative system applications were reported before the early 1970s. Although the literature on gestural mode applications has a much longer history, the bulk of work reported before the early 1960s addressed individuals with severe hearing impairments or deafness. Despite its youth, investigators have successfully validated intervention strategies to establish augmentative communication systems among toddlers with a plethora of disabilities, including those associated with pervasive developmental delay, mental retardation, severe speech and motor deficits, abuse, and neglect.

A particularly exciting area of inquiry is the preventive role that augmentative communication systems may play for young children with temporary severe respiratory impairments. The use of augmentative communication systems allows interventionists to expand a child's productive repertoire of vocabulary and communicative functions. At some later point (when the child is again able to use his or her vocal mechanisms), speech can again be added to the child's communication repertoire.

Although the instructional technology to teach augmentative communication is substantial, advances in electronic technology have vastly outstepped interventionists' abilities to use it. The efficiency of an augmentative communication system (from the user's perspective) determines, for the most part, whether the system will be used with any regularity. Advances in microcomputer technology have resulted in the potential for increased communication efficiency. Examples include the systematic miniaturization of electronic communication aids that directly influence portability. Another significant advancement is the capability to have dynamically displayed symbols. Liquid crystal screen technology allows interventionists to place virtually any type of symbol on a communication display. Furthermore, line-drawn symbols can be animated. Theoretically, this animating capability should make it easy to teach individuals to discriminate between vocabulary depicting actions and vocabulary depicting people and objects. However, limited research has explored this issue. A dynamic display of symbols also means that pages can be displayed sequentially with minimal physical effort required. This technological advance means that a vocabulary and message system can be arranged so that a master page can display major topical areas. Each symbol on the master page can be linked to other pages with more explicit symbols, which, in turn, can be linked automatically to other relevant pages of symbols. Consequently, rather than recalling from memory a sequence of two or three symbols to touch to gain access to a given message, the individual can select one symbol at a time that, in turn, will offer an array of related symbols to choose from if the individual wants to be more explicit. The resulting advantage is the use of recognition memory rather than recall memory to construct messages. Recognition memory tends to minimize errors and promotes acquisition of knowledge that can be recalled later. Recall memory should result in greater speed in selecting messages once they are acquired. Very little work has been done to examine the process that should be used to make decisions about implementing fixed and dynamic displays with augmentative system users.

One of the greatest threats to the efficiency of an augmentative communication system is the physical effort required to produce messages. As a result, augmentative system users tend to respond less often to nonobligatory conversational bids from partners than do their speaking counterparts. For many individuals with disabilities, social interaction appears to be less reinforcing than it is for typically developing individuals. A particular challenge for researchers is to parse out the relative influence and contribution of each of these variables and develop assessment and intervention strategies that will enhance opportunities for augmentative system users to maximize their social abilities.

For individuals who communicate via challenging behavior, maximizing social opportunities includes replacing socially motivated challenging behavior with acceptable communicative alternatives. Although an instructional technology exists, most of it demonstrates the efficiency of teaching the use of a communication alternative that can be reinforced whenever it is produced. Research needs to focus on the procedures necessary to minimize challenging behavior when teaching a communicative replacement that can only be reinforced under some conditions. In all likelihood, multicomponent treatments that match a combination of strategies with specific social functions of existing challenging behavior need to be designed and investigated.

CONCLUSION

Augmentative communication as a discipline is still in its infancy. Remarkable strides have been made in delineating and validating equipment and instructional technologies that have had a profound effect on the lives of individuals with developmental disabilities. To a large degree, this success has been the result of transdisciplinary study. Creating successful augmentative communication applications requires active collaboration among a wide range of disciplines, from engineering to education. The future offers great promise. As the understanding of microcomputer technology, instructional technology, and communication development grows, augmentative communication applications should become increasingly more effective, both from the perspective of the user of the technology and of the listener.

REFERENCES

Bates, E. (1976). *Language and context: The acquisition of pragmatics*. New York: Academic Press.

Bates, E. (1979). Intentions, conventions, and symbols. In E. Bates, L. Benigni, I. Bretherton, L. Camaioni, & V. Volterra (Eds.), *The emergence of symbols* (pp. 33–68). New York: Academic Press.

Bates, E., Benigni, L., Bretherton, L., Camaioni, L., & Volterra, V. (Eds.). (1979). *The emergence of symbols*. New York: Academic Press.

Bates, E., Camaioni, L., & Volterra, V. (1975). The acquisition of performatives prior to speech. *Merrill-Palmer Quarterly, 21*, 205–224.

Beukelman, D.R., & Mirenda, P. (1992). *Augmentative and alternative communication: Management of severe communication disorders in children and adults*. Baltimore: Paul H. Brookes Publishing Co.

Brady, N., & Saunders, K. (1991). Considerations in the effective teaching of object-to-symbol matching. *Augmentative and Alternative Communication, 7*, 112–116.

Carr, E.G. (1977). The motivation of self-injurious behavior. A review of some hypotheses. *Psychological Bulletin, 84*, 800–816.

Carr, E.G. (1988). Functional equivalence as a mechanism of response generalization. In R.H. Horner, G. Dunlap, & R.L. Koegel (Eds.), *Generalization and maintenance: Life-style changes in applied settings* (pp. 221–241). Baltimore: Paul H. Brookes Publishing Co.

Carr, E.G., & Durand, V.M. (1985a). Reducing behavior problems through functional communication training. *Journal of Applied Behavior Analysis, 18*, 111–126.

Carr, E.G., & Durand, V.M. (1985b). The social-communicative basis of severe behavior problems in children. In S. Reiss & R. Bootzin (Eds.), *Theoretical issues in behavior therapy* (pp. 219–254). New York: Academic Press.

Coggins, T., & Carpenter, R. (1981). The communicative intention inventory. *Journal of Applied Psycholinguistics, 2*, 213–234.

Drasgow, E., & Halle, J.W. (1995). Teaching social communication to young children with severe disabilities. *Topics in Early Childhood Special Education, 15*, 164–186.

Griffith, P., & Robinson, J. (1980). Influences of iconicity and phonological similarity on sign learning by mentally retarded children. *American Journal of Mental Deficiency, 85*, 291–298.

Guess, D., Benson, H.A., & Siegel-Causey, E. (1985). Concepts and issues related to choice making and autonomy among persons with severe disabilities. *Journal of The Association for Persons with Severe Handicaps, 10*, 79–86.

Halle, J. (1987). Teaching language in the natural environment: An analysis of spontaneity. *Journal of The Association for Persons with Severe Handicaps, 12*, 28–37.

Harding, C.G., & Golinkoff, R.M. (1979). The origins of intentional vocalizations in prelinguistic infants. *Child Development, 50*, 33–40.

Horner, R.H., & Day, H.M. (1991). The effects of response efficiency on functionally equivalent competing behaviors. *Journal of Applied Behavior Analysis, 24*, 719–732.

Horner, R.H., Day, H.M., Sprague, J., O'Brien, M., & Heathfield, L. (1991). Interspersed requests: A nonaversive procedure for reducing aggression and self-injury during instruction. *Journal of Applied Behavior Analysis, 24*, 265–278.

Horner, R.H., Sprague, J.R., O'Brien, M., & Heathfield, L.T. (1990). The role of response efficiency in the reduction of problem behaviors through functional equivalence training: A case study. *Journal of The Association for Persons with Severe Handicaps, 15*, 91–97.

Koppenhaver, D., & Yoder, D. (1992). Literacy issues in persons with severe physical and speech impairments. In R. Gaylord-Ross (Ed.), *Issues and research in special education* (pp. 156–201). New York: Teachers College Press.

Linfoot, K. (1994). *Communication strategies for people with developmental disabilities: Issues from theory and practice.* Baltimore: Paul H. Brookes Publishing Co.

Mace, F.C., & Roberts, M.L. (1993). Factors affecting selection of behavioral interventions. In J. Reichle & D.P. Wacker (Eds.), *Communication and language intervention series: Vol. 3. Communicative alternatives to challenging behavior: Integrating functional assessment and intervention strategies* (pp. 113–134). Baltimore: Paul H. Brookes Publishing Co.

McLean, J.E., & Snyder-McLean, L. (1987). Form and function of communicative behaviour among persons with severe developmental disabilities. *Journal of Developmental Disabilities, 13*(2), 83–98.

McLean, J.E., & Snyder-McLean, L.K. (1991). Communication intent and its realizations among persons with severe intellectual deficits. In N. Krasnegor, R. Schiefelbusch, & D. Rumbaugh (Eds.), *Biological and behavioral determinants of language development* (pp. 481–508). Hillsdale, NJ: Lawrence Erlbaum Associates.

McLean, J.E., Snyder-McLean, L.K., Brady, N.C., & Etter, R. (1991). Communication profiles of two types of gesture using nonverbal persons with severe to profound mental retardation. *Journal of Speech and Hearing Research, 34*, 294–308.

O'Neill, R., & Reichle, J. (1993). Addressing socially motivated challenging behaviors by establishing communicative alternatives: Basics of a general-case approach. In J. Reichle & D.P. Wacker (Eds.), *Communication and language intervention series: Vol. 3. Communicative alternatives to challenging behavior: Integrating functional assessment and intervention strategies* (pp. 205–236). Baltimore: Paul H. Brookes Publishing Co.

Owens, R.E. (1995). *Language disorders: A functional approach to assessment and intervention* (2nd ed.). Needham, MA: Allyn & Bacon.

Reich, P. (1986). *Language development.* Englewood Cliffs, NJ: Prentice Hall.

Reichle, J. (1995). *Applications in the implementation of augmentative communication systems: Case studies.* Unpublished manuscript, University of Minnesota, Minneapolis.

Reichle, J., Halle, J., & Johnston, S. (1993). Developing an initial communicative repertoire: Applications and issues for persons with severe disabilities. In A.P. Kaiser & D.B. Gray (Eds.), *Communication and language intervention series: Vol. 2. Enhancing children's communication: Research foundations for intervention* (pp. 105–135). Baltimore: Paul H. Brookes Publishing Co.

Reichle, J., Sigafoos, J., & Remington, R. (1991). Beginning an augmentative communication system with individuals with severe disabilities. In B. Remington (Ed.), *The challenge of severe mental handicap* (pp. 189–213). New York: John Wiley & Sons.

Reichle, J., York, J., & Sigafoos, J. (1991). *Implementing augmentative and alternative communication: Strategies for learners with severe disabilities.* Baltimore: Paul H. Brookes Publishing Co.

Sachs, J. (1993). The emergence of intentional communication. In J.B. Gleason (Ed.), *The development of language* (3rd ed., pp. 39–64). New York: Macmillan.

Scoville, R. (1983). Development of the intention to communicate: The eye of the beholder. In L. Feagans, C. Garvey, & R. Golinkoff (Eds.), *The origins and growth of communication.* Norwood, NJ: Ablex.

Seligman, M. (1975). *Helplessness: On depression, development, and death.* San Francisco: W.H. Freeman.

Siegel-Causey, E., & Guess, D. (1989). *Enhancing nonsymbolic communication interactions among learners with severe disabilities.* Baltimore: Paul H. Brookes Publishing Co.

Stremel-Campbell, K., Cantrell, D., & Halle, J. (1977). Manual signing as a language system and as a speech initiator for the nonverbal severely handicapped student. In E. Santag (Ed.), *Educational programming for the severely and profoundly handicapped* (pp. 335–347). Reston, VA: Council for Exceptional Children.

Sugarman, S. (1984). The development of preverbal communication. In R.L. Schiefelbusch & J. Pickar (Eds.), *The acquisition of communicative competence* (pp. 23–67). Baltimore: University Park Press.

Vygotsky, L. (1986). *Thought and language* (A. Kozulin, Ed. & Trans.). Cambridge, MA: Harvard University Press. (Original work published 1934)

Werner, H., & Kaplan, B. (1963). *Symbol formation: An organismic-developmental approach to language and the expression of thought.* New York: John Wiley & Sons.

Wetherby, A., & Prizant, B. (1989). The expression of communicative intent: Assessment guidelines. *Seminars in Speech and Language, 10,* 77–91.

Wetherby, A.M., Cain, D.H., Yonclas, D.G., & Walker, V.G. (1988). Analysis of intentional communication of normal children from the prelinguistic to the multiword stage. *Journal of Speech and Hearing Research, 31,* 240–252.

18

Facilitating Transitions Across Home, Community, Work, and School

Michaelene M. Ostrosky,
Mary M. Donegan, and Susan A. Fowler

T HIS CHAPTER DISCUSSES ISSUES RELATED to the transitions made by learners across activities and environments that influence service delivery systems. These issues are discussed as they pertain to two populations of individuals: children who are both chronologically and developmentally at the prelinguistic stage and individuals with severe developmental disabilities who do not speak. The chapter also considers strategies for promoting continuity in services and developing cross-cultural competence across learning environments. Two case studies are presented that illustrate transition issues affecting service delivery, which are followed by implications for recommended practice and directions for future research.

A *transition* is defined as a change in the delivery of services. It may involve a change in who delivers services, what services are delivered, where and when services are delivered, or how services are delivered. Transitions occur on a daily basis for everyone and may involve a change in activities (e.g., sleeping to waking), across settings (e.g., home to work), or across life events (e.g., high school to college). Planning for change is important to ensure smooth transitions.

Transition planning requires an exploration of the differences and commonalities of communicative obligations and opportunities across activities and settings. For individuals with severe developmental disabilities who do not speak and for young children who are developmentally at the prelinguistic stage, changes in the delivery of services may require particular attention. Different contexts support different types of communicative behavior (Gruenewald, Schroeder, & Yoder, 1982). For example, Coggins, Olswang, and Guthrie (1987)

The authors thank Ruth Watkins, Paula Kohler, and Suzanne Lee for their comments on an earlier draft of this chapter. Also, during the development of this chapter, the first author was a Faculty Fellow in the Bureau of Educational Research at the University of Illinois, Urbana–Champaign.

found that structured tasks worked better to elicit requests from young children, and unstructured situations were associated with greater proportions of comments. In addition, Odom and Strain (1984) noted that for very young children, sociodramatic play materials (e.g., dress-up clothes, kitchen toys) tend to facilitate conversations between children, whereas puzzles may result in limited communication between peers. For an adult with severe communication delays, an outing to a movie theater may offer limited opportunities to communicate, whereas a trip to the local bowling alley may be rich with communicative obligations and opportunities.

The optimal environment for acquiring communication skills is interactive and centered around the individual's activities and interests. In addition, the optimal environment is characterized as being responsive, nondidactic, nondirective, varied in its stimuli, and supportive while allowing for maximal independence. Furthermore, in an ideal environment, communicative partners assign meaning to early communicative attempts. For instance, if a 20-month-old infant hands his favorite bottle of bubbles to a caregiver, and she responds to the child's behavior as if it were a request for assistance, the infant is more likely to engage in communicative interactions with this caregiver in the future. If an adolescent who does not talk paces in front of a cabinet when he is hungry, and adults interpret this behavior as signaling a desire for a snack and offer choices of food items, then the adolescent may learn to approach adults when he is hungry.

Expectations and opportunities for communication vary across the environments in which individuals who do not speak participate. For young children, requests at home may be anticipated and responded to readily by parents and older siblings. However, an unfamiliar caregiver at a child care center may not provide enough time for the same child to make a communicative attempt or may not recognize an idiosyncratic gesture or a sign. Individuals who have communication delays probably have experienced some degree of failure in communicating. For instance, an adult who communicates using an augmentative and alternative communication (AAC) system may have been in situations in which his or her needs were not met because others in that environment were unfamiliar with his or her communicative system. Other children who communicate using eye gaze may not have their needs met if caregivers or peers fail to read, or if they misread, their communicative cues. If the natural contexts of a person's life have limitations for meeting individual needs and opportunities for communicative participation, then attempts should be made to modify the contexts, making the contexts more conducive to meeting needs and providing opportunities for communication and language growth (Nelson, 1993). These modifications may take the form of staff or parent training for caregivers who are unfamiliar with AAC systems, or they may necessitate restructuring the environment to provide increased opportunities for prelinguistic youngsters and individuals who do not speak to engage in positive communicative interactions with peers and adults in their environments. Restructuring may take the form of placing a highly preferred material within view but out of reach so that the individual must communicate to gain access to the desired object. Alternatively, an adult might structure an activity so that an individual who does not speak and a peer each have some materials needed to complete an activity but they must work together to complete the project (Ostrosky & Kaiser, 1991). As Warren (1988) noted, "Context is more than who is present, when, with what objects, and in what environmental setting" (p. 295). Context also includes the linguistic climate established during each interaction as well as the discourse history shared by the partners. When interactions take place in a positive linguistic climate, there is a match between the child's level of performance, the adult's support of child communicative behavior, and the new skills taught during intervention. Factors that inhibit communicative attempts by individuals who do not speak or individuals who are at a prelinguistic stage include the following: unfamiliar caregivers, caregivers who do not recognize communicative attempts, caregivers who misread communicative attempts, differences across settings in response to communicative attempts, and a history of failed communicative attempts. These factors should be considered when a change in the delivery of services is eminent. These factors are referred to throughout the remainder of the chapter.

HOW INCLUSION INFLUENCES SERVICE DELIVERY

The trend toward normalization for individuals with disabilities has gained tremendous support since the 1970s. *Normalization* is defined as the use of progressively more natural settings and procedures to establish and maintain personal behaviors that are as culturally typical as possible (Wolfensberger, 1972). According to this view, people with disabilities are expected to live and be treated like people without disabilities. The movement toward full inclusion in schools, the transition-related mandate of the Individuals with Disabilities Education Act Amendments of 1991 (PL 102-119), and the passage of the Americans with Disabilities Act (ADA) of 1990 (PL 101-336) have increased the likelihood that older children and adults who do not speak will participate in a greater variety of activities and programs, including general education classrooms, rehabilitation programs, work settings, and community-based recreation activities. Likewise, for very young children and their families, the passage of the Education of the Handicapped Act Amendments of 1986 (PL 99-457) has had a substantial impact on the availability and quality of early intervention services. Part H provides incentives to each state to develop a statewide, comprehensive, coordinated interagency system of services for eligible infants and toddlers with special needs and their families. The intent of this family-centered legislation is to coordinate existing services, which may take the form of any combination of service delivery settings, including home-based, center-based, and support services. As a result of increased participation in many environments, there is a greater likelihood that individuals who do not speak will make multiple daily transitions as they move among school, work, and recreational settings.

Changes in the work force and an increase in single-parent families have affected service delivery for individuals with disabilities, especially for families with young children. Approximately 60% of mothers of young children under the age of 5 are employed outside the home (Children's Defense Fund, 1994). For many families, there is a shortage of high-quality, affordable child care for infants and toddlers (Cost, Quality, and Outcomes Study Team, 1995). In addition, high staff turnover rates not only reduce continuity in caregivers but also pose challenges to planning staff development. Early intervention services that are part-day or located separately from child care centers necessitate additional transitions. Multiple daily transitions between environments are common when families must piece together part-day programs to meet their needs for extended child care and specialized services.

Inclusionary practices in service delivery have resulted in individuals with disabilities gaining increased access to a range of environments. However, with increased access comes multiple transitions that may place increased pressure on caregivers and service providers to carefully coordinate services.

EVALUATING TRANSITIONS TYPICALLY ENCOUNTERED BY INDIVIDUALS WITH SPECIAL NEEDS

Service delivery models have the potential to affect three types of transitions that occur routinely for many individuals with and without disabilities: 1) transitions between activities within a given setting (e.g., snack, bathroom, and outdoor play or library, lunchroom, and gym); 2) transitions between multiple settings that occur on a routine basis (e.g., home, place of employment, community recreation program); and 3) transitions between programs (e.g., when a child "graduates" or ages out of a given program, leaves one program to enter a less restrictive setting, or relocates). Factors unique to both service delivery and the individual may affect the ease of these transitions. This section discusses these three major types of transitions that face individuals with special needs and the factors that may influence the success of these transitions for individuals who do not speak.

Transitions Between Activities within a Setting

Within any given environment, frequent transitions occur between routines and activities (e.g., from a large-group lesson to snack or from outdoor play to indoors; from delivering mail to checking supplies to taking a break). During activity transitions, individuals may be required to stop what they are doing and follow new routines or adult directives or interact with new peers. During these times, an individual who does not speak is at risk for failure if he or she is overly dependent on adult support or contextual cues. The ability to make transitions between activities is considered an important skill that is required of students in general education classrooms (Sainato, 1990). It also is an expectation for young adults in the work force. However, each activity transition holds the potential for problems.

Activity transitions for young children often take more time than teachers typically plan when formulating their classroom schedules (Ostrosky, Skellenger, Odom, McConnell, & Peterson, 1994). Ostrosky and colleagues found that preschoolers spent approximately 15% of their day engaged in transition-related activities. In a review of the literature on activity transitions, Sainato (1990) demonstrated how schedules, staff assignments, and room arrangement can be changed to create smoother transitions. Planning activity transitions and assigning staff responsibilities (Hart, 1982), avoiding excess wait time (Agler, 1984), and allowing children to move freely at their own pace were found to be effective scheduling strategies. Sainato (1990) recommended staffing arrangements during activity transitions that take into account providing assistance to children with less mobility while assigning other adults a specific area of the room for monitoring groups of children. For an individual who does not speak, support provided during activity transitions may take the form of calling the individual's attention to contextual cues, providing extra time for transitions between activities, or providing additional adult or peer support. In addition, preparing children for upcoming transitions has been found to facilitate transitions between activities (Rosenkoetter & Fowler, 1986). Speech-language pathologists and classroom personnel could use activity transitions as effective natural opportunities for promoting functional communication skills by working on following directions or responding to peer comments during these times.

Children who can follow verbal directions and appropriate peer models generally experience fewer problems during activity transitions. These children are more independent and therefore rely less on adults in their environment as they make the transition from one activity to another. Peers have been used to reduce disruption during transition activities through the use of point systems (Carden-Smith & Fowler, 1984; Fowler, 1986) and buddy systems (Sainato, Strain, Lefebvre, & Rapp, 1987). Co-workers can facilitate smooth transitions for individuals who do not speak by prompting or physically guiding their peers, serving as models, or providing contextual cues.

Transitions Across Programs that Occur on a Daily Basis

Many children with special needs attend more than one program or group setting each day. A study of dual enrollment found that preschool children with special needs or who were at risk for academic failure were making an average of four transitions in the course of a day (Ostrosky & Hughes, 1994). For example, preschoolers may move from home to child care to a special education preschool then back to the child care setting before returning home. Similarly, a high school student who does not speak may make transitions daily between home, an academic setting, a vocational training program, and his or her place of employment or other community-based training site and back home again. This young adult might interact with a variety of adults during the course of a typical day, including parents, classroom teachers, related services providers, peers, co-workers, a supervisor, and a job coach. Making transitions across several part-day programs on a daily basis may become easier over time for a typically developing person; however, individuals with physical or multiple disabilities or those who do not speak may be more vulnerable to frustration due to changing or inconsistent levels of support across settings.

Although inconsistencies and natural variation may be negative or frustrating to some individuals, differences across settings may promote the acquisition of better adaptive skills for other individuals. Learning opportunities are inherent in situations in which children are exposed to different contingencies, expectations, and behaviors. Children may need to try new strategies, attend to contextual cues, and adapt to the different contingencies across settings to succeed. Making all environments consistent may not be possible or even desirable. Good communication by providers across settings may provide the key to successful transitions, especially when practitioners can share information on how a child participates and strategies for promoting participation.

For infants and toddlers who make transitions between settings in a given day, parents and caregivers may serve as liaisons between settings during drop-off and pickup times. Endsley and Minisch (1991) observed the quality and quantity of communication between parents and staff in 16 child care centers during morning and afternoon arrival and departure times and found substantial variation across centers in the likelihood of staff-initiated conversation. The mean length of conversation was 27 seconds; substantive conversation was more likely to occur with caregivers of younger children. However, parents' physical presence alone did not guarantee that communication occurred or that information was transferred. No communication occurred for 43% of the parents of preschool children. Staff were generally more available to talk in the morning; however, parents were more available in the afternoon. Such a happenstance schedule of communication creates problems for children who do not speak and who are unable to convey details of their day to parents or other care providers. Important issues and concerns may not be shared or conveyed if a scheduled time or method to exchange information is not arranged. Smith and Hubbard (1988) found that children interacted more with their teachers in settings in which staff talked more with parents and in which staff–parent relationships were balanced, warm, and reciprocal. Support personnel, such as speech-language pathologists and physical therapists, also might make use of consistent communication either in person or through notebooks as methods for sharing intervention and assessment information with families.

For preschool children with special needs enrolled in multiple settings and transported between programs by bus midday, communication between settings depends on staff. In an interview study of 24 early childhood and early childhood special education teachers who worked with preschoolers with disabilities enrolled in two or more programs, 70% of the staff reported communicating with other program staff during the course of 1 year; however, the frequency of communication varied from only one to five times during the year (Donegan, Ostrosky, & Fowler, 1996). Most teachers who communicated relied on telephone interactions. When communication took place between staff from different programs, conversations typically addressed reactions to problem behaviors rather than proactive planning. These staff cited logistics (e.g., adequate time in their schedule, parent permission, availability of money to pay for release time to visit other programs, access to a telephone) and attitudinal factors as the major barriers to communication among staff who work with children who attend multiple programs. Results suggested that few children, if any, had service providers who communicated daily with one another. For individuals who cannot communicate about events in their two (or more) programs, this arrangement can result in a failure to adequately meet their individual needs. Ostrosky and Hughes (1994) found that a number of young children who attended morning and afternoon programs in two locations missed meals and naps and that staff and parents were unaware of these omissions. In large part, these children were unable to communicate effectively about these oversights, although some children exhibited behavioral manifestations, such as fatigue, lethargy, or hunger. Teaching skills for communicating about their basic needs to individuals who do not speak should be a primary focus of intervention.

Fatigue and behavior problems have been associated with young children who experience difficulty when attending more than one program each day (Donegan et al., 1996). Staff and families may need to make arrangements and jointly plan for rest or quiet time, meals, and medication. Due to differences in behavioral expectations across settings, children may need extra adjustment time and clarification of these behavioral expectations. When children use AAC systems, staff at each program that the children attend need to be taught to use the systems. As more adults take on significant roles in the lives of individuals who do not speak, the likelihood that these adults will respond consistently to communicative attempts or understand the communication system decreases.

As with younger children, continuity between settings may not occur for older individuals who do not speak without first creating links and mechanisms for both information sharing and specific intervention planning. Sharing information is especially important given the knowledge that events that occur in a prior setting may affect behavior (Wahler & Fox, 1981). For instance, events that occurred before the school day (i.e., the number of stops being made in the vehicle in which she traveled) were found to be related to an increase in problem behavior at school by a 20-year-old woman with severe disabilities who did not speak. On days when the city route was taken (with multiple stops), problem behavior occurred more frequently than on days when a highway route (with fewer stops) was taken (Kennedy & Itkonen, 1993).

Creating mechanisms to enable individuals who do not speak to share information about their day is important. Young children who are at the prelinguistic stage of development and adults who cannot speak need a mode for communicating. Strategies such as picture books that have icons related to the various environments of an individual's day or routing notebooks in which staff in each setting and families can write about daily events or issues across settings can facilitate the sharing of information about what occurs in each setting. Adults in different environments can send newsletters home that detail the day's or week's events. These strategies are useful methods for facilitating communication across environments.

Transitions from a Concluding Program to a New Program

Transitions from a concluding program to a new program occur when an individual's enrollment in one program ends and another program begins. These transitions may be accompanied by a number of changes in service delivery, including who delivers what services, where services are provided, and the duration and intensity of services. For example, a child at age 3 years may exit a home-based early intervention program and enter a community-based preschool program. In addition to changes in the physical location of the intervention program, the curriculum (or focus of intervention) also may change somewhat (e.g., from a focus on parent–child interaction to a focus on self-care skills and peer interaction skills). In addition, the number of personnel and their roles may change. Therapists in an early intervention program may make home visits and work directly with the family. However, in elementary school settings the same professional may provide consultative services or provide direct instruction in the classroom. Consequently, as their child gets older, the family may experience a reduction in contact with service providers (Hains, Rosenkoetter, & Fowler, 1991). Parents whose child received speech therapy services at home and who participated in supporting the intervention strategies in daily routines may be left with little or no guidance on how to support communication efforts when the child begins receiving services at preschool. Failure to bridge home and school efforts may unnecessarily limit children's exposure to intervention efforts and result in a reduction in efforts or expectations at home for the children's communication skills.

Transitions in which service delivery models shift can be disruptive unless the impact that the shift has on all participants is explored. The shift from direct service delivery at home to consultation at school may not sufficiently address strategies to enhance communicative efforts across the child's day without consultation to the home and consistent exchange of information between settings. School-to-home notebooks that support the sharing of information on individual children between staff pathologists and families are important. Transfer of records and exchange of information regarding effective and ineffective strategies and child progress from the early intervention therapist to the preschool therapist are essential to ensure continuity in service delivery. Transitions between agencies can result in delayed, misplaced, or unread files; unnecessary repetition of assessments; and trial-and-error efforts at providing effective methods of speech and language therapy.

Transitions from one program to another during the secondary education years are often accompanied by an increased emphasis on job training and independent living. Postschool outcomes, including high unemployment and underemployment rates for adults with disabilities, are cause for concern for youth who do not speak (Rusch & Phelps, 1987). The Individuals with Disabilities Education Act (IDEA) of 1990 (PL 101-476) requires a statement of needed transition services in the individualized education program (IEP) by age 16 years. This guideline can be lowered to 14 years of age when appropriate. For adolescents and adults who do not speak, the importance of sharing information across programs cannot be overstated. When employers, co-workers, and job coaches engage in a trial-and-error analysis of the communication skills of an individual who does not speak, much time is wasted that could be better spent on the development of job training skills. Frustration by all parties also may result. Sharing information across sites and with families, via notebooks, telephone calls, or meetings, might alleviate some of these potential problems.

Fragmentation and Duplication of Services Across Learning Environments

When a variety of agencies are involved in service delivery, there is a greater chance for fragmentation and duplication of services as prelinguistic and non-speaking individuals make the transition from one program to another. For example, a person who does not speak cannot inform staff that vision testing was done at another program a month ago or that her teachers and therapists at the child care setting have begun honoring certain intentional idiosyncratic gestures. The transition from early intervention to preschool services and from secondary education to employment services or to postsecondary education pose special challenges for transition planning due to differences in eligibility criteria among differing administrative agencies. Dual enrollment in programs also can result in fragmentation of services if staff do not coordinate their service plans. To coordinate transitions, a systems approach is needed that involves three interrelated components: the community, the programs, and the family (Fowler & Ostrosky, 1994). Interagency agreements, developed on a local level by representatives of various programs and families, can be used to identify sources of funding, develop procedures for exchanging information, ensure familiarity with available services, and reduce gaps and miscommunication (Fowler, Hains, & Rosenkoetter, 1990). At a minimum, interagency agreements may result in an increased frequency with which staff can communicate with each other about the learners whom they both serve, the provision of release time for IEP or habilitation plan meetings, program visits, and the creation of a process for exchanging information. It is important that representation exists from various disciplines in interagency councils. Interagency agreements work best if providers with a range of discipline identities participate in their development and implementation, rather than relying solely on representation from administrative personnel from the various agencies.

Differences in Program and Staff Expectations Across Programs

Transitions from more restrictive to less restrictive environments are often accompanied by differences in program staff expectations. As children grow older or enter inclusive settings, group size generally increases. School staff typically expect higher levels of independence and thus provide decreased support. Sainato and Lyon (1989) compared characteristics of special education and general education preschool settings and found considerable differences in group size, roles of adults, and behavioral expectations of children. Children in special education programs often receive high levels of prompts and participate in more structured activities than children in general education programs. To ensure success, families need to help prepare individuals with disabilities by developing functional goals relevant to their next environment and informing new staff about supports and strategies for working with their children who do not speak. Also, program personnel can play a critical role in preparing individuals for success. For example, in light of teacher expectations for students to be able to communicate their needs and follow teacher directions, speech-language pathologists can help prepare for transitions by focusing on particular skills that are important for teacher and school success.

Lack of Communication Between Professionals

Lack of communication between sending and receiving staff has been cited as a barrier to transition planning (Fowler, Schwartz, & Atwater, 1991). To overcome this barrier, clarification of staff roles is needed. Hains, Fowler, and Chandler (1988) recommended that the responsibilities of staff from sending programs include identifying skills needed in the future environment, planning with parents to prepare the child for the next environment, and serving as a liaison to the new program. The receiving staff have the responsibility of analyzing the environment and making adaptations to support the newly enrolled child and establishing a relationship with families.

Many families desire more opportunities to plan transitions and communicate with staff before, during, and after transitions (Johnson, Chandler, Kerns, & Fowler, 1986). Although families vary in their preferred level of involvement, a focus on family needs and a clear delineation of family and staff areas of responsibility can ensure smoother transitions (Fowler, Chandler, Johnson, & Stella, 1988). As children mature, families need support in dealing with new demands created by transitions and changes in social, academic, and vocational expectations (Szekeres & Meserve, 1994).

When individuals who do not speak transfer from one program to another, they may require additional time to adjust and to understand what is expected of them in the new environment, This extra time may lead to the mistaken conclusion that an individual is not ready or is not benefiting from the new program. In some cases, an individual with special needs may fail to demonstrate previously acquired skills, leading to conclusions that he or she is not prepared to attend the new program.

Fowler (1982) recommended a three-step process that includes identifying differences in each environment, adding elements in the existing curriculum to minimize differences, and continually evaluating the effectiveness of the changes. For example, a young child with limited verbal skills who enters preschool or group care for the first time is likely to experience an environment that differs from home in many ways. To prepare the child and enhance the likelihood of adjustment, family and providers may want to consider these differences and identify which ones may be critical to the young child's adjustment. For example, separating from a parent, following new routines, making friends, communicating needs, and responding to new adults are several critical features of preschool or group child care. Having noted these differences, parents may plan opportunities at home to introduce or expand these experiences for their child. Parents can practice separation by increasing the occasions and length of time during which they leave the child under the supervision of a relative, friend, or child care provider. They can introduce the child to a neighborhood or park district parent–child playgroup to increase opportunities for their child to play in a group setting, make friends, and experience new adults. Following new instructions and routines at home may increase the child's ability to adapt to new routines at school. Before enrollment in a new program, parents may want to identify ways in which to make the school experience familiar for the child, such as making visits to explore the new environment and meet the teacher. They may want to share with the teacher information about their child's favorite stories, activities, and toys that could be introduced during the initial days of school. Finally, they may want to share the child's communication strategies with the new teacher so that he or she does not misunderstand or fail to take advantage of opportunities to respond to communicative acts.

Prelinguistic children or individuals who do not speak often use subtle or idiosyncratic cues and other means of communicating that may not be readily understood by individuals unfamiliar to them. Due to the considerable heterogeneity in both form and function of nonverbal communication produced by different individuals, the receiving program staff may spend a great deal of time initially determining the meaning of communication behaviors or cues (McLean & McLean, 1993). To maintain and support their communicative efforts, receiving staff must know and recognize the typical cues or modes of communication used by individuals with severe communication delays. Transition planning for individuals using AAC systems requires that sending staff and families work together to orient and train receiving staff, thereby facilitating the individual's adjustment to the next environment and increasing family and staff confidence. Thus, exchanging information about the child's methods of communicating is critical to promoting the child's comfort and adjustment in the new program. Parents and staff will have the opportunity to evaluate the child's accommodations to the new experiences, first when practiced at home and later when experienced at school, to determine the amount of support that the child is likely to need to feel comfortable and successful in the new program.

PROMOTING CONTINUITY IN SERVICES

Continuity between programs as well as within the components of each program in which children participate is recognized as being an essential element of quality service delivery (Bronfenbrenner, 1979; Caldwell, 1991; Kagan, 1993). However, in most situations, continuity continues to be an elusive goal. Movement away from a system of fragmented transitions requires a reconceptualization of the relationship between programs and the roles of the service providers, the family, and the child.

A Collaborative Model for Providers and Families

A commonly used model for considering the relationship between programs comprises three successive levels: cooperation, coordination, and collaboration (Kagan, 1993; Swan & Morgan, 1992). Cooperation, the easiest and most widely achieved, consists of informal relationships without any clearly defined structure. An example of cooperation between different programs that serve individuals who do not speak is sending notes or newsletters informing other programs and families of upcoming events.

Coordination involves individuals from different programs and agencies coming together to meet a shared goal. An example of coordination regarding people with disabilities is the formation of a transition team composed of representatives from sending and receiving programs and families who meet to discuss placement options and develop transition plans several months before a child's transition into a new program. Coordination is most likely to occur after programs have experienced a successful history of cooperation.

Collaboration, the most complex and most difficult level to achieve, comprises programs having joint goals and strategies with shared resources and leadership. An example of collaboration occurs when staff from each program develop a mutually agreed-upon approach to embed communication goals during snack and free-play activities in both a Head Start and child care program that serve a child with severe communication delays. When appropriate, these strategies also are used by family members so that similar expectations can be established at family mealtimes. Working together in this manner can increase the chance of developing functionally relevant goals and objectives and having families, staff, and other caregivers implement them in a consistent manner across a variety of settings throughout the day. To assess and promote the transfer of skills and expectations across settings, specific procedures may need to be implemented. Intervening in more than one setting and conducting training with more than one group of staff members are techniques used to promote generalization of behavior change (Stokes & Osnes, 1986).

To maximize an individual's use of an AAC device, interventions should be implemented in all settings in which he or she participates. To accomplish this, a working relationship must develop between the family and all significant interventionists involved with this individual in his or her educational, recreational, independent living, and vocational programming. To achieve continuity in implementation of the intervention and consistent use of the AAC system in each major setting of the individual's day, members of the educational or habilitation team must recognize one another's expertise, clarify roles and responsibilities, and develop mechanisms for information sharing. There are numerous benefits when families and staff work together. Although it takes time and effort to share expertise, the gains achieved may take the form of individuals with disabilities acquiring and generalizing new skills, staff learning new strategies for working with individuals who do not speak, and families seeing their children become more independent.

Service delivery systems often view services as being integrally linked with the place in which they are delivered. Thus, the individual is expected to move to the location of the services; previously mentioned, the result often is a lack of staff awareness of what occurs in other settings. This, in turn, leads to fragmentation and unnecessary duplication of services. To develop a coordinated service delivery system, a holistic approach to the child's day should be taken. A full-day inclusive setting with appropriate support services, in which the services are moved to the child, is an obvious approach to increasing continuity and reducing the number of transitions that a child is expected to make. Continuity between programs when a prelinguistic child or an individual who does not speak ages out or relocates can be increased by sharing information about daily routines and common activities. For example, staff and family members can share information about a child's preferred activities, effective reinforcers for desired behavior, or methods to embed communication skill training into naturally occurring routines. The following sections discuss how the staff, the child, and the family can promote continuity through sharing information about daily routines and activities.

Adults as Promoters of Continuity

The concept of team encompasses all those who work with an individual with special needs as well as the individual him- or herself. Included on the team are parents, special and general education staff, related services providers, and community agency staff. Because an individual's behavior may vary across the settings in which he or she lives, works, and plays, multiple sources of information may be needed for assessment and planning (Bailey & Wolery, 1989). For individuals who attend multiple programs each day, stress can be eased by encouraging staff to coordinate schedules to ensure opportunities for rest, adequate nutrition, medication, and socialization (Ostrosky & Hughes, 1994).

To achieve consistent patterns of communication and collaboration of effort, administrative policies are needed to support staff in communicating and planning with families and staff in other agencies. These policies might require systems change efforts. Policies should include providing staff with release time to visit programs, making time available for planning and information sharing, ensuring access to telephones, and arranging joint program in-service training. Service providers might plan ways to creatively find release time (e.g., combining classes during gym period one afternoon per month to release a staff member, making use of volunteers such as a foster grandparents program) so that staff can make telephone calls or visit programs. Increasing natural opportunities to communicate also is needed. For example, scheduling ongoing occasions for teachers and speech-language pathologists to collaborate within the classroom setting could provide direct teacher–pathologist contact with the child, thus promoting continuity in programming.

Two models for collaboration are possible: one in which an individual, either a family or a staff member, serves as the liaison or consultant among all parties to share and convey information across people and settings; and one in which opportunities are provided for staff in each program to meet in person and observe one another's program, followed by regularly scheduled communication with staff and caregivers via telephone calls and notebooks.

One medium that may be useful for bridging communication gaps across home and different programs is the use of video equipment and tapes. It has become easier and less costly to videotape children as a way of examining services received by a child who attends multiple programs. Funding for small grants might enable a school system or intervention program to purchase resources, such as video equipment. In addition, families might be willing to loan their personal equipment, or libraries might have video equipment that can be borrowed or rented for short periods of time.

Administrative support and policies may be needed to ensure that children or adults in different settings have access to equipment, curriculum, and instructional methods that support and promote their communicative efforts. For example, limiting the use of sign language to one program or segment of the day because some staff are not comfortable signing is unlikely to improve the quality of an individual's communication or life. Instead, it imposes a dual system of communicating: one in which the individual has opportunities to convey needs, likes, dislikes, and abilities and one in which the individual does not.

Children as Promoters of Continuity

Children can be given a role in creating links across settings. Notebooks, in which staff, families, and caregivers record data-based and anecdotal observations of child behavior, can be transported in a child's book bag. For example, written correspondence between settings about the form or function of a particular gesture will help ensure or promote consistent responding across settings. Children also can transport graphic mode communication systems between settings. Families, caregivers, and related services staff can be enlisted to ask individuals with special needs about events of the day by prompting them with specific questions or comments. For example, encouraging a prelinguistic individual to select a piece of artwork or other permanent product made at one setting to take to the other setting might provide increased opportunities for this preschooler to initiate interactions with peers and adults. An adult from the first setting could write a "story" of what the artwork is about to assist adults at the second setting in initiating a meaningful conversation. This type of strategy would enable the adult in the second setting to "read" the story with the child or to make comments or ask questions about the artwork.

Families as Promoters of Continuity

Parents can serve as catalysts for initiating communication between programs. Requests by parents for communication to occur between programs can cause formerly independent programs to cooperate with one another and increase consistency by sharing goals and instructional strategies for working with individuals with special needs. Because staff and family concerns regarding confidentiality issues may serve as a barrier in some situations (Donegan et al., 1996), programs need to obtain parent permission to share information. Parents may initiate consent for release of information and may stimulate cross-program communication by inviting staff from other programs to attend meetings and by requesting that information sharing be specified on a child's IEP. In addition, putting a notebook in a child's book bag to be shared by families and staff in each setting will serve as a reminder to staff to communicate with home and staff at other programs.

IMPACT OF CULTURAL DIFFERENCES ON TRANSITIONS

The cultural background of families of individuals with disabilities can have a profound impact on many aspects of service delivery (e.g., family–professional relationships, family expectations). Cultures regulate the behavior of individuals through creating, organizing, and maintaining roles within the larger group. All cultures have developmental expectations that influence the amount of support provided by families and communities. These expectations typically are tied into the chronological age of an individual rather than the developmental level. Regardless of culture, an incongruence between caregivers' expectations and children's abilities may result in feelings of failure or in frustration by both the caregivers and the individuals with disabilities.

Cultural sensitivity and respect for the cultural differences of families are crucial to the successful delivery of services to both families and children

(Bowe, 1995). Service delivery is affected when the language spoken by the professionals differs from that of the individual who does not speak and his or her family. A family's ethnic, racial, and cultural identification strongly influence their values and beliefs regarding the meaning of a disability, education, healing and health care, child rearing, and the perceived importance of family involvement in interventions (Hanson, Lynch, & Wayman, 1990; Harry, 1992). The long-term expectations each family has for an older individual with disabilities also may vary depending on their culture of origin.

Cultural differences may impede the development of collaborative relationships between professionals and the family. To overcome these barriers, staff training may be needed to develop cross-cultural competence, through awareness of one's own cultural limitations (i.e., understanding one's beliefs and values and how these will differ from others'); openness, appreciation, and respect for cultural differences; a view of intercultural interactions as learning opportunities; the ability to use cultural resources in interventions; and acknowledgment of the integrity and value of all cultures (Lynch & Hanson, 1992).

IMPLICATIONS FOR EDUCATIONAL PRACTICE

The case studies presented in this section illustrate transition-related issues affecting transition for a prelinguistic child and for a young man who does not speak. These two individuals, who participate in various educational and community settings, are described to illustrate several factors that affect transitions for nonspeaking individuals, regardless of their age.

Marie

Marie is a 3-year-old with multiple disabilities, including Down syndrome. She lives in a foster home with three other children, all of whom have disabilities. One foster sibling ambulates using a wheelchair; the other two walk. The children range from 3 to 12 years of age, and all four have significant developmental delays. Marie's foster mother is employed as a speech-language therapist in a high school special education program.

Although Marie is just learning to walk with the aid of a walker, she is able to move quickly from one location to another by scooting. She has a motorized wheelchair that she is learning to operate independently. Marie's attention span is short. She typically attends to an activity for less than 3 minutes. Marie is nonverbal and is learning to use an electronic communication aid. In addition, she is learning to speak for one communicative function, social greetings.

Marie recently completed the transition from a birth-to-3 early intervention program to a public preschool special education program. Services through the early intervention program were provided in the home with a child development specialist, a speech-language therapist, and a physical therapist making home visits at least once a week. The composition of Marie's preschool program includes 15 other children, 5 with identified developmental delays or disabilities and 10 who are at risk for academic failure. Four adults are in the classroom: an early childhood special education teacher, two teaching assistants, and a one-to-one assistant assigned to Marie. Marie's typical half-day preschool program includes group time, learning centers, gym or outdoor play, snack, a bathroom break, and a story.

Marie currently has more than 50 line-drawn symbols on her electronic communication aid; however, her selection of communicative responses typically appears haphazard and not contextually related to ongoing activities. Marie often will select the same message repeatedly, yet she appears uninterested if offered the materials requested or if taken to the activity selected. Staff in the preschool environment do not know all of the symbols on the electronic communication aid and frequently use a "cheat sheet" in an attempt to communicate with Marie. They have stated repeatedly that they are uncomfortable using the electronic communication aid and that they consider it bulky and distracting to Marie. Marie frequently arrives at large-group activities without her communication device because staff believe that she plays with it or selects inappropriate messages during these activities.

Transitions between daily activities are difficult for Marie, especially if she is not given adequate time to make the transition independently from one environment to another or if activities require her to sit passively for extended periods of time. Marie also has a difficult time interacting with her peers as a result of her severe communication delays. Staff have begun prompting Marie to verbally greet her peers when she enters the preschool program each morning. However, staff are unsure how best to support peer interaction given Marie's AAC system. Peers in Marie's environment have been instructed not to touch her device because "it is very expensive, and they could break it."

In addition to the transitions between activities within the preschool environment that Marie makes on a regular basis, she also makes a transition by bus to a family child care setting for 4 hours each afternoon. In this environment, Marie is the youngest of three children, including two girls who are 4 and 5 years of age. The child care provider had never worked with a child with disabilities before Marie came to her home; however, she is eager to learn instructional strategies and techniques to facilitate Marie's development. When Marie arrives at the family child care home, she often appears irritated and fussy, and her communicative responses often are unclear because she does not have programmed utterances that can be used to respond to questions asked by her child care provider. Communication among caregivers at Marie's preschool, her child care setting, and the foster home is limited.

Several service delivery issues appear to affect Marie's fluency at communicating in different environments. First, staff across all environments are not comfortable using the electronic communication aid. Training needs to be provided in the use of this AAC system. In addition, specific training in Marie's use of the system and in adaptations to the preschool, child care, and home environments needs to be addressed. This training could take the form of hands-on experience with the electronic communication aid for staff from the various settings, sharing videotapes of Marie using the electronic communication aid in the different environments, or demonstrations with Marie present during which various individuals interact with her and her electronic communication aid. Staff across environments also should continue to support Marie's verbal communication skills by prompting her to greet peers and staff when she arrives at each setting.

The second service delivery issue affecting Marie's fluency at communicating is the inconsistent use of the electronic communication aid across environments. Marie would benefit from staff discussing together her entire day and delineating when and how the electronic communication aid could be incorporated into naturally occurring routines and planned activities across all contexts. Staff could assist one another in planning ways to use the device during various activities.

The third service delivery issue affecting Marie is her limited interactions with peers across environments. Service providers report that Marie seldom initiates or responds to peers; therefore, strategies are needed to support positive peer interaction using the electronic communication aid. Peers and adults need to use the device for Marie, who needs augmented input. Staff can model ways for peers to interact with Marie and prompt them to engage in social interaction with her. In addition, staff can arrange for small groups to meet during which social interaction is facilitated by the adults and her peers are taught specific strategies to use with Marie.

Marie's fatigue is the fourth service delivery issue affecting her behavior. Marie may need to nap or be provided with some quiet time upon arrival at the child care setting. Having an area with a bean bag chair, a mat, or a cot where she could relax for a short time may result in increased engagement during other periods of the day. The final service delivery issue affecting Marie is the lack of communication across the three environments where she spends the majority of her day: home, the early childhood special education preschool program, and the family child care setting. Developing a consistent mechanism for communicating across these environments is necessary. Marie's foster mother, in partnership with her other caregivers, can determine the best method for communicating as well as the desired frequency. Increased communication will enable all significant caregivers to become more aware of Marie's behavior across environments and become more cognizant of the effects of each environment on Marie's overall behavior.

Alexander

Alexander is a 21-year-old male who lives at home with his parents and two high school–age siblings. He takes medication to control his seizures, which occur one to two times per week. These seizures often leave Alexander exhausted and needing a quiet place to rest. Both of Alexander's parents work full time, and their dream for Alexander is that one day he will be able to live in a small group home or in a supervised apartment.

Much of Alexander's speech is unintelligible. He typically communicates by tapping others on the shoulder to get their attention, grunting, using gestures (e.g., waving his arm, extending his hand), or answering yes/no questions. He does not use an AAC system. Alexander enjoys being around other people and is generally an even-tempered, happy-go-lucky young man. However, when frustrated he will, on occasion, fall to the ground, scream out, or hit others.

Alexander works part time at a fast-food restaurant and part time in a sheltered workshop. At the fast-food restaurant he is responsible for cleaning tables, floors, and the bathrooms and for monitoring the status of the condiments and eating utensils. Because Alexander has been employed in the community for only 1 month, a job coach works closely with him. At the sheltered workshop, Alexander typically assembles automobile parts for a large automobile company in town. The 20 employees with disabilities at the sheltered workshop are supervised by three staff members. Alexander works at both employment sites Monday through Friday; his job coach transports him daily from the sheltered workshop to the fast-food restaurant. Alexander brings his lunch each day and frequently eats it with his job coach at the sheltered workshop or en route to the fast-food restaurant. Occasionally the job coach and Alexander eat lunch together at a local pizza parlor.

During a typical week, Alexander makes many transitions between his two employment sites, at which he interacts regularly with his job coach, co-workers, and supervisors. Also, he frequently attends activities at the church where his mother works, and he visits the car dealership where his father is employed. Alexander's social activities include attending many athletic events at the high school where his brother plays basketball, baseball, and football. He also enjoys going to the movies at the theater where his sister is an usher.

Issues that affect Alexander's life as he makes the transitions between environments include the lack of a consistent system for communicating across settings and his challenging behaviors. Alexander's aggression often occurs when he is tired or not feeling well, when he has had a seizure, when he needs a break, or when he is bored. Due to his limited communication skills, he often becomes frustrated and resorts to aggression in an attempt to get others to understand his wants and needs. Convening a team meeting with Alexander's family and the primary players in his work and social settings to determine a method for staff to communicate across environments would be useful. Having a notebook float between environments in Alexander's backpack would be one method for alerting others to such issues as medical concerns or fatigue. Alexander could be instrumental in sharing this communicative device by including pictures as a means of communicating. A discussion about Alexander's idiosyncratic communicative behavior and its meaning would be helpful as all staff could become more aware of the interpretation of this behavior by others who have a longer history of interacting with Alexander (e.g., his parents) as well as the perspectives of individuals from varied environments (i.e., home, work, social). A consistent communicative mode to help Alexander become more independent and have more control of his environment is needed. Teaching him to ask for a break from work using a picture symbol or gesture that is honored across settings might be a first step. The availability of assistive technology to support Alexander's communication skill development also should be investigated. Improved communication skills might result in increased independence in living skills (e.g., independent traveling abilities) and decreased problem behavior. Working with Alexander's co-workers to teach them strategies for communicating with Alexander would support communication skill development and the development of increased social relationships with peers with and without disabilities.

IMPLICATIONS FOR FUTURE RESEARCH

Service delivery issues that affect transitions have implications for prelinguistic youngsters and individuals who do not speak. A careful examination of topics, such as recognizing and responding to communicative attempts, supporting communication within and across environments, establishing consistency within and across settings, determining staff development needs, and increasing awareness of what occurs across all phases of an individual's daily life, is necessary.

Future research efforts should address several areas. First, research is needed to study the effect of increased consistency within and across programs for nonspeaking individuals and their families, particularly as it relates to fostering and supporting specific child or student behaviors, especially communication efforts. Studies that evaluate student outcomes when consistency within and across settings is a focus of programming can assist professionals and families in determining the best strategies to support this consistency and, therefore, support communication efforts by individuals who do not speak. For instance, in Marie's case, research investigating the impact of consistent access to her electronic communication aid in preschool, child care, and home might identify the environmental cues that foster Marie's use of the device and the form and consistency of responses by her listeners. The quality and range of responses by significant others to her communicative attempts are likely to be factors influencing her communicative efforts.

A second area requiring empirical scrutiny involves identifying components of service delivery models that are most effective in meeting the needs of prelinguistic children or individuals who do not speak. One service delivery model does not meet the needs of all people with communication delays or disabilities as this is not a homogeneous group. However, an increased awareness of all phases of a person's daily life might facilitate the development of a systematic method for determining the array of service delivery variables that best meet the needs of individuals who do not speak at certain chronological and developmental levels. For instance, in Alexander's case, research investigating the effects of increased communication across significant others who interact with him might identify strategies to facilitate collaboration in program planning and implementation.

Finally, research examining staff development models for facilitating communication and continuity across settings by caregivers should be investigated. Staff development efforts ideally should be aimed at teams of professionals who frequently work together in partnership with the families of individuals who do not speak. Needs assessments must be conducted to determine individual as well as programmatic needs when individuals who do not speak are the focus of intervention efforts. Follow-up and individual coaching for staff might be necessary when the focus of staff development includes such topics as recognizing communicative attempts by youngsters at a prelinguistic level of communication. Staff development efforts can support consistency and continuity within and across programs by raising awareness of issues surrounding the communicative behavior of individuals who do not speak and the potential for challenging behaviors to develop.

CONCLUSION

Young prelinguistic children and individuals who are unable to speak present unique challenges to service providers. First among these challenges is determining ways to serve these individuals in a manner that fosters, recognizes, and respects communicative attempts. A significant focus of service delivery should be directed at facilitating and enhancing the communicative interaction between nonspeaking individuals and significant others in their environment. A second challenge is coordinating the flow of information about the individual's daily events and goals across settings and significant others so that important information, typically conveyed by an individual who can speak, can be shared. A third challenge is coordinating services across settings and providers to ensure that services are integrated so that providers are working in concert and not in isolation or competition in meeting the learning and life skill needs of these individuals.

We are excited by the dramatic improvements that have been made in the ability of professionals to provide inclusive educational services. However, we are constantly cognizant of the improvement that remains to be made. Facilitating transitions across home, community, work, and school remains an area that should be a primary focus of efforts to further streamline service delivery.

REFERENCES

Agler, H.A. (1984). Transitions: Alternatives to manipulative management techniques. *Young Children, 39,* 16–25.

Americans with Disabilities Act (ADA) of 1990, PL 101-336, 42 U.S.C. §§ 12101 *et seq.*

Bailey, D.B., & Wolery, M. (1989). *Assessing infants and preschoolers with handicaps.* Columbus, OH: Charles E. Merrill.

Bowe, F.G. (1995). *Birth to five: Early childhood special education.* New York: Delmar Publishers.

Bronfenbrenner, U. (1979). *The ecology of human development: Experiments by nature and design.* Cambridge, MA: Harvard University Press.

Caldwell, B. (1991). Continuity in the early years: Transitions between grades and systems. In S.L. Kagan (Ed.), *The care and education of America's young children: Obstacles and opportunities. The Nineteenth Yearbook of the National Society for the Study of Education* (pp. 69–90). Chicago: The University of Chicago Press.

Carden-Smith, L.K., & Fowler, S.A. (1984). Positive peer pressure: The effects of peer monitoring on children's disruptive behavior. *Journal of Applied Behavior Analysis, 17,* 213–227.

Children's Defense Fund. (1994). *The state of America's children: Yearbook 1994.* Washington, DC: Author.

Coggins, T.E., Olswang, L.B., & Guthrie, J. (1987). Assessing communicative intents in young children: Low structured or observation tasks? *Journal of Speech and Hearing Disorders, 52,* 44–49.

Cost, Quality, and Outcomes Study Team. (1995). Cost, quality, and child outcomes in child care centers: Key findings and recommendations. *Young Children, 50*(4), 40–44.

Donegan, M.M., Ostrosky, M.M., & Fowler, S.A. (1996). Children enrolled in multiple programs: Characteristics, supports and barriers to teacher communication. *Journal of Early Intervention, 20*(2), 95–106.

Education of the Handicapped Act Amendments of 1986, PL 99-457, 20 U.S.C. §§ 1400 *et seq.*

Endsley, R.C., & Minisch, P.A. (1991). Parent–staff communication in day care centers during morning and afternoon transitions. *Early Childhood Research Quarterly, 6,* 119–135.

Fowler, S.A. (1982). Transition from preschool to kindergarten for children with special needs. In K.E. Allen & E.M. Goetz (Eds.), *Early childhood education: Special problems, special solutions* (pp. 309–334). Rockville, MD: Aspen Publishers, Inc.

Fowler, S.A. (1986). Peer-monitoring and self-monitoring: Alternatives to traditional teacher management. *Exceptional Children, 52,* 573–581.

Fowler, S.A., Chandler, L.K., Johnson, T.E., & Stella, E. (1988). Individualizing family involvement in school transitions: Gathering information and choosing the next program. *Journal of the Division for Early Childhood, 12,* 208–216.

Fowler, S.A., Hains, A.H., & Rosenkoetter, S.E. (1990). The transition between early intervention services and preschool services: Administrative and policy issues. *Topics in Early Childhood Special Education, 9*(4), 55–65.

Fowler, S.A., & Ostrosky, M.M. (1994). Transitions to and from preschool in early childhood special education. In P.L. Safford, B. Spodek, & O.N. Saracho (Eds.), *Early childhood special education: Yearbook in early childhood education* (Vol. 5, pp. 142–164). New York: Teachers College Press.

Fowler, S.A., Schwartz, I., & Atwater, K.J. (1991). Perspectives on the transition from preschool to kindergarten for children with disabilities and their families. *Exceptional Children, 58,* 136–145.

Gruenewald, L., Schroeder, J., & Yoder, D. (1982). Considerations for curriculum development and implementation. In B. Campbell & V. Baldwin (Eds.), *Severely handicapped/hearing impaired students: Strengthening service delivery* (pp. 163–180). Baltimore: Paul H. Brookes Publishing Co.

Hains, A.H., Fowler, S.A., & Chandler, L.K. (1988). Planning school transitions: Family and professional collaboration. *Journal of the Division for Early Childhood, 12*, 108–115.

Hains, A.H., Rosenkoetter, S.F., & Fowler, S.A. (1991). Transition planning with families in early intervention programs. *Infants and Young Children, 3*, 38–47.

Hanson, M.J., Lynch, E.W., & Wayman, K.I. (1990). Honoring the cultural diversity of families when gathering data. *Topics in Early Childhood Special Education, 10*(1), 112–131.

Harry, B. (1992). Making sense of disability: Low-income, Puerto Rican parents' theories of the problem. *Exceptional Children, 59*, 27–40.

Hart, B. (1982). So that teachers can teach: Assigning roles and responsibilities. *Topics in Early Childhood Special Education, 2*(1), 1–8.

Individuals with Disabilities Education Act (IDEA) of 1990, PL 101-476, 20 U.S.C. §§ 1400 *et seq.*

Individuals with Disabilities Education Act Amendments of 1991, PL 102-119, 20 U.S.C. §§ 1400 *et seq.*

Johnson, T.E., Chandler, L.K., Kerns, G.M., & Fowler, S.A. (1986). What are parents saying about family involvement in school transitions? A retrospective transition interview. *Journal of the Division for Early Childhood, 11*, 10–17.

Kagan, S.L. (1993). The research–policy connection: Moving beyond incrementalism. In B. Spodek (Ed.), *Handbook of research on the education of young children* (pp. 506–518). New York: Macmillan.

Kennedy, C.H., & Itkonen, T. (1993). Effects of setting events on the problem behavior of students with severe disabilities. *Journal of Applied Behavior Analysis, 26*, 321–327.

Lynch, E.W., & Hanson, M.J. (Eds.). (1992). *Developing cross-cultural competence: A guide for working with young children and their families.* Baltimore: Paul H. Brookes Publishing Co.

McLean, L.K., & McLean, J.E. (1993). Communication intervention for adults with severe mental retardation. *Topics in Language Disorders, 13*(3), 47–60.

Nelson, N.W. (1993). *Childhood language disorders in context.* Columbus, OH: Charles E. Merrill.

Odom, S.L., & Strain, P.S. (1984). Classroom-based social skills instruction for severely handicapped preschool children. *Topics in Early Childhood Special Education, 4*(3), 97–116.

Ostrosky, M.M., & Hughes, M. (1994, October). *Now where am I going? Issues surrounding multiple placements of young children.* Session presented at the annual Division for Early Childhood of the Council for Exceptional Children Conference, St. Louis, MO.

Ostrosky, M.M., & Kaiser, A.P. (1991). Preschool classroom environments that promote communication. *Teaching Exceptional Children, 23*(4), 6–10.

Ostrosky, M.M., Skellenger, A.C., Odom, S.L., McConnell, S.R., & Peterson, C. (1994). Teachers' schedules and actual time spent in activities in preschool special education classes. *Journal of Early Intervention, 18*, 25–33.

Rosenkoetter, S.E., & Fowler, S.A. (1986). Teaching mainstreamed children to manage daily transitions. *Exceptional Children, 19*, 20–23.

Rusch, F., & Phelps, L.A. (1987). Secondary special education and transition from school to work: A national priority. *Exceptional Children, 53*, 487–492.

Sainato, D.M. (1990). Classroom transitions: Organizing environments to promote independent performance in preschool children with disabilities. *Education and Treatment of Children, 13*(4), 288–297.

Sainato, D.M., & Lyon, S.R. (1989). Promoting successful mainstreaming transitions for handicapped preschool children. *Journal of Early Intervention, 13*(4), 305–314.

Sainato, D.M., Strain, P.S., Lefebvre, D., & Rapp, N. (1987). Facilitating transition times with handicapped preschool children: A comparison of peer-mediated and antecedent prompt procedures. *Journal of Applied Behavior Analysis, 20*, 285–291.

Smith, A.B., & Hubbard, P.M. (1988). The relationship between parent/staff communication and children's behavior in early childhood settings. *Early Child Development and Care, 35*, 13–28.

Stokes, T.F., & Osnes, P.G. (1986). Programming for the generalization of children's social behavior. In P.S. Strain, M.J. Guralnick, & H.M. Walker (Eds.), *Children's social behavior: Development, assessment, and modification* (pp. 407–443). Orlando, FL: Academic Press.

Swan, W.W., & Morgan, J.L. (1992). *Collaborating for comprehensive services for young children and their families: The local interagency coordinating council*. Baltimore: Paul H. Brookes Publishing Co.

Szekeres, S.F., & Meserve, N.F. (1994). Collaborative intervention in schools after traumatic brain injury. *Topics in Language Disorders, 15*(1), 21–36.

Wahler, R.G., & Fox, J.J. (1981). Setting events in applied behavior analysis: Toward a conceptual and methodological expansion. *Journal of Applied Behavior Analysis, 14*, 327–338.

Warren, S.F. (1988). A behavioral approach to language generalization. *Language, Speech, and Hearing Services in Schools, 19*, 292–303.

Wolfensberger, W. (1972). *Normalization: The principle of normalization in human services*. Toronto, Ontario, Canada: National Institute on Mental Retardation.

Author Index

Subject Index

Page numbers followed by "t" denote tables; those followed by "f" denote figures

ABC, *see* Autism Behavior Checklist
Activity transitions, 440–441
ADA, *see* Americans with Disabilities Act (ADA) of 1990 (PL 101-336)
Adult responsivity to child behavior, 39–55, 286, 421
  affective attunement and selective attunement, 120–121
  clinical implications of, 50–54
    cross-cultural differences, 52–54
    limitations of social responsivity in facilitating early language development, 51–52
    compared with Milieu Language Teaching, 51–52, 369–370
  definition of, 40
  developmentally sensitive model of, 50–51
  directions for future research on, 54–55
  forms of, 40
  functional classification of, 40–43
    linguistic contingent responses to child's communicative act, 42–43
    linguistic contingent responses to child's focus of attention, 42
    nonlinguistic contingent responses, 40–42
  immediacy of, 40
  literature on linguistic contingent responses to child's communicative act, 47–48
    limited evidence of generalization, 47
    stronger evidence of generalization, 47–48
  literature on linguistic contingent responses to child's focus of attention, 45–47
    limited evidence of generalization, 45–46
    stronger evidence of generalization, 46
  literature on nonlinguistic contingent responses, 44–45
    limited evidence of generalization, 44–45
    stronger evidence of generalization, 45
  literature on studies that do not allow specification of type of responsivity, 48–50
    limited evidence of generalization, 48–50
    stronger evidence of generalization, 50
  mothers of children with developmental disabilities, 421–422
  readiness for linguistic communication related to, 396–399
  scope of review of, 43–44
    evidence of generalization demonstrated in studies, 44
    experimental and longitudinal correlational studies, 43–44
AEPS, *see* Assessment, Evaluation, and Programming System for Infants and Children
Affect

joint attention and, 118–119
  nonverbal communication skills and, 118–127
Affective attunement, 120–121
Affective sharing, 116, 122
Ages & Stages Questionnaires, 271
Aggressive behavior, *see* Challenging behaviors
ALB, *see* Assessing Prelinguistic and Early Linguistic Behaviors in Developmentally Young Children
American Sign Language, 62, 417
Americans with Disabilities Act (ADA) of 1990 (PL 101-336), 439
Analogue assessments, 274
Apraxia of speech, 106
Assessing Prelinguistic and Early Linguistic Behaviors in Developmentally Young Children (ALB), 240–241
Assessment, 6–8
  analogue, 274
  clinical, 233–255; *see also* Clinical assessment of emerging language
  of communicative production, 249–250, 250*t*
  critical features of, 288–289
  definition of, 233, 253
  dynamic, 7, 241–242, 274–275, 285–307; *see also* Dynamic assessment
  of emerging comprehension, 247–249, 248*t*
  functional, 7, 290–291, 317–331, 343–344; *see also* Functional assessment
  of gestures, 64–66, 81
  of graphic symbols, 206
  judgment-based, 275
  limitations of traditional methods for, 239–245, 288–289
    performance variability, 244–245
    predictive validity of assessment results, 242–244
    reflection of clinical research, 240–241
    representativeness of assessment conditions, 241–242
  of nonverbal communication skills, 113–118
  of play, 186–187
  role of caregivers in, 261–279; *see also* Caregivers
  static, 289–290
Assessment, Evaluation, and Programming System (AEPS) for Infants and Children, 252–253, 271
Attachment
  assessed by "strange situation" procedure, 126–127
  joint attention and, 125–127
  nonverbal communication skills and, 112
  secure, 41